Color Duplex Sonography

Color Duplex Sonography

Principles and Clinical Applications

Edited by
Karl-Jürgen Wolf
and Franz Fobbe

with contributions by
F. Fobbe, P.-M. Klews
R. Kubale, P. Landwehr
and J. Siegert

467 illustrations, most in color

1995
Georg Thieme Verlag
Stuttgart · New York

Thieme Medical Publishers, Inc.
New York

Cover design: *Renate Stockinger*, Stuttgart

Translated by Terry C. Telger
6112 Waco Way
Fort Worth, TX 76133
USA

Library of Congress Cataloging-in-Publication Data

Color duplex sonography : principles and clinical applications / edited by Karl-Jürgen Wolf and Franz Fobbe : with contributions by F. Fobbe... [et al] ; [translated by Terry C. Telger].
p. cm.
Includes bibliographical references and index.
ISBN 3-13-100351-0 (GTV, Stuttgart). – ISBN 0-86577-542-7 (TMP, New York)
1. Duplex ultrasonography. I. Wolf, Karl-Jürgen, II. Fobbe, Franz.
[DNLM 1. Ultrasonography–methods. WB 289 C719 1994]
RC78, 7. U4C64 1994
616.07 543–dc20
DNLM/DLC
for Library of Congress 94-23586
CIP

This book is an authorized, updated and revised translation of the German edition published and copyrighted 1993 by Georg Thieme Verlag, Stuttgart, Germany. Title of the German edition: Farbkodierte Duplexsonographie

Any reference to or mention of manufacturers or specific brand names should not be interpreted as an endorsement or advertisement for any company or product.

Typesetting by Druckhaus Götz GmbH,
D-71636 Ludwigsburg
(typeset on CCS-Textline [Linotronic 630])
Printed in Germany by Appl, D-86650 Wemding

ISBN 3-13-100351-0 (GTV, Stuttgart)
ISBN 0-86577-542-7 (TMP, New York) 2 3 4 5 6

Important Note:

Medicine is an ever-changing science undergoing continual development. Research and clinical experience are continually expanding our knowledge, in particular our knowledge of proper treatment and drug therapy. Insofar as this book mentions any dosage or application, readers may rest assured that the authors, editors and publishers have made every effort to ensure that such references are in accordance with the state of knowledge at the time of production of the book.

Nevertheless this does not involve, imply, or express any guarantee or responsibility on the part of the publishers in respect of any dosage instructions and forms of application stated in the book. Every user is requested to examine carefully the manufacturers' leaflets accompanying each drug and to check, if necessary in consultation with a physician or specialist, whether the dosage schedules mentioned therein or the contraindications stated by the manufacturers differ from the statements made in the present book. Such examination is particularly important with drugs that are either rarely used or have been newly released on the market. Every dosage schedule or every form of application used is entirely at the user's own risk and responsibility. The authors and publishers request every user to report to the publishers any discrepancies or inaccuracies noticed.

Foreword

This book on color duplex sonography covers the most important indications for color duplex ultrasound excluding echocardiography. The chapters are organized with a description, the most common uses, examination techniques, and, finally, a discussion of the value of the method in the clinical setting. There is also a chapter about basic techniques and several chapters discussing the principles of pulsed and color duplex and ultrasound. There is even a chapter on its use with ultrasound contrast agents.

The authors have had extensive experience in utilizing color duplex equipment, both techniques and interpretation. Color duplex imaging is one of the most rapidly growing areas of ultrasound, not only in Europe but throughout the world. The German edition was a success, and the English translation should fare similarly. This book is one of the first that covers this field in a broad, well-organized fashion. It should appeal to both physicians and non-physicians throughout the world. In addition, this English edition has been updated to include new material and references.

Barry B. Goldberg, M.D.
Professor of Radiology
Director, Division of Diagnostic Ultrasound
Thomas Jefferson Medical School and Hospital
Philadelphia, Pennsylvania

Preface

Color duplex sonography is a relatively new procedure that has been available since 1986. It combines two different technologies–Doppler ultrasound and gray-scale ultrasound–in a way that ideally provides simultaneous, real-time visualization of soft tissue structures and blood flow over the entire scan field. As a result, the examiner must process considerably more information in a shorter time than with conventional ultrasound techniques. The accurate interpretation of this information requires a knowledge of pathology and pathophysiology, as well as a basic understanding of the technical principles of color duplex imaging. The book is therefore divided into three parts: The first part (Chapters 1–4) reviews the basics of color duplex sonography, the bioeffects of ultrasound, hemodynamic principles, and general problems relating to instrument settings and examination technique. In the second part (Chapters 5–15) the main areas of application of color duplex sonography (excluding cardiology) are described for specific body regions. All these chapters follow the same format, proceeding from normal anatomy and the most common pathologic findings to a discussion of the diagnostic value of color duplex in relation to other diagnostic procedures. This discussion emphasizes that color duplex sonography is not an "add-on" study, but can actually replace more costly and invasive procedures. The third part of the book (Chapters 16–18) first deals with ultrasound contrast agents and presents initial clinical experience with contrast-enhanced color duplex imaging. This chapter was included in the belief that contrast agents will greatly expand the diagnostic capabilities of ultrasound in the future. The book concludes with a detailed chapter on the physical principles of ultrasound and a glossary. The interested reader can explore technical details of ultrasound physics that go well beyond the information covered in the first chapter.

Color duplex sonography is a relatively new, but very promising and exciting diagnostic procedure. The present book provides an up-to-date review based on the experience of the authors and published reports.

Berlin, Spring 1995

Karl-Jürgen Wolf
Franz Fobbe

Addresses

F. Fobbe, M.D.
Ass. Prof.
Free University of Berlin
Universitätsklinikum Benjamin Franklin
Radiologic Clinic
Hindenburgdamm 30
12200 Berlin
Germany

P.-M. Klews, Ph.D.
Philips Medical Systems
Röntgenstr. 24
22335 Hamburg
Germany

R. Kubale, M.D.
University Clinic Homburg/Saar
Diagnostic Radiology Clinic
Oscar-Orth-Str.
66424 Homburg/Saar
Germany

P. Landwehr, M.D.
University Clinic Cologne
Institute for Diagnostic Radiology
Joseph-Stelzmann-Str. 9
50931 Cologne
Germany

J. Siegert, M.D.
APOGEPHA Arzneimittel GmbH
Medical Research
Kyffhäuser Str. 27
01309 Dresden
Germany

K.-J. Wolf, M.D.
Professor
Free University of Berlin
Universitätsklinikum Benjamin Franklin
Radiologic Clinic
Hindenburgdamm 30
12200 Berlin
Germany

Contents

5 Carotid and Vertebral Arteries ... 45

P. Landwehr

6 Extremity Arteries ... 68

P. Landwehr

7 Hemodialysis Shunt 92

P. Landwehr

8 Peripheral Veins 110

F. Fobbe

9 Aorta and its Symmetrical Branches 126

R. Kubale

10 Splanchnic Arteries 141

R. Kubale

11 Abdominal Veins, Portal Venous System, and Liver 155

R. Kubale

12 Renal Transplants 183

F. Fobbe

1 Introduction to Color Duplex Sonography (CDS)

P.-M. Klews

Color duplex sonography (CDS), also referred to as color flow mapping (CFM), or technically not quite correct color Doppler, has become an essential modality in medical diagnostic imaging. To interpret CDS images correctly it is essential to have at least a basic understanding of ultrasound imaging in general and of the Doppler effect in particular.

In this chapter the reader is introduced to the basic physical and technical principles governing CDS. A more in-depth and explicit introduction to the physics and technology of color duplex sonography is presented at the end of this book, in Chapter 17. Readers who are further interested in the "whys" and "hows" of CDS, are referred to that chapter.

1.1 Introduction

A CDS image is composed of a gray-scale and a color part. The gray-scale part of the image contains information on the morphology of the object under investigation. The color part of the image indicates movement within the image field. Usually the movement pertains to the flow of blood. Any particle movement or density variations within the fluid or the displacement of tissue can be detected and color-encoded. Flow information and morphologic information are gathered in completely different ways. Both parts of the CDS image are governed by completely different laws. Following a general review of the physics and technology involved in CDS, a closer look at the various imaging modalities is presented. How Doppler spectrum analysis works will also be explained because this method is often used. An understanding of Doppler frequency analysis is helpful in working with color duplex sonography.

A static image is only of little help in visualizing blood flow dynamics. CDS, with its ability to provide a virtually real-time depiction of blood flow, can display dynamic events while they are occuring. The speed of sound of 1,540 m/s is assumed to be constant in all cases. This implies certain restrictions that should be known to the medical user. Often an improvement in one area leads to a disadvantage in another. For instance, a higher frequency resolution leads to a proportionally lower temporal resolution or, to take another example, a higher line density automatically reduces the image repetition frequency or frame rate by the same amount.

1.2 General Physics

The propagation of sound is dependent on the elastic properties of the medium in which the sound wave propagates. Sound waves fall into the category of elastic waves. Particles are excited to mechanial vibrations around their center of gravity or equilibrium position. These temporally periodic vibrations propagate through the medium (Fig. 1.**1**). In wave motion, energy and momentum are transferred from one particle to the next. In this case kinetic energy—energy of motion—is of main concern. The vibrating particles themselves do not move along with the wave. Only the state of motion of the matter itself propagates from one particle to the next. In general, the spatial propagation of a periodic disturbance with no net transport of the material of the medium is called a wave. In the case of sound, matter is alternately compressed and decompressed. A sound wave represents a periodic temporal and spatial change of pressure (or density). The stronger the bonding between the particles of the medium, the faster the propagation of the change of state, i.e., the higher the speed of sound within the medium. In the case of sound (as far as it is of concern here), particles vibrate parallel to the direction of propagation of the wave. This type of wave is called a longitudinal wave.

If the particles are vibrating at a rate of 20,000 to 1 billion times per second around their center of gravity, this is within the frequency range of ultrasound. The unit for frequency f is hertz, Hz = 1/s. The frequency range from 2 to 10 MHz and lately up to 30 MHz is used in medical diagnostic imaging.

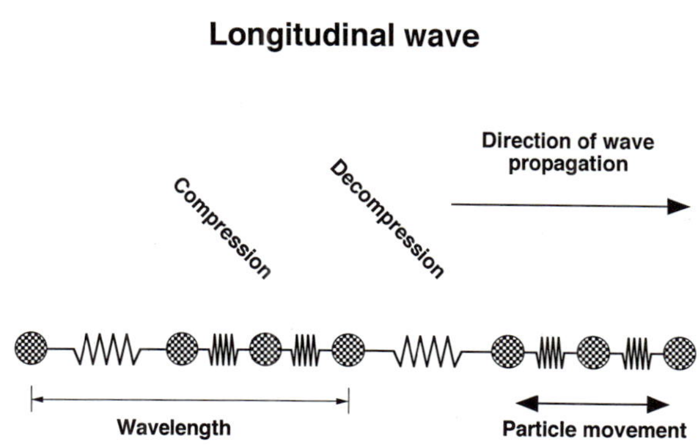

Fig. 1.**1** Longitudinal wave propagation

The fundamental relationship governing rectilinear motion is also valid in wave propagation. That means that the quotient of the (average) displacement (distance traveled) per unit time λ divided by the time interval *t* is equal to a constant *c*. The wavelength λ is the distance between two consecutive particles in the same state of motion (phase) along a straight line in the direction of propagation of the wave. The constant *c* is the speed of sound. Another way of expressing the above relationship is: the product of the wavelength λ times the frequency *f* is equal to the speed of sound *c*. In medical ultrasound diagnostics, the speed of sound is taken to be constant, i.e., tissue independent, and equal to 1,540 m/s. With this knowledge the ultrasound wavelength at a given frequency can immediately be calculated. Different cases are listed in Table 1.**1**.

Table 1.**1** Frequencies and wavelengths when the speed of sound is equal to **c** = 1,540 m/s

Frequency (MHz)	Wavelength (mm)
2.0	0.77
3.5	0.44
5.0	0.31
6.5	0.24
7.5	0.21
10.0	0.15

All currently used ultrasound imaging methods rely on the transmission of a short ultrasound pulse and the continuous reception of the returning ultrasound echoes. Echoes originate at the interface between two different media. The magnitude (amplitude, intensity) of the echo depends on how easily the wave can traverse the boundary between two media. This depends on the physical properties of the media. A term called acoustic impedance is used in this case. The impedance is equal to the product of the true speed of sound in the material times the density of the medium. An echo is created when the acoustic impedances of the two adjacent media differ. The greater the difference in impedances, the greater the magnitude of the returning echo and the smaller the amplitude of the transmitted wave into the second medium. This immediately leads to the conclusion that all ultrasound gray-scale images only display the interfaces between different media within the image field. If there are no interfaces, there can be no echoes. Logically, the ultrasound image of a tank of degased and nonmoving water is a black screen because there are no interfaces present.

The physical laws related to optics are in general also valid in acoustics. In both cases we are dealing with wave propagation. Reflection, scattering, refraction, interference, diffraction, and absorption all exist in ultrasound.

Reflection and scattering of sound waves occur, according to Figure 1.**2**, at the surface between two (different) media. When the surface structures are smaller than the wavelength, scattering is the dominant effect. In the opposite case, when the surface structures are much larger than the wavelength, reflection will mostly occur. Reflection is directed in a specific direction but scattering at first sight is not. The angle of incidence between the direction of propagation of the incident wave and the normal to the surface and the angle of reflection between the direction

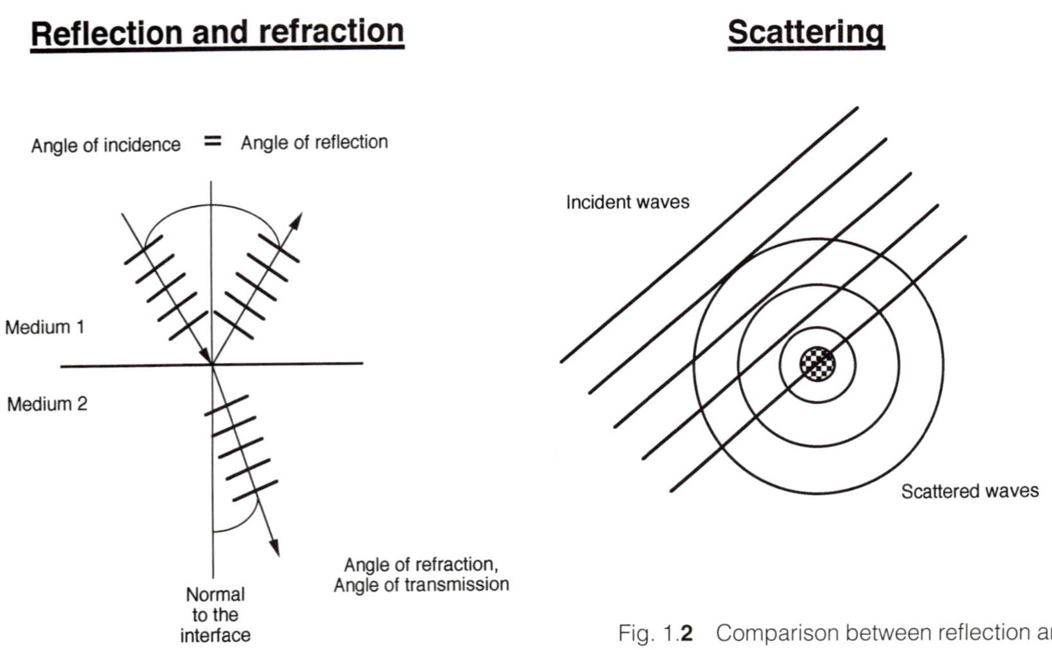

Fig. 1.**2** Comparison between reflection and scattering

of propagation of the reflected wave and the normal to the surface are identical. For this reason vessel walls running perpendicular to the direction of flight of the ultrasound pulse light up very brightly in the ultrasound image. In this special case the total reflected ultrasound intensity is reflected back to the transducer. The scattered waves, on the other hand, diverge in all directions away from the scattering particles with a slight predominance of the backscattered component.

The wave transmitted into the second medium is refracted at the interface. Depending on the relation of the respective speed of sound in the two media, the refracted wave is either refracted toward the normal to the surface or away from it.

The interaction of two or more waves with one another is called interference. Depending on the momentary state (phase) of the waves, the interference may be either destructive or constructive. In other words, the net signal is either amplified or diminished. Local interference is largely responsible for the appearance of the gray-scale image.

Diffraction at the edges of obstacles with dimensions comparable to the wavelength of the sound wave, i.e., nonrectilinear wave propagation, makes it possible for an ultrasound signal to be generated behind an object.

Finally, absorption takes place when a sound wave travels through tissue. Absorption exponentially reduces the intensity of the signal with increasing image depth.

Absorption is frequency-dependent. It increases almost linearly with frequency. Scattering, on the other hand, increases with the fourth power of the frequency. This is the reason why the penetration depth of high-frequency transducers is higher than would be expected when only absorption is taken into account.

As a general assumption the total round-trip attenuation from all effects combined amounts to about 1 dB/MHz cm. The loss of intensity must be compensated by a depth-dependent amplification because equal impedance jumps must result in equal image brightness at all depths.

1.3 Imaging with Ultrasound in General

All ultrasound imaging methods used today work by transmitting a short ultrasound pulse followed by the reception of the returning echoes. This is called a pulse–echo system. One or more pulse–echo cycles generate one ultrasound scan line of the image. A two-dimensional ultrasound image is comprised of many ultrasound scan lines next to one another (Fig. 1.**3**). There are many more video lines than ultrasound scan lines in one image.

Except for mechanical sector transducers, all standard transducers are made up of a linear assembly of piezoelectric elements. Applying an electric AC-voltage to the elements creates a forced mechanical vibration of the elements. In this way a proportional change of pressure is created in the surrounding area. These pressure changes, called sound waves, propagate away from the transducer into the tissue. While the echoes are being received, the piezoelements act as pressure sensors. The pressure changes at the piezoelements generate an electric voltage that can be measured with the help of an appropriately designed electronic circuit.

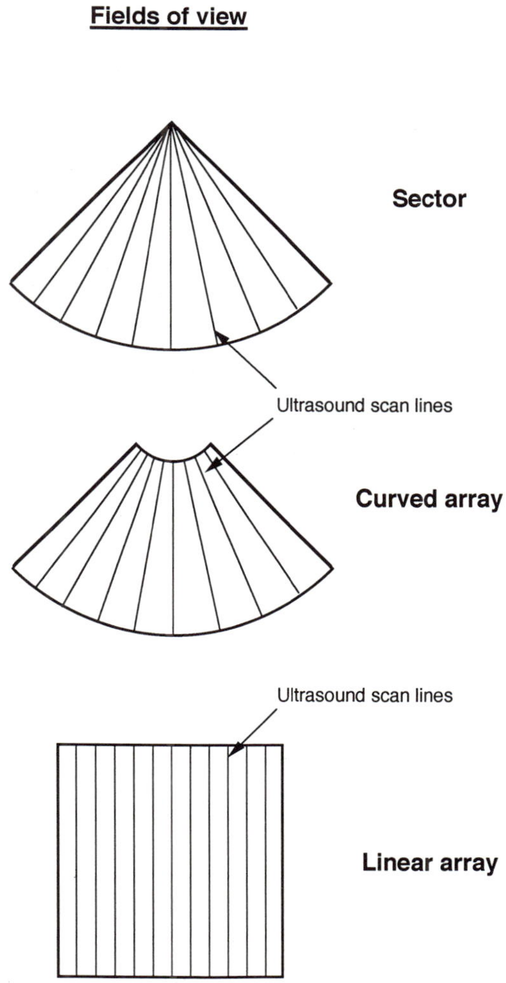

Fig. 1.**3** Sector, convex (CA) and linear transducers have different fields of view. The ultrasound scan lines are directed radially away from the transducer

The display of echo amplitudes over time is called an A(amplitude)-mode image. Since the speed of sound in human tissue is almost constant, the distance from the transducer, where the echoes were generated, can be calculated directly from the time of flight of the pulse–echo system. The time of flight measured is scaled into a distance traveled to the origin of the echo by the ultrasound pulse.

In the case of a B(brightness)-mode image, many successive A-mode lines next to one another are

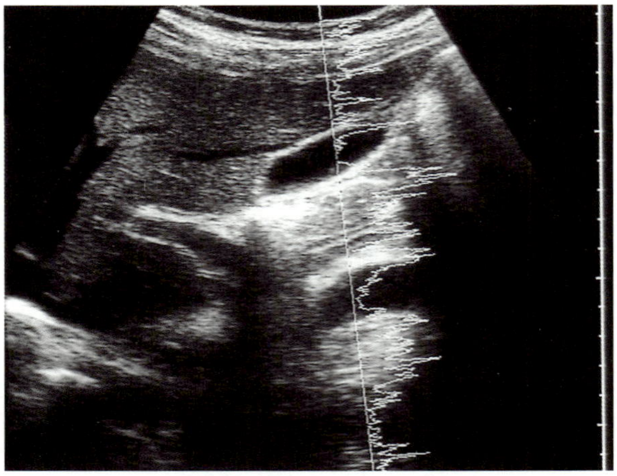

Fig. 1.**4** B-mode image of a liver and gall bladder. One scan line is displayed in A-mode

needed. The amplitudes are translated into shades of gray. The larger the amplitude, the brighter the corresponding point in the image. Since the lateral ultrasound scan line separation is known and also, at the same time, the distance of the echo-generating structure from the transducer is known from the pulse–echo time of flight, a geometrically correct two-dimensional image can be created on the image screen. Figure 1.**4** shows the B-mode image of a liver and a gall bladder. One ultrasound scan line is displayed in A-mode.

Next to the A-mode display and the B-mode image there exists still another gray-scale image format: the M-mode image (motion, time–motion). In the case of an M-mode image all ultrasound pulses are transmitted in the same direction chosen by the user. That means that the same ultrasound scan line is continuously used. The information gathered along the chosen direction over time is displayed laterally line by line on the image screen. This type of display is mostly used to visualize highly dynamic processes in the heart such as the movement of valves.

The ultrasound scan lines are always directed vertically away from the transducer except in the case of beam steering or phased-array transducers. This is the reason why the shape of the image field depends on the shape of the transducer (Fig. 1.**3**).

A phased-array transducer consists of a flat (in one plane) linear array of piezoelements. These elements are electrically excited with certain time delays relative to one another. The sum signal of all elementary waves coming from all piezoelements can be steered in specific directions by precise time control. In this way a sector- or trapezoid shaped image is created.

The same type of steering as just described in the case of phased arrays is called beam steering when facilitated on linear arrays. This method is used here in order to create a more advantageous angle of incidence during spectral Doppler analysis as well as in color encoding.

Mechanical sector transducers are divided into two groups: single-element fixed-focus transducers and multielement annular-array transducers. Annular-array transducers are composed of a number of concentric, ring-shaped piezoelements. A sector-shaped image is automatically created by stepwise rotation of the piezoelements for each pulse–echo cycle. Mechanical transducers are seldom used in CDS.

Ultrasound imaging is a real-time modality. Based on the relatively low speed of sound in tissue of 1,540 m/s only a small number of true ultrasound scan lines per image can be used in order to ensure a close to real-time image display. The emission of an ultrasound pulse from the transducer must be delayed until after the arrival of the echo from the previous pulse coming from the greatest possible distance. Otherwise the echoes cannot be uniquely related to a specific pulse or depth.

In CDS more than one pulse–echo cycle per ultrasound scan line is needed (see Section 1.**7**). For this reason it is up to the user to determine the width of the color part of the image.

Another problem in this respect is posed by the use of multiple transmit pulses focused at different depths. Each transmit pulse can be focused at only one selected depth. This automatically means that an optimal spatial resolution can only be achieved around the specially selected distance from the transducer. To compensate for this, often more than one pulse–echo cycle per ultrasound scan line is used, with each transmitted pulse being focused at different depths. Every ultrasound scan line is then pieced together to achieve optimal spatial resolution throughout the whole field of view. In the simplest case the time needed to create an ultrasound image is increased by the number of transmit focal zones used. The frame rate is reduced accordingly.

On electronic transducers transmit and receive focusing in the direction parallel to the long axis of the transducer is done by precise time control of the individual elements used for transmit and receive. Transmit focusing in this direction is achieved by delaying the excitation of the individual piezoelements relative to one another by a short well-calculated period of time. Receive focusing in this direction is done by temporally correct summation of the signals picked up by the individual transducer elements within a certain period of time. In the direction parallel to the short axis of the transducer, focusing is accomplished with the help of an acoustic lens. The focus position in this direction cannot be changed by the user.

The spatial resolution, i.e., the size of the objects that can be detected within the image, depends partially on the position of the object in the image. As can be seen in Figure 1.**5** in the case of a linear array transducer the resolution varies in x, y, and z directions. The spatial resolution in z direction depends on the pulse length. The resolution in y direction depends on electronic focusing and on the distance from the transducer. The resolution in x direction depends on the focusing capabilities of the acoustic lens as well as on

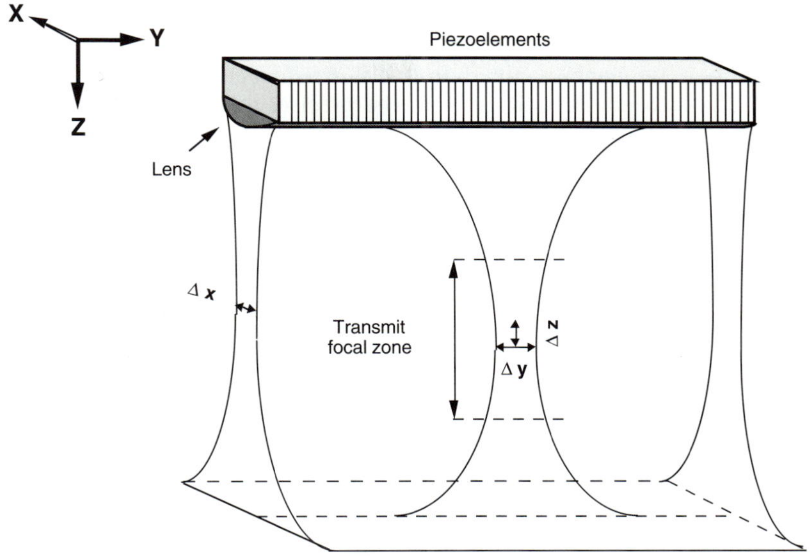

Fig. 1.**5** Overall sound field and spatial resolution Δx, Δy, and Δz of a linear-array transducer

the position in the image. The spatial resolution in *x* direction is also termed slice thickness.

Almost all modern ultrasound systems employ dynamic receive focusing. The receive focus is continuously (or in small steps) shifted as the transmitted pulse travels away from the transducer. This method does not lead to any reduction in frame rate.

1.4 The Doppler Effect

This effect was discovered by Christian Doppler in 1842. He realized that the wavelength recorded by an observer depends on the movement of the source and the observer relative to one another.

To gain a better understanding of this effect, imagine, for example, that a fly is traveling (as an unknown passenger) along in a car. The fly believes that it and the driver are not moving and that the people on the sidewalk are speeding past the car in a certain direction at velocity v. Someone standing on the sidewalk believes he is not moving but that the car with the fly is moving at velocity v in exactly the opposite direction. If the fly is flying through the car from the front to the back, it could think that the pedestrians have slowed down during its flight. This shows that the measurement of velocity and the direction of movement depend on the frame of reference.

This example will now be applied to the analysis of blood flow. The transducer emits an ultrasound pulse that encounters moving scatterers in the blood. Let us assume that the blood cells are moving toward the transducer at a constant velocity. The wavelength was defined in Section 1.1 as the shortest distance between two consecutive particles in the same state of motion (phase) along a straight line in the direction of wave propagation. It takes a certain amount of time for the wave to propagate a distance equal to one wavelength. But in this case, the blood cells are traveling in a direction opposite to the direction of wave propagation. The scatterers (blood cells) take less time to cover the distance of one wavelength than it would take for the wave to travel one wavelength past a stationary object. Since distance is equal to the product of time and velocity (Section 1.2), and the speed of sound is constant, different distances are measured. A shorter wave length would be measured from the perspective of the moving object than from the perspective of the stationary object. In other words, the frequency measured in the frame of reference of the moving object is higher than that measured in the stationary frame of reference. As a result, the frequency as seen by the moving object is shifted to a higher value.

If the blood cells and the transducer are moving away from each other, the frequency is shifted to a lower value. If the transmitted frequency is known, it is possible to calculate the velocity and the direction of movement of the objects relative to one another with the help of a frequency measurement.

It might be said that in the measurement of blood flow the effect takes place twice. The transducer emits ultrasound with a certain frequency. The moving blood cells “measure” a different frequency and “send” back an echo with that frequency. The transducer itself receives a signal (echo) from moving scatterers (transmitter) and, depending on the direction of blood flow, measures an even higher or lower frequency.

The mathematical formulation of the Doppler effect described above is called the Doppler equation or Doppler formula:

$$f_d = 2f_0 \frac{v}{c} \cos(\alpha)$$

or solving for v

$$v = \frac{f_d}{2f_0} \frac{c}{\cos(\alpha)}$$

where v = blood flow velocity
f_d = measured Doppler frequency shift
f_0 = frequency emitted from the transducer (center frequency or, to be precise, the Doppler reference frequency used)
c = speed of sound in tissue
α = angle between the direction of blood flow and the direction of propagation of the sound wave

The Doppler frequency shift is usually just called Doppler shift and the angle α is called Doppler angle for short. In order to correctly interpret Doppler spectra and CDS images, knowledge of the Doppler equation is mandatory. In medical ultrasound diagnostics the transducer and the direction in which the sound pulses are transmitted into the body are the points of reference for all evaluations concerned with the direction of blood flow and blood flow velocity.

It follows from the Doppler equation that a Doppler shift does not occur at a Doppler angle of 90°. At this flow angle the blood–transducer distance is constant. Blood is then flowing parallel to the transducer and not away from or toward it. Only the velocity component parallel to the direction of propagation of the sound wave can be measured directly. The true flow velocity can only be calculated after measuring the Doppler angle.

The difficulty in the interpretation of the Doppler signal shall be explained for the case of a 5.0-MHz transducer. In Figure 1.**6** the Doppler shift versus blood flow velocity has been plotted. It is evident that at constant velocity the Doppler shift increases with decreasing Doppler angle. Failure to take note of the angle dependency of the Doppler shift can lead to serious diagnostic errors, especially in CDS.

Every ultrasound machine has a specific frequency resolution. With the help of a user-variable high-pass filter, called wall filter in medical ultrasound, the lowest possibly detectable frequency shift can be defined. In Figure 1.**7** the Doppler shift has again been plotted as a function of blood flow velocity. This time, emphasis has been put on the detection of low flow velocities at different wall filter settings. The lower the choice of the wall filter, the lower the measurable flow velocities. The closer the blood flow comes to flowing directly toward or away from the transducer, the lower the detectable flow velocities regardless of the wall filter used.

From Figure 1.**8** it becomes evident that the detection of slow flow velocities improves when high-frequency transducers are used. The measured Doppler shift caused by a certain flow velocity is higher when using high-frequency transducers than with lower-frequency transducers. On the other hand, with low-frequency transducers higher velocities are measurable at the same Doppler shift.

From the above explanations it is obvious that stating the measured Doppler shift alone yields no or only little information on blood flow. Only after measuring the Doppler angle and also stating the reference frequency of the transducer used along with the Doppler shift does a statement on blood flow become of value. However, naming the blood flow velocity alone is a relevant statement. The pulsatility index (PI) and the resistance index (RI) for instance are relative and not absolute quantities (see Chapter 3). These indices are, at least theoretically, angle independent.

The often stated "magic" Doppler angle of 60° at which a Doppler examination should be conducted is of no significance. There is one single advantage in using this angle: The cosine of 60° is 0.5. This only simplifies the calculation. In order to minimize the error caused by an incorrect angle measurement a Doppler angle as close to 0° as possible should be used.

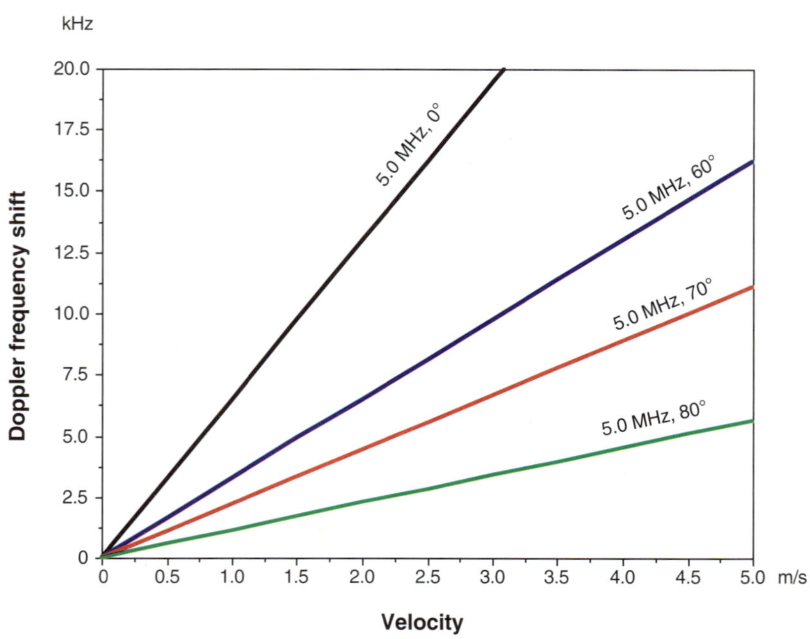

Fig. 1.**6** Doppler frequency shift vs. blood flow velocity at different Doppler angles in the case of a 5.0-MHz transducer

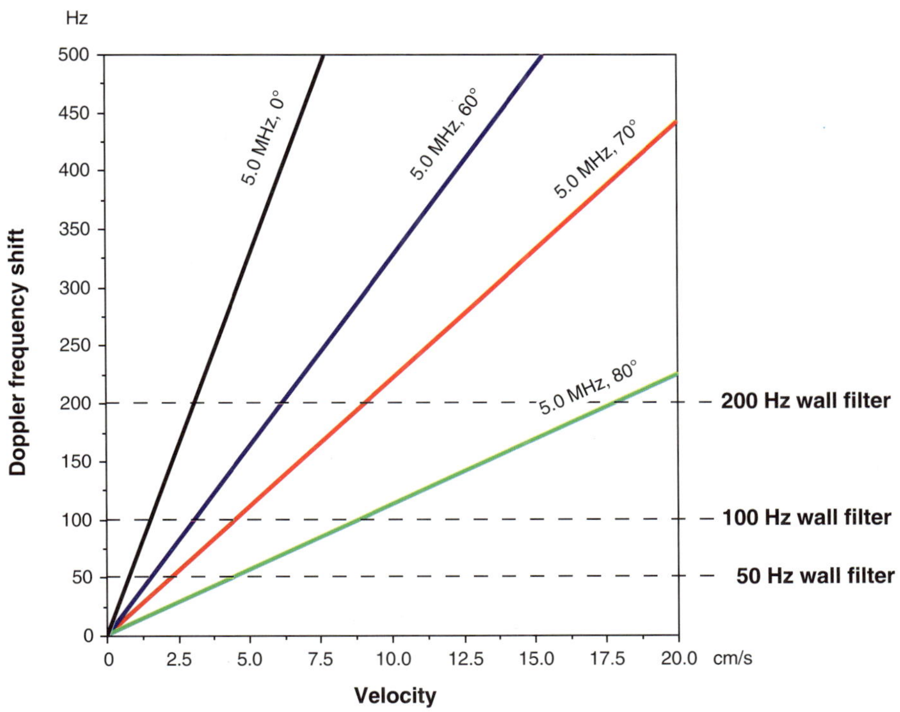

Fig. 1.**7** Resolution of low Doppler frequency shifts vs. blood flow velocity at different Doppler angles in the case of a 5.0-MHz transducer using different wall filters

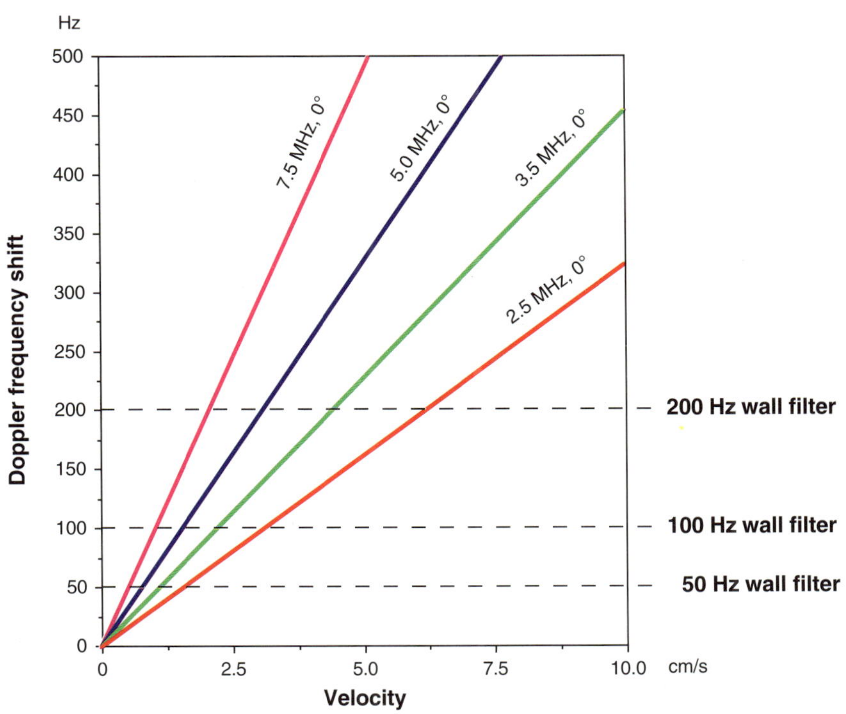

Fig. 1.**8** Resolution of low Doppler frequency shifts vs. blood flow velocity at a Doppler angle of 0° using different wall filters on a number of different transducers

1.5 The Doppler Frequency Spectrum

The first question that arises is: What is a spectrum? A look at Figure 1.**9** will help clarify this. A handful of marbles are rolled across the floor. Suppose that at the beginning at time t_0 all marbles are rolling at the same speed. The velocities of the marbles are then measured a short time later at time t_1. Owing to friction, the marbles are now rolling at different velocities. The possible velocity range is divided into equal-sized velocity increments (steps, boxes). The number of marbles having velocities that fall into each individual velocity increment are counted. The distribution of the number of marbles over all velocity increments is called the velocity spectrum of the marbles at time t_1. At time t_2 the measurement is performed again. A different velocity spectrum is the result.

If the velocity of the marbles were measured with ultrasound, the Doppler shifts caused by the moving objects could be evaluated. The Doppler frequency distribution at specific individual points in time are the Doppler (frequency) spectra of the rolling marbles. Equally, this model can be used as an aid in understanding the velocity distribution of the erythrocytes in the blood.

The term Doppler spectrum in medical ultrasound has a somewhat different "colloquial" meaning than in physics. Many individual, consecutive Doppler spectra gathered over time and displayed one time increment apart, one after the other, comprise a medical Doppler spectrum. For a better understanding look at Figure 1.**10**. A medical Doppler spectrum is displayed in a somewhat unusual manner. The length of the time increments correspond to the amount of time it takes to gather all the information needed for one physical Doppler spectrum (velocity distribution within the time increment). In the case of pulsed Doppler, 32, 64, or 128 pulse–echo cycles are generally used. The size of the time increment therefore depends directly on the image depth from which the spectral data is being gathered. The size of the frequency increments is equal to the pulse repetition frequency divided by the number of pulse–echo cycles used for one spectrum (see Section 17.3.**3**). The gray and chequered boxes represent the amplitudes of the individual Doppler frequencies within each spectrum. Normally the amplitudes are displayed in different shades of gray. Higher amplitudes of the respective Doppler frequencies are designated by a lighter shade of gray.

The following conclusions on the medical Doppler spectrum can be drawn from the above (a method called scrolling FFT [fast Fourier transform] is not included):

- The frequency resolution of the Doppler spectrum is equal to the pulse repetition frequency divided by the number of pulse–echo cycles used for one spectrum.
- The temporal resolution depends on the number of pulse–echo cycles used for one physical Doppler spectrum and therefore depends directly on the image depth from which the data is gathered.
- An improvement in frequency resolution automatically lowers the temporal resolution and vice versa.
- By reducing the pulse repetition frequency, the frequency resolution in the low-frequency range can be improved, but at the same time the ability to uniquely measure high Doppler frequencies is sacrificed by the same factor (aliasing).
- The often repeated question about the time it takes the computer to calculate a Doppler spectrum is meaningless for the user of modern pulsed Doppler systems because the computation time does not in-

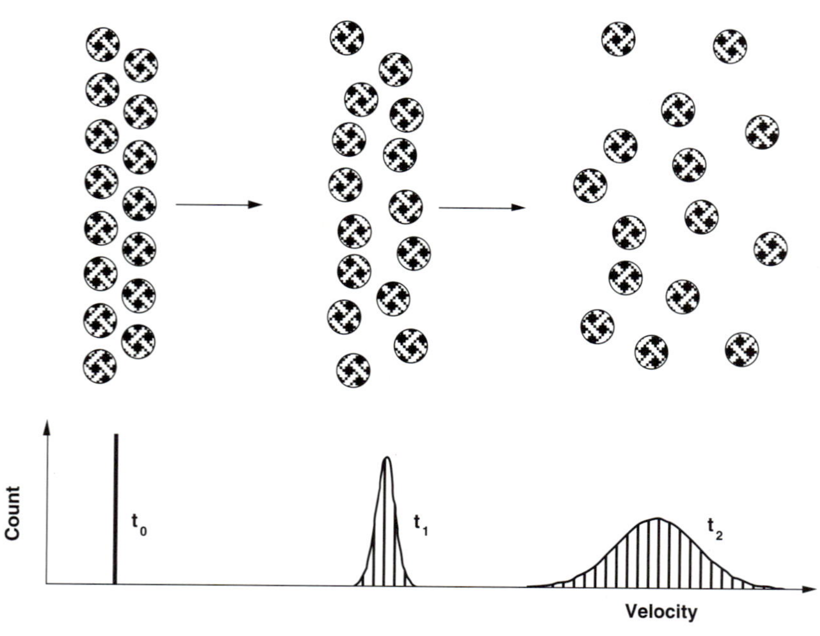

Fig. 1.**9** A number of rolling marbles have different velocity distributions or velocity spectra at different points in time t_0, t_1, and t_2

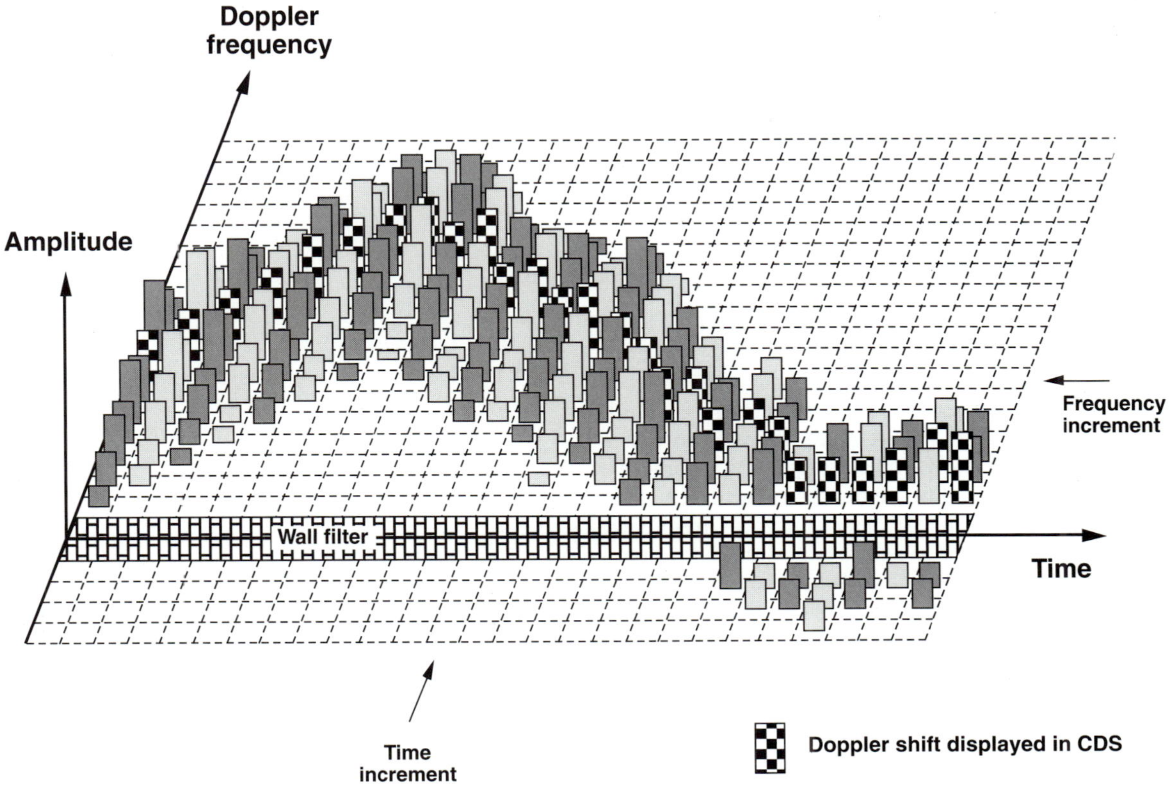

Fig. 1.10 A "medical" Doppler spectrum is made up of many individual consecutive "physical" Doppler spectra. The heights of the boxes correspond to the amplitudes of the respective Doppler frequencies. Usually the amplitudes are displayed in different shades of gray. The chequered boxes represent the Doppler shifts (velocities) shown in color in CDS imaging if both methods had the same spatial and temporal resolution, which in reality they do not

fluence the temporal resolution. Whether the computer waits for data either 10% or 90% of the time is irrelevant.

1.5.1 Acquiring the Doppler Spectrum

According to the Doppler equation, the velocity measured depends on the frequency shift of the transmitted signal. Depending on the direction of blood flow, the frequency shift can be either negative or positive. The frequency shifts are of the order of magnitude of hertz or kilohertz and are in the range of human hearing. However, the center frequency of the transmitted signal is in the megahertz region. Technically the frequency shifts around the frequency of the transmitted signal must be isolated and displayed in some way or made audible.

A common device capable of doing this very reliably already exists, namely the radio. It receives radio stations with a frequency (carrier frequency) in the megahertz range and via loudspeaker it sends out signals within a frequency range that the ear can hear. At the radio station the carrier (MHz) is modulated with a frequency shift (music). In connection with radio the term FM (frequency modulation) is well known. This is exactly what happens in case of a Doppler signal. The ultrasound wave is frequency modulated. The ultrasound signal has to be demodulated in order to extract the Doppler signal, i.e., the carrier has to be removed from the signal (echo). How this is done technically is described in Section 17.3.4.

After the carrier has been removed, and a few other manipulations performed, the pure Doppler signal is isolated. It can be sent directly to a loudspeaker. The ear can hear frequencies in a range up to about 20 kHz. One has only to listen to a concert to be convinced that it is an excellent spectrum analyzer. Usually one would like to document the Doppler frequency spectrum and might possibly also want to mathematically or graphically evaluate it. The spectrum must in some way be displayed on a monitor or in CDS, a color-encoded value representing a certain blood flow velocity or Doppler shift has to be presented.

The isolated Doppler signal has to be analyzed according to its spectral (frequency) distribution. It is assumed that the amplitudes of the individual frequencies composing the Doppler signal correspond in magnitude to the velocity distribution of the blood flow.

The method of choice used in frequency analysis is based on a mathematical algorithm called fast Fourier transform, or FFT for short. In order to do this, the Doppler signal has to be converted to a digital format. With this method the amplitudes of certain discrete frequencies are calculated. The amplitudes are displayed in shades of gray in the graphic representation of the Doppler spectrum on the monitor. In the case of CDS a different approach is used (see Section 1.**7**).

There is a distinction between CW (continuous wave) Doppler and PW (pulsed wave) Doppler:

CW Doppler comes closest to radio. In CW Doppler, sound transmission and echo reception go on continuously. That is why CW Doppler has no depth resolution, i.e., it is not known from which image depth the signal is coming. Theoretically there is no upper limit to the detectable Doppler frequency. In practice there does exist a limit to the maximum uniquely definable Doppler frequency since digital frequency analysis (FFT) is used to acquire the frequency spectrum (analog zero-crossing detectors are outside the scope of this book). The reason for this is explained in the next chapter and in more depth in Section 17.3.1. CW Doppler will not be described further because in color encoding a pulsed signal is mandatory. Depth resolution is a must in CDS.

PW Doppler has depth resolution. Demodulation is done pulse by pulse. Each echo yields after demodulation the phase of the Doppler signal at a specific point in time. The phase is the instantaneous state (of motion) of the signal (see Section 17.3.2). The complete Doppler signal is constructed in this way point by point. What happens between the individual pulses/echoes is unknown. This is equivalent to the fact that high frequencies above a certain limit with a very quick change in phase cannot be measured. Once the Doppler signal has been pieced together, FFT analysis is used to generate a Doppler spectrum displaying the amplitude distribution and frequency components of the signal.

1.6 The Problem with Sampling: Aliasing

Both CDS and PW Doppler display spatial resolution. The axial spatial resolution relies on the emission of a short ultrasound pulse. The pulse length together with the sample gate length defines the axial resolution. This imposes some drawbacks in evaluating the Doppler signal. The Doppler signal is because of pulsing not a continuous signal but composed of individual samples. The temporal distance between samples is equal to the temporal separation of the pulses or pulse interval. This is equal to the reciprocal of the pulse repetition frequency f_{PRF}. Thus, it is not possible to measure frequencies beyond a certain limit (Fig. 1.**11**). The low-frequency Doppler signal is composed of many individual measurements or samples. The curve between the samples is interpolated. The true shape of the curve is not known.

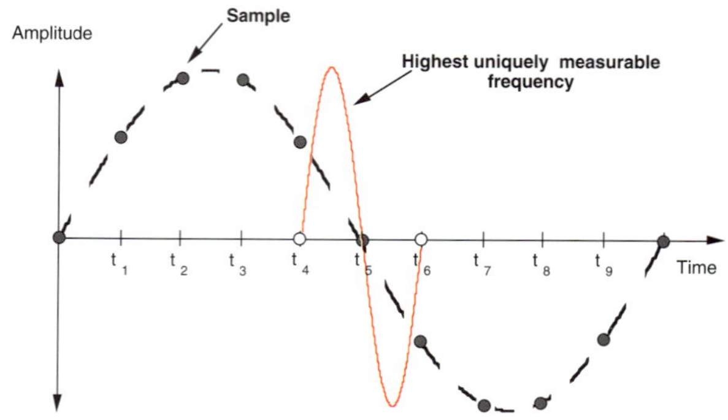

Fig. 1.**11** The Doppler signal is composed of a number of individual samples. The temporal distance of the samples is equal to the temporal pulse interval, which is equal to the reciprocal of the pulse repetition frequency

The highest frequency that can possibly be measured is slightly (infinitesimally) less than half the pulse repetition frequency. At higher Doppler frequencies not enough samples are available to correctly construct the signal. If the frequency were two or four times as high as the highest possible uniquely detectable frequency shown in Figure 1.**11** (red), the samples would have the same values. One could not distinguish the frequencies from one another, and there is no reason to assume that they should be higher than half the pulse repetition frequency.

The Doppler frequency shift can be positive or negative. Both cases are separated electronically and evaluated separately. For this reason the unambiguous frequency range in which the Doppler shift is uniquely defined is equal to the pulse repetition frequency. This unambiguous frequency range extends from $-f_{PRF}/2$ to $+f_{PRF}/2$.

Suppose, as in Figure 1.**12a**, that a particle is continuously speeding up, i.e., is under constant acceleration. The Doppler shift would increase continuously over time. The Doppler shift that would actually be measured and displayed by a pulsed system in such a case has been drawn in Figure 1.**12b**. First of all the non-baseline shifted case shall be compared with the true Doppler shift.

From the start until reaching half the pulse repetition frequency, the displayed Doppler shift in both cases follows the same track. After reaching $f_{PRF}/2$ the measured and displayed Doppler shift jumps to the greatest possible negative Doppler shift $-f_{PRF}/2$. From then on the displayed Doppler shift increases parallel to the true Doppler shift until $f_{PRF}/2$ is reached again before returning once more to a value of $-f_{PRF}/2$. This erroneous display of the Doppler frequency is called aliasing. The jumps result from a pulse repetition frequency that is too low. It is not always possible to increase the pulse repetition frequency because above a certain value range ambiguity will occur.

A helpful but limited possibility of avoiding aliasing exists. The user can decide that in some specific case no negative (positive) Doppler shifts exist and

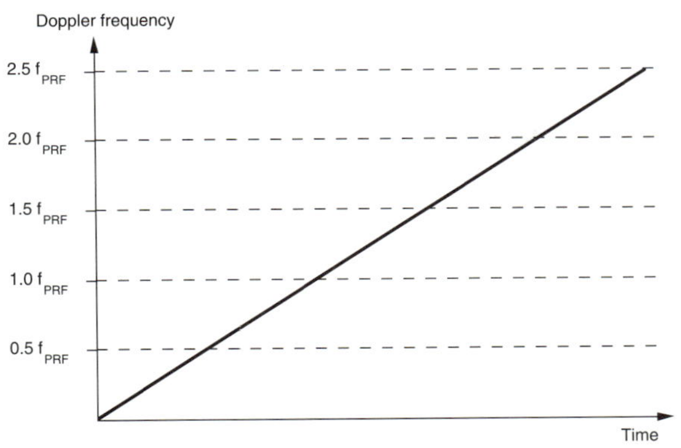

Fig. 1.**12a** Doppler signal of a continuously accelerated particle vs. time

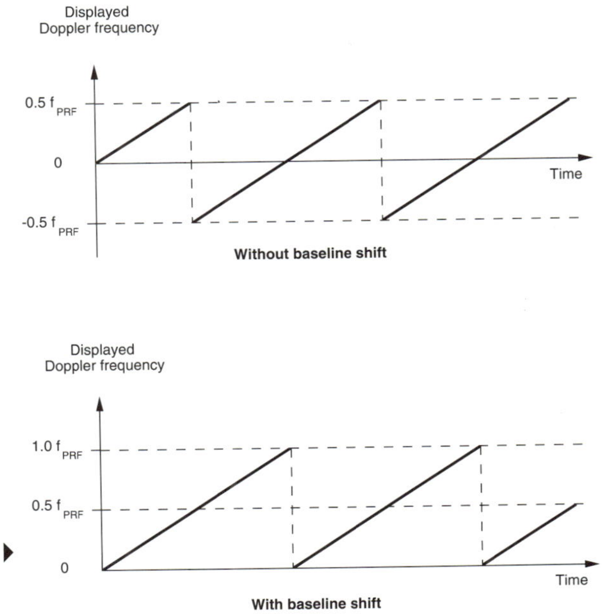

Fig. 1.**12b** The actual Doppler frequency shift of a continuously accelerated particle vs. time measured by pulsed Doppler—in the lower graph after a baseline shift

can then manually implement a baseline or zero-point shift. The size of the unambiguous frequency range in which the Doppler shift can be uniquely measured is not increased by this process but is only shifted. Enlarging the positive frequency range automatically reduces the negative frequency range by the same amount and vice versa. In this way, depending on the direction of the baseline shift, higher positive or negative Doppler frequency shifts can be measured resulting in the ability to determine higher flow velocities in a specific direction.

The above discussion is equally valid in color encoding because these methods are also based on the evaluation of multiple pulse–echo cycles. Aliasing also occurs in the case of time-of-flight analysis (time domain processing) of the non-demodulated RF signal. The reasons for it are different but the resulting effect and consequences for the user are the same.

1.7 Methods of Color Encoding

Three different methods for calculating the mean or intensity-weighted average flow velocity used in color encoding are implemented on commercially available ultrasound systems today. All of them differ very much from the FFT method used in spectrum analysis.

Usually 64 or 128 pulse–echo cycles are used in Doppler frequency analysis as described above. FFT frequency analysis results in 64 or 128 values per time interval. The time needed for data acquisition over a whole image field composed of 128 ultrasound scan lines with 64 or 128 pulse–echo cycles each, would rule out real-time imaging completely. The number of pulse–echo cycles per line has to be reduced. The frequency resolution of FFT analysis is equal to the pulse repetition frequency divided by the number of samples used for one time line of the spectrum. A reduction to 8 samples per line, for example, would lead to an unacceptable loss of frequency resolution. In CDS only one velocity value for each picture element is needed. For that reason it is not necessary to perform a full spectrum analysis. Averaging methods can be used that deliver only one precise value.

All CDS methods have in common the use of fewer ultrasound scan lines than in B-mode imaging. In some cases only every fourth ultrasound scan line is subjected to color flow analysis. The values in between these lines result from interpolation.

Two of the most common methods have been explicitly published in technical literature. These are the autocorrelation method (3,4) first developed in Japan and the cross-correlation method (time domain processing, time-of-flight analysis) (1,2) developed in Paris, France. The method developed in the USA utilizing discrete Fourier analysis has, up to now, not been published in detail.

The autocorrelation method is based on the comparison of the demodulated Doppler signal over different time intervals with itself. The less variability in the flow velocity over time, the better the method works. An advantage of the method that was first introduced to cardiology is that the calculation of variance is an integral part of it. Variance is equal to the square of the standard deviation and represents the error of measurement. This is usually added in green to the shades of red and blue used in color encoding. The more green added, the greater the possible error. In medicine this is often looked upon as an indicator of turbulance.

The discrete Fourier analysis method is also based on the evaluation of the demodulated Doppler signal. The method works best if there is little variability in flow velocity over time, as in vessels. Variance is not automatically calculated as is the case in autocorrelation. This is a low-resolution spectrum analysis method based on only a few pulse–echo cycles per line because real-time imaging is mandatory in CDS. The method relies on digital filtering. By utilizing highly efficient averaging methods it is very effective in calculating the intensity-weighted average Doppler frequency. After all, only one flow value per pixel is needed in CDS and not a complete spectrum.

Time domain processing of Doppler signals is based on measuring the difference in the time of flight of two pulse–echo cycles. Due to the flow of blood, the time of flight of two consecutive pulse–echo cycles related to the same scatterers differ. The difference in the time of flight is proportional to the blood flow velocity. The advantage of this technically very sophisticated method lies in the direct evaluation of the high-frequency signals without demodulation. The blood flow velocity (still being angle dependent) is calculated directly and not the Doppler frequency shift. The method can be described in short as a kind of pattern recognition method. The calculation of variance is not an integral part of this method.

The Doppler shift or the blood flow velocity resulting from the use of all of these methods is difficult, if not impossible, to derive from the Doppler spectrum. One reason for this is that completely different time intervals are being looked at. In Doppler spectrum analysis the time increment is longer by a factor of about 7 to 26 depending on the number of points used in the FFT analysis compared with the different CDS methods. Also, the flow velocity is not identical over the whole sample volume. The calculated blood flow velocity value depends on the velocity distribution within the sample volume. The derived velocity is in all cases the mean or intensity-weighted average velocity averaged over the total sampling time and sample volume. The displayed velocity depends on the amplitudes and the width of the spectral distribution of the Doppler signals coming from the sample volume (Fig. 1.**10**).

1.8 Interpretation of CDS Images

A CDS image is composed of a gray-scale and a color part. The gray-scale part coincides with the normal B-mode image. It is used to evaluate structural characteristics of tissue. The brighter and darker parts of the image designate organs and blood vessels as well as spaces filled with fluid, like the bladder or the gall bladder. Structural changes such as cysts or solid masses can be recognized by the typical distribution of gray-scale values in the region of interest.

Color encoding indicates movement within the image field. Usually blood flow characteristics are examined. Color is integrated into the gray-scale image. A pixel (picture element) can receive either a gray-scale or a color value. If movement is detected in a cer-

a

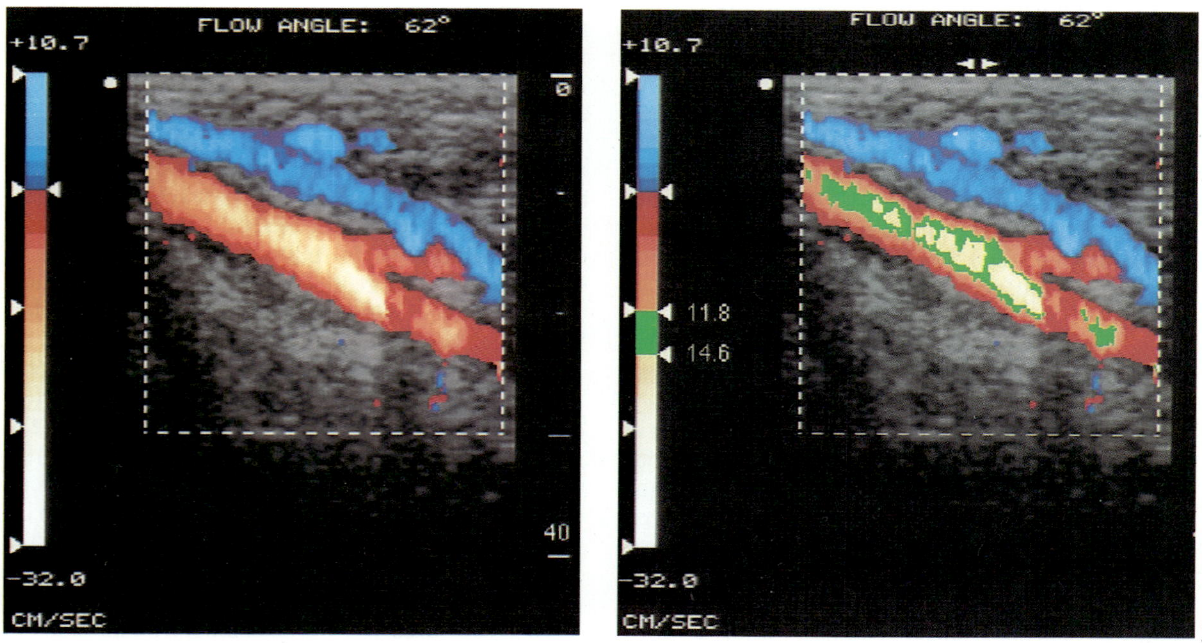

b

Fig. 1.**13** Bifurcation of a normal brachial artery (red) with parallel running vein (blue) in CDS

a The colors blue and red indicate the direction of flow (toward or away from the transducer, respectively). The higher the Doppler shift, the brighter the hue of the color (center of the vessel) and the lower the Doppler shift, the darker the shade of the color (flow near the vessel walls)

b If the flow angle is known, a velocity range can be marked in a separate color (green tag) in the real-time image (in this example the green-tagged flow velocities range from 11.8 to 14.6 cm/s, see color bar on the left) tain part of the image, the related pixels are displayed in color. The local gray value is not displayed in this case. That means color has a write priority.

Most machines display blood flow in different hues of red and blue. The lower the color saturation, i.e., the whiter the color displayed at a certain position in the image, the higher the Doppler shift or, after angle correction, the higher the blood flow velocity at that point. One color represents flow toward the transducer and the other color flow away from the transducer. The choice of colors is usually left up to the user to decide. As can be seen in Figure 1.**13** there is usually some kind of color bar representing the displayed flow velocities for reference. Above and below the color bar the highest Doppler shifts or, after angle correction, the highest velocities measurable in the image in each direction are displayed. The pulse repetition frequency is usually equal to the sum of these two Doppler frequency values.

In some cases green is added to the red and blue values as a qualitative indicator of variance. Variance is equal to the square of the standard deviation and defines the magnitude of the possible error of the displayed flow value. In medicine it is assumed that green indicates a certain amount of turbulance at that position in the image.

Green is also used as a velocity marker for either individual velocities or a range of blood flow velocities. The green-tagged color region is manually defined by the user, and the numerical values of the velocities or Doppler shifts are displayed.

1.9 References

1 Bonnefous, O., P. Pasqué: Time Domain Formulation of Pulse-Doppler Ultrasound and Blood Velocity Estimation by Cross Correlation, Ultrasonic Imaging, Vol. 8, Academic Press (1986) 73–85

2 Bonnefous, O., P. Pasqué, X. Bernard: A New Velocity Estimator for Color Flow Mapping. IEEE Ultrasonics Symposium (1986) 855–860

3 Kasai, C., K. Namekawa: Real-Time Two-Dimensional Blood Flow Imaging using an Autocorrelation Technique. IEEE Ultrasonics Symposium (1985) 953–985

4 Kasai, C., K. Namekawa, A. Koyano, R. Omoto: Real-Time Two-Dimensional Blood Flow Imaging using an Autocorrelation Technique. IEEE Transactions on Sonics and Ultrasonics, Vol. SU–32 (1985) 458–463

2 Biological Effects of Ultrasound

P.-M. Klews

2.1 Introduction

This chapter deals with some general aspects of the biological effects of ultrasound at intensities commonly used in diagnostic equipment. Therapeutic sound intensities like those used in shock-wave lithotripsy are substantially higher.

The energy of diagnostic ultrasound enters the body in the form of a pressure pulse, and the returning pressure waves, or echoes, are evaluated according to various criteria. A portion of the energy that does not leave the body as echoes is absorbed by tissue. One cannot simply measure the total applied energy and use that to assess the biological effects of ultrasound. For example, one could stroke a dog with the palm of the hand for an hour and the absorbed energy per unit time would not be high enough to injure the animal. But if the same energy were absorbed through a small area in one millisecond, a potentially lethal "bioeffect" could result. The energy of a gentle stroke administered with a sharp blade would likewise produce a traumatizing effect. These unusual examples illustrate the principle that a great many separate factors must be taken into account before it can be determined whether a procedure is safe or harmful.

2.2 Definition of Intensity

The term intensity is commonly used. Here it shall be defined as it pertains to ultrasound. Only harmonic, longitudinal sound waves will be considered. First the nature of a sound wave will be reviewed briefly.

What is it that propagates in a sound wave? Particles (atoms or molecules) oscillate around their resting or equilibrium position (center of gravity). But in the time-average, the particles do not move from their equilibrium position; that is, they do not travel with the wave. Only a state of motion propagates with the wave. Thus the wave carries energy and momentum, not matter, from one place to another. Because of particle motion, sound waves represent a mechanical transfer of energy and momentum.

A change of pressure (the pressure gradient) leads to an acceleration of particles. In the case of a harmonic wave, the pressure fluctuates uniformly around a mean value. During compression of the sound-conducting medium, an increased or higher than normal pressure prevails at a given site at a given point in time. During rarefication a decreased or lower than usual pressure (negative pressure or rarefication pressure) prevails at a given site and time. This time-varying pressure is logically termed the alternating sound pressure, designated $p(t)$, or simply the acoustic or sound pressure. It represents the difference between the pressure that prevails at a given instant (instantaneous pressure) and the equilibrium (steady-state) pressure that ordinarily prevails. This difference corresponds to the pressure pulse that is emitted by the ultrasound transducer.

The displacement of the oscillating particles from their equilibrium position, termed the amplitude $A(t)$ in Section 17.3.2, is a time-varying quantity. The displacement may be positive or negative, i.e., in the direction of motion or opposite to it. The largest displacement is designated A_0.

The particles move at a velocity v relative to their equilibrium position. The velocity v of particle motion in the sound wave corresponds to the temporal change in amplitude $\left(v = \frac{dA}{dt}\right)$ and is termed the particle velocity. The particle velocity itself is time-varying, because the particles are alternately accelerated and decelerated as they oscillate back and forth around their equilibrium position. In the case of a harmonic wave, the maximum particle velocity is $v_0 = 2\pi f A_0$ (f = frequency). This differs from the speed of sound c, which is the velocity of propagation of the wave, or the speed at which a sound wave moves through a medium. The speed of sound is equal to the phase velocity of the longitudinal wave and is a material constant. The speed of sound c is equal to the product of the wavelength λ times the frequency f. Group velocity and signal velocity are subjects best explored in physics texts (see for example [1]).

It shall now be attempted to explain the concept of sound intensity without referral to explicit computations (the precise calculation can be found in [2] and [9]). A sound (pressure) pulse is generated at the surface of the ultrasound transducer. The transducer elements exert a force upon the medium, and thus incite a displacement of the particles, which move at the particle velocity $v(t)$. The instantaneous energy that is applied per unit area, also called the instantaneous energy density, is the product of the particle velocity and the applied sound pressure $p(t)$. It is assumed that particle motion (velocity) and the applied pressure are in phase. The sound intensity I is the temporal average of the instantaneous energy density or the average energy flow per unit area. Averaging over time leads to the equation:

$$I_{ave} = 2\varrho c\pi^2 f^2 A_0^2 = \frac{1}{2}\varrho c v_0^2 = \frac{p_0^2}{2\varrho c} \quad (2.1)$$

where ϱ = specific density of the medium
f = transducer center frequency
A_0 = maximum particle displacement
v_0 = maximum particle velocity
p_0 = maximum pressure

The sound intensity, then, increases with the square of the transducer center frequency and with the square of the maximum particle displacement. The maximum instantaneous sound intensity is two times greater than the time-averaged sound intensity noted above.

2.3 Commonly Used Average Intensity Definitions

The ultrasound user should have at least a working knowledge of the various terms used to designate intensity. Since these terms sometimes appear in the operating instructions furnished by equipment manufacturers and suppliers, they should be mentioned here. The following definitions are based on FDA guidelines (7) and refer to terms that are important in assessing the power output of ultrasound transducers. Some of these terms are illustrated in Figure 2.**1**. For clarity, amplitude variations rather than intensity variations are plotted in the figure as a function of time. The intensity is always positive, of course, and is proportional to the square of the amplitude, as stated in equation 2.1.

The maximum sound intensity I_m is defined as the highest intensity of the sound pulse time-averaged over one pulse half-cycle (one half of a wavelength). The measurement is made at the site where the sound intensity is highest—generally at the focus of the transducer. The maximum local intensity at the time of the highest amplitude I_{SPTP} (spatial peak–temporal peak intensity) corresponds to the highest pressure amplitude in the acoustic field. The spatial peak of the temporal average intensity, averaged over the pulse interval t_{PRF}, is designated as I_{SPTA} (spatial peak–temporal average intensity). This is the value most commonly used in describing ultrasound intensity. The temporal average intensity averaged over the pulse cross-sectional area is designated as I_{SATA} (spatial average–temporal average intensity). This is the lowest of the above intensity values. Spatial averaging is done over the cross-sectional area of the sound pulse and over time. This is defined as the area in which the individual local intensities are no less than 25% of the maximum intensity (actually 25% of the maximum pulse intensity integral). Temporal averaging is done over the scan interval—the time needed to complete one complete scan, equal to the reciprocal of the frame rate. The spatial peak of the pulse average intensity is designated as I_{SPPA} (spatial peak–pulse average intensity). The pulse is time-averaged over the duration of one pulse. The pulse duration, or the time from the beginning to the end of a pulse, is defined as 1.25 times the time period during which the value of the time integral over the intensity lies between 10% and 90% of the total value. The pulse duration divided by the temporal pulse interval (t_{pulse}/t_{PRF}) yields the "duty factor", or the fraction of time that the sound is "on".

The pulse repetition frequency at a given site can be very low on pure gray-scale scanners, because only

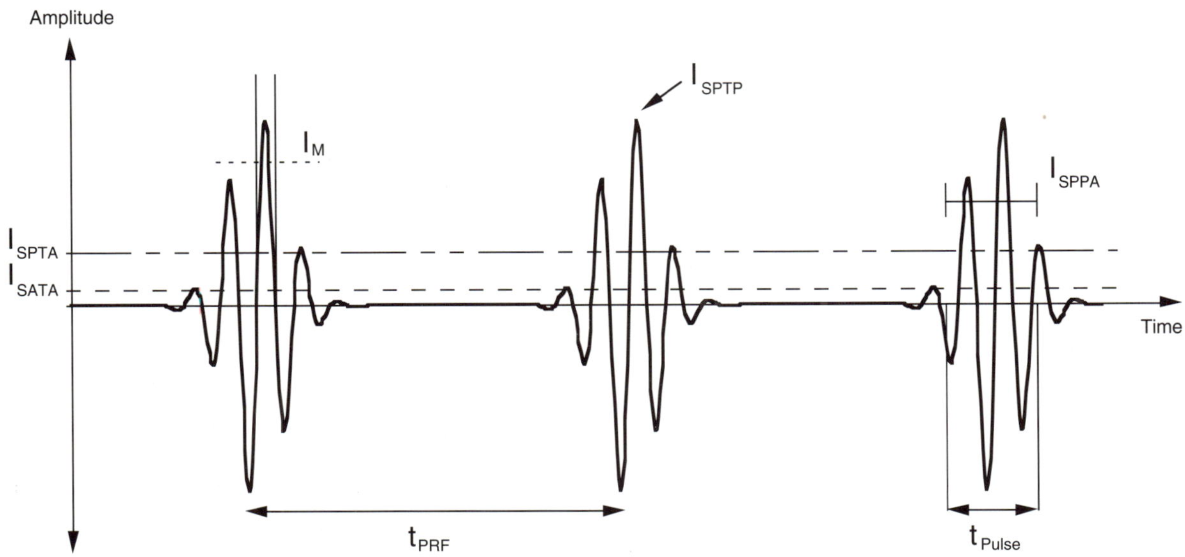

Fig. 2.**1** The various definitions of intensity are explained in the text. The intensity levels and pulse length t_{pulse} are shown only in approximation and are not drawn to scale

one pulse may be required per ultrasound scan line. The pulse repetition frequency may be equal to the frame rate. For this reason alone, the SPTA intensity is significantly higher on Doppler systems for a given maximum amplitude than on other types of systems. A Doppler system may be operated at the highest pulse repetition frequency that will still allow for unambiguous Doppler evaluation. In HPRF-Doppler-mode the pulse repetition frequency will even exceed this limit.

All of these intensity values can be measured in water using a hydrophone. Of course, the intensity values in water I_{water} are substantially higher than in tissue due to the greater attenuation of sound in tissue. Unfortunately, the intracorporal ultrasound intensities $I_{in\ situ}$, the only really relevant values, cannot be measured directly, but can only be estimated from the measured water values using the following formula (7):

$$I_{in\ situ} = I_{water} e^{-0.23afz} \qquad (2.2)$$

where a = attenuation coefficient at 1MHz (in $^{dB}/_{MHz\ cm}$)
f = transducer center frequency in MHz
z = distance from the transducer

The following attenuation coefficients (in $^{dB}/_{MHz\ cm}$) are assumed for various soft tissues (7):

Brain	0.53 ± 0.3
Heart	0.66 ± 0.26
Kidney	0.79 ± 0.15
Liver	0.43 ± ?
Muscle	0.55 ± ?

Detailed information on methods of intensity measurement and on other data can be found in (8) and (12). Intensity values measured in water along with the in situ values are listed in Table 2.**1** for two ultrasound systems having a number of different transducers and capable of operating in different modes.

New national (USA) AIUM/NEMA guidelines for the display of thermal and mechanical acoustic output indices were published in 1992 (4) and will be discussed shortly at the end of this chapter. A new international standard (IEC 1157) for the declaration of the acoustic output of medical diagnostic ultrasound equipment was also published in 1992 (11). This will also be discussed in Section 2.6. The national (USA only) guidelines and the international standard have somewhat different viewpoints.

Table 2.**1** As an example the intensity values measured in water along with the calculated in situ values are listed for two ultrasound systems (A and B) having a number of different transducers and capable of operating in different modes. The I_M values are as a rule of the thumb about twice as high as the I_{SPPA} values. LA, linear array; CA, curved array; EV, endovaginal curved array

Transducer Systems A and B	Intensity	Units	B-mode in water/in situ	M-mode in water/in situ	PW Doppler or color-M-mode in water/in situ	CDS-mode in water/in situ
LA 3.5 MHz (A)	I_{SPTA}	mW/cm²	54/ 16	80/ 25	620/ 74	290/ 87
	I_{SPPA}	W/cm²	200/ 60	200/ 60	64/ 7.7	350/110
LA 3.5 MHz (B)	I_{SPTA}	mW/cm²	18/ 6	89/ 31	552/243	209/ 72
	I_{SPPA}	W/cm²	226/ 91	226/ 91	76/ 34	270/ 92
CA 3.5 MHz (A)	I_{SPTA}	mW/cm²	35/ 9	66/ 17	920/ 74	130/ 57
	I_{SPPA}	W/cm²	130/ 32	130/ 32	91/ 9	200/ 57
CA 3.5 MHz (B)	I_{SPTA}	mW/cm²	146/ 64	155/ 58	1237/446	149/ 74
	I_{SPPA}	W/cm²	347/152	473/176	230/ 83	313/171
LA 5.0 MHz (A)	I_{SPTA}	mW/cm²	140/ 62	200/ 87	840/ 81	210/ 85
	I_{SPPA}	W/cm²	310/140	310/140	110/ 13	400/170
LA 5.0 MHz (B)	I_{SPTA}	mW/cm²	10/ 4	35/ 10	351/206	117/ 30
	I_{SPPA}	W/cm²	191/ 72	168/ 49	101/ 59	326/ 72
LA 7.5 MHz (A)	I_{SPTA}	mW/cm²	110/ 51	150/ 69	280/ 84	78/ 35
	I_{SPPA}	W/cm²	300/170	300/170	190/ 54	310/140
LA 7.5 MHz (B)	I_{SPTA}	mW/cm²	26/ 13	81/ 31	1756/961	153/ 78
	I_{SPPA}	W/cm²	570/213	491/188	419/230	384/197
EV 6.5 MHz (A)	I_{SPTA}	mW/cm²	64/ 30	74/ 36	250/ 81	160/ 72
	I_{SPPA}	W/cm²	130/ 61	130/ 61	100/ 34	200/ 92
EV 6.5 MHz (B)	I_{SPTA}	mW/cm²	5/ 2	18/ 9	77/ 32	54/ 18
	I_{SPPA}	W/cm²	69/ 25	90/ 42	22/ 9	197/ 66

2.4 Statements on Ultrasound Safety

The biological safety of ultrasound is of central importance. The assumption that ultrasound is not harmful to patients at diagnostic levels is based largely on the statement issued by the Biological Effects Committee of the American Institute of Ultrasound in Medicine (AIUM) in 1978 (3):

> **Statement of Mammalian in Vivo Ultrasonic Biological Effects**
> October 1978
>
> In the low megahertz frequency range there have been as of October, 1978, no confirmed significant effects in mammalian tissues exposed to intensities* below 100 mW/cm². Furthermore, for ultrasonic exposure times ** less than 500 seconds and greater than one second, such effects have not been demonstrated even at higher intensities, when the product on intensity * and exposure time ** is less than 50 joules/cm².
>
> * Spatial peak, temporal average as measured in free field in water.
>
> ** Total time: this includes off-time as well as on-time for a repeated-pulse regime.

The above statement indicates that the I_{SPTA} may exceed 100 mW/cm². Exposure to an intensity of 100 mW/cm² for 500 seconds yields a total of 50 Ws/cm² (1 joule = 1 Ws). Thus, if the transducer output is equal to 500 mW/cm², for example, the exposure time should not exceed 100 seconds. While this precaution does not limit technical progress in diagnostic ultrasound, it does oblige the examiner to complete the examination in a minimum amount of time when higher intensities are employed.

The AIUM issued another important statement on clinical safety in 1983 (14):

> **Statement on Clinical Safety**
>
> No confirmed biological effects on patients or instrument operators caused by exposure at intensities typical of present diagnostic ultrasound instruments have ever been reported. Although the possibility exists that such biological effects may be identified in the future, current data indicate that the benefits to patients of the prudent use of diagnostic ultrasound outweigh the risks, if any, that may be present.

In conceding the possibility of bioeffects, the AIUM acknowledges the fact that, practically speaking, the biological safety of diagnostic ultrasound cannot be absolutely assured. Nevertheless, the advantages for the patient outweigh the possibly existing risks. For this reason the examiner should always apply the **ALARA principle** (*A*s *L*ow *A*s *R*easonably *A*chievable) by using the lowest ultrasound intensity that is sufficient to make a diagnosis and by keeping the examination as brief as possible. Careful patient selection when doing ultrasound examinations is just as important as when using any other diagnostic method. This particularly applies to Doppler examinations.

Finally, it should be emphasized that no adverse biologic effects from exposure to diagnostic ultrasound have ever been reported anywhere in the world.

2.5 Cavitation and Heat Production

The current debate on the safety of diagnostic ultrasound centers on two effects: cavitation and local heat production. Some physical aspects related to these effects will be considered here. It is not intended to present a complete and thorough analysis of the problems.

Cavitation generally refers to the formation or growth of gas bubbles in a liquid medium. How does a gas-filled space form within a liquid? Thermodynamics can give the answer. The phenomenon can be understood in terms of general thermodynamic principles illustrated by analogies drawn from everyday experience. The precise definitions of the very complex thermodynamic functions will not be given (see for example [10]).

Cavitation is based upon a phase transition from a liquid to a gaseous state. Figure 2.**2** shows the pressure–temperature phase diagram of an arbitrary material. A substance exists in a particular phase or state: solid, liquid, or gaseous. A change of state from the liquid phase to the gas phase, for example, can be achieved by lowering the ambient pressure while keeping the temperature constant. An ultrasound pulse is a pressure pulse or local change of pressure. It disrupts the equilibrium of the system. A substantial negative pressure (lower than in the steady state) develops in the rarefication phase of the pressure pulse, and this may be sufficient to incite a phase transition from liquid to gas. The pressure pulse adds energy to the system; this energy enables the phase transition. This transition is not associated with a rise in temperature (isothermal growth). As can be seen

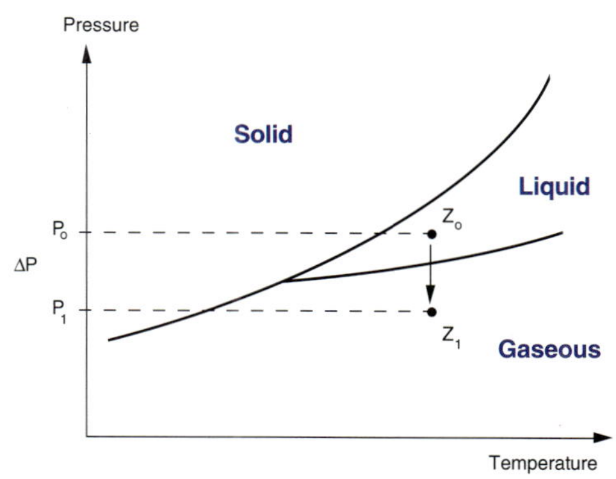

Fig. 2.**2** Pressure–temperature phase diagram. A phase transition from the liquid state (Z_0) to the gaseous state (Z_1) can occur without a rise in ambient temperature

from the phase diagram, incidentally, washed and frozen laundry can dry in the wintertime at subfreezing ambient temperatures as the water (ice) transforms directly from the solid to the vapor state.

Once a gas bubble has formed, depending on its size, it will grow or collapse. This is governed by various parameters such as the duration of the ultrasound exposure, i.e., the pulse length, the surface area of the newly created bubbles, and the volume of the bubbles. There is a critical size beyond which bubbles tend to grow rather than collapse. The decisive thermodynamic quantity is the free energy of the bubble. This has both a volume component and a surface area component. Every object tends to minimize its surface area for a given volume, i.e., objects tend to minimize their free energy. This is why soap bubbles are round, for example. If the surface term is greater than the volume term, the gas bubble will collapse; if not, it will remain stable.

Stable gas bubbles do not pose a problem. But when a bubble collapses, all of its energy is released at the site of the bubble, causing a marked local rise in temperature. In a special case Apfel et al. (5) calculated a significant temperature increase associated with the collapse of gas bubbles up to 3 μm in size.

When speaking of temperature elevation induced by ultrasound, generally, the possible rise in temperature caused by cavitation is not meant. In this case heating is caused by the absorption of the energy introduced into the body by the ultrasound pulse. Only a small fraction of the applied ultrasound energy leaves the body in the form of echoes. Most is lost through absorption. As noted earlier, an incident pressure wave displaces particles and lets them oscillate around their equilibrium position. They return to that position after the pressure wave has passed. The associated kinetic energy is released to the environment in the form of heat. Under extreme conditions, Carnes et al. (6) observed temperature elevations of 1 to 4 °C in fetal mice.

A good review of ultrasound bioeffects can be found in Wells (13). Articles on this subject are frequently published in *Ultrasound in Medicine and Biology.*

2.6 New Guidelines for the Declaration of Acoustic Output

In 1992 two new guidelines for reporting the acoustic output of medical diagnostic ultrasound equipment were published. One guideline was developed for the USA by the American Institute of Ultrasound in Medicine (AIUM) together with the National Electrical Manufacturers Association (NEMA). It is called the "Standard for Real-Time Display of Thermal and Mechanical Acoustic Output Indices on Diagnostic Ultrasound Equipment" (ODS) (4). The other was developed by the International Electrotechnical Commission as an international standard and is called the IEC 1157 or "Requirements for the Declaration of the Acoustic Output of Medical Diagnostic Ultrasound Equipment" (11).

A basic look at the two guidelines based on a random example is presented here. Interested readers are referred to the published guidelines. Surprisingly, both guidelines have very little in common. According to IEC 1157 the I_{SPTA}, peak-negative acoustic pressure, output beam intensity, and other values measured directly in water must be stated. The AIUM/NEMA guidelines call for the publication of special unitless indices based on derated values such as a number of thermal indices and the mechanical index. IEC 1157 asks for data that can be readily measured in a water tank, whereas AIUM/NEMA ask for the water tank measurements to be derated and then inserted into a special formula to calculate the respective index. In situ measurement is in general not possible. That means that all measurements must be conducted in either case in water using special calibrated hydrophones. According to AIUM/NEMA, all measured data must be derated with the help of a special derating factor. This is a "multiplicative factor applied to acoustic output parameters intended to account for ultrasonic attenuation of tissue between the source and the particular location in the tissue. The average ultrasonic attenuation is assumed to be 0.3 dB/MHz cm along the beam axis in the body."

IEC 1157, for example, asks that the non derated peak-negative or peak-rarefication acoustic pressure P_r measured directly in water (in MPa) be stated. AIUM/NEMA on the other hand, ask for the mechanical index MI, which also is based only on the measurement of p_r to be displayed. The mechanical index is defined as (4):

$$MI = \frac{P_{r.3}(Z_{sp})}{\sqrt{f_c}}$$

where $P_{r.3}(Z_{sp})$ = peak-rarefication acoustic pressure derated by 0.3 dB/MHz cm
f_c = center frequency in MHz

Now, derating of the amplitude is accomplished by inserting the measured water value of $p_r = p_{water}$ into a slight modification of equation 2.2 (12):

$$P_{r.3}(Z_{sp}) = p_{water}\ e^{-0.115\,afz}$$

where $a = 0.3$ = attenuation coefficient at 1 MHz (in dB/MHz cm),
$f = f_c$ = transducer center frequency in MHz,
$z = Z_{sp}$ = distance from the transducer where the derated pressure is highest

The above equation for the MI would not be unitless. Making the mechanical index unitless calls for (4) the above equation to be multiplied by $\frac{\sqrt{1 MHz}}{1 MPa}$

It is difficult to compare the MI and p_r. The distance Z_{sp} from the transducer where the derated peak-rarefication pressure is measured may be different from the distance z at which the nonderated peak-rarefication pressure is located. The thermal indices also require a lot of arithmetic.

In attempting a numerical comparison between the two guidelines it will be supposed that the distances Z_{sp} are practically the same. Taking the MI to be equal to 1 and looking at a 3.5 MHz transducer having its maximum peak pressure at a depth of 12 cm leads to a derated peak-negative pressure $p_{r.3}$ of 1.87 MPa. The pressure p_r actually measured in water with a hydrophone would be 7.97 MPa. Similar results are achieved when looking at the SPTA intensity. According to NEMA (12) equation 2.2 must be used in this case. Imagine the derated $I_{SPTA.3}$ at a depth of 12 cm using the same 3.5 MHz transducer would be 100 mW/cm^2. Inserting these values into equation 2.2 leads to a nonderated I_{SPTA} of 1,814 mW/cm^2 or 1.8 W/cm^2. Of course, these numerical comparisons are not absolutely correct because of the reasons stated above but it is close enough in order to get a general impression of the differences between the two guidelines. The true in situ pressure or intensity is always unknown during an actual examination. They are patient-and scan-plane-dependent. Derated values are an educated guess.

The objective of both guidelines is to provide maximum information to the user and the patient while minimizing the patient's exposure to ultrasound. Both guidelines are in use. Obviously much more can be said about both guidelines. It is definitely not the aim of this book to decide which guideline is of more help to the user and the patient. The existence of two guidelines is, regrettably, often not known.

2.7 References

1 Alonso, M., E. Finn: Fundamental University Physics, Vol. 2. Addison-Wesley (1975) 704–706

2 Alonso, M., E. Finn: Fundamental University Physics, Vol. 2. Addison-Wesley (1975) 694–697

3 American Institute of Ultrasound in Medicine (AIUM)/National Electrical Manufacturers Association (NEMA): Safety Standard for Diagnostic Ultrasound Equipment, Standards Pub. No. UL 1-1981. J. Ultrasound Med. (Suppl.) 2, No. 4 (1983) 20

4 American Institute of Ultrasound in Medicine (AIUM)/National Electrical Manufacturers Association (NEMA): Standard for Real-Time Display of Thermal and Mechanical Acoustic Output Indices on Diagnostic Ultrasound Equipment (1992)

5 Apfel, R. E., C. K. Holland: Gauging the likelihood of cavitation from short-pulse, low-duty cycle diagnostic ultrasound. Ultrasound Med. Biol., 17, No. 2 (1991) 179–185

6 Carnes, K. I., J. L. Drewniak, F. Dunn: In utero measurement of ultrasonically induced fetal mouse temperature increases. Ultrasound Med. Biology. 17, No. 4 (1991) 373–382.

7 510(k) Guide for Measuring and Reporting Acoustic Output of Diagnostic Ultrasound Medical Devices, Dec. 1985. Center for Devices and Radiological Health

8 Duck, F. A.: The measurement of exposure to ultrasound and its application to estimates of ultrasound "dose". Phys. Med. Biol. 12, No. 3 (1987) 303–325

9 Gerthsen, C., H. O. Kneser, H. Vogel: Physik, 12th ed. Springer-Verlag (1974) 187–188

10 Huang, K.: Statistische Mechanik, Vol. 1. Bibliographisches Institut, Hochschultaschenbücher Verlag (1964)

11 International Electrotechnical Commission: International Standard (IEC 1157), Requirements for the Declaration of the Acoustic Output of Medical Diagnostic Ultrasound Equipment, 1st ed. (1992–07)

12 National Electrical Manufacturers Association (NEMA): Acoustic Output Measurement Standard for Diagnostic Ultrasound Equipment, Standard Pub. No. UD 2, 1992, 46, § 5.4.13 (MI), 47, § 5.4.21, and 5.4.26 (I_{SPTA})

13 Wells, P. N. T.: Biomedical Ultrasonics. Academic Press (1977)

14 Wells, P. N. T. (Ed.): The safety of diagnostic ultrasound. Brit. J. Radiol. (Suppl.) 20 (1987) 26

3 Basic Hemodynamics

P. Landwehr

3.1 Introduction

Just as hydrodynamics describe the motion of fluids, especially of water, and the interactions of the fluid with its boundaries, hemodynamics are concerned with the flow characteristics of blood. Blood is a mixture of plasma and cellular constituents, mostly erythrocytes. Hydrodynamic principles are applicable to blood vessels that are normally accessible to duplex sonography (larger than 1 mm in diameter) (10).

The flow velocity profile has been thought of as being basically parabolic with the streamlines in normal vessels running parallel to one another and also parallel to the vessel walls. Based on more precise evaluation methods, often using ultrasound, the concept of spiral flow is emerging. The flow profile in systole displayed in figure 17.4, for example, can well be explained when using this concept. If this proves to be true, it will have a strong impact on the quantitative evaluation of flow. Nevertheless the basic qualitative concepts and methods described in this chapter remain valid.

Like all fluids, blood exhibits the physical property of viscosity (based on internal friction), which determines the force needed to move adjacent fluid layers relative to one another. The viscosity of blood is determined mainly by its hematocrit. Its viscosity remains constant up to a hematocrit of about 10. Above that value it increases exponentially according to an empirical equation. Besides depending on the volume of the red blood cells, the viscosity of blood also depends on the viscosity of plasma and the diameter of the blood vessel. There is a substantial decrease of blood viscosity in the terminal capillary bed due to a deformation of the erythrocytes.

3.2 Continuous Flow

3.2.1 Preliminary Remarks

The ideal conditions enabling continuous laminar flow (see section 3.2.3) are rare in the human body. The flow velocity profile, or distribution of flow velocities across the vessel lumen, can vary greatly due to the elasticity of the vessel walls, the pulsatility of the flow, and the vessels curvature and branching. Nevertheless, an analysis of the physical principles governing continuous flow is helpful in understanding flow phenomena associated with pulsatile flow and stenotic vascular lesions and their visualization by color duplex sonography (CDS).

3.2.2 Physical Aspects

Flow, which is the movement of a fluid (or of particles) in a certain direction, can arise only when a force is exerted upon the fluid. The flow velocity in continuous flow is independent of time. The relationship between the flow volume per unit time q, viscosity η, length of the vascular segment l, vessel radius r, and the pressure difference $P_2 - P_1$ between two different points along the segment of interest is described by the Hagen–Poiseuille equation:

$$P_2 - P_1 = \frac{8 \cdot l \cdot \eta \cdot q}{\pi \cdot r^4}$$

By analogy with Ohm's law in electricity

$$U = R \cdot I$$

where U = potential difference (voltage, electromotive force) (corresponds to $P_2 - P_1$),
R = resistance,
I = current (corresponds to q)

the resistance to flow can be calculated from the Hagen-Poiseuille equation:

$$R = \frac{8 \cdot l \cdot \eta}{\pi \cdot r^4}$$

This means that decreasing the vessel radius by one-half, for example, increases the flow resistance by a factor of 16. The major part of the total resistance of the vascular system originates from the arterioles (3)—the part of the arterial vascular tree with the largest capacity for vasomotor regulation (Fig. 3.**1**). This fact must be considered in all Doppler examinations, since the peripheral vascular resistance can (and usually does) affect all flow phenomena observed by

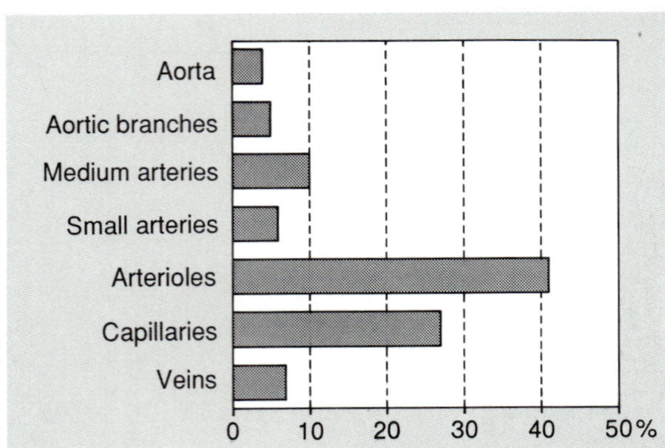

Fig. 3.**1** Relative flow resistance in different parts of the vascular system (3)

Doppler spectrum analysis or color duplex sonography.

3.2.3 Flow Velocity Profile in a Straight Vessel with a Uniform circular Cross-Sectional Area

The flow velocity profile in a central longitudinal section of a straight, rigid vessel with a uniform, circular cross-sectional area will be approximately parabolic. The flow velocities are highest at the center of the vessel, while the fluid layers in contact with the vessel walls are assumed to have zero flow velocity. This "laminar" flow pattern can be visualized in a simplified way as being created by a stack of concentric hollow cylinders (laminae) moving along smooth paths in the same direction at different velocities relative to one another (2) (Fig. 3.2**a, b**). The velocities are inversely proportional to the distance of the cylinder from the center of the vessel. The velocity gradient (velocity difference over distance between adjacent laminae) depends on the viscosity of the fluid. The shape of the flow profile is influenced by viscosity (internal friction), cohesion (the tendency of bodies of like composition to hold together as a result of intermolecular attractive forces), and adhesion of the fluid to the vessel walls (responsible for external friction). Flow is usually laminar when it is directed parallel to the vessel walls.

In CDS imaging a laminar flow velocity profile is present when the lightest shades of a color are located along the center of a vessel, indicating central high-velocity flow. At the same time, flow close to the vessel walls is coded in darker shades of the same color representing lower flow velocities (Fig. 3.4**b, c**).

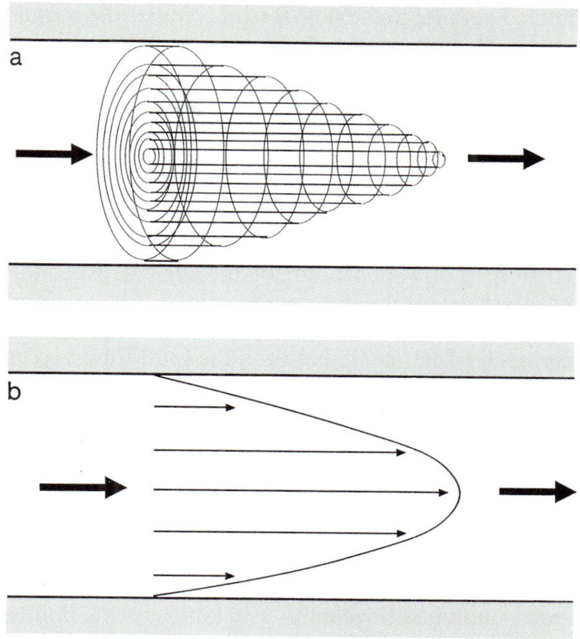

Fig. 3.2**a, b** Principle of laminar flow in a vessel with a circular cross section
a The flow velocity within individual fluid layers (concentric cylinders) increases with distance from the vessel wall
b Laminar flow velocity profile in longitudinal section. The tips of the individual velocity vectors describe a parabola. Flow velocities are highest at the center of the vessel

3.2.4 Effects of Geometric Changes of the Lumen Cross-Sectional Area on the Flow Velocity Profile

The mean flow velocity of a fluid originating from a reservoir or a vessel with a larger diameter in comparison to the mean flow velocity in a more distal segment with a reduced diameter will be lower than in the distal segment due to the reduction in cross-sectional area. This effect is based on the principle of continuity, i.e., there is no loss or gain of fluid volume (volumetric flow is independent of the vessel cross-sectional area). The flow velocity profile in the initial portion of the segment is very flat ("entrance effect, plug flow") except for a large velocity gradient in the boundary layer along the vessel walls. Farther along the distal segment the flow gradually reaches its steady-state parabolic velocity profile.

The opposite effect occurs when there is a sudden increase in the cross-sectional vessel area ("exit effect"). The flow velocity profile elongates as the velocity gradient between the central and peripheral laminae increases. Eventually the parabolic flow velocity profile will be restored. The more drastic the increase in lumen diameter, the greater the likelihood of flow separation near the vessel walls. This is characterized by localized zones of flow reversal—intrinsically laminar eddy currents. This must be differentiated from turbulence (see section 3.2.5). This type of physiological flow separation occurs, for example, in the carotid bulb where the common carotid artery bifurcates into the internal and external carotid arteries. Flow separation is also commonly observed distal to a vascular stenosis, especially when there is a sudden increase in vessel diameter (Fig. 3.**9**). Localized flow reversal is visualized in CDS by pixels near the vessel walls, which are encoded in a color opposite to that of the main flow direction.

3.2.5 Disturbed Flow and Turbulence

Depending on the viscosity and density of the fluid as well as the cross-sectional area of the vessel lumen, the volume flow rate increases proportionally as predicted by the Hagen–Poiseuille law when the pressure difference along the vascular segment is increased. If the cross-sectional area of the lumen remains constant, for example, the flow velocity must increase. If the flow velocity is increased beyond a certain value, the initially laminar flow is destabilized. At first the fluid laminae are no longer continually directed parallel to the vessel walls. Wave-like irregularities develop in the laminae, creating a pattern known as "disturbed flow". As the flow velocity continues to increase, vortices may form near the vessel walls. Since the Doppler angles related to the individual fluid particles are no longer identical, an inhomogeneous distribution of different shades of color appears in the CDS image across the vessel lumen. Some pixels may undergo a complete color flip, even in disturbed flow, depending on the angle between the total flow vector (vector sum of all the flow vectors) and the direction of the ultrasound beam. This will only occur if the angle between the total flow vector and ultrasound beam is close to 90°. A Doppler angle close to 90° is unfavorable for all angle-dependent Doppler ultrasound techniques and should be avoided if possible by repositioning the transducer or by electronically steering the ultrasound beam at another angle.

When the flow velocity exceeds a critical value, the entire lumen is filled with fluid components whose individual velocity vectors are randomly aimed in all directions. This "chaotic" flow pattern is the result of turbulence (2) (Fig. 3.**9**). The total velocity vector, however, still points in the main flow direction. The flow velocity profile in a region with turbulent flow is very flat, resulting in a large velocity gradient near the vessel walls. Turbulent flow can be recognized in CDS by a mixture of different color pixels next to one another representing flow in different directions.

The existence of turbulent flow depends on the vessel diameter $d = 2r$ (r = radius), the average flow velocity v across the vessel lumen, the density of the fluid ρ, and the viscosity η of the fluid. Using these variables the Reynolds number—named after Osborne Reynolds who first described this phenomenon—can be calculated:

$$\mathrm{Re} = \frac{v \cdot 2 \cdot r \cdot \rho}{\eta}$$

The Reynolds number is dimensionless. A value of approximately 2000 is generally defined as the critical value for the transition from laminar to turbulent blood flow (11). In the presence of stenotic vascular lesions, however, the critical value of Re can be much lower. It is not necessary to know the particular Reynolds number for a stenosis in order to understand how the stenosis affects blood flow and how the hemodynamics are displayed in color duplex imaging. Nevertheless, a knowledge of the factors influencing the development of turbulent flow is helpful in understanding hemodynamic phenomena arising in certain situations (see section 3.4.3).

As an additional feature on some diagnostic ultrasound systems a special color (green) is added to the existing colors to encode the degree of local variance of the average flow velocity ("velocity variance mode", sections 1.8 and 17.4.1). This reportedly enables a more sensitive detection of disturbed flow (16) (Fig. 3.**10**, see also Chapter 4).

3.3 Pulsatile Flow

3.3.1 Preliminary Remarks

Compared with continuous flow, the analysis of discontinuous, pulsatile flow is considerably more complex. To keep the thematic scope of this book within reasonable limits, the reader is referred to McDonald (12) for a detailed discussion of the boundary conditions of pulsatile flow. However, a brief review of some specific aspects of this type of flow is given.

3.3.2 Origin of Pulsatile Flow Patterns

On account of the pulsatile pumping action of the heart, flow in the arterial vascular system is characterized by alternating phases of acceleration and deceleration. The heart creates both pressure and volume changes. Anatomic and physical circumstances modulate the original intraventricular pressure and volume-flow curves. Whereas large pressure amplitudes develop in the left ventricle during each cardiac cycle, the aorta and large vessels reduce the pressure amplitudes that are transmitted to the arterial tree (Windkessel effect, aortic compliance). The large vessels constitute a reservoir that is sufficiently compliant to store some of the pulsatile energy of the heart and allow for a more continuous flow than that created by the left ventricle alone. The magnitude of the continuous flow component within the pulsatile flow cycle depends on the peripheral vascular resistance to flow. Flow resistance, especially at the arteriolar level, gives rise to reflections of varying intensity that influence the flow velocity waveforms. These different boundary conditions result in two basic types of Doppler waveform representing pulsatile flow: high-resistance flow and low-resistance flow.

The flow waveforms recorded in the peripheral arteries at rest (Figs. 3.**3a**, 3.**4a–g**) are an example of flow under high peripheral resistance. Since only a low flow rate is required at rest in these vessels, the arterioles are mostly vasoconstricted. The time–velocity curves, or Doppler spectra, typically exhibit a sharp systolic rise up to peak systole, followed by a quick drop in flow velocity. In early and mid-diastole a significant reverse flow is detected followed by a second, small forward-flow component in late diastole. This constitutes the typical triphasic flow pattern seen when the body is at rest, in arteries that mainly supply the muscles and skin with blood and not the inner organs (e.g., the arteries of the arms and legs, the external carotid artery, the penile arteries, and to a limited degree the mesenteric artery). Physiological conditions that increase the peripheral circulatory demand (e.g., muscular work, tumescence, digestion) as well as pathological conditions (e.g., local inflammation, sepsis, poststenotic situation) tend to lower the peripheral vascular resistance both through central regulatory mechanisms (increased heart rate, stroke volume, and blood pressure) and by vasodilata-

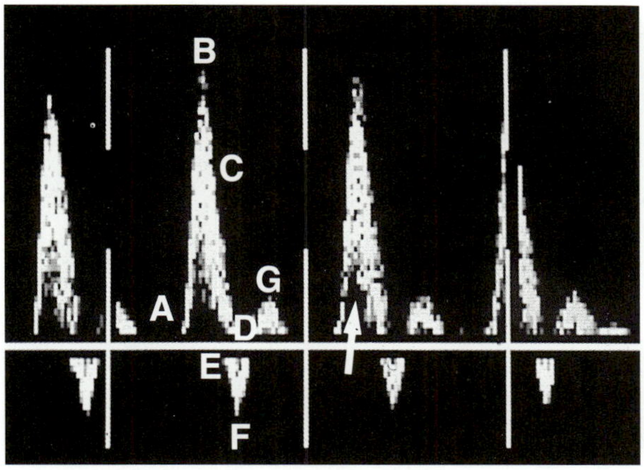

a

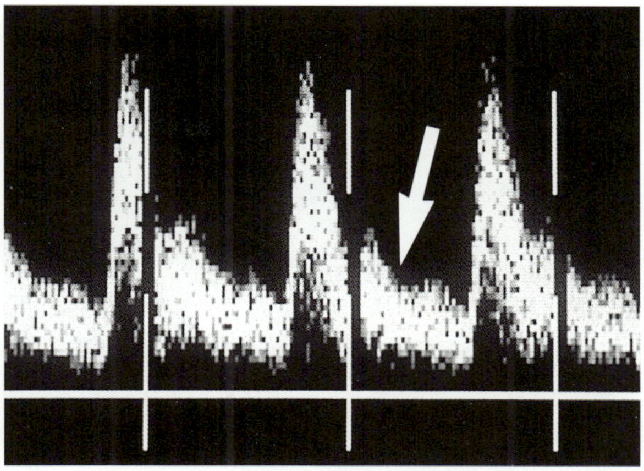

b

Fig. 3.**3a–c** Influence of the peripheral flow resistance on Doppler spectra recorded from the brachial artery (**a**, **b**) and internal carotid artery (**c**) in a healthy subject
a Triphasic spectrum at rest. High peripheral vascular flow resistance (peripheral-artery pattern) with a sharp systolic velocity increase (A–B), a rapid drop in velocity in late systole (C–D), diastolic flow reversal (E–F), and late-diastolic forward flow (G). Note the spectral window below the systolic peak (white arrow)
b After exercise (10 tight fist clenchings), a pronounced forward-flow component appears in diastole (white arrow) due to the decrease in peripheral flow resistance. The spectral pattern is intermediate between **a** and **c**
c Low peripheral vascular flow resistance. The spectrum displays a high diastolic forward flow and less pulsatility than in **a** and **b** (parenchymal artery pattern). The empty systolic window (arrow) indicates undisturbed flow. Periodic refreshing of the color duplex image creates a brief, intermittent void in the spectral waveform (*)

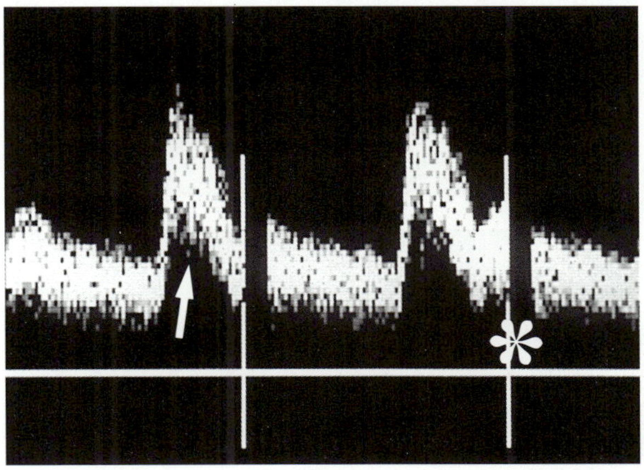

c

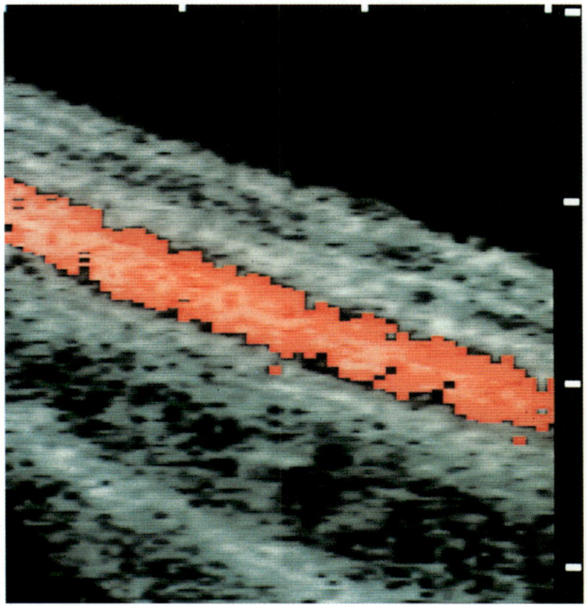

a

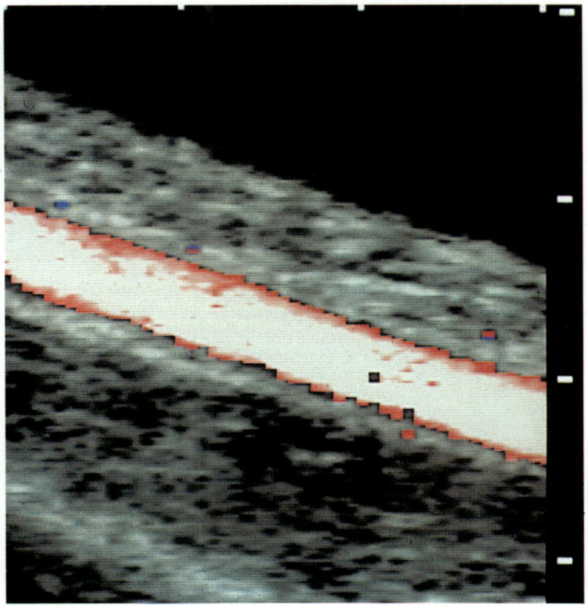

b

Fig. 3.**4a–g** Color duplex image series displaying pulsatile flow in the brachial artery. Phases A–G correspond to the points marked in the spectrum of Fig. 3.**3a**. The flow direction is from left to right

a Early systolic phase with low flow velocities (dark red)
b The systolic peak is marked by high flow velocities, especially at the center of the vessel (encoded light red or white)

Fig. 3.**4c–g** ▸

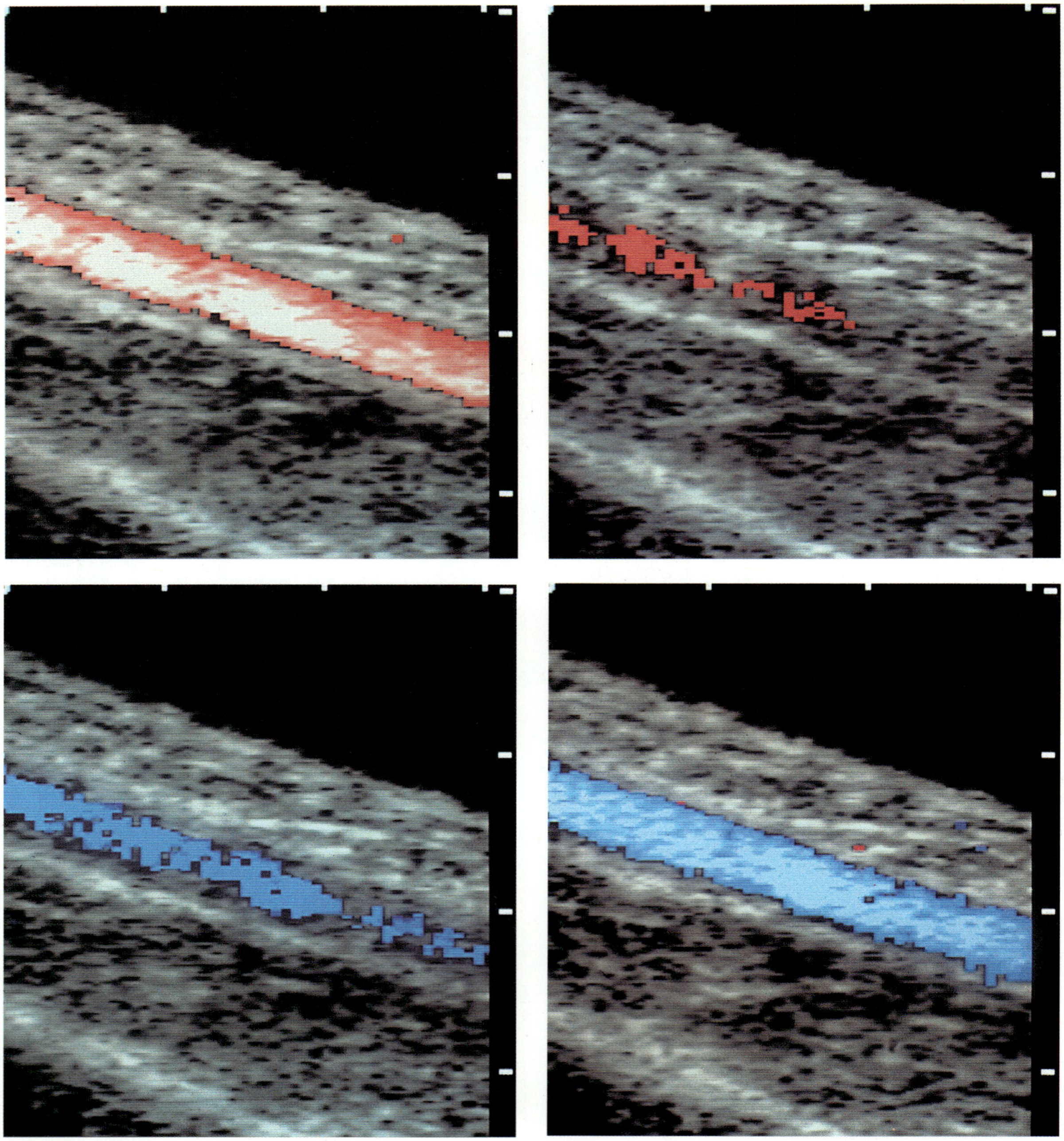

c d e f

Fig. 3.**4 c–f**

c The midsystolic phase shows a drop in flow velocities (darker red)

d A few scattered color signals in late systole indicate a virtual absence of flow

e The beginning of reverse flow in early diastole is marked by signals of opposite color (here, blue) that are diffusely distributed within the vessel but do not completely fill the lumen

f With diastolic flow reversal fully developed, the lumen is filled in completely with blue-encoded signals

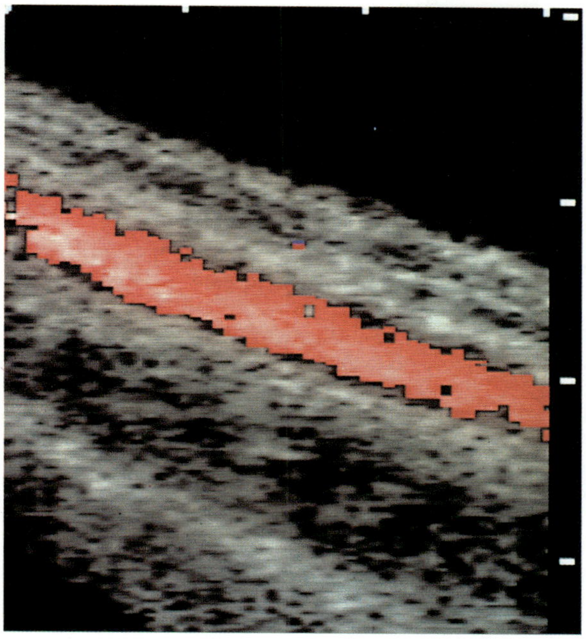

g The third phase of the cycle later in diastole is marked by the reestablishment of antegrade flow (red)

tion, especially of the arterioles. As the diastolic flow volume rises, this leads to a significant increase in the integral flow rate (Fig. 3.**3**). This manifests itself in the time–velocity waveforms or Doppler spectra by the appearance of a substantial forward flow component in diastole. The time–velocity waveforms resemble those recorded in arteries supplying parenchymatous organs.

The "parenchymal artery" type of flow pattern is characteristic of arteries that supply parenchymatous organs or organ systems. In particular, the arteries supplying the kidneys, liver, spleen, and brain exhibit a more continuous flow pattern than the demand-oriented vessels that supply the peripheral muscles. The peripheral resistance in the arterial system of the organs is low in order to maintain a constant perfusion. A significant antegrade flow even in diastole maintains a high integral volume flow rate (Fig. 3. **3**).

Depending on the amount of flow carried to parenchymal or peripheral arteries in relation to the total volume flow of the vessel, the time–velocity waveform patterns or Doppler spectra are more similar to one type or the other. Under pathological conditions, for example, a parenchyma-supplying artery may yield a Doppler spectrum very similar to that of a peripheral artery. This is illustrated by the altered Doppler spectrum in the arteries of a renal transplant undergoing acute rejection. Among other things, the pattern of the Doppler spectra makes it possible to draw important diagnostic conclusions with respect to the peripheral vascular resistance and possible pathological changes. Specific diagnostic applications are discussed in the chapters dealing with specific vessel systems.

3.3.3 Peripheral Vascular Resistance Indices

Calculating a resistance index is a semiquantitative adjunct to the qualitative description of a Doppler spectrum. Such an index describes the pulsatility of blood flow. As noted earlier, pulsatility depends on multiple factors. In practice, the indices discussed here are used mainly for assessing the peripheral vascular resistance.

Various indices have been defined in the literature. They are based on flow velocities or Doppler frequency shifts derived from the Doppler spectrum. All indices are practically independent of the Doppler angle, so a good-quality Doppler spectrum is all that is required. Generally the indices are calculated using the maximum velocity/frequency envelope (see Sect. 3.4.5.2) of the Doppler spectrum.

The most commonly used indices are:

a) The pulsatility index (PI) (5)

$$PI = \frac{V_{max} - V_{min}}{V_{avg}}$$

V_{max}: maximum systolic frequency shift/flow velocity during a cardiac cycle

V_{min}: minimum frequency shift/flow velocity during a cardiac cycle

V_{avg}: frequency shift/flow velocity averaged over a cardiac cycle

b) The resistance index (RI; Pourcelot index) (15)

$$RI = \frac{V_{max} - V_{min}}{V_{max}}$$

Unlike the Pourcelot index, the pulsatility index is dependent on the complete spectral waveform because of the averaging of all frequency shifts throughout a cardiac cycle. This implies a theoretical advantage of the pulsatility index, although in practical use the Pourcelot index can be calculated more quickly and is less susceptible to artifacts than the PI, which additionally requires a computer-based integration of the frequency shifts. It is more important, however, to always use the same index in clinical applications when making intraindividual or interindividual comparisons.

3.3.4 Pulsatile Flow Velocity Profile

In principle, pulsatile flow is laminar. However, the flow velocity profile of pulsatile blood flow is subjected to extensive changes during the cardiac cycle. The reason for this is that blood flow is opposing a resistance based on inertial forces (law of inertia or Newton's first law) which damp quick pulsatile changes of motion. The flow velocity profile is flat during the acceleration phase and approximates a parabolic shape only as long as some forward flow persists after the acceleration phase ends. If transient flow reversal occurs (especially in arteries of the upper and lower extremities), it begins near the vessel walls, where the lowest flow velocities prevail during antegrade flow, and propagates toward the center of the vessel (14). The flow is particularly unstable during this phase, and turbulence can develop even at very low Reynolds numbers (13).

3.3.5 Turbulence

As in continuous flow, the change from laminar to turbulent flow is marked by transitional phenomena referred to as "disturbed flow" (see Sect. 3.2.5). Unlike continuous flow, the Reynolds number in pulsatile flow varies over the cardiac cycle due to changes in flow velocity and vessel diameter. Even under physiologic conditions, this can give rise to periodic turbulence during certain parts of the cardiac cycle. The development of turbulence in pulsatile flow is also influenced by the shape of the flow velocity profile and the heart rate.

3.4 Hemodynamics at Stenoses

3.4.1 Preliminary Remarks

A basic understanding of blood flow dynamics at stenoses is essential for the correct interpretation of most phenomena encountered in Doppler studies of the arterial system. Prestenotic, intrastenotic, and poststenotic changes in absolute and relative flow velocities and flow patterns are the variables that lead to a correct diagnosis and permit a quantitative assessment of pathologic findings, regardless of the Doppler technology used.

3.4.2 Principle of Continuity in Assessing the Severity of Stenoses

Volume flow (flow rate per unit time) in a particular vessel remains constant in any given segment of the vessel (Fig. 3.5), except at sites where part of the flow volume is diverted from the original channel at an arterial branching of the vessel. Volume flow q is expressed by:

$$q = A \cdot v$$

where q = volume flow per unit time
A = cross sectional area of the vessel
v = average flow velocity in a given cross section of the vessel

If the vessel has a circular cross section the above equation changes to:

$$q = \pi \cdot r^2 \cdot v$$

where r = vessel radius

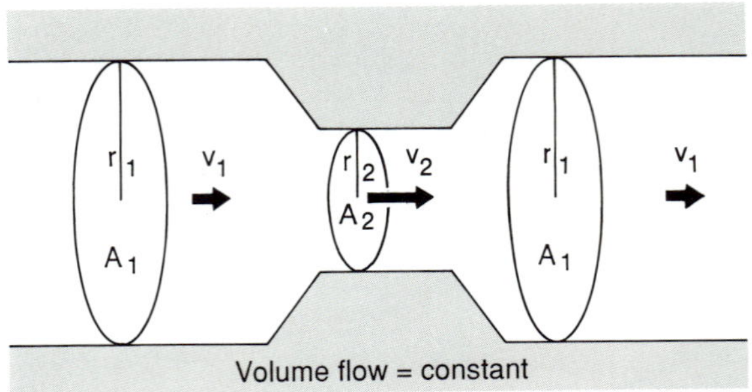

Fig. 3.**5** The principle of continuity. The flow velocity $v_{1,2}$ changes according to the variations in the cross-sectional area $A_{1,2}$ of the vessel. The flow volume in the vessel remains constant at all positions. Thus, the increase in flow velocity can be used in determining the reduction in patent luminal cross-sectional area and calculating the degree of stenosis (see text)

The principle of continuity is expressed by the continuity equation:

$$q_1 = q_2$$
$$q = A_1 \cdot v_1 = A_2 \cdot v_2$$

or

$$\frac{A_1}{A_2} = \frac{v_2}{v_1}$$

where $q_{1,2}$ = volume flow per unit time at position 1 and 2
$A_{1,2}$ = cross-sectional areas of a vessel at position 1 and 2
$v_{1,2}$ = average flow velocities in a given cross section of the vessel at position 1 and 2

A reduction in the lumen diameter necessarily leads to an increase in flow velocity. For example, a 50% reduction in diameter corresponding to a 75% reduction in area leads to an increase in flow velocity by a factor of 4. Based on the relative increase in flow velocity, the degree of stenosis can be calculated as far as the continuity equation is valid:

$$X = 100\,(1 - \frac{100}{Y})$$

where X = degree of stenosis in percent (relative area reduction)
Y = relative velocity increase in percent

$$X = 100\,(1 - \frac{v_1}{v_2})$$

or

where v_1 = prestenotic velocity and
v_2 = intrastenotic velocity

Thus the detection and determination of the severity of vascular stenoses with Doppler ultrasound is based on recording the relative velocity increase or Doppler frequency shift that is produced by the stenosis. It is pointless to base the severity of a stenosis on

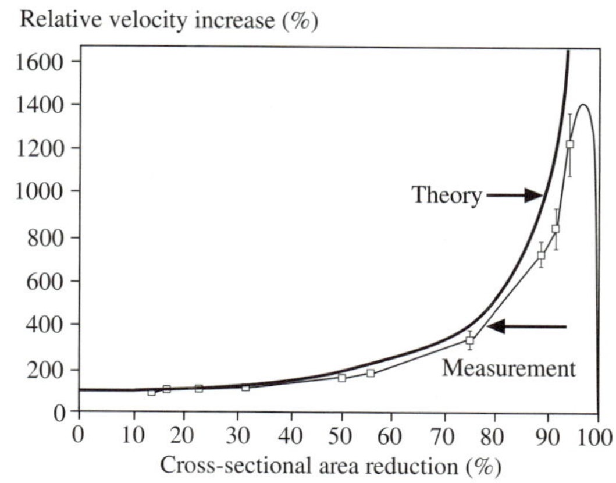

Fig. 3.**6** Relative increase in flow velocity versus degree of stenosis. Theoretical values were calculated with the help of the continuity equation. Duplex measurements were performed in experimental models with various degrees of stenosis. In case of a severe stenosis, the measured values are below the predicted values due to the conversion of energy to heat caused by friction

the absolute values of maximum intrastenotic frequency shifts or flow velocities alone, because absolute velocities depend not only on the degreee of stenosis but also on the prestenotic flow velocity. Very severe, flow rate-limiting lesions can reduce the intrastenotic flow velocity to such a degree that the absolute intrastenotic flow velocity is less than that associated with a moderate, non-flow-reducing stenosis. Using the absolute intrastenotic velocity in the case of a severe stenosis would lead to an underestimation of the degree of stenosis. Calculations based on the relative velocity increase avoid this error.

Based on a stenosis model, Figure 3.**6** shows the dependence of the intrastenotic velocity increase on the degree of stenosis. As the degree of stenosis increases, the velocities measured by Doppler frequency analysis are lower than theoretically predicted as a consequence of intrastenotic energy losses due to friction that was neglected in the above equations.

During hemodynamic evaluation of the severity of stenoses by duplex sonography it is presumed that the vascular segment of interest can be visualized in longitudinal section. The scan-plane must pass precisely through the center of the prestenotic and intrastenotic areas to ensure that maximum flow velocities are obtained for use in the calculation. Prominent vascular calcifications, intervening gas or bone, and obesity are physical obstacles that can prevent direct visualization of the stenotic area. In these cases duplex ultrasound permits only an approximate, indirect assessment of the severity of the vascular obstruction (see section 3.4.5). Aliasing can also make it impossible to quantify the flow velocity and thus the severity of the stenosis. By using the maximum Doppler shift or flow velocity displayed in color by the ultrasound system or the maximum velocity that is uniquely determinable by spectrum analysis (upper limit of the frequency/velocity axis) the flow velocity that is definitely exceeded when aliasing occurs can be determined. This is at least helpful in estimating the minimum degree of stenosis present.

In vessels that do not show significant branching in the area near the stenosis, flow velocities should be measured at the intrastenotic and immediate prestenotic levels for quantifying a stenosis. Although the continuity equation is still valid, the relative distribution of volume flow is unpredictable if the stenosis is located at a bifurcation (e.g., origin of the internal carotid artery) or at an arterial branching. The degree of stenosis can be determined from velocity measurements only by measuring both the intrastenotic flow velocity and the flow velocity at a more distal site in a segment having normal lumen size, well away from the stenotic jet or turbulence. Alternatively, the degree of a proximal stenosis of the internal carotid artery can be estimated from empirically derived ratios of the maximum systolic velocities at the prestenotic and intrastenotic levels (see Chapter 5).

There are two basic methods in duplex sonography for determining the severity of a stenosis on the basis of flow velocities (9):

1. By Doppler spectrum analysis (Fig. 3.**7c –e**)
2. By evaluation of the color-encoded flow velocities in CDS (Fig. 3.**7a, b**).

As a basic rule, the maximum flow velocity in a given vascular segment should be measured at the time of maximum systolic forward flow. The maximum flow velocity can be derived from the Doppler spectrum or determined by using a special color in the color duplex image to tag the highest flow velocities (9). The use of maximum systolic velocities permits the most accurate assessment of the degree of stenoses (9). If time-averaged velocities are used, the severity of the lesion will be underestimated due to entrance effects and changes in the flow velocity profile during the pulse cycle.

It must be pointed out again that it is absolutely mandatory to perform a Doppler angle correction when flow velocities are calculated from the Doppler frequency shift (see the Doppler formula in sections 1.4, 17.3 or Chapter 4). It is only possible to use the

a
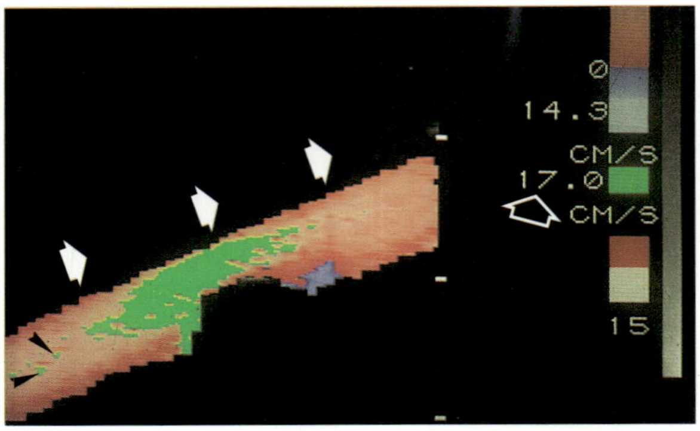

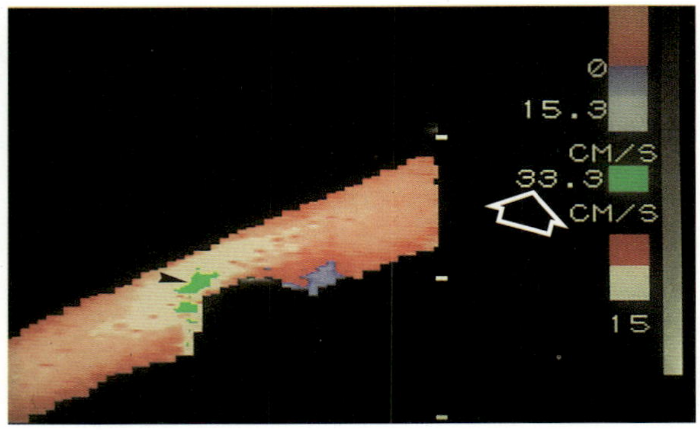

b

c
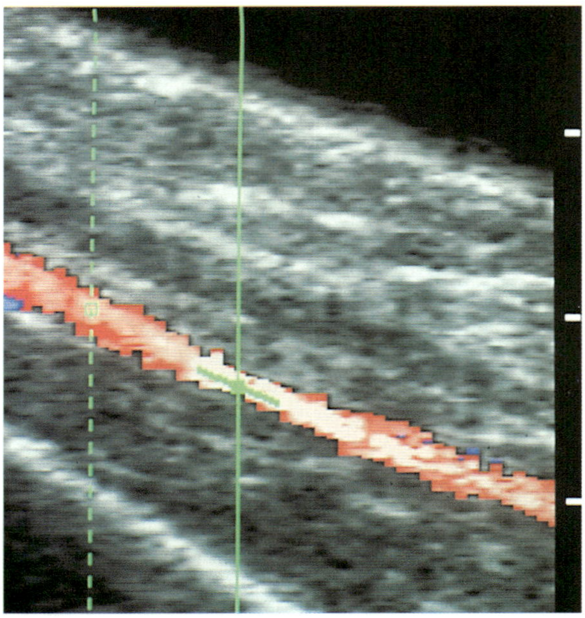

d
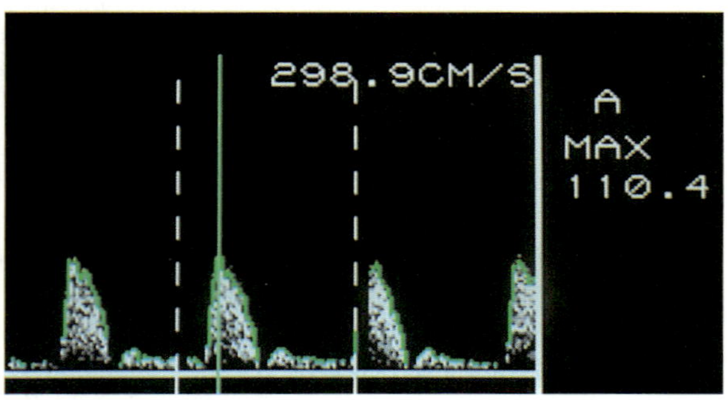

e
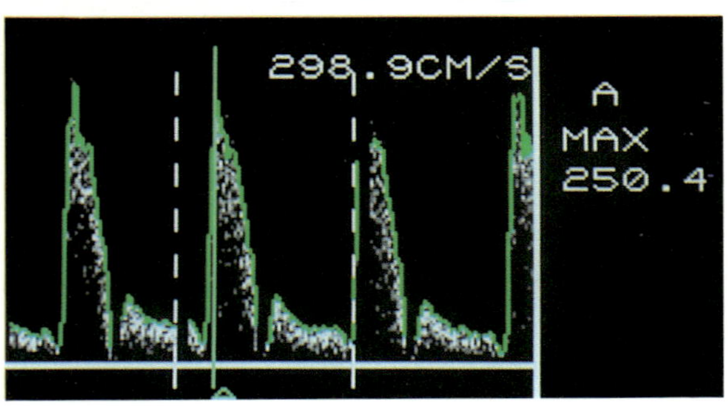

Fig. 3.**7a–e** Measurement of the degree of stenosis in a vascular phantom (**a**, **b**) and in a superficial femoral artery (**c**–**e**):

a Eccentric stenosis with a 50% luminal cross-sectional area reduction displayed at peak systole. The flow direction is from left to right. The displayed flow velocities are angle-corrected. The image was recorded at maximum systole. Maximum prestenotic flow velocity (open arrow) = 17 cm/s (the instrument is set so that flow velocities of 17 cm/s and higher are tagged green). The blue pixels just after the stenosis indicate flow reversal near the wall

b This image was recorded at the same point in time as **a**, but threshold for green tagging was raised to the maximum intrastenotic (black arrow) flow velocity of 33.3 cm/s (open arrow). The continuity equation indicates a 49% stenosis

c Concentric stenosis of the superficial femoral artery. Flow direction is from left to right. Intrastenotic and poststenotic flow velocities are increased (light color encoding). Broken green line = prestenotic sample volume site, solid green line = intrastenotic sample volume site for Doppler frequency analysis (**d**, **e**). Angle-correction was based on the longitudinal vessel axis in the region of interest (= intrastenotic green cursor)

d Prestenotic Doppler spectrum. The maximum systolic velocity at peak systole proximal to the stenosis measures 110.4 cm/s (vertical green line)

e Intrastenotic Doppler spectrum. The velocity increases to 250.4 cm/s, corresponding to a 56% stenosis (area reduction). At this moderate degree of stenosis, there is still an empty systolic window and no significant decrease in pulsatility

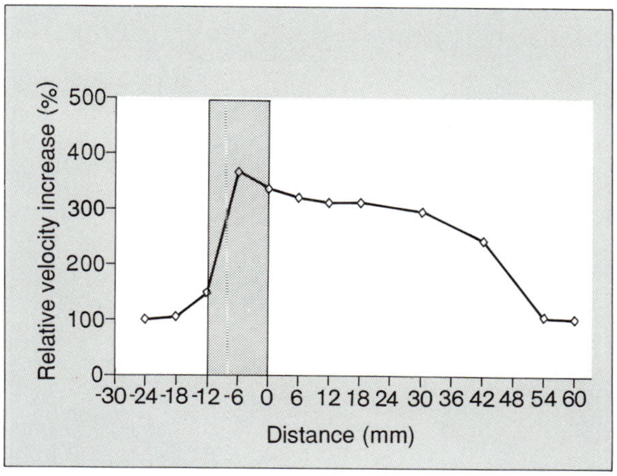

Fig. 3.**8** Measurement of the flow velocities across a stenosis causing a 75% concentric area reduction (= 50% diameter reduction) in a vascular phantom. Luminal diameter is 6 mm proximal and distal to the stenosis. Length of the stenosis is 12 mm. The shaded box indicates the vicinity of the stenosis (– 12 to 0 mm). The Doppler sample volume was positioned mid-stream, and the velocities were calculated from the Doppler spectrum (maximum systolic velocity). The graph shows a typical progression of velocity changes across the stenosis (relative to the prestenotic value). The relative velocity increase does not quite reach the theoretically predicted value of 400% due to frictional losses. The poststenotic jet extends several centimeters distally past the stenosed segment

Doppler frequency shift in calculating the degree of stenosis if the crossover angle (Doppler angle) between the longitudinal vessel axis and the individual ultrasound beams are the same in both positions.

3.4.3 Intrastenotic and Poststenotic Flow Changes

Due to the increased flow velocity, the intrastenotic Reynolds number can rise tremendously in the case of severe lesions. This may lead to disturbed flow or even turbulence within the stenosis. Distal to the stenosis, the maximum flow velocity continues to be elevated (poststenotic jet), at least in certain zones of the vascular cross section (Figs. 3.**8**, 3.**11**), with "exit effects" playing a significant role. Zones of retrograde, inherently laminar flow can develop near the vessel walls distal to a stenosis (flow separation, flow reversal) (Figs. 3.**9a–e**, 3.**11a, b**). These stationary eddy currents close to the vessel walls may propagate distally depending on the flow velocity and degree of stenosis (1, 17). The poststenotic Reynolds number may far exceed the intrastenotic Reynolds number as the flow enters the poststenotic lumen at elevated velocities. This may cause marked turbulence to develop in the poststenotic segments in addition to zones of flow reversal along the vessel walls (Figs. 3.**9**, 3.**11**). This may extend distally for a distance several times the

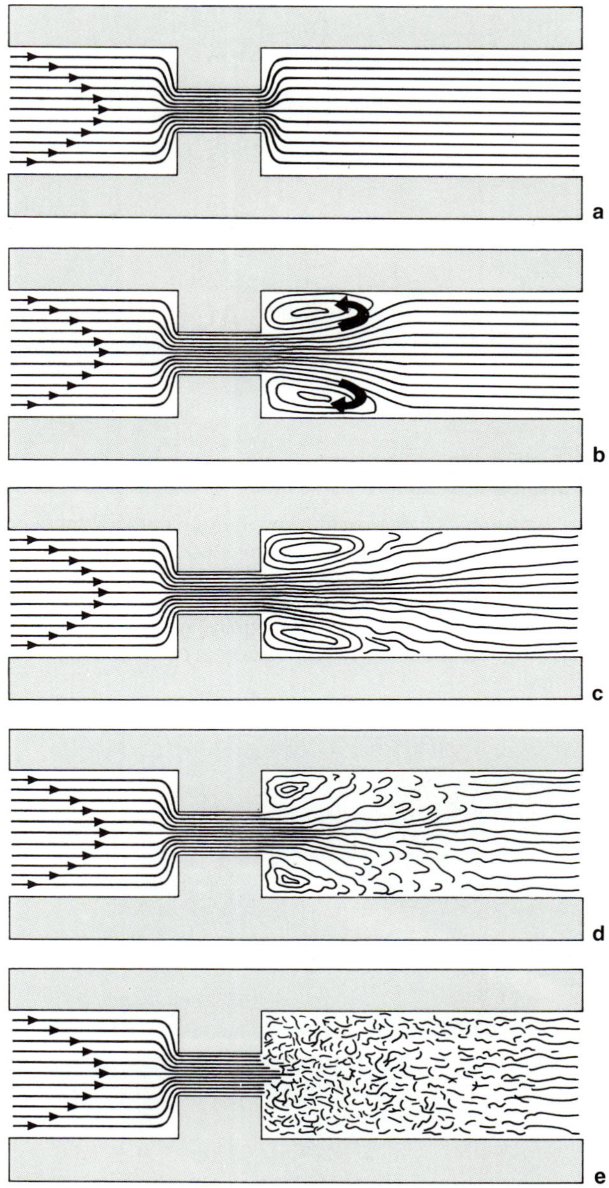

Fig. 3.**9a–e** Schematic representation of poststenotic flow changes as a function of physical boundary conditions. The prestenotic flow velocity increases from **a** to **e** while the degree of stenosis remains constant. In principle, the progression of changes from **a** to **e** is characteristic of all factors that would produce an increase in the Reynolds number

a Low prestenotic flow velocity. There are no poststenotic flow disturbances

b With a slight increase in prestenotic flow velocity, zones of flow reversal (curved arrows) develop near the vessel walls, but the flow remains generally laminar, and there is no turbulence

c When the prestenotic flow velocity is increased further, wave-like irregularities develop in the laminae (disturbed flow) in addition to flow reversal

d At a high prestenotic flow velocity, turbulence develops distal to the stenosis from the zones of flow reversal. Flow is still disturbed at some distance from the stenosis

e A very high prestenotic flow velocity is associated with severe poststenotic turbulence

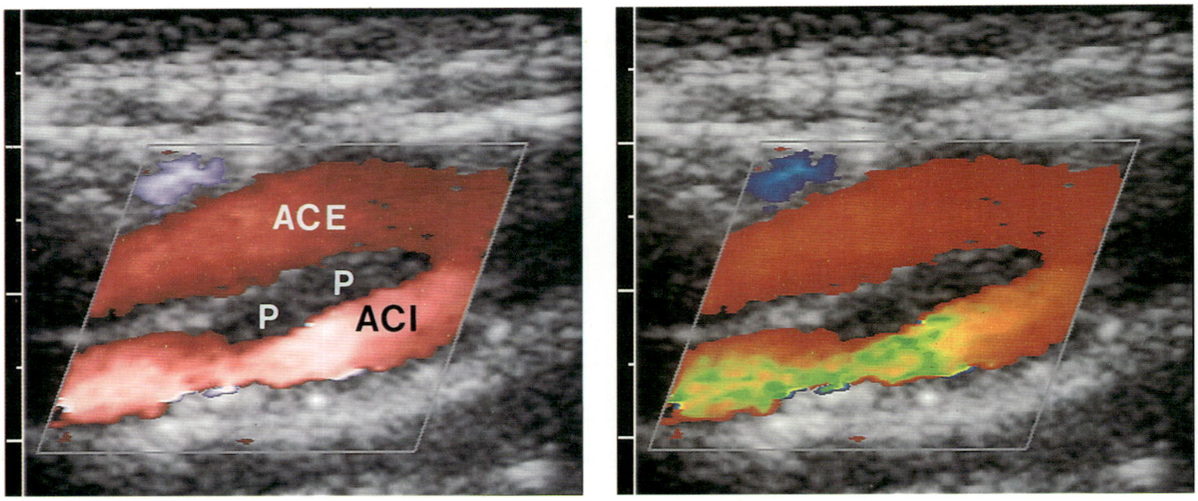

a b

Fig. 3.**10 a, b** CDS images of an internal carotid stenosis without and with velocity–variance encoding

a In the "normal" color image, blood flow in the area of the stenosis is encoded light red to indicate its high velocity. There is no red–blue color mix signifying turbulence. ACI = Internal carotid artery, ACE = external carotid artery, P = plaque

b Imaging in the velocity–variance mode can demonstrate even slight flow irregularities by adding green to the basic colors. In the present example this indicates disturbed flow within and distal to the stenosis

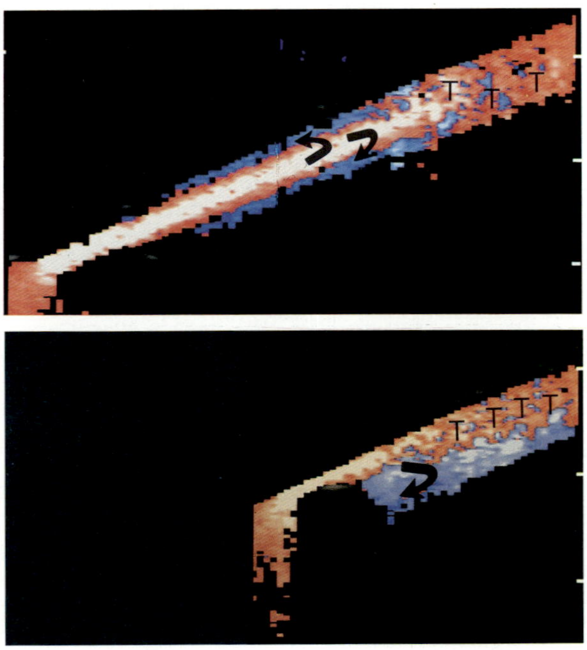

a b

Fig. 3.**11 a, b** CDS display of stenotic flow changes in a vascular phantom. Flow direction is from left to right. The diameter of the phantom vessel is 6 mm in its nonstenosed region

a Concentric stenosis causing an 88% cross-sectional area reduction. There is a marked intrastenotic and poststenotic velocity increase (light red/white). Poststenotic zones of flow reversal (blue, curved arrows) give way to turbulence (T) farther downstream. All poststenotic changes are approximately concentric, reflecting the geometry of the stenosis

b Eccentric stenosis causing a 92% cross-sectional area reduction. There are pronounced eccentric zones of poststenotic flow reversal (curved arrows) and turbulence (T)

normal vessel diameter (9). Besides the pressure drop across the stenosis, turbulence is partially responsible for the energy loss resulting in a volume flow reduction associated with severe stenoses.

Turbulence and flow reversal are easily recognized in color duplex imaging (see section 3.2.5) (Fig. 3.**11**). Using Doppler frequency analysis, turbulent flow produces a broadening of the Doppler spectrum (increased low-frequency shifts that may completely fill in the systolic window beneath the spectrum envelope [see section 3.4.5.3]) and the simultaneous occurrence of positive and negative Doppler frequency shifts (simultaneous forward and reverse flow components within the sample volume).

The location and extent of local flow reversals and turbulence depend in a complex way on the geometry of the stenosis, the degree of stenosis, the surface structure of the vessel walls, the prestenotic flow velocity, the viscosity of the blood, and the pulsatility of the flow. There are no general rules for determining the severity of stenosis from the length and extent of the flow reversals and turbulence. The main value of a color-coded presentation of these phenomena is that it permits the identification of vascular stenoses when the lesion itself is obscured by vessel–wall calcifications or calcified plaque.

3.4.4 Hemodynamic Significance of a Stenosis

In a strict sense, any stenosis is "hemodynamically significant" because it produces a measurable change in local hemodynamics. From a clinical viewpoint, however, a lesion is hemodynamically significant only if it causes a reduction in the volume flow rate leading to a peripheral perfusion deficit during rest or exercise. The higher the degree of a stenosis and the greater its length, the greater the pressure drop across the lesion. Beyond a critical degree of stenosis there is a reduction of volume flow throughout the vessel. This critical value depends strongly on the peripheral vascular resistance. When peripheral vessels are dilated, as during muscular exercise, a stenotic lesion may cause the perfusion pressure to fall enough to result in a condition of relative or absolute ischemia. A 50% reduction in peripheral artery vessel diameter (i.e., a 75% area reduction) is generally acknowledged as the critical threshold. This empirical threshold is useful only as a general point of orientation. The "critical" value in a given patient will depend on the prestenotic and poststenotic cardiovascular performance and the extent of collateralization.

3.4.5 Interpretation of Doppler Spectra in the Presence of Stenoses and Occlusions

A significant advantage of CDS over conventional, single-gated duplex sonography is that it greatly simplifies the identification of blood vessels and vascular pathology. Stenosing plaques are easily identified by the narrowing of the perfused vessel lumen and the typical stenotic flow abnormalities described above. The total occlusion of a vessel is manifested by the complete absence of a color flow signal. The quantification of vascular stenoses can be accomplished with the help of the color-coded image alone by noting the relative intrastenotic velocity increase. As stated above, however, scanning conditions are not always ideal (complete visualization of the stenotic area, no aliasing, absence of a large vessel branching off just proximal to the stenosis). When conditions are less than ideal, Doppler frequency analysis must additionally be used to estimate the severity of a lesion.

3.4.5.1 System Settings

In the recording of Doppler spectra as well as in CDS imaging, the operator must use an appropriate pulse repetition frequency (PRF) and must choose a suitable baseline setting to avoid aliasing (see sections 1.6, 17.3.1, 17.3.3 and Chapter 4). Given the significantly higher acoustic intensities that are transmitted into the tissue in pulsed Doppler mode in spectrum analysis (see Chapter 2), the power output should be set at the lowest level possible for obtaining an adequate spectrum. The gain setting should be adequately adjusted while still minimizing electronic noise. This is best accomplished by acquiring a calibration spectrum in a healthy vascular segment and adjusting the gain to produce a well-defined spectral waveform with an empty systolic window. According to the flow velocity profile discussions (see section 3.2), the sample volume in Doppler spectrum analysis must be positioned at the center of a vessel, unless the observed stenosis is an eccentric stenosis producing an off-axis jet also visualized in the CDS image.

3.4.5.2 Envelope Traces of the Doppler Spectrum

So called "envelopes" are commonly used in a simplified description of spectral waveforms and in the measurement of flow velocities. The traces or curves may be drawn by the machine itself, or traced manually. An envelope is obtained by drawing a trace along the time axis connecting the selected displayed Doppler frequency shifts that satisfy a particular criterion, yielding an envelope that plots frequency shifts over time. The most commonly used envelopes trace the maximum and mean frequencies over time. Various envelopes in Doppler spectrum analysis are used, as defined below:

- Maximum frequency shift (F_{max}): The highest Doppler frequency shift at each moment in time (within each time increment) in the Doppler spectrum. In order to eliminate noise, generally the frequency below which a certain percentage (e.g., 95%) of all measured frequency shifts fall is selected as F_{max} (Fig. 3.**7d, e**).
- Mean frequency shift (F_{mean}): The arithmetic mean of all Doppler frequency shifts at each moment in time (within each time increment) in the Doppler spectrum.
- Mode frequency shift (F_{mode}): The Doppler frequency shift that exhibits the greatest intensity of all frequency shifts at each moment in time (within each time increment) in the Doppler spectrum.
- Minimum frequency shift (F_{min}): The lowest Doppler frequency shift at each moment in time (within each time increment) in the Doppler spectrum.

3.4.5.3 Systolic Window

When in Doppler spectrum analysis no frequency shifts are detected within a certain range of frequencies this region remains "black" in the conventional gray-scale display of the Doppler spectrum. The "systolic window" is said to be "empty" or "clear". The systolic window in a Doppler spectrum represents the frequencies below the minimum detected Doppler frequency shift whithin each time increment. When a small sample volume is used, the size of the systolic window indicates the degree of laminar flow present. The larger the bandwidth of the measured Doppler frequency shifts, the smaller the systolic window. An increased bandwidth of the Doppler frequencies characterizes an increasing degree of flow disturbance based on nonuniform orientations of the velocity vectors of the individual flow elements in the sample volume. Especially in poststenotic spectra, the window may be completely filled in, i.e., nonexistent

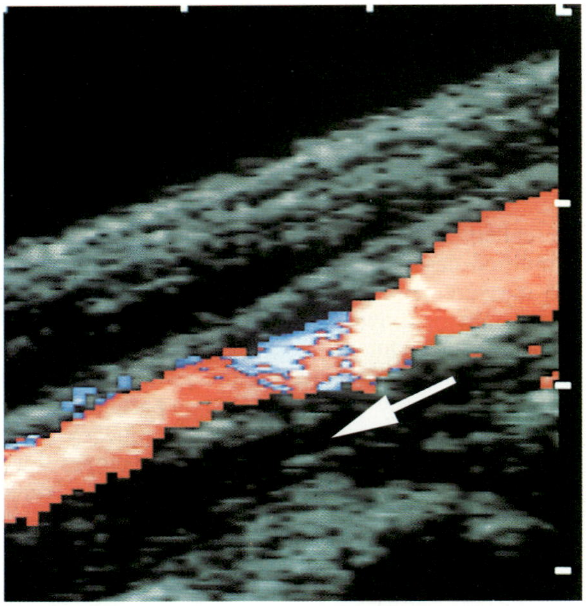

a

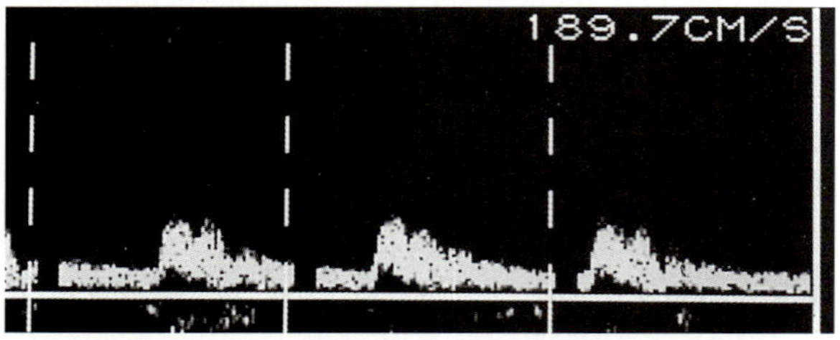

b

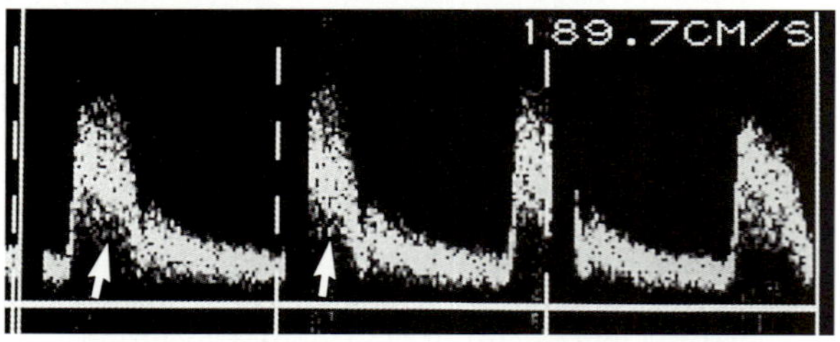

c

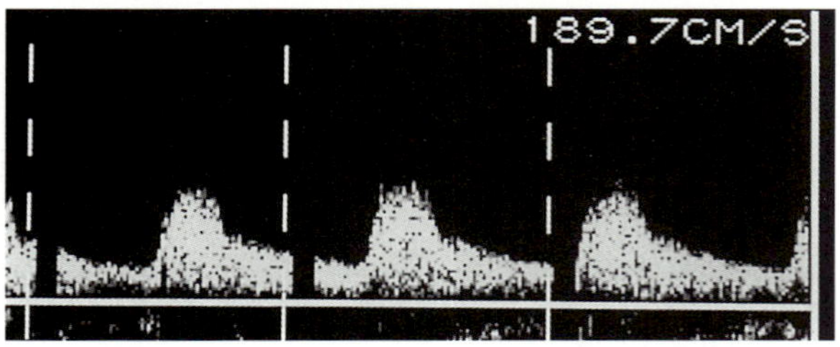

d

Fig. 3.**12a–d** Doppler spectral changes associated with a stenosis of the internal carotid artery near the carotid bulb
a CDS image of the stenosis (flow direction from right to left = arrow) demonstrates an intrastenotic velocity increase (light red/white), poststenotic flow reversal, and mild turbulence
b Prestenotic spectrum from the common carotid artery
c Intrastenotic spectrum shows a marked elevation of flow velocity, but the systolic window is still empty (arrows)
d Poststenotic spectrum shows filling in of the systolic window (= greater prevalence of lower frequency shifts due to flow disturbances), a rounded systolic peak, and an increased systolic rise time compared with **b** and **c**

(Fig. 3.**12a–d**). The following equation may be used to calculate the size of the systolic window, which can either be determined at the point of maximum systolic flow or integrated over the complete systolic phase of the cardiac cycle:

$$\text{Systolic window} = \frac{F_{min}}{F_{max}} \cdot 100\ (\%)$$

As stated above, filling-in of the systolic window, or "spectral broadening", is most often detected in the poststenotic vessel segment. For this reason, several attempts have been made to define indices related to spectral broadening that are useful in determining the severity of a stenosis (such as the SBI or spectral broadening index, see Chapter 5). While such indices correlate well with the degree of stenosis, the problem is to define the optimum poststenotic sampling site for the acquisition of the spectral data needed, since the flow changes on which the measurement is based exhibit a very complex spatial distribution (7).

3.4.5.4 Evaluation of the Doppler Frequency Spectrum

The influence of the peripheral vascular resistance on the Doppler frequency spectrum and the description of the spectrum with the help of angle-independent indices was discussed in Sect. 3.3.2 and 3.3.3. This section deals with the principal changes in the Doppler frequency spectrum associated with arterial obstructions.

Numerous factors influencing the arterial Doppler spectral waveform must be taken into account, which in some cases depend on the position of the Doppler sample volume:

- Cardiac output (e.g., reduction of the systolic amplitude in the Doppler frequency spectrum caused by cardiac insufficiency)
- Aortic valve function (e.g., reduced systolic acceleration caused by an aortic valve stenosis, enlarged systolic–diastolic amplitude due to aortic valve incompetence)
- Changes in compliance of the aorta and outflow from the aorta (Windkessel function)
- Course of the vessel (e.g., spectral broadening due to tortuosity)
- Surface structure of the intima (e.g., surface irregularities that increase stenotic flow disturbances)
- Degree of lumen reduction
- Collateralization
- Peripheral vascular resistance

Given these factors, it is not possible to postulate general valid rules for spectral waveform interpretation. All of the above factors should be checked for relevance in any given case. Also, spectra should be obtained at multiple proximal and distal sites in the vascular system and compared with one another.

Only severe obstructive lesions (= hemodynamically significant stenosis exceeding 75% area reduction, occlusions) will produce obvious spectral changes proximal to the lesion, especially when collateralization is poor and the spectrum is recorded close to the lesion itself. Pulsatility is increased due to the high flow resistance induced by the vascular obstruction. A reduction in flow volume is connected with a reduced systolic amplitude, but the steepness of the systolic acceleration slope generally remains unchanged. The systolic peak is followed by a steep deceleration slope to the zero baseline and in some cases by a phase of diastolic reverse flow. With an acute occlusion, the (ineffectual) pulsations of the preocclusive vascular segment may be transmitted to the occluded area, occasionally producing narrow, almost streak-like Doppler signals of very low frequency that do not represent true flow.

The principal intrastenotic waveform changes in the originally biphasic or triphasic Doppler frequency spectrum of a peripheral artery include high frequencies that may exceed the maximum unambiguously detectable Doppler frequency shift, resulting in aliasing, and a decreased pulsatility of the flow within and just distal to a hemodynamically significant stenosis. The latter feature is due mainly to the high pressure gradient across the relatively short segment of luminal narrowing. Additionally, spectral broadening reduces the size of the systolic window as noted above, which is initially seen poststenotically but may also occur within the stenosis if the reduction of the patent lumen area is severe. In the case of turbulence, Doppler frequencies below the zero baseline will be displayed and the systolic window will disappear.

Spectral broadening can persist for a considerable distance distal to the lesion and is a useful clue to the presence of a proximal stenosis that cannot be directly visualized. Two additional waveform changes indicating a proximal flow obstruction are typically present in this situation. Similar to an aortic valve stenoses, a vascular stenosis tends to slow down the systolic pressure rise distal to the lesion. There is less systolic blood flow acceleration, and the acceleration slope in the Doppler spectrum is less steep leading to a delayed systolic peak (Fig. 3.**13a–c**). Besides measuring the interval from the start of the antegrade systolic flow to the systolic peak, this change in the pattern of the Doppler frequency spectrum can be easily recognized by comparing proximal and distal Doppler spectra. Another sign of a significant proximal obstruction is decreased pulsatility caused by a reduced peripheral vascular flow resistance in response to the perfusion deficit (Fig. 3.**14**).

A very severe proximal flow obstruction can produce a markedly flattened spectral waveform with a rounded systolic peak. This pattern is influenced by the peripheral collateral circulation and the factors noted above. The different lengths of the various collateral channels result in different distances traveled by the individual pulse waves. If the collaterals reenter the main vessel distal to the stenosis or occlusion, the individual systolic peaks of the pulse waves are time-shifted relative to one another in a manner

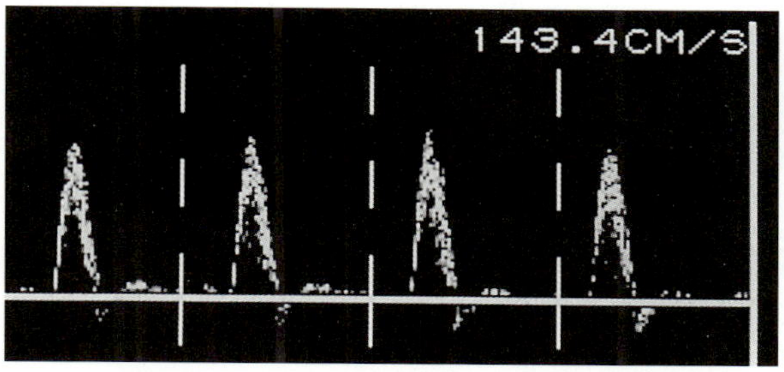

a

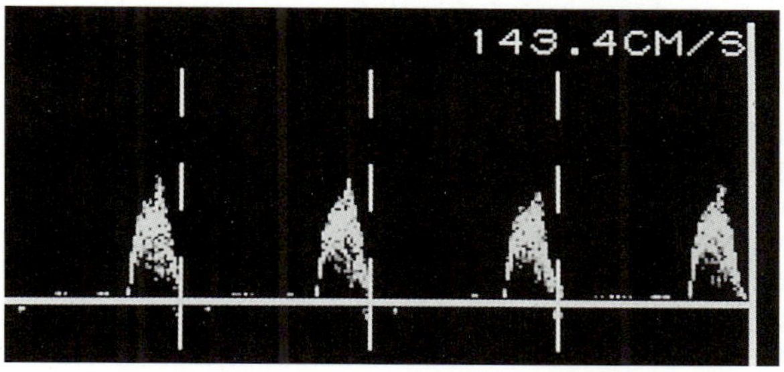

b

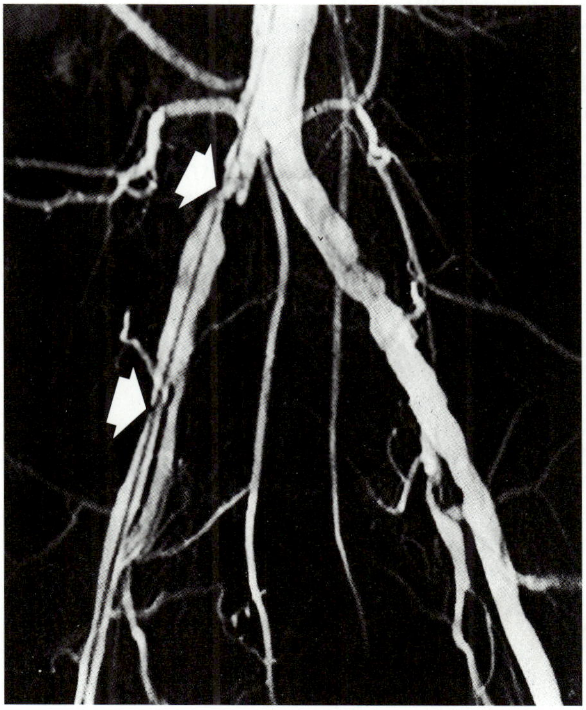

c

Fig. 3.**13a–c** Hemodynamically significant stenoses of the right iliac arteries detected indirectly by comparing the Doppler spectra of both common femoral arteries

a Normal triphasic spectrum recorded from the left common femoral artery

b The spectrum from the right common femoral artery shows a delayed and reduced systolic peak compared with the opposite side, decreased pulsatility (absence of diastolic flow reversal), and a reduced systolic window relative to the left side

c Intra-arterial DSA demonstrates significant stenoses in the right common and external iliac arteries (arrows) with severe arteriosclerosis

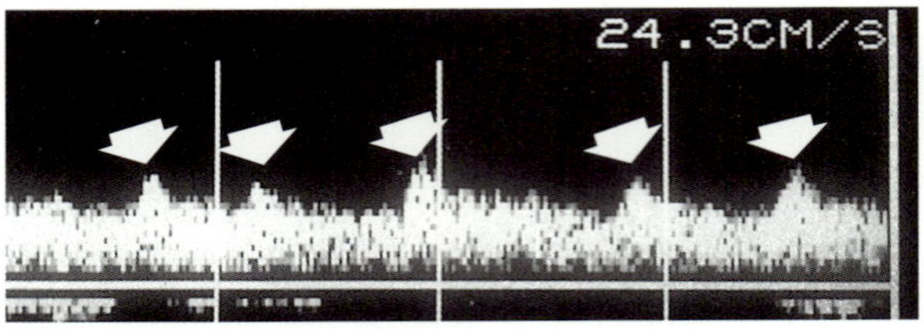

Fig. 3.**14** Doppler frequency spectrum from the posterior tibial artery in a patient with a fresh, poorly collateralized occlusion of the superficial femoral artery. There is an almost complete loss of normal flow pulsatility with minimal systolic peaks (arrows). Arrhythmia is also present

that produces rounded systolic peaks in the Doppler frequency spectrum (Fig. 3.**14**).

Given the various factors listed above, it is impossible to quantify a vascular lesion on the basis of proximal and distal spectra alone. These are helpful only in a gross interpretation of the findings. On the whole, the more pronounced the spectral abnormalities are and the greater the distance between the lesion and the sampling site where they can still be detected, the greater the likelihood that a hemodynamically significant vascular lesion is present. If an unchanging spectral pattern can be recorded along the course of a vessel, it is reasonable to exclude the presence of a hemodynamically significant lesion.

3.4.6 Practical Recommendations on the Quantitative Assessment of Arterial Stenoses

The quantification of a vascular stenosis is usually time-consuming and is not always necessary. In selecting patients for angioplasty, for example, it is generally sufficient to correlate clinical findings, Doppler blood pressure ratios, and the detection of a localized, hemodynamically significant stenosis. A basic problem in determining the severity of a stenosis in the vicinity of a branching vessel or bifurcation relates to the definition of the nonstenosed vascular segment. For example, is the point of reference for calculating the degree of a proximal internal carotid stenosis:

- the carotid bulb?
- the prebulbar segment of the common carotid artery?
- the poststenotic segment of the internal carotid artery?
- the local outer vessel wall diameter in the stenotic area?

Unfortunately there is no single, standard nomenclature that permits the results of different studies to be compared. It is imperative, however, for the examiner and therapist to agree upon a protocol and consistently maintain that routine in follow-up examinations. They must also decide whether to express the degree of stenosis in terms of percentage diameter reduction or area reduction. It is not the object of this book to define a standard in this respect.

Whenever CDS is used for the quantification of stenoses, every effort should be made to obtain a direct image of the stenotic area. In accordance with the principles outlined above, the severity of a stenosis should be determined by measuring the relative velocity increase between the prestenotic and the intrastenotic segments. This leads to the percentage of area reduction. If the prestenotic velocity cannot be unambiguously determined, it is acceptable to measure the poststenotic velocity instead, as long as there is no evidence of distal turbulence and there are no large branching vessels between the stenosis and the sampling site.

If the stenotic area is accessible to ultrasound imaging, a geometric measurement may be conducted to supplement findings based on hemodynamic criteria. This is done by imaging the stenosed area in the transverse plane and determining the ratio of the area of the perfused lumen and the total cross-sectional vessel area (outer vessel contour). CDS is ideal for this purpose, because the color-encoded image and grayscale image portray the true local degree of stenosis. The problem related to the geometric measurement of a stenosis is that the calculated degree of stenosis is usually based on an expected circular cross-sectional area of the lesion.

Additionally, a precise cross-sectional image plane implies a 90° Doppler angle that is unfavorable for demonstrating flow. Nevertheless, the plausibility of the hemodynamic severity of a stenosis should be tested whenever possible by performing a geometric measurement. Compared with Doppler sonography, the geometric method tends to overestimate the degree of stenosis because the area measurement is usually based on the measurement of the outer diameter of the vessel and disregards the physiologic thickness of the vessel walls.

Besides calculating the degree of the stenosis by utilizing hemodynamic principles as described above, it is advisable to classify the stenosis of a carotid artery or peripheral artery as belonging to one of several categories based on empirical studies. These categories are described in the pertinent chapters. Empirical data are particularly useful in classifying the severity of proximal internal carotid stenoses, since the continuity equation cannot be accurately applied at sites near vessel branchings (see Sect. 3.4.2).

If there is no significant branching vessel close to the stenosis, then the degree of stenosis can be grossly classified by determining the ratio of the maximum prestenotic and intrastenotic systolic velocities (Table 3.**1**). This correlation is based both on the value predicted by the continuity equation and on experi-

Table 3.**1** Classification of the severity of arterial stenoses based on the continuity equation and experimental data using duplex sonography. This table is valid for all arterial stenoses that are not located near a bifurcation. The correlation of area reduction and diameter reduction is based on the assumption of a concentric stenosis. Possible aliasing associated with severe stenoses is disregarded

Degree of stenosis Area reduction	Diameter reduction	V_{max}(intra)/V_{max}(pre) Theory	In vitro
≥ 50%	≥ approx. 30%	≥ 2	≥ approx. 1.8
≥ 75%	≥ 50%	≥ 4	≥ approx. 3.6
≥ 85%	≥ approx. 60%	≥ 6.6	≥ approx. 6.3
≥ 95%	≥ approx. 80%	≥ 20	≥ approx. 15

Table 3.**2** Classification of the severity of internal carotid arterial stenoses near the carotid bulb using duplex sonography (see section 5.4.3.1 for details). The indicated values are valid only if the external carotid artery has normal patency (ICA = internal carotid artery, CCA = common carotid artery)

Degree of stenosis Area reduction	Diameter reduction	V_{max}(ICA)/V_{max}(CCA)
≥ 75%	= 50%	≥ 1.5
≥ 85%	≥ approx. 60%	≥ 1.8
≥ 90%	≥ approx. 70%	≥ approx. 2.5
≥ 95%	≥ approx. 80%	≥ 3.7

mental results in model stenoses (9), also taking intrastenotic frictional losses into account (Table 3.**2**). If the stenosed section of the vessel cannot be visualized, Doppler frequency analysis should be used to check for indirect signs of stenosis as described in Sect. 3.4.5.2.

3.5 Integral Flow Velocity and Volume Flow Measurements

CDS, with its simultaneous measurement of flow velocities in each pixel of the image, permits quantification of the integral flow velocity averaged over the cross section of the vessel. In conventional duplex sonography, where flow velocities only within a single sample volume of variable size are determined by frequency analysis, the flow velocity profile is not measured.

Determination of the integral flow velocity with CDS is accomplished not by spectrum analysis of the Doppler signal originating from a specific location but by evaluation of the color-coded image. All frequency shifts along a user-defined line in the color-coded image are integrated (Fig. 3.**15 a, b**). Following angle correction, a time–velocity trace is plotted and used to calculate the weighted time-averaged integral flow velocity V_{avg}. By additionally determining the vessel radius r and by using the equation

$$q_{avg} = V_{avg} \pi r^2$$

the volume flow rate q_{avg} averaged over the vessel cross section and over time can be calculated.

At present, only a few manufacturers of CDS systems offer software for computing the flow volume by the above method. If this option is not available, the approximate integral flow velocity can be determined by Doppler frequency analysis using one of two methods:

- Selection of a large Doppler sample volume (size must correspond to the transverse vessel diameter); determination of the time-averaged F_{mean} (see section 3.4.5.2) or V_{mean} after angle correction.
- Choice of a small Doppler sample volume positioned exactly in the center of the vessel; determination of the time-averaged F_{max} (see section 3.4.5.2) or angle-corrected V_{max}. The integral flow velocity is approximately equal to one half the flow velocity measured at the center of the vessel (assuming a parabolic flow velocity profile).

Quantification of the integral flow velocity is highly error-prone and requires optimum examination conditions. These include:

- The use of a high-frequency transducer (5 MHz or preferably 7 to 7.5 MHz) to achieve a high spatial resolution.
- Optimum adjustment of the image with optimal color saturation and no aliasing.
- Use of a relatively small Doppler angle (65° or less, if possible) and selection of a straight vascular segment to minimize the effects of faulty angle determinations (see sections 1.4, 17.3, and Chapter 4).
- Application of only a light transducer pressure to avoid a distortion of the vessel shape (volume flow formula is valid only for vessels of circular cross section).

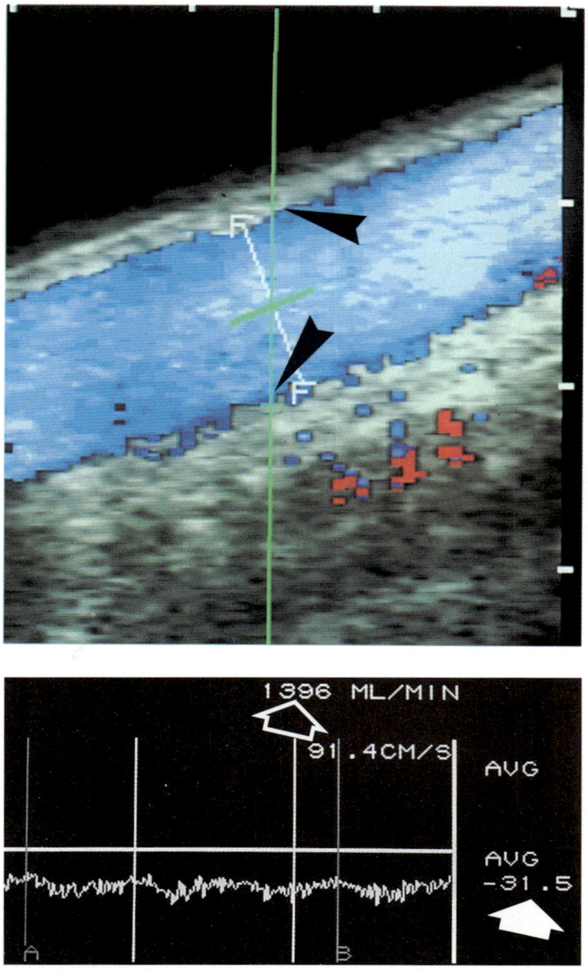

a

b

Fig. 3.**15a, b** The principle of integral volume flow measurement by CDS in a Brescia–Cimino hemodialysis shunt in the upper arm

a The two diameter markers are positioned on the vessel wall (arrowheads). The green angle-correction cursor is in line with the longitudinal axis of the vessel. The transverse diameter of the vessel (white line) is equal to 9.7 mm

b Integrated flow–velocity curve. The average flow velocity over the total cross section of the vessel over several pulse cycles (between points A and B) is 31.5 cm/s (filled arrow). The integral flow volume is 1396 mL/min (open arrow)

- Selection of an optimum scan-plane along the maximum transverse diameter of the vessel in longitudinal section (off-center scanning leads to underestimation).
- Absence of turbulence and vortices (angle-correction must be correct for all pixels along the selected line of measurement at any given moment).
- Accurate determination of the transverse vessel diameter (ideally, a time-averaged M-mode measurement, if available; otherwise a distance measurement along the line selected for flow velocity measurement; measurement of the maximum systolic diameter introduces a small systematic error but is most reproducible).
- When a Doppler technique is used, measurement of superficial vessels only; the Doppler frequency shift depends not only on the flow velocity and beam angle but also on the distance of the transducer from the backscattering particles (see Chapters 1 and 4).

The results of the volume flow measurements are very accurate under ideal laboratory conditions (8). Since optimal examination conditions are required for integral volume flow measurements, a meticulous examination technique must be used. Volume flow measurements are limited to superficial vessels only for the reasons stated above.

The measurement of volume flow rates in hemodialysis shunts has acquired considerable clinical importance (see Chapter 7) (Fig. 3.**15**). The quantification of shunt flow in traumatic a–v fistulae is another application of clinical importance (see Chapter 6).

3.6 References

1 Azuma, T., Fukushima, T.: Flow patterns in stenotic blood vessel models. Biorheology 13 (1976) 337–355

2 Burns, P. N.: Hemodynamics. In Taylor, K. J. W., P. N. Burns, P. N. T. Wells (Eds.): Clinical Applications of Doppler Ultrasound. Raven Press, New York (1988) 46–75

3 Burton, A. C.: Physiology and Biophysics of the Circulation, 2nd ed. Yearbook Medical Publishers, Chicago (1972)

4 Douville, Y., K. W. Johnston, M. Kassam: Determination of hemodynamic factors which influence the carotid Doppler spectral broadening. Ultrasound Med. Biol. 11 (1985) 417–423

5 Gosling, G., D. King: Arterial assessment by Doppler-shift ultrasound. Proc. roy. Soc. Med. 67 (1974) 447–449

6 Hutchinson, K. J., E. Karpinski: Stability of flow patterns in the in vivo poststenotic velocity field. Ultrasound Med. Biol. 14 (1988) 269–275

7 Khalifa, A. M. A., D. P. Giddens: Characterization and evolution of poststenotic flow disturbances. J. Biomech. 14 (1981) 279–296

8 Landwehr, P., W. Dölken, K. Lackner: In-vitro-Messung des intravasalen Blutflusses mit der Farb-Doppler-Sonographie. Fortschr. Röntgenstr. 150 (1989) 192–197

9 Landwehr, P., R. Schindler, U. Heinrich, W. Dölken, Th. Krahe, K. Lackner: Quantification of vascular stenoses with color Doppler flow imaging: in vitro investigations. Radiology 178 (1991) 701–704

10 McDonald, D. A.: The viscous properties of blood. In McDonald, D. A. (Ed.): Blood Flow in Arteries, 2nd ed. Edward Arnold, London (1974) 55–70

11 McDonald, D. A.: Steady flow of a liquid in cylindrical tubes. In McDonald, D. A. (Ed.): Blood Flow in Arteries, 2nd ed. Edward Arnold, London (1974) 17–54

12 McDonald, D. A.: Blood Flow in Arteries, 2nd ed. Edward Arnold, London (1974)

13 McDonald, D. A.: Turbulence and disturbed flow patterns in the circulation. In McDonald, D. A. (Ed.): Blood Flow in Arteries, 2nd ed. Edward Arnold, London (1974) 71–100

14 McDonald, D. A.: The velocity profile in pulsatile flow. In McDonald, D. A. (Ed.): Blood Flow in Arteries, 2nd ed. Edward Arnold, London (1974) 101–117

15 Pourcelot, L.: Applications cliniques de l'examen Doppler transcutané. Les Colloques de l'Institut National de la Santé et de la Recherche médicale. INSERM 34 (1974) 213–240

16 Trattnig, S., B. Schwaighofer, P. Hübsch, F. Kainberger, D. Pötzleitner: Velocity-Variance-Funktion: Zusatzinformation in der farbkodierten Doppler-Sonographie der Karotiden. Fortschr. Röntgenstr. 153 (1990) 663–668

17 Yonchareon, W., Young, D. F.: Initiation of turbulence in models of arterial stenoses. J. Biomech. 12 (1979) 185–196

4 System Settings and Examination Technique

F. Fobbe, P.-M. Klews, R. Kubale, P. Landwehr

An accurate diagnosis is based on the evaluation of the patient's history and requires the use of an examination technique that is most appropriate for the specific inquiry. The ultrasound equipment must be adjusted to its optimum. Ultrasound systems coming from different manufacturers have different strengths and weaknesses. The examination of a particular organ requires the adaptation of the examination technique according to system requirements. In CDS blood flow is displayed in color and simultaneously organ morphology is displayed in gray scale, all in one image. This presents the examiner with considerably more information than in gray scale imaging alone. Also, to a great extent the examiner must be able to evaluate the CDS images immediately while the examination is being carried out. This requires the user to have a much higher degree of skill and training than in B-mode imaging alone.

It is not possible to give general recommendations regarding system settings, examination technique, and image interpretation. But it is important to take note of some fundamental problems. In this chapter we shall only address basic principles pertaining to instrument settings and the examination technique used, while pointing out common sources of error. Details on specific examinations are presented in subsequent chapters.

A CDS examination, like any ultrasound examination, begins with the optimum adjustment of the gray scale image. The focus or focuses are positioned at the desired depths. In particular, the patient-dependent power level setting (if changeable) and time gain compensation (TGC, DGC) adjustments must be optimized. After the power level has been set to the lowest possible level, the TGC controls are adjusted to obtain a balanced image. If this does not produce optimum results, the power level may be increased. The color display tends to influence the operator in putting less stress on gray scale image quality. It must always be kept in mind that the B-mode image forms the foundation of every examination, with color-encoded flow providing only additional (though important) information.

The power level affects not only the quality of the gray scale image but also the quality of the color-encoded information on flow. When the ultrasound system is properly adjusted, the lumen of a normal blood vessel is completely filled with color during systole. When axial laminar flow is present, brighter colors appear at the center of the vessel (larger Doppler shift, higher velocity) than along the vessel walls (smaller Doppler shift, lower velocity). Color pixels should not be visible outside the vessel lumen. If the transmit power is set too high, for example, some scattered blue pixels may appear even in a vessel with laminar flow being displayed in shades of red. Additionally, color tends to "bleed" into the B-mode image (usually on the far side of the vessel). The Doppler spectrum (frequency analysis over time) will appear obscured, also lacking a systolic window and displaying an additional mirror image of the spectral waveform on the opposite side of the zero baseline. Correct adjustment of the system will eliminate these artifacts (Fig. 4.**1a, b**), which may be confused with aliasing or small eddy currents caused by wall irregularities. The color shift associated with aliasing (Fig. 4.**2a, b**) generally shows up only during systole and is concentrated along the center of the vessel. True wall irregularities (Fig. 4.**3a, b**) are manifested by circumscribed color changes confined to the vessel walls.

On most instruments three parameters controlling the color information are user adjustable: (1) the intensity threshold, (2) the lower limit of the color-coded frequency shift (wall filter, see section 1.4), and (3) the maximum frequency shift that can be detected without aliasing (see Sections 1.6 and 17.3.1). The upper limit depends on the pulse repetition frequency used.

Threshold defines the signal intensity above which echo signals are processed for color encoding. It is used for noise suppression and looks similar to the gain function in gray scale imaging. In reality it removes signals below a user-defined intensity level from color processing. The threshold should be set to a level where no color pixels appear outside the vessel while the transducer is held stationary.

The Doppler frequency range (points 2 and 3 above) is adjusted according to the anticipated blood flow velocity, choosing settings that will detect all relevant motion with a minimum amount of artifacts (aliasing) (Fig. 4.**2a, b**). On some instruments the upper and lower frequency limits can be adjusted separately and on others both are adjusted concurrently. When examining a region with low-velocity flow, as in veins, the wall filter should be adjusted to detect relatively slow-moving blood in the target structure. Signal interference from an adjacent structure, such as a parallel running artery exhibiting more rapid flow, must be

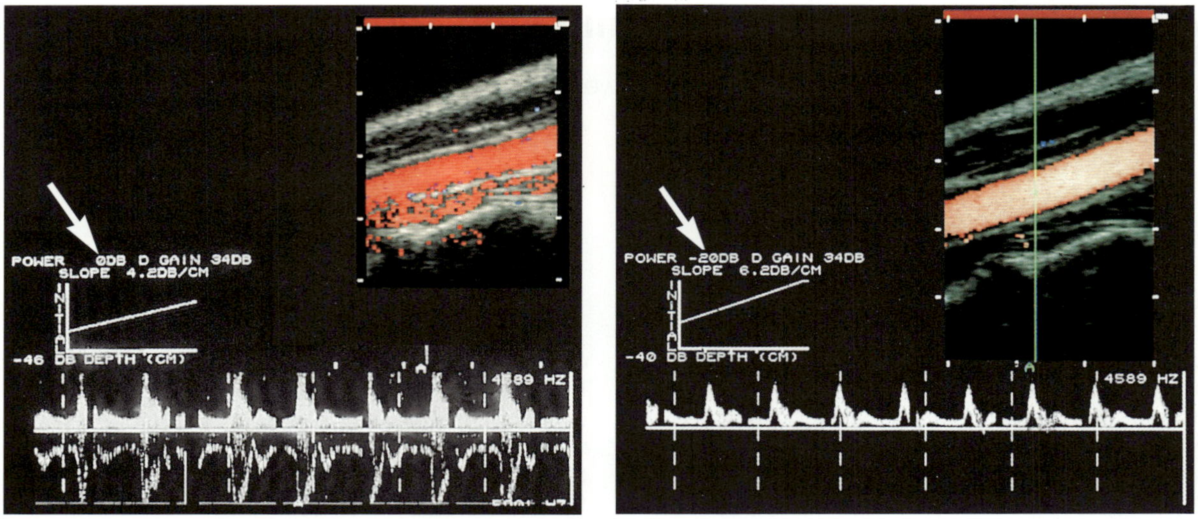

a b

Fig. 4.**1 a, b** Influence of the transmit power on the quality of the color-encoded image and the displayed Doppler spectrum (normal common carotid artery)
a Transmit power setting (= 0 dB, arrow) is too high: Scattered blue pixels appear within the predominantly red-encoded systolic flow. Additionally, color pixels are visible on the far side of the vessel, i. e., outside the vessel lumen. The spectral waveform is blurred and a systolic spectral window nonexistent. A mirror image of the spectrum waveform is visible below the zero baseline
b Using lower transmit power (– 20 dB, arrow), the artifacts disappear. The color is homogeneous and confined to the vessel lumen. The spectrum is clean, there is a clear systolic window visible, and there is no mirror image of the spectrum waveform visible below the zero baseline

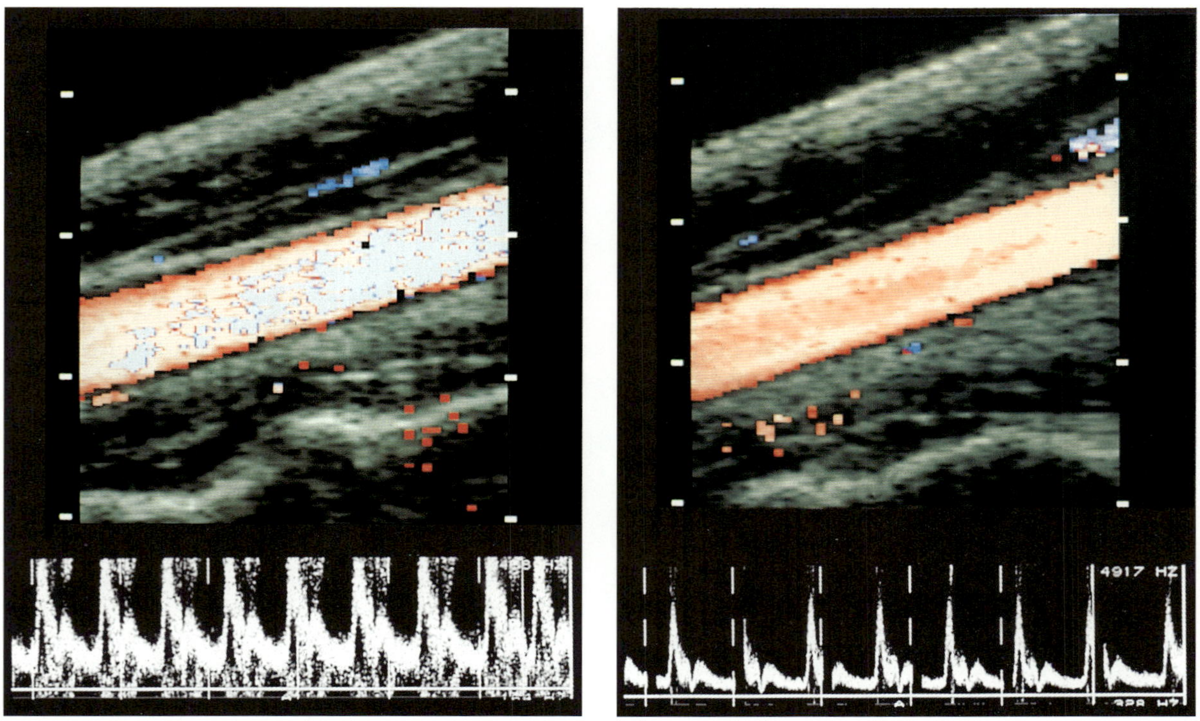

a b

Fig. 4.**2 a, b** Influence of the pulse repetition frequency (PRF) on the quality of the color-encoded image and the displayed Doppler spectrum (normal common carotid artery)
a PRF setting is too low: During systole there is a clear red-to-blue color flip at the center of the vessel (aliasing). Due to aliasing the systolic peaks in the Doppler spectrum transcend the display area and appear below the baseline; the maximum frequency shift cannot be determined
b Correct PRF setting: Flow is encoded in color (red). The very light shade of red at the right of the image signifies a higher velocity (systole) than the darker color at the left (still diastole). The Doppler spectrum is displayed correctly

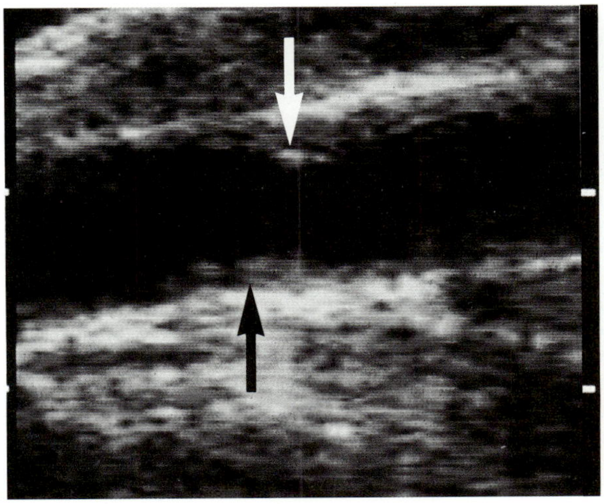
a

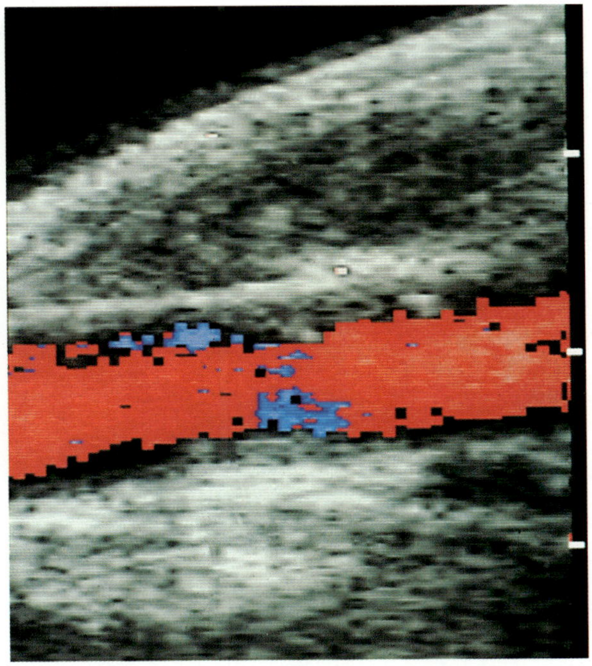
b

Fig. 4.**3 a, b** Wall irregularities in a common carotid artery
a The gray-scale image shows hyperechoic band-shaped plaque along the vessel walls (arrows) creating only a slight reduction in luminal diameter
b CDS shows a disturbance of the laminar flow caused by wall irregularities (areas where the color is changed from red to blue)

surpressed (e.g., veins: 5-MHz transducer, wall filter setting ≥ 50 Hz; testis: 7.5-MHz transducer, wall filter setting ≥ 40 Hz). It should be possible to detect frequency shifts up to 10 kHz (5-MHz transducer) without aliasing when examining blood flow in arteries with high flow velocities (carotids, arteries of the extremities). In all cases the user should consult the operating instructions that are supplied with the equipment.

If the appropriate transducer is used for the specific application and the system is correctly adjusted, a color change within a vessel is indicative of pathology. Zones of turbulence form distal to a hemodynamically significant stenosis. They can be detected in a real-time color-encoded image. In a typical case, the increased flow velocity in the stenosis will appear almost "white" on the CDS image, while the poststenotic flow disturbances are displayed as a mixture of "red" and "blue" colors. The detection of poststenotic turbulence in the CDS image can also be used for the indirect evaluation of vascular segments that cannot be directly visualized due to heavy calcification of the vessel walls (Fig. 4.**4 a–c**).

On some systems a so-called "turbulence indicator" (Fig. 3.**10 a, b**) is implemented. It is designed to facilitate a simplified recognition of disturbed flow, usually by adding green to the different shades of red and blue. Turbulence can be recognized in the usual two-color display by a rapid color change from "red" to "blue" or vice versa. The amount of "green" mixed with the "red" and "blue" is proportional to the square of the standard deviation (variance) of the measured Doppler frequency shifts (see Section 17.4.1). The more green added, the greater the potential error. A pure green pixel means that any frequency shift is possible in that area. Opinions vary regarding the practical value of the turbulence indicator. Presumably, its usefulness is influenced by the sensitivity (spatial resolution) of the system for normal color encoding and by the constancy of the blood flow during the sampling interval.

Most systems can be used with transducers that have either a flat (linear array) or convex (curved array) surface. Soft-tissue compression is accomplished more easily with a curved array transducer, especially in obese patients. Curved array transducers have a disadvantage in CDS imaging that can be annoying and even misleading. Due to the continuous change of the flow direction relative to the direction of the individual ultrasound beams (i.e., a continuous change in Doppler angle), there is a change in the brightness of the color and sometimes even a color flip from "red" to "blue" or vice versa although the blood is flowing at constant velocity (see Section 17.3). When examining vessels in the scan plane running parallel to the transducer, this kind of color reversal can be misleading and even result in an erroneous diagnosis (Figs. 4.**5 a, b**, 17.**39 a, b**). The use of linear transducers for the examination of peripheral arteries is therefore highly recommended.

The major vessels of the neck and extremities are mostly aligned parallel to the skin. Thus, when a linear transducer is used, the Doppler angle between the moving blood and the incident sound waves is equal to or near 90°. According to the Doppler formula, frequency shifts cannot be measured at this

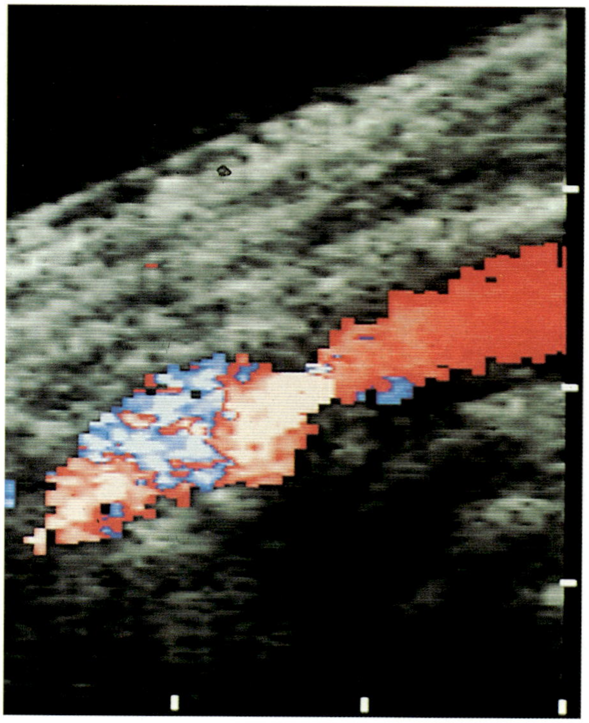

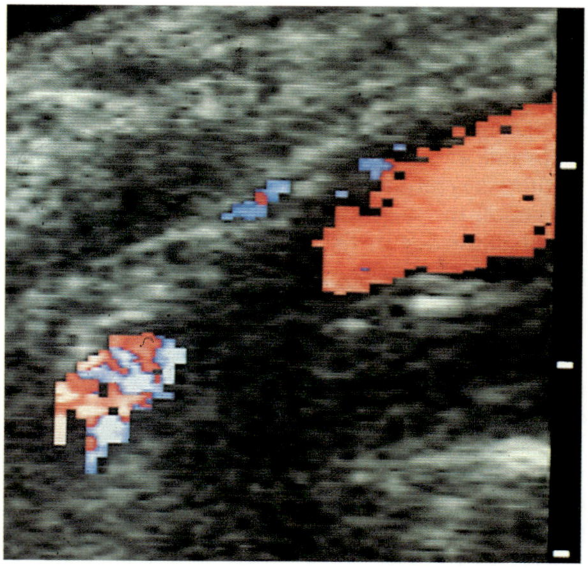

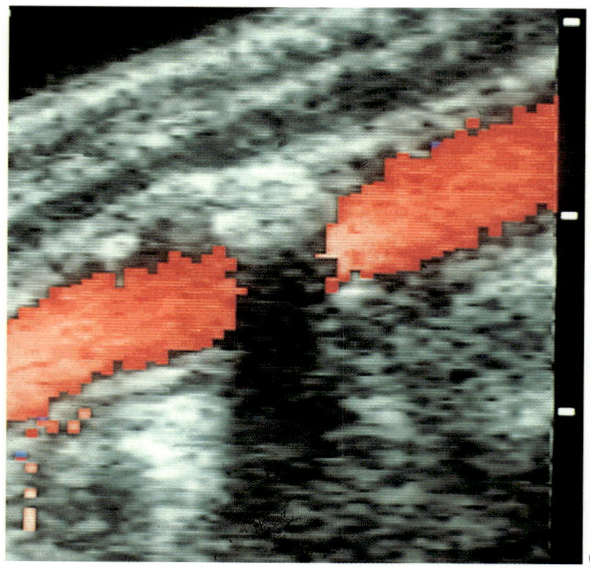

Fig. 4.**4a–c** Narrowing of the vessel lumen and post-stenotic flow turbulance

a More than 50% lumen reduction in a common carotid artery. In systole the signals are coded almost white, indicating a high-velocity flow. The mixed red and blue colors indicate turbulence (eddy currents) in the widened post-stenotic segment

b Pronounced circumferential vessel–wall calcification causing acoustic shadowing. The mixed red and blue signals indicate turbulance (eddy currents) cranial to the calcification (left side of image), confirming a hemodynamically significant stenosis in the calcified area

c Pronounced circumferential vessel–wall calcification with acoustic shadowing. In this case, however, laminar flow is detected proximal and distal to the calcified area (uniform red coloration), thereby excluding a hemodynamically significant stenosis in the calcified area

angle (see Sections 1.4 and 17.3). Manufacturers of ultrasound systems offer two solutions for this situation: a wedge-shaped standoff or electronic beam steering (Fig. 4.**6a–c**). Using a wedge-shaped standoff is disadvantageous in that it slightly degrades the quality of the gray scale image due to the oblique angle of incidence of the sound waves. On the other hand it is advantageous to use a wedge-shaped standoff in that it permits a color-encoded display over the entire image. Beam steering can reduce the available color-encoded area by up to 50% depending on the selected angle and the skin–vessel distance. According to our experience, the wedge-shaped standoff is preferable to beam steering for examinations of peripheral vessels. Color encoding over the entire image field permits the assessment of a larger area and in this way shortens the examination time. Additionally, the near-field image quality is improved by increasing the distance between the transducer and the skin. The evaluation of vessels close to the skin is also improved.

The Doppler angle is also of significant importance when examining vessels in cross section. If the

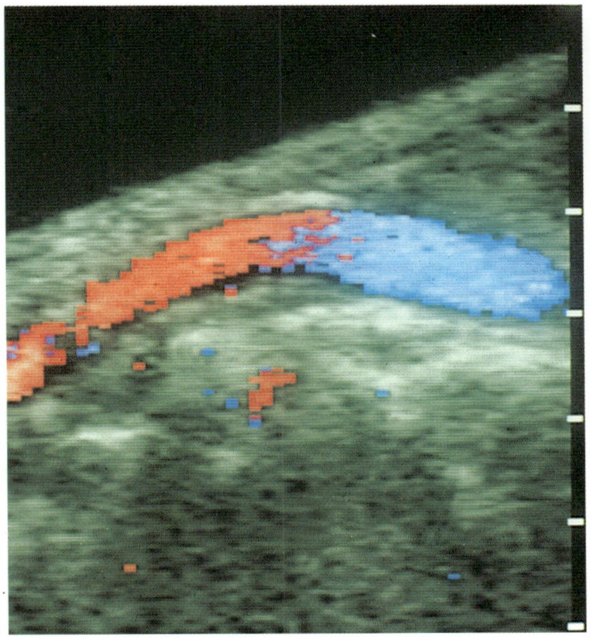

a

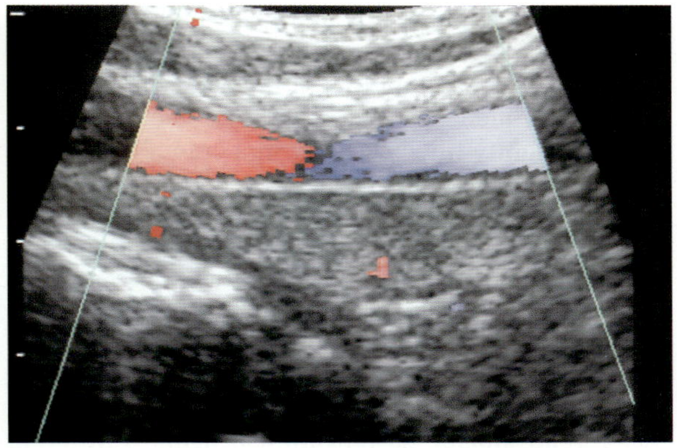

b

Fig. 4.**5a, b** Directional dependence of color assignment (see also Fig. 17.**39a, b**)
a Tortuous segment of a common carotid artery examined with a linear-array transducer using a wedge-shaped standoff. Blue-to-red color flip at the apex of the arch
b In a straight segment of a common carotid artery examined with a curved-array transducer, a similar red-to-blue color flip occurs opposite the apex of the transducer surface

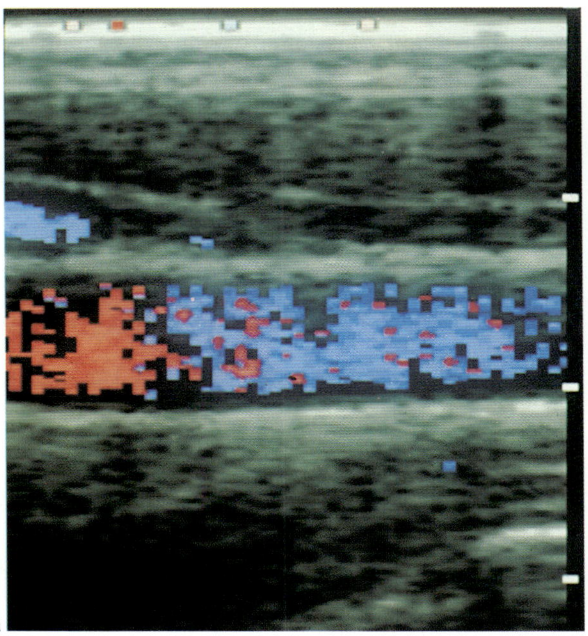

a

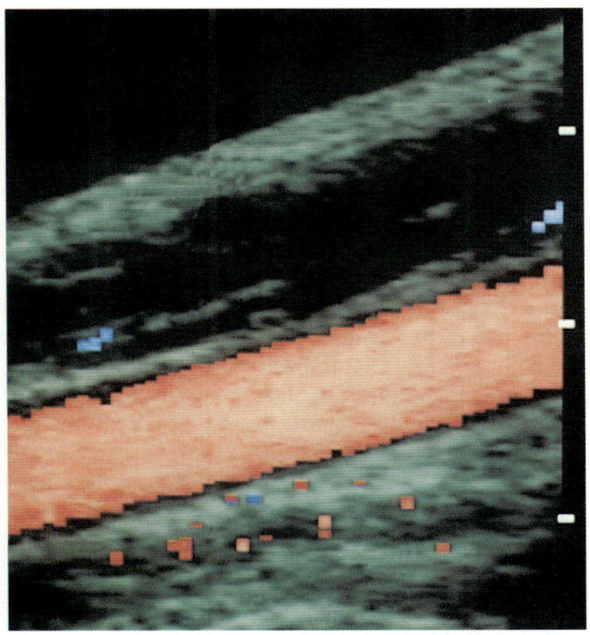

b

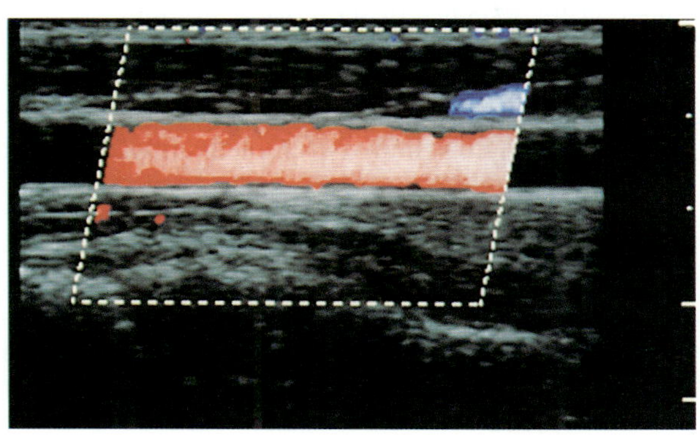

c

Fig. 4.**6a–c** Examination of a vessel running parallel to the skin (normal common carotid artery)
a Without a wedge-shaped standoff, there are only scattered (red and blue) color pixels displaying undefined flow in the lumen (Doppler angle = 90°)
b When a wedge-shaped standoff is used (Doppler angle ≠ 90°), the lumen is uniformly filled with color (red) denoting a well-defined flow direction
c Beam steering (electronic deflection of the sound waves) also produces good color filling of the lumen, but the frequency shifts on the right and left sides of the image cannot be determined

vessel runs parallel to the skin and the transducer is held in a perpendicular position to the vessel, the resulting 90° Doppler angle will preclude the measurement of frequency shifts. Therefore the transducer must be slightly tilted (usually in a cranial direction). An angle of 10° – 15° is generally sufficient. Angling the transducer too far from the vertical will result in significant degradation of the B-mode image quality.

Vessels may also run parallel to the transducer surface during examination of parenchymatous organs. Because it is not possible to measure a Doppler frequency shift in this region, the erroneous diagnosis of a circumscribed perfusion defect may result. The area should always be reexamined using a different transducer position (different acoustic window, probe angulation). If no perfusion at all is detected in an organ, the possibility of a faulty system setting or an equipment malfunction (check by scanning an adjacent vessel) should be considered.

The width of the color-encoded area of the CDS image determines the frame rate. This is usually not a problem when a narrow, high-frequency transducer is used for examining superficial structures. But if the image width of the transducer and the penetration depth are large (e.g., a 3-MHz transducer in abdominal sonography), color encoding over the entire image width can lead to a significant reduction in frame rate. This relates to the image generation process and the physical properties of the sound waves (see Sections 1.3 and 17.2.2). The broader and deeper the imaged area, the more time is needed to generate an image. The frame rate can be increased by reducing the width of the color-encoded area. All manufacturers offer the possibility of reducing the size of the "color window." This option is particularly useful for abdominal examinations. Using transducers having a wide field of view and a high penetration depth leads to a very slow frame rate (2 to 3 frames per second) when extending the color window over the whole image width at maximum imaging depth. This frame rate is unsuitable for the examination of dynamic processes. The frame rate can be considerably raised, for example, by reducing the color window to one-half the width of the image field.

On some systems, switching on the color mode can cause a significant deterioration in the quality of the gray-scale image. These instruments enhance the Doppler frequency resolution of the color-encoded image at the expense of the gray scale image quality (see Section 17.2.4, Spatial and Frequency Resolution). When using such a system, the user should first examine the organ of interest completely in the pure gray scale imaging mode before activating the color mode.

The documentation of CDS images is basically the same as in gray scale ultrasound; the organ or vessel of interest should be documented in two planes. Additionally, all pathologic findings must be recorded. Principally, this rule cannot be followed in the case of peripheral vessels. Image documentation must then be supplemented by a detailed description of the findings, which must also be transferred to a schematic drawing on the report form. Particularly in CDS imaging, the diagnosis is based on the conclusions arrived at during real-time imaging. Only the result of the diagnosis made during the examination should be documented. This is much more important than in B-mode imaging. Many hemodynamic processes cannot be sufficiently evaluated on a static image.

Neglect of the Doppler angle in the "Doppler formula" is a frequent cause of misdiagnoses. According to this formula, the measured frequency shift must be multiplied by the cosine of the angle between the blood flow direction and the incident ultrasound beam in order to calculate the blood flow velocity. The reference frequency of the transducer must also be taken into account. Several examples are presented to underscore the importance of these variables in calculating the blood flow velocity (see Section 1.4 or 17.3):

"Doppler-formula"

$$f_d = 2f_o \frac{v}{c} \cos(\alpha)$$

$$\rightarrow \quad v = \frac{f_d}{2f_o} \frac{c}{\cos(\alpha)} \quad \left(\frac{Hz \cdot \frac{cm}{s}}{Hz} = cm/s \right)$$

$$c = 1540 \text{ m/s} = 154\,000 \text{ cm/s}$$

It is assumed in the first three examples that a reference frequency f_0 of 3 MHz is used and a Doppler frequency shift f_d of 4000 Hz is measured.

Example 1: Doppler angle α between incident sound wave and the direction of motion:
$\alpha = 0° \rightarrow \cos\alpha = 1$

$$v = \frac{4000 \cdot 154\,000}{2 \cdot 3\,000\,000 \cdot 1} = \frac{616}{6} = \mathbf{103\ cm/s}$$

Example 2: Doppler angle $\alpha = 40° \rightarrow \cos\alpha = 0.7660$

$$v = \frac{4000 \cdot 154\,000}{2 \cdot 3\,000\,000 \cdot 0.766} = \frac{616}{4.6} = \mathbf{134\ cm/s}$$

Example 3: Doppler angle $\alpha = 80° \rightarrow \cos\alpha = 0.1736$

$$v = \frac{4000 \cdot 154\,000}{2 \cdot 3\,000\,000 \cdot 0.1736} = \frac{616}{1.0416} = \mathbf{591\ cm/s}$$

Example 4: Doppler angle α as in example 3 (80°), but using a reference frequency f_0 of 5 MHz.

$$v = \frac{4000 \cdot 154\,000}{2 \cdot 5\,000\,000 \cdot 0.1736} = \frac{616}{1.736} = \mathbf{355\ cm/s}$$

As can be seen in examples 1 through 3, when the angle changes from 0° to 80° the calculated velocity increases by almost a factor of 6, while the frequency shift remains constant! The closer the angle approaches 90°, the greater the velocity difference. Even a small change in angle will lead to a large change in velocity (see Fig. 17.**41**). Simply changing the reference frequency from 3 MHz (example 3) to 5 MHz (example 4) decreases the computed velocity by almost a factor of ½. Consequently, there is gener-

Table 4.**1** Common causes of color artifacts and recommended corrective actions

Appearance	Causes	Corrective actions
1. Well-defined vessel having normal diameter in B-mode image. Displaying a mixture of red and blue pixels plus color pixels outside of the vessel lumen in CDS	a) Transmit power setting too high b) PRF too low (aliasing) c) Lower frequency limit for color-encoded frequency shifts (wall filter) too low	a) Reduce transmit power b) Increase PRF (if possible) or shift baseline or change beam angle (bring Doppler angle closer to 90°) or use lower frequency transducer c) Raise wall filter
2. Little or no color encoding	a) Transmit power setting too low b) PRF too high c) Wall filter too high d) Doppler angle close to 90° e) System defective	a) Increase transmit power setting b) Decrease PRF c) Lower wall filter d) Use wedge-shaped standoff or beam steering
3. Constant or varying "color cloud" (mixture of red and blue) in and surrounding the vessel lumen (Fig. 4.**7**)	a) Vibration of soft tissue near a tight stenosis or a–v fistula b) Very high blood flow (dialysis shunt) c) "Pseudostenosis" caused by excessive probe pressure d) Ambient noise (intestinal peristalsis, cardiac pulsations, muscular tremor)	a, b) Reduce blood flow by manual compression of feeding artery proximal to the examination site c) Reduce exerted probe pressure d) Immobilize the bowel (e. g., with anticholinerc drugs), decrease the color-encoded area ("color window"), try a different acoustic window

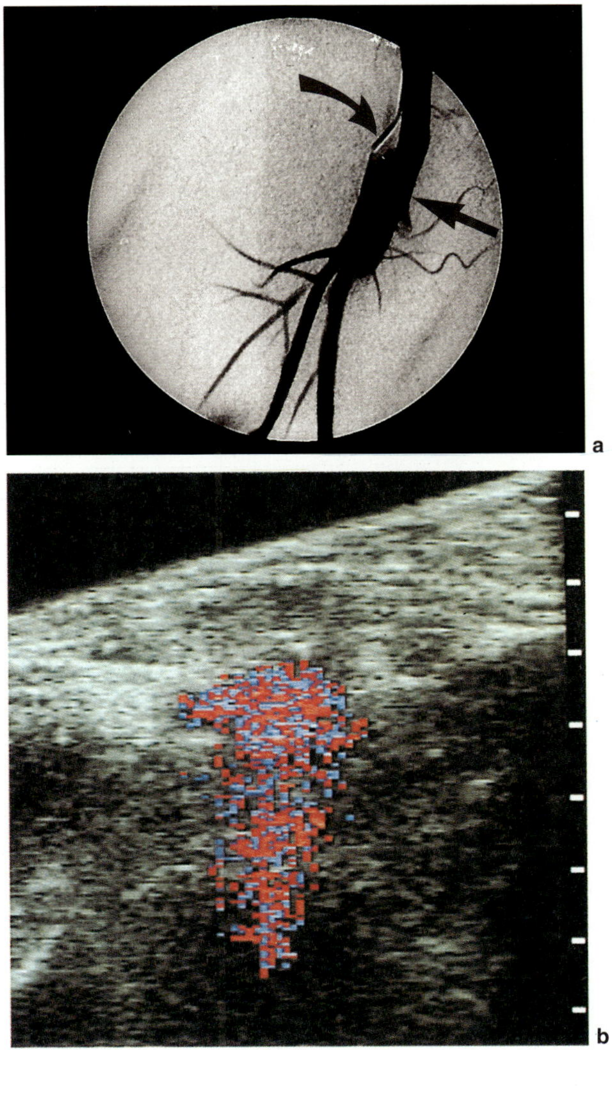

Fig. 4.**7a, b** Fistula between the right common femoral artery and vein following arterial puncture
a Angiography: Puncture of the contralateral femoral artery with the catheter tip (curved arrow) positioned in the distal external iliac artery. Injected contrast medium immediately displays the femoral vein (straight arrow) along with the deep and superficial femoral arteries
b CDS shows a typical circumscribed "cloud" of mixed red and blue pixels. The cloud obscures the vessels and the fistula itself, which cannot be identified. The rapid flow across the fistula produces tissue vibrations that are detected and color encoded by the ultrasound system

ally no point in reporting a Doppler frequency shift without noting the Doppler angle and the reference frequency. Moreover, a change in the brightness level of color pixels can be caused simply by a change in the orientation of the vessel (see Fig. 17.**40a, b**). Essentially flow evaluation should only be done after angle correction.

Absolute measurements in ultrasound, whether of velocities, volumes, or distances, should always be checked for plausibility before they are assumed to be true. The importance of the angle factor in velocity measurements has already been pointed out. But there are a number of other factors that influence absolute measurements in ultrasound. Only three others will be discussed here:

1. Distances in ultrasound images are calculated from the time of flight of the emitted ultrasound pulse and the returning echo. A fixed speed of sound in tissue is assumed. Regrettably, the speed of sound varies in different tissues and regions of the body. This effect is negligible when measuring objects close to the transducer. But the magnitude of the error increases with the distance from the transducer.
2. The energy of the sound wave is partially attenuated as it passes through tissue. This attenuation is frequency dependent, and higher frequencies are attenuated more than lower frequencies. This introduces another source of error into the calculation of flow velocity: the velocity of flow directed away from the transducer is overestimated while the velocity of flow directed toward the transducer is underestimated. This error is particularly significant in the examination of abdominal regions far away from the transducer.
3. The accuracy of the measurement depends directly on the accurate placement of the sample volume and on the position of the blood vessel (beam – vessel angle). The greater the distance between the transducer and the vessel, and the lower the transducer operating frequency (lower spatial resolution), the more difficult it is to obtain a reliable measurement. For example, when positioning the sample volume at a distance of 10 cm from the transducer, a deviation of 1° corresponds to a lateral error of position of 1.7 mm.

When ratios are calculated (e.g., the pulsatility index), it must be kept in mind that in multiplication and division errors of measurement are multiplied and not merely added. Stating ratios with an assumed precision of 1% error, implies an accuracy that cannot realistically be attained either by the examiner or by the method of measurement. Despite these limitations, which are based on the physics of ultrasound, measurements, in particular relative measurements, are still possible with the help of ultrasound. This is especially true when measurements are used for interindividual comparisons and regular checkup examinations.

Ultrasound, and CDS especially, is a fascinating diagnostic modality. The optimum utilization of ultrasound requires that both its capabilities and limitations be known.

5 Carotid and Vertebral Arteries

P. Landwehr

5.1 General

Although the incidence of stroke has declined significantly in recent years (9, 20), it remains a leading cause of death in industrialized countries. Approximately one-third of acute cases have a fatal outcome. Many survivors of stroke face prolonged and often irreversible disability. The paralysis that follows stroke frequently leads to a complete reliance on nursing care and permanent speech disorders that hamper the patient's ability to communicate.

Untreated patients who have experienced a transient ischemic attack (TIA) or stroke with persistent neurologic deficits have an approximately 15–20 times higher risk of sustaining a new cerebrovascular insult than the asymptomatic population (24, 46). The spontaneous risk of stroke following a previous TIA is 4–10% per year.

Thrombembolism from the heart is responsible for only one-fifth of cases of transient or permanent brain ischemia. Four-fifths of ischemic insults are due to atherosclerosis. The great majority of these lesions involve the extracranial cerebral arteries, and they are especially prevalent at the carotid bifurcation. This makes the surgical treatment of atherosclerotic lesions feasible. The procedure of choice is open thromboendarterectomy (TEA), which may involve the use of a venous or synthetic patch graft. Whereas balloon dilatation is rarely possible for nonulcerating stenoses in the area of the carotid bifurcation and internal carotid artery (28), stenoses of the subclavian artery and innominate artery are a particularly favorable indication for percutaneous transluminal angioplasty (PTA) (12).

The debate concerning the role of open surgery in the treatment of asymptomatic carotid stenoses is still partly unresolved due to the significant operative morbidity and mortality, the availability of conservative treatment with platelet aggregation inhibitors and coumarins, and the significant long-term risk of myocardial infarction. The benefit of surgical treatment in symptomatic patients is well established, however. The incidence of stroke can be markedly reduced compared with patients not receiving surgical treatment (50). Two current randomized studies on the efficacy of carotid TEA (50, 51) for symptomatic, high-grade stenoses of the carotid artery (70–99% diameter reduction) clearly document a benefit for surgically treated patients compared with conservatively managed cases, whereas patients with low-grade stenoses (< 30% diameter reduction) do not benefit from surgery (50). The benefit in patients with moderate carotid stenosis (30%–69% diameter reduction) is unclear, and further long-term studies are needed to determine whether surgery is preferable to medical treatment with platelet aggregation inhibitors in this population (14, 50, 51).

The extracranial distribution of the majority of cerebrovascular lesions makes them accessible to ultrasound examination. The major questions to be addressed with diagnostic ultrasound are the nature, location, and extent of the disease. The territory of the carotid arteries is a classic area of application for Doppler ultrasound. Before the advent of duplex technology, diagnosis was based on the analysis of CW Doppler spectral waveforms recorded by examination of the carotid artery and the periorbital arteries using compression tests (19). CDS allows for the simultaneous visualization of vascular pathology in the gray-scale image (plaque, stenosis, occlusion) and associated flow abnormalities in the color-encoded image (intrastenotic velocity increase, poststenotic flow disturbances, absence of flow due to occlusion). The goal is to utilize the results of the imaging procedure as a basis for making a clinically oriented diagnosis. The present chapter deals with the anatomic, pathologic, pathophysiologic, and clinical principles that must be known in order to interpret the findings of color duplex sonography.

5.2 Normal Anatomy, Common Variants, and Examination Technique

5.2.1 Preliminary Remarks

Brain tissue is very sensitive to ischemia and thus to hypoxia. This low tolerance for ischemia is reflected in the copious blood supply to the brain, which is derived from four major arteries. When the supply from one artery is lost, the remaining arteries may be able to compensate through collateral pathways and ward off neurologic deficits.

5.2.2 Vessels Arising from the Aortic Arch

The brain normally derives its blood supply from the two internal carotid arteries and the two vertebral arteries, the vertebral arteries uniting at the inferior border of the pons to form the basilar artery. The supply is not entirely symmetrical, as the left common carotid artery and left subclavian artery generally branch separately from the aortic arch, while the right common carotid artery and right subclavian artery arise by a common origin, the brachiocephalic (innominate) artery (Fig. 5.**1**). The classic anatomy of the aortic arch is present in about 70% of the population. Variations in the supra-aortic arteries, which develop from the branchial arches, are fairly common and chiefly involve the vessels arising from the aortic arch. For example, all the arterial branches of the aortic arch, including the vertebral arteries, may arise separately from the arch, or there may be a single trunk from which all of the brachiocephalic vessels arise (27).

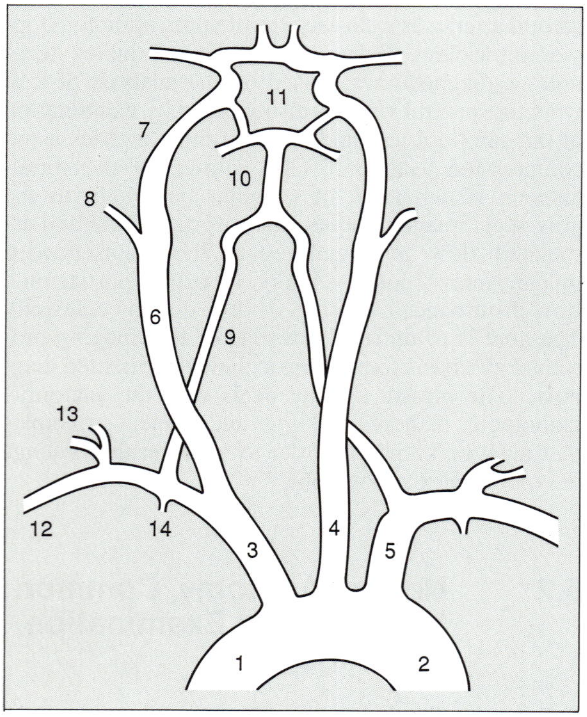

Fig. 5.**1** Schematic representation of the normal anatomy of the origins of the aortic arch branches and their principal divisions. 1 = Ascending thoracic aorta, 2 = descending thoracic aorta, 3 = brachiocephalic (innominate) artery, 4 = left common carotid artery, 5 = left subclavian artery, 6 = right common carotid artery, 7 = right internal carotid artery, 8 = right external carotid artery, 9 = right vertebral artery, 10 = basilar artery, 11 = circle of Willis, 12 = right subclavian artery, 13 = thyrocervical trunk, 14 = internal thoracic artery

5.2.3 Common Carotid Artery and Carotid Bifurcation

The right common carotid artery arises from the brachiocephalic artery behind the sternoclavicular joint. The left common carotid artery arises at a more posterior level and springs directly from the aortic arch. Each common carotid artery ascends to the neck behind the medial third of the clavicle, under cover of the sternocleidomastoid muscle, and runs lateral to the posterior part of the thyroid gland in the lower portion of the neck, accompanied by the vagus nerve and the internal jugular vein, which is anterolateral to the artery. The upper part of the common carotid artery and the carotid bifurcation are located in the carotid triangle, bounded by the sternocleidomastoid muscle, the posterior belly of the digastric muscle, and the superior belly of the omohyoid muscle. At this level the neurovascular bundle runs along the anterior border of the sternocleidomastoid muscle. The cervical portion of the common carotid artery divides into the internal and external carotid arteries (Fig. 5.**2**). The carotid bifurcation can occur at various sites but generally is located at the level of the fourth through sixth cervical vertebrae. With aging, the bifurcation tends

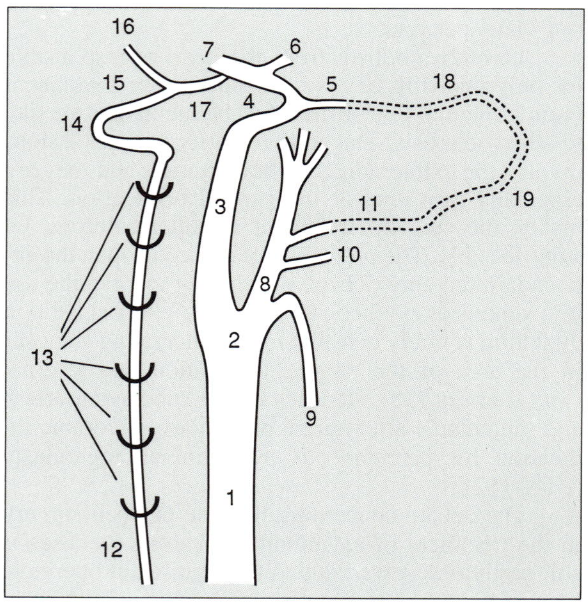

Fig. 5.**2** Schematic representation of the normal anatomy of the extracranial cerebral arteries on the right side. 1 = Common carotid artery, 2 = carotid bulb, 3 = internal carotid artery, 4 = carotid siphon, 5 = ophthalmic artery, 6 = anterior cerebral artery, 7 = middle cerebral artery, 8 = external carotid artery, 9 = superior thyroid artery, 10 = lingual artery, 11 = facial artery, 12 = vertebral artery, 13 = transverse foramina of the cervical spine, 14 = atlas loop of the vertebral artery, 15 = basilar artery, 16 = posterior cerebral artery, 17 = posterior communicating artery, 18 = branches of ophthalmic artery (e.g., supraorbital artery, supratrochlear artery), 19 = angular artery

to descend to a slightly lower position in the neck. Within the carotid bifurcation is a chemoreceptor, the carotid body, which normally is too small to be defined with ultrasound.

5.2.4 Internal and External Carotid Arteries

The internal carotid artery lies posterior to the external carotid artery in approximatly 90% of cases, showing a slight medial or lateral deviation. In about 10% of cases the internal carotid is medial to the external carotid. Very rarely the internal carotid artery runs anteromedial to the external carotid (35). Typically the area of the bifurcation is markedly expanded in relation to the terminal segment of the common carotid artery. This dilatation, called the carotid bulb, usually includes the origin of the internal carotid artery, especially in its posterior portion. The internal carotid artery passes through the carotid canal of the skull base and enters the cranium without giving off any side branches (98% of cases). The external carotid artery, however, divides at once into numerous branches (Fig. 5.**2**) that supply the external soft tissues of the cranium, face, and neck (47).

5.2.5 Collateral Connections between the Internal and External Carotid Arteries

Several collateral pathways exist between the territories of the internal and external carotid arteries. The most important route is through the ophthalmic artery (branch of the internal carotid) and the facial or maxillary artery (branches of the external carotid) by way of the periorbital arteries and angular artery (Fig. 5.**2**). This collateral circulation, which may be activated by vascular pathology, formed the basis for the first diagnostic applications of CW Doppler ultrasound in the carotid artery (22).

5.2.6 Vertebral Artery

The two vertebral arteries, each arising from the ipsilateral subclavian artery, are partly intraosseous as they ascend from the sixth cervical vertebra to the atlas, passing through the transverse foramina of the corresponding vertebrae (Fig. 5.**2**). As a result, only certain segments of the vertebral artery are accessible to ultrasound imaging. Variations of vessel caliber are much more common in the vertebral arteries than in the carotids. Unilateral hypoplasia or aplasia of a vertebral artery is generally associated with compensatory hypertrophy of the contralateral vessel to ensure maintenance of the basilar supply. The vertebral artery may arise separately from the aortic arch, as noted above.

5.2.7 Circle of Willis

The uniqueness of the cerebral blood supply is exemplified by the circle of Willis, a ring-like arterial anastomosis at the base of the brain that connects all of the arteries supplying the brain. When the circle of Willis is fully developed, cross-collateralization can even occur by way of the anterior and posterior communicating arteries. It is very common, however, for portions of the arterial circle to show some degree of hypoplasia (in about 80% of cases) (21), so certain portions of the brain may receive an atypical supply even in healthy individuals (e.g., flow from the internal carotid artery to the territory of the posterior cerebral artery), and—in cases of vascular disease—certain collateral pathways may become unavailable.

5.2.8 Examination Technique

5.2.8.1 Preliminary Examinations

Before the cerebral arteries are examined by CDS, a detailed history should be obtained along with arterial blood pressure measurements. Right–left discrepancies of up to 10 mmHg in the systolic pressures are considered normal (17). Larger discrepancies may indicate a hemodynamically significant flow obstruction in the brachiocephalic artery, subclavian artery, or thoracic aorta between the origins of the brachiocephalic artery and left subclavian artery that may underlie a symptomatic steal syndrome or brachial claudication.

5.2.8.2 Ultrasound Instrumentation

We recommend that only linear transducers be used for examinations of the cervical arteries. An acceptable Doppler angle can be achieved with a standoff wedge or beam steering. A 5-MHz transducer is essential and will adequately demonstrate the cervical arteries even in obese patients. A 7.5-MHz transducer is useful for achieving higher spatial resolution and when examining very thin patients or children (see Chapter 4).

First the instrument is adjusted to optimize the gray-scale and color flow images. Color pixels should completely fill the vessel of interest, at least in systole, and there should be no extraluminal color bleed. The flow image should be free of aliasing (no red-to-blue color shift). For more rapid orientation, the examination should start imaging in the color duplex mode; this is particularly helpful for identifying the carotid bifurcation. Alternating use of the gray-scale and color flow modes is recommended only if an instrument is used in which the color encoding significantly degrades the gray scale quality compared with gray-scale imaging alone.

5.2.8.3 Position of the Patient and Examiner

The patient is placed in the supine position. The upper body may be slightly elevated if desired. The head should be hyperextended by placing a small pad or roll beneath the neck to assist visualization of the soft tissues at the mandibular angle. The patient should be comfortably positioned with the head resting on the table surface to avoid neck muscle tension that would hamper penetration of the ultrasonic sound waves. The patient's arms are adducted and extended with the shoulders relaxed. The examiner may sit on the patient's right side as in abdominal sonography, or behind the patient's head. The advantage of sitting at the patient's side is that it provides a spatial orientation identical to that in most other types of ultrasound examination. It is also advantageous when working in small rooms.

For the examination of specific vessels, the patient is told to turn the head to the opposite side while keeping the neck relaxed. It is best to scan the left side of the neck first so that the patient can watch the initial part of the examination on the monitor. The patient is told not to speak, to breathe quietly and evenly, and to swallow as little as possible to avoid motion artifacts. The transducer should press very lightly on the skin to respect the pressure sensitivity of the cervical soft tissues and laryngeal area; also, excessive transducer pressure on the carotid bifurcation could evoke a vagal response by irritating the carotid sinus receptors (carotid sinus syndrome).

5.2.8.4 Examination Protocol

CDS examination of the carotid arteries begins by imaging the common carotid artery and carotid bifurcation in transverse section (Fig. 5.**3a–c**). The transducer may be applied more from the anteromedial or lateral side of the sternocleidomastoid muscle, depending on the relation of the arteries to the muscle. The vessels can also be clearly imaged through the muscle itself (Figs. 5.**3**, 5.**4a–e**). Generally, the lower

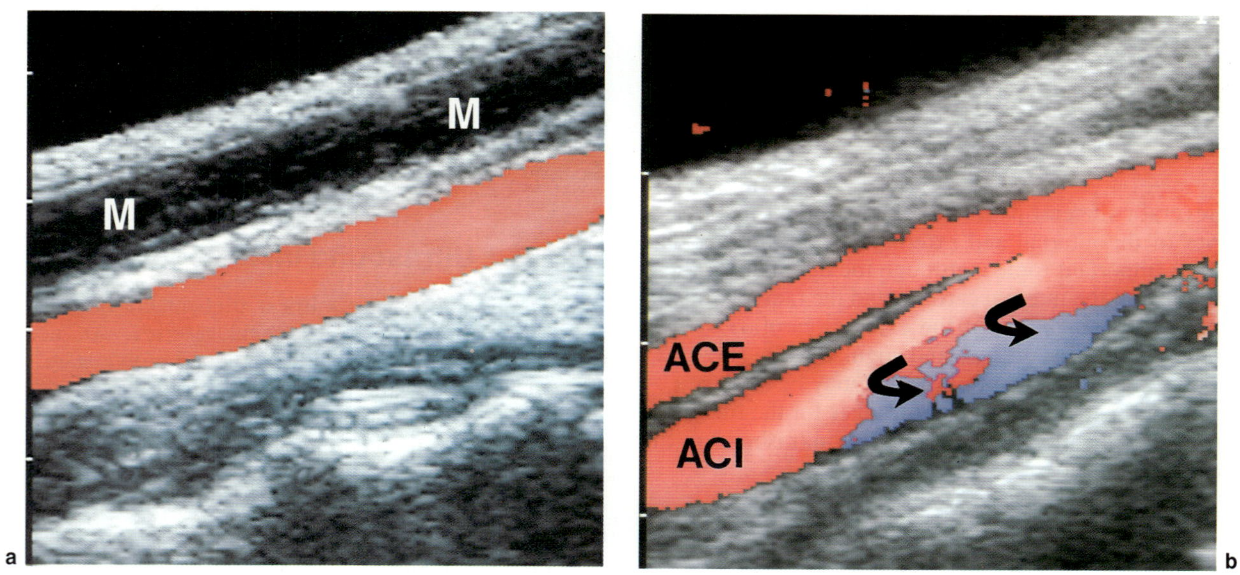

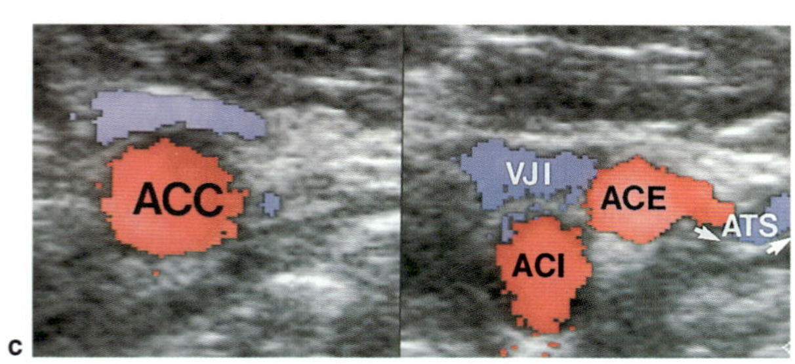

Fig. 5.**3a–c** Normal CDS findings in the right carotid artery. ACC = Common carotid artery, ACI = internal carotid artery, ACE = external carotid artery, VJI = internal jugular vein

a Longitudinal image of the normal common carotid artery. Flow direction is from right to left. There is homogeneous color saturation consistent with laminar flow, with slightly lighter shades of red (higher velocity) at the center of the vessel and darker red at the periphery. M = Sternocleidomastoid muscle

b Longitudinal image of the normal carotid bifurcation. Areas of physiologic flow reversal are apparent at the origin of the internal carotid artery (arrows)

c Transverse images of the normal carotid bifurcation. The scan planes pass through the carotid bulb (left) and through the origin of the superior thyroid artery (ATS, arrows) (right). The internal jugular vein is anterior to the common carotid and internal carotid arteries. The internal carotid artery runs laterally above the level of the bifurcation.

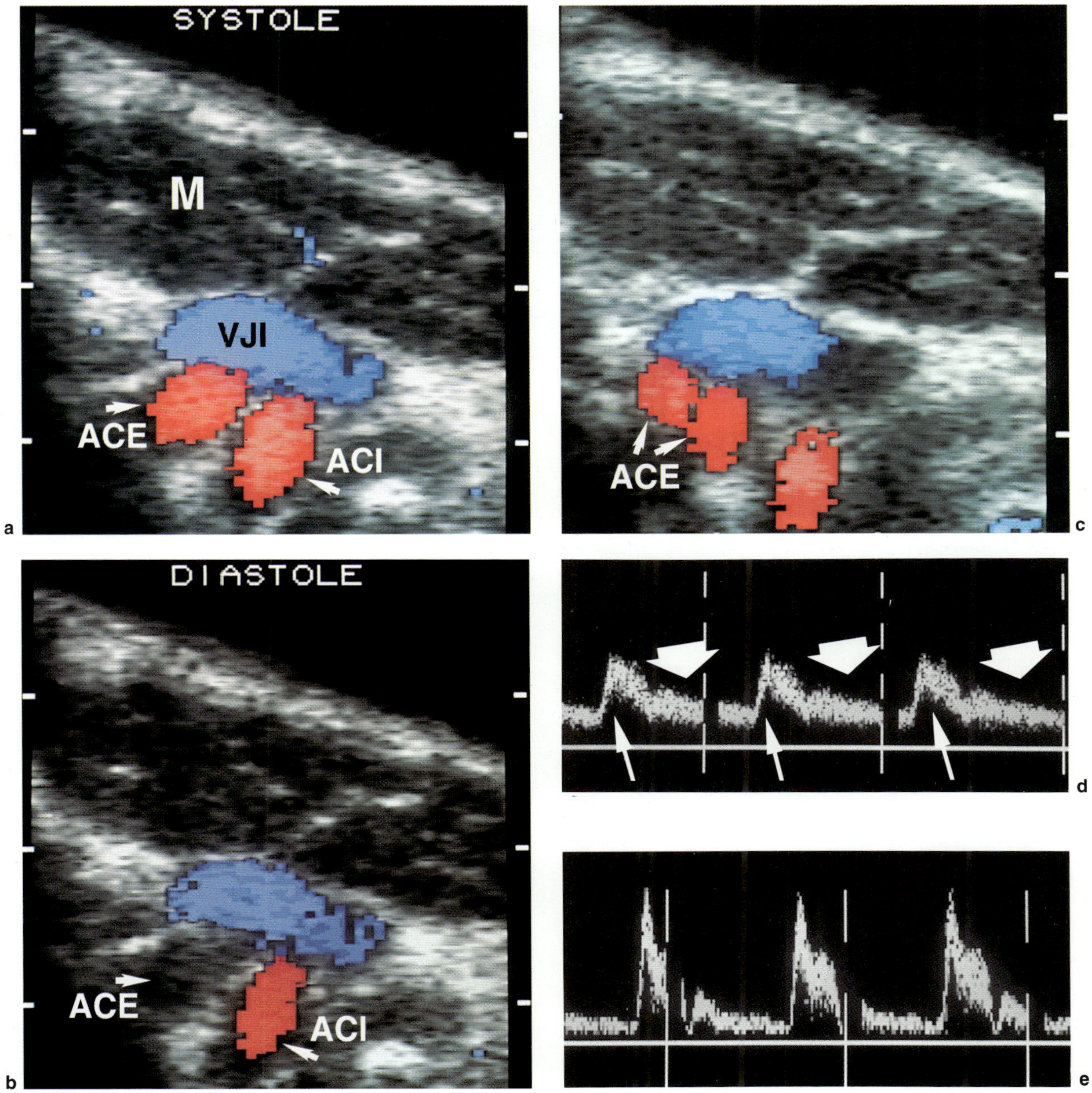

Fig. 5.**4a–e** Differentiation between the normal internal and external carotid arteries (left side) in the color duplex image. ACI = Internal carotid artery, ACE = external carotid artery, VJI = internal jugular vein, M = sternocleidomastoid muscle

a Transverse image just above the carotid bifurcation. Flow is evident in both the internal and external carotid arteries during systole

b Same plane as in **a**. In diastole, flow persists in the internal carotid artery but is absent in the external carotid artery due to the high peripheral resistance in the supply region of the external carotid artery

c When the image plane is moved 1 cm cephalad from **a** and **b**, the external carotid artery is clearly identified by the origin of the lingual artery (arrows)

d Doppler spectrum from the internal carotid artery shows persistence of antegrade flow in diastole (wide arrows, parenchymal artery pattern) and a clear spectral window (thin arrows)

e Doppler spectrum from the external carotid artery shows a marked reduction of diastolic flow compared with the internal carotid artery (**d**) (extremity artery pattern)

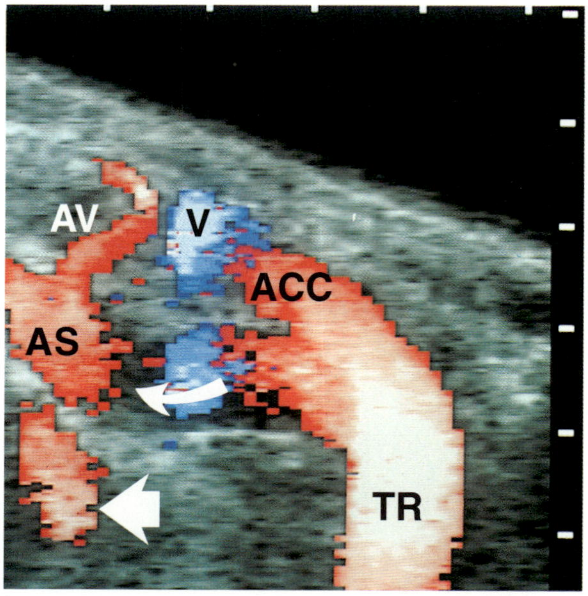

a

Fig. 5.**5 a–c** Normal CDS findings in the vertebral artery
a At the origin of the right vertebral artery (AV), blood flow in the subclavian artery (curved arrow) is initially shown in blue because it is directed away from the transducer in that area. Artifactual color encoding (red, short arrow) represents a mirror artifact of the subclavian artery from the pleura. TR = brachiocephalic artery, ACC = common carotid artery, AS = subclavian artery, V = internal jugular vein
b Longitudinal image of the cervical portion of the vertebral artery. Asterisks mark the acoustic shadows caused by the transverse processes of the vertebral bodies. V = Internal jugular vein
c Normal Doppler spectrum from the vertebral artery shows relatively high antegrade diastolic flow comparable to that in the internal carotid artery (parenchymal pattern)

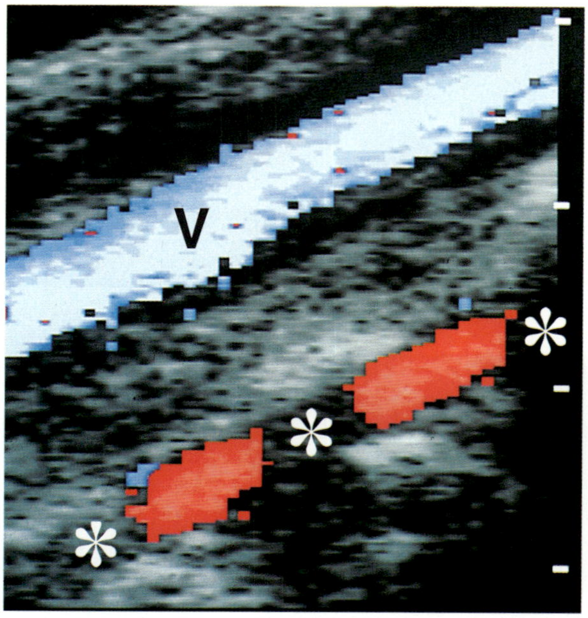

b

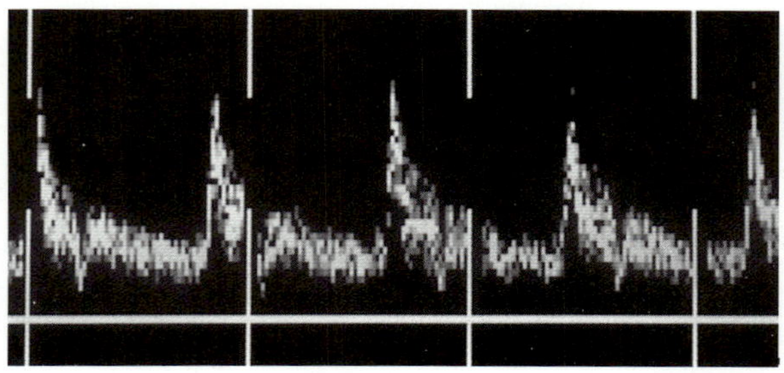

c

portions of the vessels are defined better from the medial aspect, while the upper portions, and especially the internal carotid artery, are seen more clearly from an anterolateral or posterolateral approach. For transverse imaging, the transducer should be angled slightly to obtain a satisfactory Doppler angle. Individual anatomy and topography are rapidly surveyed by proceeding cephalad with the transverse examination along the course of the cervical arteries. Most abnormalities can already be appreciated in the transverse survey. The division of the brachiocephalic artery into the common carotid artery and subclavian artery can usually be identified on the right side (Fig. 5.**5**). Rarely, it may be possible to demonstrate the origins of the aortic arch branches if the arch is elongated or ectatic.

The internal and external carotid arteries are imaged concomitantly in the transverse plane (Figs. 5.**3 b, c**, Fig. 5.**4 a–e**), and the internal carotid artery is traced as far cephalad as possible to determine the individual course of the vessel (straight, S-shaped, looped, or coiled) for the subsequent longitudinal examination. Next the common carotid artery, carotid bifurcation, internal carotid artery, and external carotid artery are imaged in longitudinal section. A beam–vessel angle appropriate for detection of a Doppler shift should always be maintained (generally 50°–70°). The scan should simultaneously define the outer and

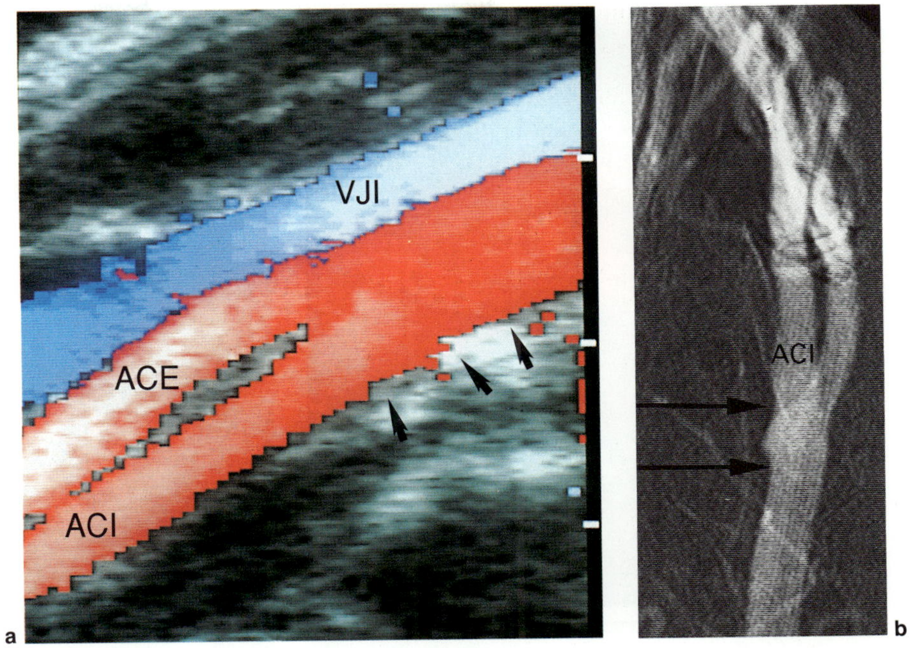

Fig. 5.**6 a, b** Flat atherosclerotic plaque in the left carotid bulb without a hemodynamically significant stenosis. ACI = Internal carotid artery, ACE = external carotid artery, VJI = internal jugular vein
a Longitudinal CDS image shows a flat vessel-wall thickening of mixed echogenicity (arrows). The flow reversal normally present at the origin of the internal carotid artery is not visible. There are no flow abnormalities characteristic of stenosis
b Intra-arterial DSA of the same lesion (aortic arch injection) demonstrates wall irregularities caused by atherosclerotic plaques (arrows)

inner vessel walls and the perfused lumen, underscoring the importance of optimizing the gray-scale and color images. Meanwhile the examiner observes the color flow pattern for signs of abnormality. The recording of Doppler spectra in a vessel that can be clearly imaged in two planes serves only as confirmation of the color findings.

Calcified plaque in the near wall of a vessel can produce a total reflection of the incident ultrasound waves (Fig. 5.**7 a**). In this case the examiner should try to find a different insonation window to project the calcification in an altered position so that the perfused lumen can be evaluated. This is not possible with a circumferential calcification, however. If calcification prevents flow evaluation in the affected segment, the diagnosis must rely on the color flow images and Doppler spectra immediately proximal and distal to the segment (Fig. 4.**4**, 5.**7 a, b**).

While CW Doppler relies on the sampling of vessels interconnecting the internal and external carotid systems (especially the periorbital arteries) aided by compression tests (22), these vessels are of minor importance in CDS. The retrobulbar portion of the ophthalmic artery can be demonstrated by placing the transducer on the closed eye. One edge of the transducer should rest against the glabella to assist control of the transducer and relieve pressure on the eye.

The vertebral arteries are first imaged in longitudinal section because of their smaller caliber and their less favorable course for ultrasound imaging. Because of the deeper position of the vessels compared with the common carotid artery and their somewhat lower flow velocities, different instrument settings are required than in carotid examinations and the gain, TGC, and color flow parameters should be adjusted accordingly. Examination of the vertebral artery begins by obtaining a longitudinal image of the common carotid artery with the transducer positioned anterolaterally. The image plane is then shifted laterally and angled slightly medially and posteriorly to demonstrate the transverse processes of the cervical vertebrae and the intervening segments of the vertebral artery (Fig. 5.**5**). Alternatively, after obtaining the longitudinal image of the caudal common carotid artery from the front, the transducer is only angled laterally until the vertebral artery is visible. Not infrequently, the vertebral vein is simultaneously visualized. The transducer can then be shifted caudad to image the proximal part of the vessel and may occasionally demonstrate its origin from the subclavian artery (Fig. 5.**5 a–c**). The image plane can be shifted cephalad and angled obliquely to define the atlas loop.

Stress-induced subclavian steal in patients with antegrade vertebral flow at rest can be demonstrated clinically by placing a blood pressure cuff on the upper arm and inflating it to a suprasystolic pressure while imaging the ipsilateral vertebral artery. After 3 minutes the cuff is deflated, allowing a reactive hy-

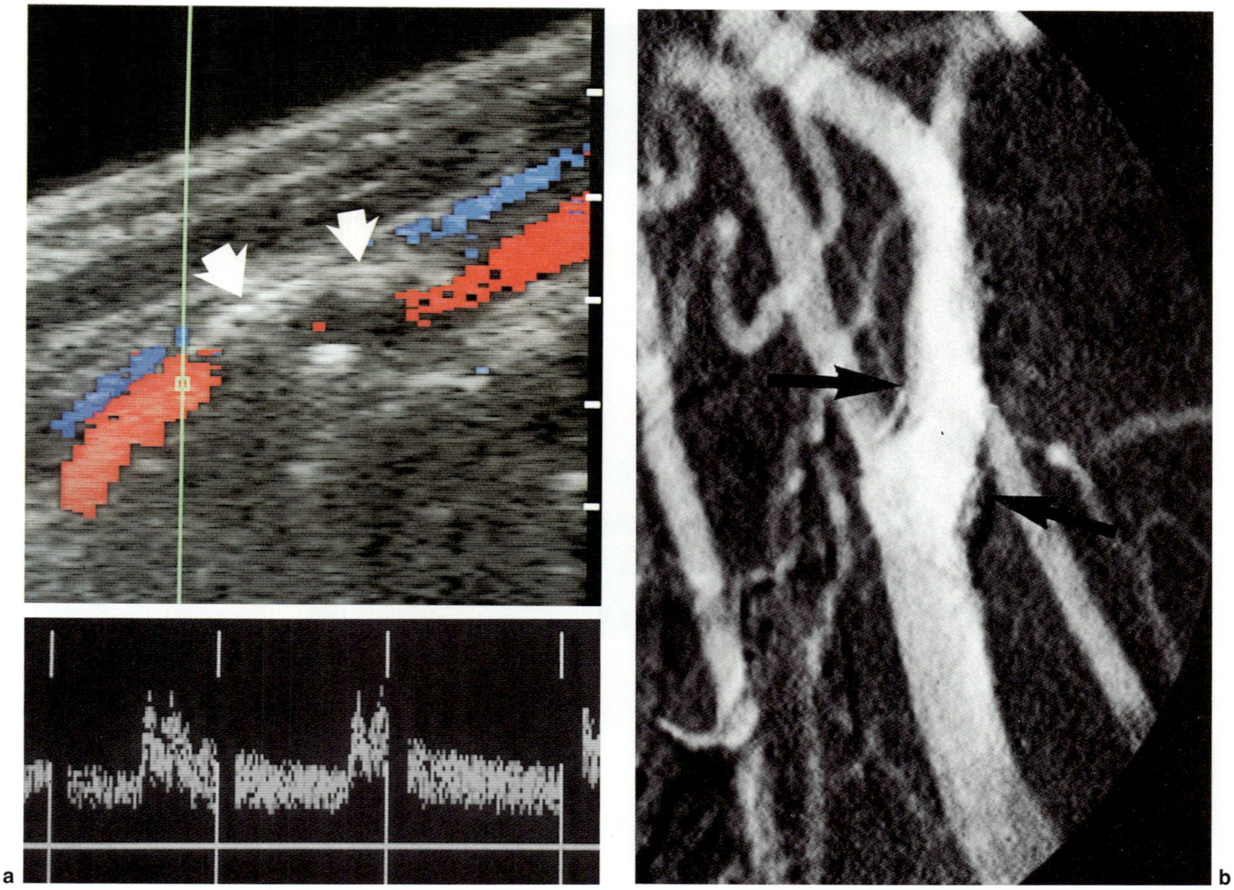

Fig. 5.7 **a, b** Pronounced wall calcification at the origin of the left internal carotid artery
a CDS shows acoustic shadowing behind the wall calcification (arrows). The blood flow cannot be evaluated in this approximately a 2-cm long segment of the vessel. The cranial portion of the vessel shows homogenous color-encoded flow with normal Doppler spectral features = no indirect signs of stenosis
b Intra-arterial DSA confirms the segmental wall calcification at the origin of the internal carotid artery (arrows = subtraction artifacts caused by pulsation of the calcified wall) with no associated stenosis

peremia to develop in the periphery of the arm. If a hemodynamically significant obstruction is present in the subclavian or brachiocephalic artery, reverse flow will be observed in the ipsilateral vertebral artery, possibly accompanied by clinical symptoms of vertebrobasilar insufficiency.

Besides the vessels themselves, the nonvascular soft tissues should be examined for relevant associated findings, giving particular attention to hyperperfused focal lesions (suggestive of thyroid adenoma) or diffuse thyroid abnormalities (suggestive of hyperthyroidism) (see Chapter 15).

5.2.8.5 Documentation

CDS findings should be documented both with representative real-time sequences (digital or analog video recordings) and with individual representative sonograms. All sequences and individual frames should be clearly labeled to facilitate demonstration and review. The minimum documentation of a complete CDS examination of the carotid and vertebral arteries should include the following:

- A longitudinal image and Doppler spectrum (angle corrected) of the common carotid artery on each side
- A longitudinal and transverse image of the carotid bifurcation on each side
- A longitudinal image and Doppler spectrum of the internal carotid artery, external carotid artery, and vertebral artery
- If pathologic findings are noted: a longitudinal and transverse image of the abnormal area with associated spectra combined with measurement of peaksystolic flow velocities caudal to and within the abnormal area.

Written documentation is also provided. This may be a descriptive narrative concluding with the diagnosis, or pathologic findings may be recorded in schematic outline drawings on a report form (similar to the diagrams in Figs. 5.**1** and 5.**2**).

5.3 Normal Findings

The luminal diameter of the common carotid artery is constant up to the level of the carotid bulb (Fig. 5.**3a**). The artery normally presents a mixed type of flow pattern (see Chapter 3) since it supplies parenchymatous organs (brain, thyroid gland, salivary glands) as well as muscles and skin. This can be appreciated both in the color flow image (identical colors in systole and diastole whose brightness varies with the phase of the pulse cycle) and in the spectral waveform, which shows marked pulsatility with a moderate forward flow component in diastole.

The carotid bulb appears as a club-like dilatation in the area of the carotid bifurcation. One effect of this dilatation is a physiologic slowing of the blood flow, manifested by a darkening of the color shade in the color-encoded image and a reduced peak systolic velocity in the spectral trace. Additionally, the "exit effect" of the dilatation causes areas of flow separation to develop near the wall of the carotid bulb (see Chapter 3). These areas are opposite in color to the main flow direction (i.e., blue when the main flow direction is encoded red) and are visible in both longitudinal and transverse views. The zones of flow separation almost always occur on the side of the bulb opposite the origin of the external carotid artery (i.e., generally on the posterior side) and usually extend past the bifurcation into the proximal internal carotid artery (Fig. 5.**3b**). The zone of retrograde flow may continue directly onto the posterior wall of the internal carotid artery, it may separate from the posterior wall of the bulb and reattach to the superficial wall of the internal carotid artery, or it may do both. Flow separation is most pronounced in early and mid (peak) systole and occasionally may persist into early diastole. The percentage of a pulse cycle in which flow reversal can normally be demonstrated at the carotid bulb and bifurcation is highly variable. Middleton (31) found that the average period of flow separation accounts for 22% of the total cycle length, with a range from 8–80%. The length of flow separation measured in longitudinal section (average = 14 mm with a range of 6.1–22 mm) and the planimetrically measured cross sectional area of flow separation relative to the total area of the carotid bulb (average = 33% with a range of 8–64%) are likewise subject to large interindividual variations. The essential point, however, is that flow separation can always be demonstrated in normal individuals when proper examination technique is used. Absence of flow separation provides early evidence for the presence of atherosclerotic plaque in the carotid bulb. The site of physiologic flow separation forms a site of predilection for plaque formation, although the pathophysiology of this process is not fully understood (increased platelet aggregation? altered metabolic exchange between the slow-moving blood and vessel wall?).

The internal and external carotid arteries are easily distinguished from each other in normal individuals. Usually the color-encoded flow image is sufficient to make this distinction based on the different flow patterns produced by the different peripheral resistances in the vessels (see Chapter 3, Fig. 3.**4 a–g**). While the internal carotid artery exhibits a more continuous pattern with marked antegrade flow in diastole, there is less diastolic flow in the external carotid artery, and there may be a brief interval of diastolic reverse flow. The vessel identities can be confirmed by sampling their Doppler spectra. Typical spectral patterns are illustrated in Fig. 5.**4d, e**. The external carotid artery can also be identified by the modulation of its Doppler spectrum induced by sharp, rhythmic tapping of the ipsilateral temporal artery. Other differentiating features are the caliber of the vessel, its course, and the demonstration of side branches (see Table 5.**1,** Fig. 5.**3c**, Fig. 5.**4c**).

The carotid bulb, internal carotid artery, and external carotid artery cannot always be imaged simultaneously on the same longitudinal plane, but this is not essential since an image depicting all structures may not represent an accurate longitudinal section of either artery. It is quite acceptable to obtain a longitudinal view of both vessels, along with the contiguous bulbar segment of the common carotid artery, and examine them for abnormalities. Depending on the level of the bifurcation and the thickness of the cervical soft tissues, this view may demonstrate 1–4 cm of the internal carotid artery above its origin. The more cranial parts of the internal carotid artery are then visualized in the transverse plane. The entrance effect (see Chapter 3) may alter the internal carotid spectral waveform

Table 5.**1** Criteria for differentiating the internal and external carotid arteries with CDS (in normal individuals)

	Internal carotid artery	External carotid artery
Flow pattern	More continuous	More pulsatile
Branching vessels	None from the bifurcation to the skull base	Superior thyroid artery, facial artery, maxillary artery, etc.
Luminal size	Larger than the external carotid artery	Smaller than the internal carotid artery
Relation to the internal jugular vein	Usually runs adjacent to the internal jugular vein	More distant from the internal jugular vein

for a considerable distance, so a classic internal carotid spectrum may not be recorded until flow is sampled 1–2 cm cranial to the origin of the artery.

The external carotid artery tapers markedly as it ascends, due to its numerous side branches. Sometimes its main trunk is very short and can be defined for a distance of about 1 cm.

The vertebral artery cannot be imaged in continuity because portions of the artery are intraosseous. The segments between the transverse processes can always be defined in normal individuals (41, Fig. 5.**5b**). The origin of the vessel can be imaged in approximately 90% of cases on the right side (Fig. 5.**5a**) and 67% on the left side (41). The atlas loop can be visualized in only about 75% of cases. The vertebral artery displays a flow pattern similar to that of the internal carotid artery due to their similar peripheral resistances.

5.4 Pathologic Findings

5.4.1 Preliminary Remarks

Central ischemia may result from a reduction of blood flow in portions of the arterial supply system or from the embolization of thrombotic material. Whereas emboli often tend to cause transient or permanent neurologic symptoms due to cerebrovascular occlusion, the clinical impact of a reduction in regional blood flow (e.g., due to carotid artery stenosis) depends on the functional competence of anatomic (circle of Willis, external-to-internal carotid collaterals) and physiologic (autoregulation of cerebral perfusion by vasodilatation and increased diastolic flow) compensatory mechanisms.

5.4.2 Clinical Manifestations of Cerebrovascular Insufficiency

Ischemic cerebrovascular disease can remain in the asymptomatic stage (stage I disease) for a long time even when significant pathologic changes are present (stenosis, occlusion). When symptoms of cerebrovascular insufficiency arise, they are determined by the location of the deprived brain area. Ischemia in areas supplied by the internal carotid artery most commonly lead to monocular visual disturbances, speech disturbances (with involvement of the dominant cerebral hemisphere), impairment of consciousness, facial paresthesias, hemiparesis, and hemiplegia. Symptoms of vertebrobasilar insufficiency include binocular visual disturbances, dizziness, alternating hemiparesis, quadraparesis/quadraplegia, paresthesia, and ataxia.

The neurologic deficits may be transient, progressive, or permanent. Stage II disease is characterized by intermittent symptoms of cerebrovascular insufficiency. The deficit may take the form of transient ischemic attacks (TIAs), lasting seconds or minutes but no more than 24 hours, or a "prolonged reversible ischemic neurologic deficit" (PRIND) lasting up to 3 weeks. Stage IIa is said to be present if the symptoms resolve completely, and stage IIb if mild neurologic deficits persist. Stage III represents a progressive stroke and stage IV an established, "completed" stroke. A partial or almost complete regression of symptoms may occur during the weeks or months following a completed stroke.

5.4.3 Ischemia Due to Nonembolic Arterial Obstruction

The most common cause of nonembolic blood flow disturbances is atherosclerotic luminal narrowing in the setting of a stenosis or occlusion. Atherosclerosis is promoted by risk factors such as arterial hypertension, diabetes mellitus, hypercholesterolemia, smoking, and genetic predisposition, with overlapping risk profiles for cerebrovascular and ischemic heart disease (48). While atherosclerotic lesions can develop anywhere in the cerebrovascular circulation, they are most prevalent at sites where the vessel wall is exposed to increased stresses, i.e., at bifurcations (e.g., the carotid bifurcation) and in strongly curved vascular segments. Even moderate luminal narrowing leads to hemodynamic changes such as increased blood flow velocity and poststenotic vorticity. But a stenosis does not become "hemodynamically significant" until the residual lumen is so small that it causes a reduction in volume flow. Generally this is assumed to occur when the cross-sectional area is reduced by 75% or more (29). In these cases a correlation exists between the degree of stenosis and the incidence of stroke (6). A hemodynamically significant lesion, such as a carotid stenosis, does not become clinically significant until the foregoing anatomic and physiologic compensatory mechanisms have failed as a result of additional stenoses, for example, involving contralateral or intracerebral vessels. Even when there is a functioning collateral circulation, an initially compensated stenosis or occlusion can still lead to neurologic deficits in patients whose cardiac output is temporarily reduced due to blood pressure fluctuations or cardiac arrhythmias (7, 15, 37). Over time, a hemodynamically nonsignificant stenosis can progress to a flow-reducing stenosis or complete occlusion due to progressive atherosclerosis, intraplaque hemorrhage, or local thrombosis.

Rare causes of arterial lumen reduction leading to cerebral ischemia include various forms of arteritis, moyamoya disease (5), spontaneous and traumatic dissections (23, 34), radiation-induced atherosclerosis (25), fibromuscular dysplasia (26), and vascular compression or infiltration by tumors.

5.4.3.1 Stenoses and Occlusions of the Carotid Artery

The hemodynamic significance of a carotid stenosis depends less on its pathogenesis than on its local extent and its association with other lesions. In this sense the discussions on the CDS features of atherosclerotic stenoses and occlusions are applicable to other, far less common causes of vascular obstruction.

The detection of carotid stenoses and occlusions with CDS relies largely on the combination of B-mode and color-encoded flow imaging, which are excellently suited for evaluation of the sonographically accessible carotid vessels. The B-mode image defines the outer boundary of the vessel wall and lumen-reducing material while the color image demonstrates the associated flow pattern (Fig. 5.**10**). Doppler frequency analysis serves merely to confirm the imaging findings and may be necessary for quantification. It is also useful in cases where certain vascular segments are not clearly defined by the color-encoded image.

The majority of stenoses are demonstrated at the origin of the internal carotid artery, but many atherosclerotic lesions additionally involve the carotid bulb and the origin of the external carotid artery, resulting in a true bifurcation stenosis. Isolated stenoses of the external carotid artery also may occur. Since most isolated external carotid stenoses have no clinical significance, positive confirmation of vessel identity is essential in all cases.

The most subtle atherosclerotic vascular lesion is a circumscribed plaque with a smooth surface that blends smoothly with the adjacent, healthy vessel wall. These early changes can be observed in the posterior part of the carotid bulb, for example (30). Characteristic features include slight wall thickening and an absence of normal flow reversal near the wall (Fig. 5.**6a, b**). The slight lumen reduction implies a local increase in flow velocity, but this is usually so small that it is within the range of peak systolic velocity fluctuations that occur normally in the carotid bulb. A flat plaque of this kind would not be expected to produce distal flow changes such as turbulence or circumscribed flow reversal.

Higher degrees of luminal narrowing produce the typical flow abnormalities associated with stenosis: intrastenotic velocity increase, poststenotic flow separation and reversal, poststenotic disturbed flow, and turbulence (13, 30, 39, 45). The CDS diagnosis of a stenosis is generally based on the obvious narrowing of the perfused lumen and the flow abnormalities described above (Figs. 5.**10**, 5.**11**–5.**13**). Imaging in longitudinal and transverse planes can establish the position, length, and geometry (predominantly eccentric or concentric) of the stenotic lesion. These images also permit a rough estimation of the degree of lumen reduction, as in the subjective interpretation of angiograms.

The principles involved in the quantification of stenoses were discussed in Chapter 3. The problem of defining a "normal" reference point is especially challenging in the area of the carotid bifurcation (Fig. 5.**8**).

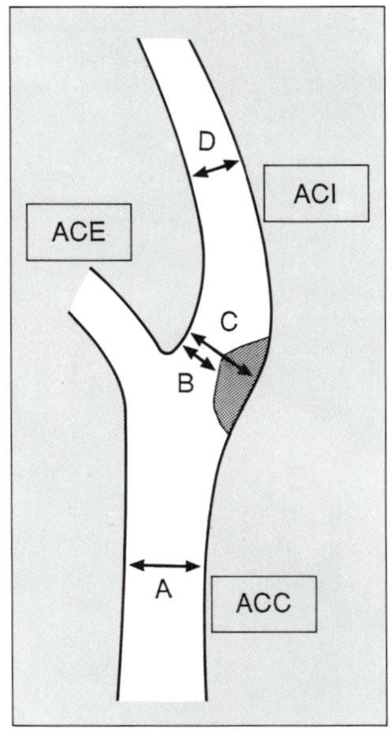

Fig. 5.**8** Problem of grading a stenosis in the area of the carotid bifurcation, illustrated for the case of diameter reduction. The degree of stenosis depends in part on how a normal vessel diameter is defined. An ideal solution is to state the *local degree of stenosis* $[(1 - B/C) \cdot 100\%]$ (geometric determination). But the local degree of stenosis cannot be measured on the basis of hemodynamic factors. Doppler criteria can furnish only the *proximal degree of stenosis* $[(1 - B/A) \cdot 100\%]$ and, in the absence of turbulence, the *distal degree of stenosis* in the poststenotic segment $[(1 - B/D) \cdot 100\%]$. ACC = Common carotid artery, ACI = internal carotid artery, ACE = external carotid artery

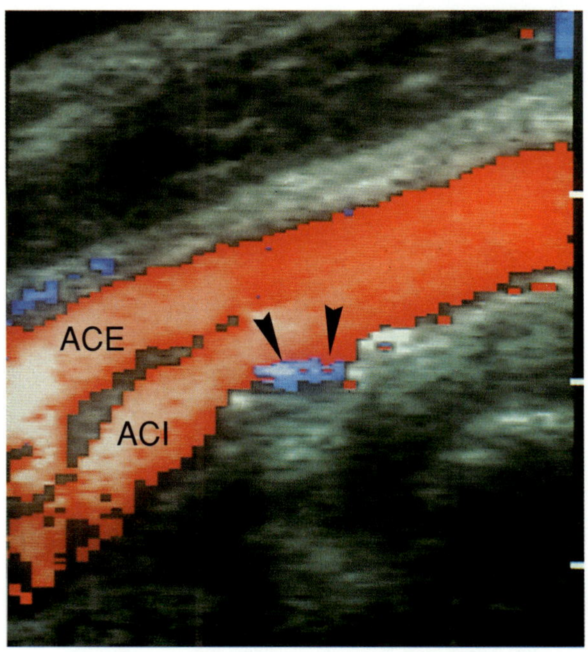

Fig. 5.**9** Ulcerated plaque at the origin of the internal carotid artery (confirmed at operation) in a patient with recurrent TIAs. A crater-like defect is visible in the plaque (arrowheads). ACE = External carotid artery, ACI = internal carotid artery

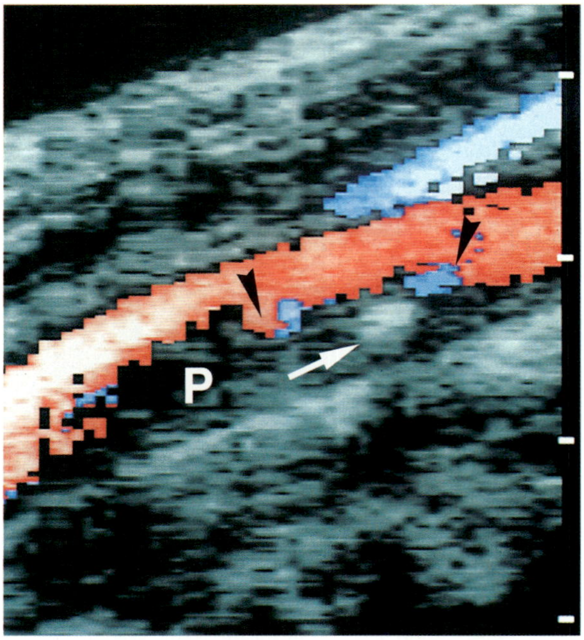

Fig. 5.**10** Eccentric, hemodynamically significant stenosis of the common carotid artery causing greater than 75% area reduction. Longitudinal CDS scan shows inhomogeneous hypoechoic plaque (P) with a small calcification (white arrow) and foci of superficial plaque ulceration (arrowheads)

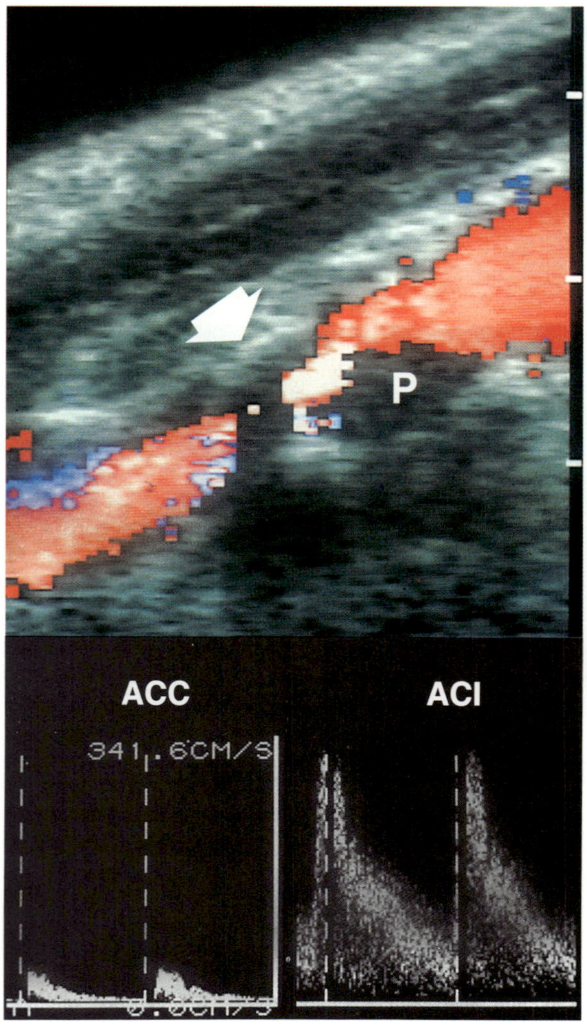

a

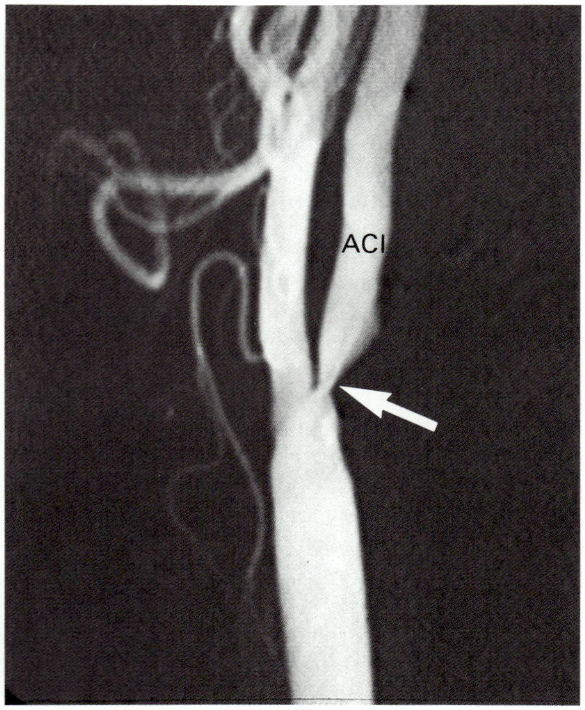

b

Fig. 5.**11 a, b** High-grade proximal stenosis of the right internal carotid artery

a Longitudinal CDS image shows hypoechoic plaque at the origin of the internal carotid artery (P), and a small wall calcification (arrow). The white color encoding indicates a marked intrastenotic velocity increase. The peak systolic velocity in the common carotid artery (ACC, prebulbar segment) is 54 cm/s compared with 340 cm/s at the stenosis in the internal carotid artery (ACI). According to Table 3.**2**, this correlates with a greater than 95% degree of luminal area reduction. There is only moderate poststenotic turbulence and flow reversal due to the flow-restricting effect of the very high-grade stenosis

b The same lesion demonstrated by intra-arterial DSA (arrow)

If a proximal stenosis of the internal carotid artery is graded geometrically (by measurement of cross-sectional area), then either the local degree of stenosis or the degree of stenosis relative to the common carotid artery should be calculated. If the stenosis is graded hemodynamically on the basis of the continuity equation, then the maximum systolic velocity in the carotid artery should be measured at the prebulbar and intrastenotic levels. Duplex studies have confirmed the inherent validity of this approach for evaluating carotid stenoses (2, 3, 10, 49). These studies have proven that systolic velocity indices correlate with degree of stenosis even in low-grade and moderate lesions (< 75% area reduction), whereas the detection of poststenotic flow phenomena (spectral broadening, window fill-in, spectral broadening index) is not useful for the identification of low-grade stenoses (38, 49). In higher-grade stenoses as well (> 75% area reduction), the correlation of relative velocity indices with degree of stenosis is higher than in the evaluation of poststenotic spectral changes (10). This is consistent with experimental data acquired in model stenoses (see Chapter 3).

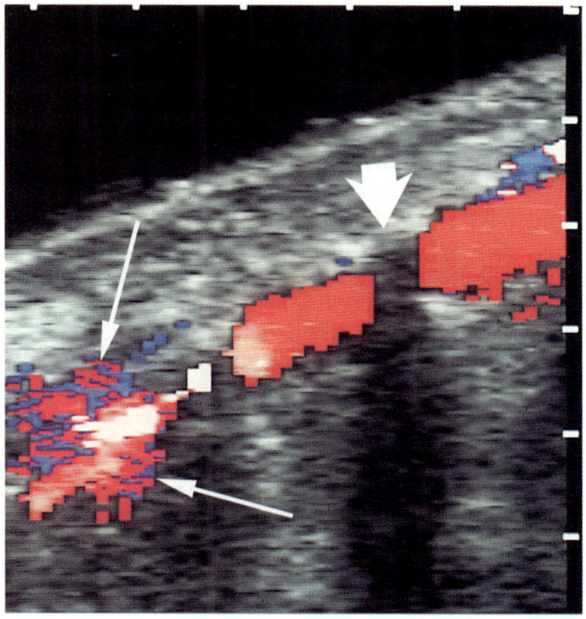

Fig. 5.**12** High-grade concentric stenosis of the internal carotid artery. The cloud-like color-encoded mosaic transcending the poststenotic vessel wall is caused by vibration of the soft tissues (thin arrows). A nonstenosing wall calcification (thick arrow) appears proximally

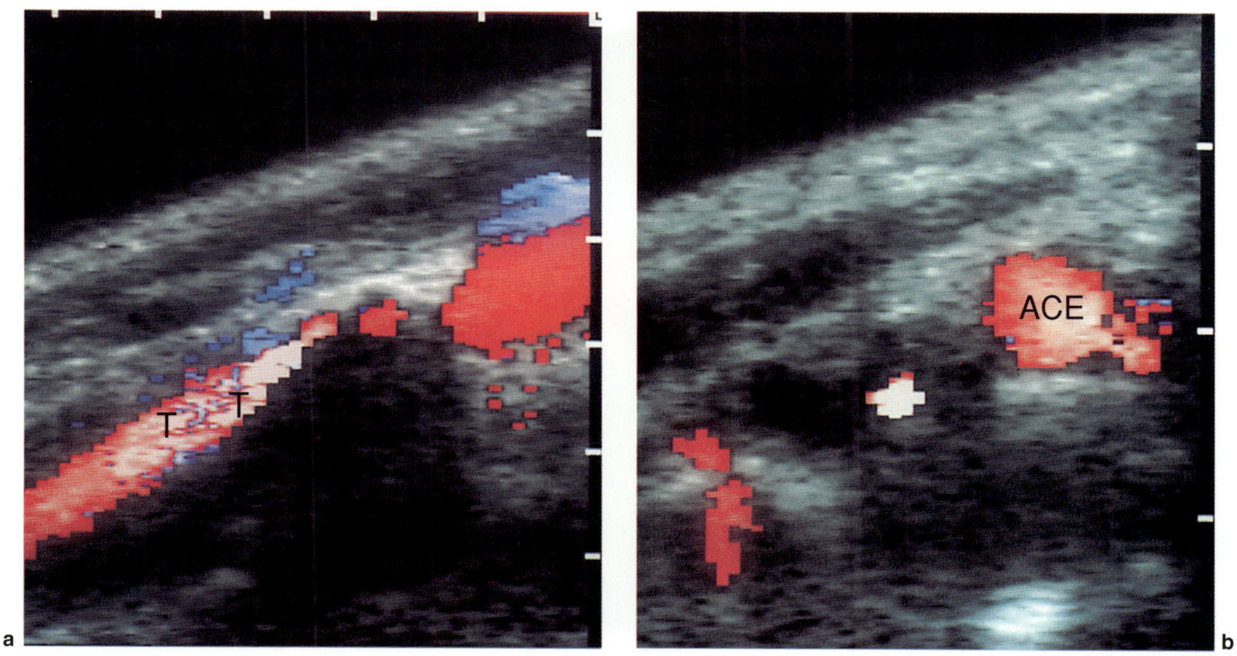

Fig. 5.**13a, b** High-grade stenosis of the right internal carotid artery

a Calcifications partially obscure the stenosed segment on the longitudinal image. There is conspicuous poststenotic turbulence (T, mixture of red and blue-encoded signals)

b Transverse image at the center of the stenosis shows luminal narrowing by hypoechoic, partially calcified plaques. ACE = External carotid artery

Due to the problem of branched flow in the carotid bifurcation described above, the simplified assumption of the continuity equation must be modified for the quantification of a proximal internal carotid stenosis. Moreover, a rough classification of the degree of stenosis is generally acceptable for clinical purposes. Comparisons of angiography and duplex sonography have shown that a ratio ≥ 1.5 of maximum systolic velocity in the internal carotid artery to maximum systolic velocity in the prebulbar segment of the common carotid artery implies an internal carotid stenosis equal to 75% in area reduction (50% diameter reduction) with a diagnostic accuracy of 90% (10). An index > 1.8 characterizes stenoses exceeding about 85% in area reduction (60% diameter reduction), while an index ≥ 3.7 indicates a stenosis exceeding about 95% in area reduction (80% diameter reduction) (49). Assuming an exponential course of the velocity index curve depending on the degree of stenosis, an internal carotid/common carotid peak systolic velocity index of more than about 2.5 indicates a stenosis of more than 70% diameter reduction. According to the latest studies (50, 51) this represents the cutoff value for a significant benefit from endarterectomy. This index cannot be calculated for very high-grade stenoses when aliasing is present, however. In this case it would still be possible to quantify the stenosis by using image-guided CW Doppler, which is not susceptible to aliasing.

The above velocity indices are used only for proximal stenoses of the internal carotid artery. With a more cranial internal carotid stenosis or an infrabulbar stenosis of the common carotid artery, a sufficiently long prestenotic vascular segment is generally available for velocity measurement, and the continuity equation can be used to grade the stenosis as described in Chapter 3.

If the stenotic area cannot be directly visualized, the diagnosis must rely strictly on indirect signs of stenosis. Assuming that a short vascular segment is obscured by circumferential calcifications, the absence of a pathologic flow pattern in the color-encoded image and Doppler spectrum just distal to that region is sufficient to exclude a significant stenosis (Figs. 4.**4**, 5.**7a, b**). If the image shows only small zones of flow separation and the spectral window just distal to the lesion (Doppler sample volume outside the separation zone!) is preserved or shows only moderate filling-in with low frequencies, the degree of stenosis will generally be less than 75% area reduction. But if a jet is found projecting from the obscured region along with markedly disturbed flow, turbulence, large zones of flow separation, and significant ($>$ 50% bandwidth relative to peak systolic velocity) or complete fill-in of the spectral window, it is certain that a hemodynamically significant stenosis is present (4). Another indirect sign of a high-grade carotid stenosis is a flattened systolic peak of reduced amplitude in the spectrum distal to the lesion. This change might also signify a very proximal stenosis of the common carotid artery or innominate artery.

A right–left discrepancy between the spectra recorded from the prestenotic vascular segment and a normal contralateral segment can provide a sensitive

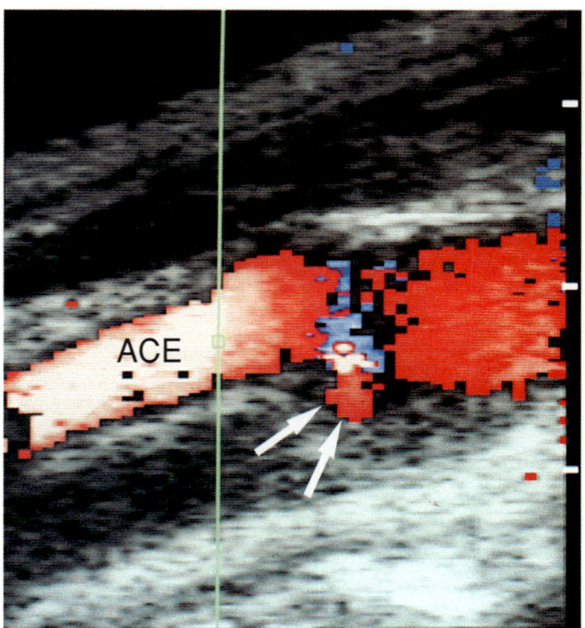

a

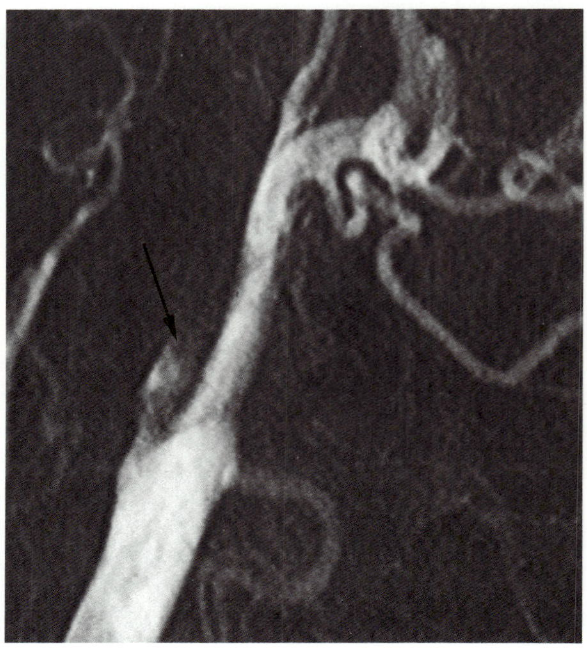

b

Fig. 5.**14a, b** Occlusion of the right internal carotid artery
a CDS shows the short perfused stump of the vessel at the origin (arrows). The external carotid artery ACE is prominently displayed
b Intra-arterial DSA also demonstrates the proximal occlusion and the small residual perfused stump (arrow)

but somewhat nonspecific sign of high-grade stenosis. The diastolic forward-flow component in the common carotid artery is markedly reduced or abolished on the side where the high-grade internal carotid artery stenosis is present. This criterion also aids in the detection of more distal high-grade internal carotid stenoses that are located too high for direct visualization. This assessment requires comparative spectral sampling from both internal carotid arteries.

A special case of high-grade internal carotid stenoses involves lesions that cause such extreme flow reduction that there is only a trickle of residual flow. These lesions may exhibit none of the typical intrastenotic or poststenotic flow abnormalities, and they can mimic an occlusion when the poststenotic flow velocity is below the sensitivity range of the instrument. If color-encoded flow signals are not detected in the internal carotid artery, the instrument sensitivity should be increased by switching the pulse repetition frequency (PRF) and filter frequency to the lowest settings. With the latest generation of CDS instruments, a very high-grade stenosis (usually $>98\%$ area reduction) should be reliably distinguished from an occlusion (39, 45).

A complete vascular occlusion is characterized by the absence of a flow signal in the vessel lumen, which can be obliterated by hypoechoic thrombotic material (Figs. 5.**14a, b**, 5.**15a–c**). Due to the absence of branching vessels, an occlusion of the internal carotid artery always extends to the vessel's origin at the carotid bulb. Especially in acute cases, a patent vascular stump several millimeters in length can often be demonstrated, as in an angiogram (Fig. 5.**14a, b**). Even in longer-standing cases, it is usually possible to demonstrate a considerable length of the occluded lumen with ultrasound. This can be difficult in very old occlusions due to scar contraction of the vessel, but diagnosis is often aided in these cases by the detection of vascular calcifications. It is very important to differentiate clearly between the occluded and the residual carotid artery. With an internal carotid occlusion that is receiving sufficient external-to-internal carotid collateral flow, the spectral features of the external carotid artery can very closely approximate the typical internal carotid spectrum due to the altered conditions of peripheral resistance. Positive identification of the external carotid artery is then accomplished by the demonstration of branching vessels or by percussion of the superficial temporal artery.

While occlusions of the internal carotid artery can be functionally compensated by flow through the circle of Willis or by ipsilateral external-to-internal carotid collaterals, occlusions of the common carotid artery can be collateralized by external-to-external carotid connections from the opposite side. In this case an occlusion of the common carotid artery does not necessarily occlude the internal carotid artery if the latter is being supplied by retrograde flow in the ipsilateral external carotid artery (Fig. 5.**15a–c**) (40). Because surgical intervention is an option in this kind of situation, the duplex instrument should be set to maximum sensitivity to check for collateral inflow at the level of the carotid bulb whenever a common carotid occlusion is detected.

Table 5.**2** Significant indirect signs of stenosis

Degree of stenosis (area reduction)	CDS
< 50%	– Possible absence of physiologic flow reversal in the carotid bulb – Poststenotic flow reversal near the wall
< 75%	– Poststenotic flow reversal – Short poststenotic jet – Slight broadening of immediate poststenotic spectrum (slight fill-in of spectral window)
> 75%	– Marked poststenotic flow separation, jets, and turbulence – More than 50% fill-in of poststenotic spectral window
> 95%	– Massive turbulence, possibly with perivascular vibration artifacts – Complete fill-in (disappearance) of poststenotic spectral window – no (or only slight) cyclic changes in the poststenotic vessel
Subtotal occlusion	– Major reduction of poststeonotic flow relative to healthy side – Moderate poststenotic turbulence
Occlusion	– No flow signal; in acute cases, pulsations of the thrombotic material can simulate minimal alternating flow

5.4.3.2 Kinking and Coiling of the Internal Carotid Artery

Besides plaque formation, possible morphologic signs of atherosclerosis include dilatation and elongation of the affected vessel. Tortuosity of the internal carotid artery is a particularly common finding in older patients. The hemodynamic significance of complete coiling of the vessel (Fig. 5.**17a, b**) and kinking is still unclear. Color-encoded flow imaging in mutiple planes usually permits an accurate analysis of the situation. Each segment of the coiled vessel should be scrutinized for pathologic flow patterns, however. As of this writing, there has been no systematic research to show whether the detection or exclusion of disturbed or turbulent flow in a uniform vascular loop correlates with the clinical prognosis and might thus affect the selection of patients for operative treatment.

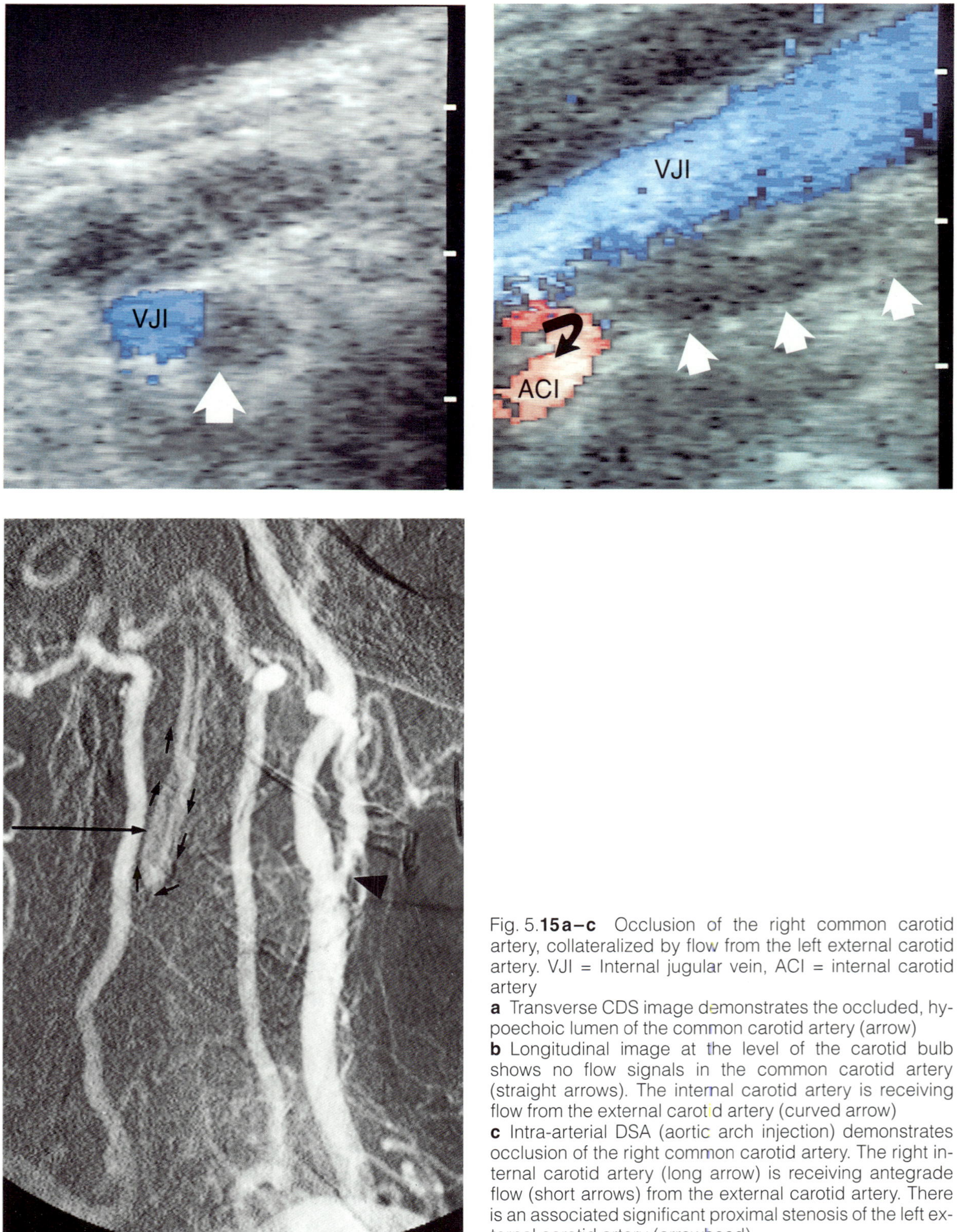

a b c

Fig. 5.**15 a–c** Occlusion of the right common carotid artery, collateralized by flow from the left external carotid artery. VJI = Internal jugular vein, ACI = internal carotid artery

a Transverse CDS image demonstrates the occluded, hypoechoic lumen of the common carotid artery (arrow)

b Longitudinal image at the level of the carotid bulb shows no flow signals in the common carotid artery (straight arrows). The internal carotid artery is receiving flow from the external carotid artery (curved arrow)

c Intra-arterial DSA (aortic arch injection) demonstrates occlusion of the right common carotid artery. The right internal carotid artery (long arrow) is receiving antegrade flow (short arrows) from the external carotid artery. There is an associated significant proximal stenosis of the left external carotid artery (arrowhead)

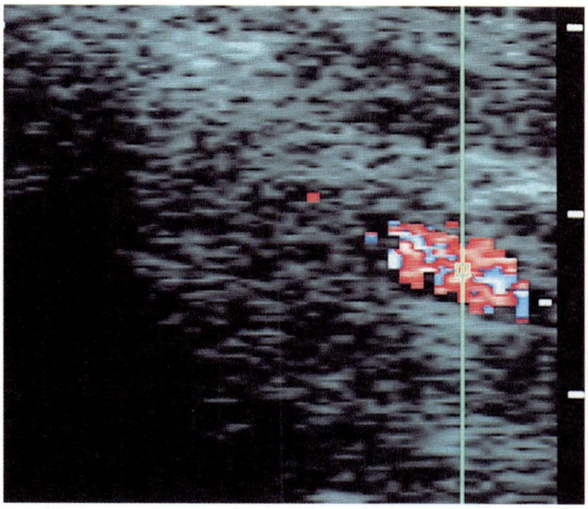

a

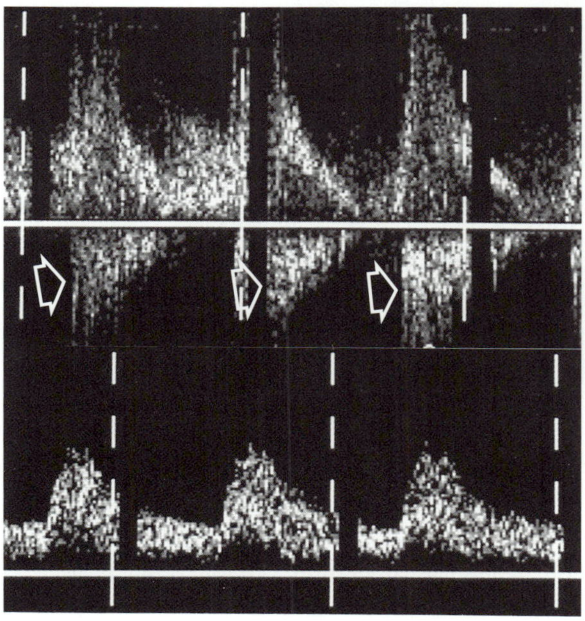

a

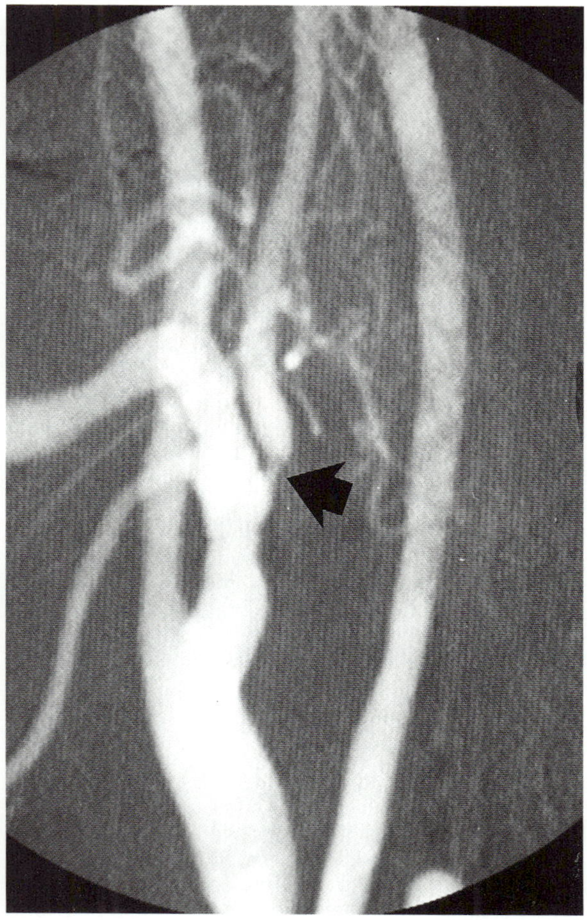

b

Fig. 5.**16a–c** High-grade proximal stenosis of the right vertebral artery (same patient as in Fig. 5.**18**)
a Indirect detection of the stenosis with CDS: The origin of the vertebral artery cannot be seen, but marked turbulence (mixed red and blue) is apparent at a slightly more cranial level. Doppler spectral analysis (center) confirms the turbulent flow (distribution of values above and below [arrows] the baseline, closed spectral window). A clear spectral window reappears in the cranial part of the vessel (lower spectrum), but the systolic peak is still rounded (see Fig. 5.**5**) as an indirect sign of the proximal stenosis
b Intra-arterial DSA demonstrates a high-grade proximal vertebral stenosis (arrow) with occlusion of the left subclavian artery, see also Figure 5.**18**

5.4.3.3 Stenoses and Occlusions of the Vertebral Artery

Basically the same principles apply to the detection of stenoses and occlusions in the vertebral artery as in the carotid vessels. However, since not all parts of the vertebral artery can be visualized, and since most stenoses occur at the origin of the vertebral artery from the subclavian, the diagnosis is based far more often on indirect signs of stenosis (Fig. 5.**16a, b**). Given the relative frequency of anatomic variations in the vertebral system, it may occasionally be necessary to differentiate a proximal stenosis from hyperplasia when a right–left perfusion discrepancy is noted. Hypoplasia is evidenced by preservation of the spectral waveform (possibly with a reduced diastolic forward-flow component) with a clear spectral window, no signs of turbulence anywhere in the vessel, and marked dilatation

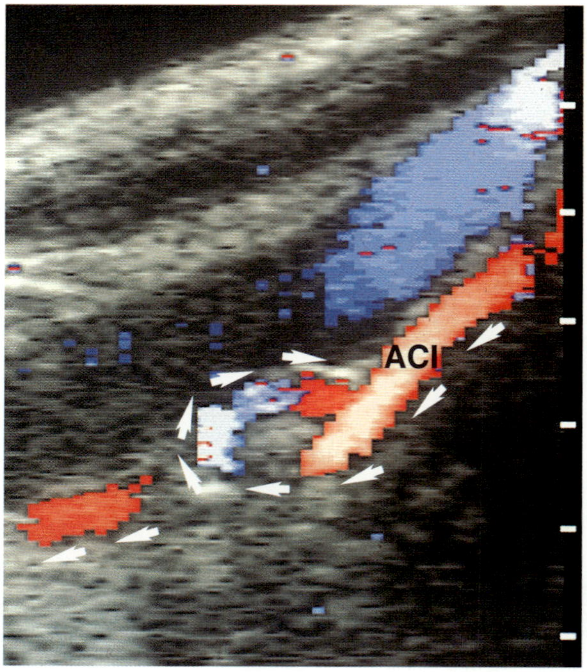

a

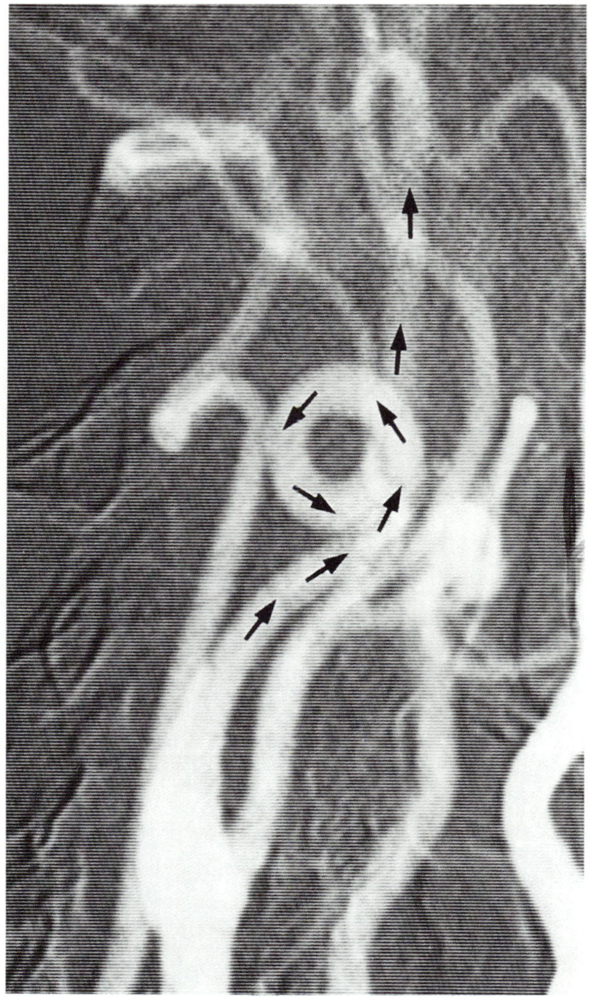

b

Fig. 5.**17a, b** Coiling of the right internal carotid artery
a With CDS, the blue color encoding in the vascular loop represents flow toward the transducer. In segments devoid of color flow signals, the blood is flowing parallel to the transducer face. ACI = Internal carotid artery
b Intra-arterial DSA confirms 360° coiling of the right internal carotid artery

of the contralateral artery. CDS can differentiate aplasia from occlusion by showing an absence of flow in the color-encoded image combined with well-defined vertebral arterial walls in the gray-scale image (44). Occlusion of the vertebral artery may be evidenced by the appearance of a small, ineffectually perfused vascular stump branching from the subclavian artery. The diagnosis of occlusion is considered established if the vessel becomes totally obstructed after it has already been defined as open in a previous examination.

5.4.4 Ischemia Due to Arterial Embolism

Arterial emboli may originate in the heart or from an atherosclerotic artery. Cardiac thrombi can form in association with valve defects (e.g., mitral stenosis), myocardial infarction with or without aneurysm formation, cardiac arrhythmias, or endocarditis and can embolize to any part of the arterial circulation. The concurrence of cerebral ischemic symptoms with a peripheral embolism (extremity arteries, renal arteries, mesenteric system) suggests a cardiac origin. A crossed embolism involves the blockage of a systemic artery by a venous thrombus passing through a patent foramen ovale. Similar clinical presentations can result from emboli arising in aneurysms or dissections of the ascending aorta, or from aortic dissections that cause branch-vessel obstruction at various levels.

The second major source of cerebrovascular emboli is atherosclerotic disease, which may generate recurrent emboli as a result of surface characteristics or geometry. Stenoses that are "nonsignificant" by hemodynamic criteria alone (non-flow-reducing) may well become a source of clinically significant embolization. Subintimal hemorrhage into atherosclerotic plaque that appears heterogeneous in the B-mode image can lead to defects (ulcerations) in the plaque (Figs. 5.**9**, 5.**10**) and the dislodgment of atherosclerotic material (8, 16). Plaque surface irregularities, plaque ulcerations, and poststenotic "dead-water zones" of flow reversal and diminished flow velocity create sites of predilection for local platelet aggregation. If these small thrombi are not eliminated by endogenous lysis, they can detach from the wall and embolize. Hypercoagulability, abnormally increased platelet aggregation, and an elevated hematocrit are factors that increase the risk of local thrombosis, while medical treatment with platelet aggregation inhibitors or coumarins can decrease the risk.

No prospective studies have yet been done on the relationship between specific flow patterns defined by CDS (e.g., isolated poststenotic flow separation) and the risk of cerebral embolism. In any case, there is no ultrasound technique that can directly identify thrombi at risk for embolism, because even thromboemboli in the millimeter or submillimeter range are capable of producing significant clinical effects.

5.4.4.1 Plaque Ulcerations

Plaque ulcerations generally appear as crater-like defects on sonographic images. The sensitivity of ultrasound detection is poor, however (33% for ulcers smaller than 2 mm, 58% for ulcers larger than 2 mm) (18). It is unclear whether CDS will provide greater accuracy in the detection of plaque defects (Figs. 5.**9**, 5.**10**) or whether a definite clinical correlation exists between ulcer size and location and the propensity for embolization.

5.4.5 Subclavian Steal Syndrome

Subclavian steal syndrome is a special form of cerebrovascular insufficiency in which a stenosis or occlusion of the subclavian artery proximal to the origin of the vertebral artery (or an occlusion of the brachiocephalic artery) leads to vertebrobasilar ischemia during exercise of the ipsilateral arm. A drop of poststenotic perfusion pressure in the subclavian artery distal to the lesion, either present at rest or precipitated by an increased demand in the peripheral vessels of the arm, evokes a flow reversal in the ipsilateral vertebral artery. Assuming a competent circle of Willis, the upper extremity in this situation will draw its blood supply from the cerebrovascular circulation, and neurologic deficits can result.

Like obstructions of the carotid and vertebral arteries, the subclavian steal phenomenon does not necessarily lead to clinical complaints. But if the pathologic and pathophysiologic aspects of subclavian steal create a significant perfusion deficit in the territory of the basilar artery, the patient may experience dizzy spells, binocular visual disturbances, headache, and possible sensorineural hearing loss during exercise of the affected extremity. The symptoms increase with the extent of the exercise and decrease or subside when the arm is rested.

The diagnosis of subclavian steal syndrome by CDS is based on the demonstration of retrograde flow in the vertebral artery on the affected side (Fig. 5.**18 a, b**) and by the analysis of poststenotic or postocclusive Doppler spectra recorded from the subclavian artery distal to the stenosed or occluded segment. With a moderate subclavian stenosis, the associated pressure drop may be so small at rest that the arm must be exercised in order to evoke retrograde flow down the ipsilateral vertebral artery. Examination at rest may disclose alternating vertebral flow or a significantly attenuated antegrade flow in relation to the opposite side. Provocative tests (see section 5.2.8.4) can be used to establish the diagnosis of a stress-induced subclavian steal syndrome.

5.4.6 Postoperative Follow-up

Just as CDS can be used to diagnose primary stenoses and occlusions, it is useful for the detection or exclusion of recurrent disease following carotid endarterectomy, patch grafting, and bypass surgery (43). Even when a patch graft is not applied, marked bulbar dilatation with potentially significant flow separation can be demonstrated in about one-fourth of endarterectomized carotid bifurcations (43). The prognostic significance of this observation with regard to the development of recurrent stenosis is unclear. Following a vascular transposition or bypass procedure (e.g., carotid–subclavian transposition or bypass), color duplex is generally very useful for evaluating the anastomoses and bypass material and checking for luminal narrowing and hemodynamic abnormalities.

5.4.7 Miscellaneous Findings

Traumatic stenoses and occlusions of the carotid and vertebral arteries show basically the same B-mode and color-encoded flow characteristics as atherosclerotic lesions. CDS is particularly valuable in multiple-injury patients, as it permits a rapid, noninvasive, and reliable diagnosis.

The B-mode image can demonstrate spontaneous dissections, traumatic dissections, and dissections originating from the aortic arch. Careful scanning can demonstrate the intimal flap as an echogenic intraluminal septum that oscillates with each cardiac cycle. With CDS it may be possible to differentiate the true lumen from the false lumen (often perfused by slower flow) by a comparative analysis of the flow patterns. In a dissection of the common carotid artery, it should be noted whether the luminal division continues into the internal carotid artery. CDS can detect thrombosis in one of the two lumina by the absence of a flow signal.

True and false aneurysms are easily detected with CDS by the circumscribed vascular dilatation and by the demonstration of flow within the aneurysm (42). A hypoechoic rim with no flow signal indicates mural thrombosis.

Arteriovenous fistulae, which usually have a traumatic etiology, can be directly visualized in accessible regions of the neck. The high flow velocity at the fistula often induces a vibration of the vessel walls and adjacent soft tissues. These vibrations, which are both palpable and audible, generate strong artifacts

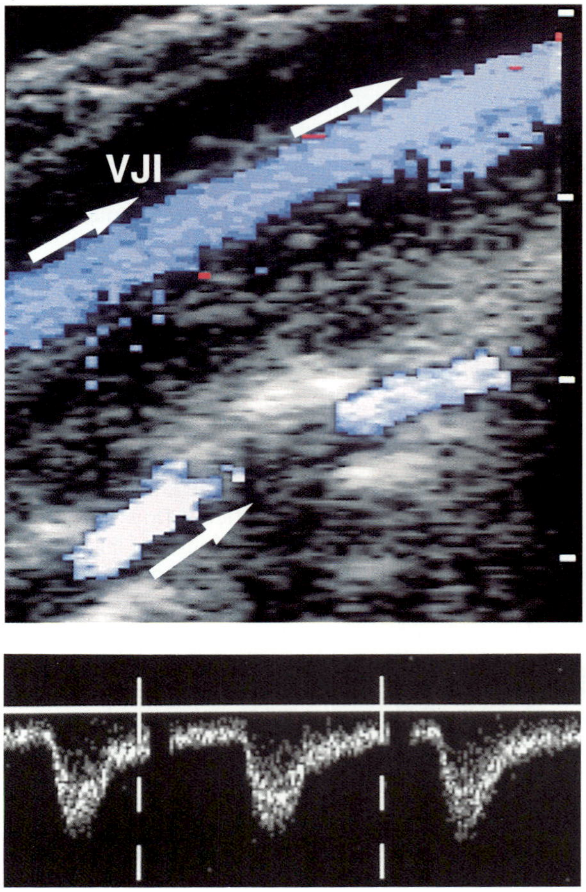

a

Fig. 5.**18a, b** Subclavian steal syndrome due to occlusion of the left subclavian artery (same patient as in Fig. 5.**16**)

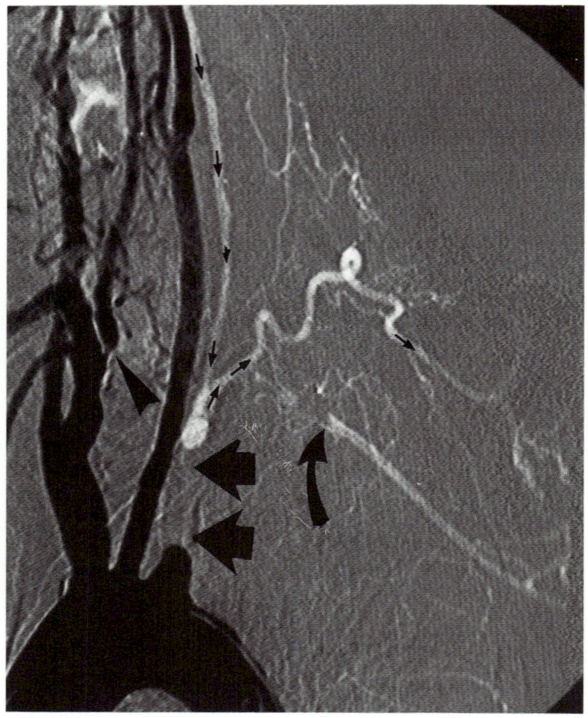

b

a CDS demonstrates retrograde flow in the left vertebral artery (blue color encoding) parallel to that in the internal jugular vein (VJI)
b Intra-arterial DSA shows retrograde perfusion of the left vertebral artery (small arrows) secondary to a proximal occlusion of the ipsilateral subclavian artery (wide arrows). The middle third of the subclavian artery (curved arrow) is supplied by branches of the thyrocervical trunk (small lateral arrows). A proximal stenosis of the right vertebral artery is also demonstrated (arrowhead) (see Fig. 5.**16**)

that are portrayed in the CDS image as a conspicuous, mosaic-like "color cloud" in the fistulous region (see Fig. 4.**7a, b**). The color cloud transcends the vessel lumen and obscures the actual fistulous communication. Rarely, such artifacts may also develop in association with high-grade arterial stenosis. But in these cases the a–v fistula is easily distinguished from a stenosis by the Doppler spectrum recorded proximal to the lesion. The pulsatility of the blood flow proximal to an a–v fistula is decreased due to the diminished peripheral vascular resistance, whereas the flow proximal to a high-grade stenosis shows increased pulsatility. These same criteria also apply in principle to congenital a–v malformations.

The cervical tumors that most commonly lead to arterial involvement are lymph node metastases from head and neck tumors. CDS is excellent for demonstrating the spatial relationship of the tumor to the vessels and for identifying the vessels involved (Fig. 5.**20**). Tumor-related arterial stenoses and occlusions, unlike thrombosis of the internal jugular vein, are quite rare, but the same criteria apply as those described for the recognition of arterial stenoses. A tumor can compromise blood flow by compression or infiltration of the vessel wall. The ability of CDS to provide additional information on the extent of vessel wall infiltration remains to be determined.

Carotid body (glomus) tumors (= paraganglioma) are very heavily vascularized neoplasms arising from the chemoreceptor at the carotid bifurcation. The associated mass effect produces a splaying of the bifurcation that is detectable by CDS imaging, which can also demonstrate the multiple small tumor vessels (49) arising mostly from the external and occasionally from the internal carotid artery (Fig. 5.**19a, b**). Low pulsatility in the external carotid artery in an otherwise normal vessel strongly suggests a highly vascularized tumor near the base of the skull (e.g., a glomus jugulare tumor).

5.4.8 Common Pitfalls

The most common error in carotid examinations is assigning a stenosis or occlusion to the wrong artery. But the clinically important differentiation of the internal and external carotid arteries can almost always be

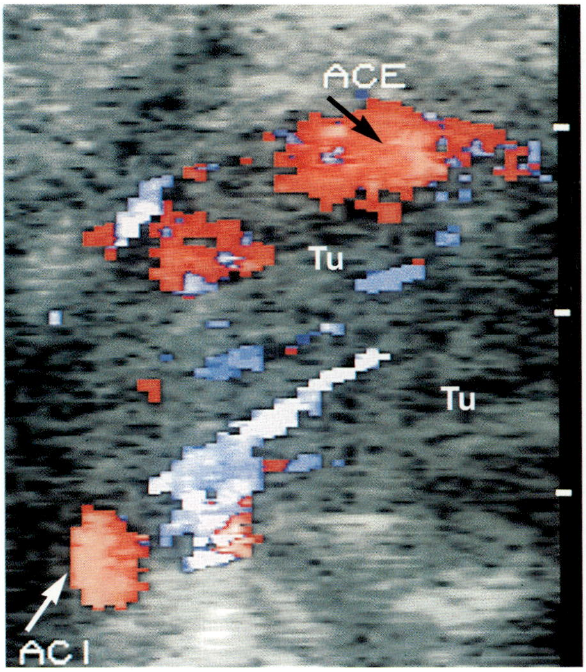

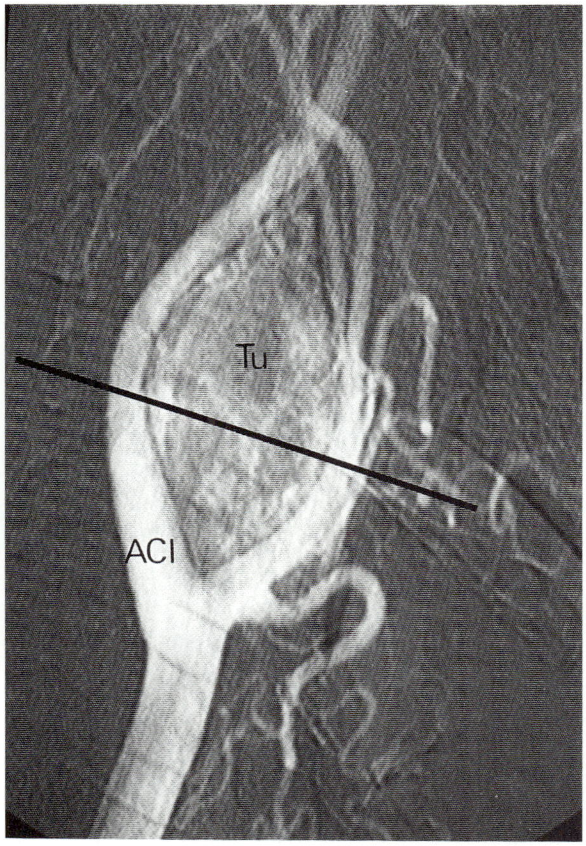

Fig. 5.**19** Right-sided carotid body tumor
a Transverse CDS image above the carotid bifurcation (scan plane indicated in **b**) shows separation of the internal and external carotid arteries by a hypoechoic, strongly perfused tumor (Tu). ACE = External carotid artery, ACI = internal carotid artery

b Intra-arterial DSA confirms a richly vascularized mass in the area of the carotid bifurcation. The solid line indicates the scan plane in **a**

accomplished by a systematic analysis of all the differentiating criteria noted above.

A second error of equal clinical significance involves mistaking a subtotal stenosis for an occlusion. This can be avoided, as noted earlier, by using the highest instrument sensitivity for the examination of a suspected occlusion.

In postoperative evaluations of the carotid bifurcation, the sound attenuation caused by hematomas or air inclusions in the immediate postoperative period can lead to false-positive results unless this problem is taken into account.

In examinations of the vertebral artery, small branches of the thyrocervical trunk may run close to the vertebral artery and be mistaken for the artery itself. This can be avoided by recording Doppler spectra and by tracing the course of the imaged vessel caudad and cephalad.

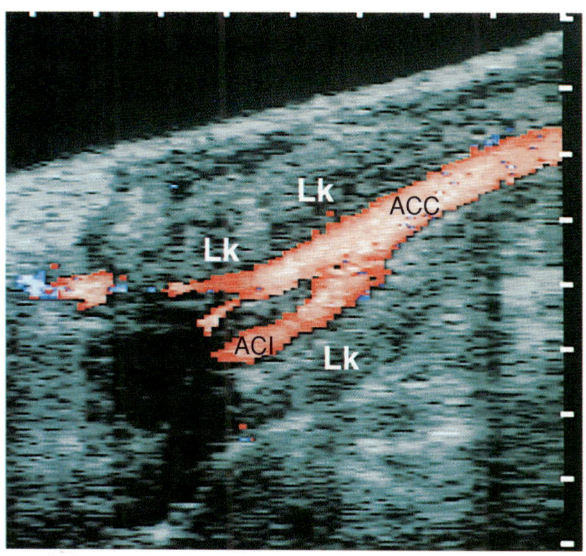

Fig. 5.**20** Encasement of the carotid bifurcation by extensive lymph node metastases (Lk) from a squamous cell carcinoma. ACC = Common carotid artery, ACI = internal carotid artery

5.5 Diagnostic Value of Color Duplex Sonography in Relation to Other Diagnostic Procedures

Selective angiography is the standard by which all noninvasive procedures for evaluating the cervical arteries are judged (33). It must be considered, however, that even angiographic methods can fall short in the grading of stenoses, since angiography demonstrates only the perfused lumen and not the vessel wall itself. This inherent advantage of color duplex sonography can be utilized in selected cases for the critical evaluation of angiographic findings.

Contrast angiography is inherently advantageous over sectional ultrasound imaging in its continuity, scope, and ease of demonstration. As in all ultrasound techniques, the result of the sonographic examination depends strongly on the diligence and experience of the examiner.

In studies comparing CDS imaging and angiography, CDS has shown a sensitivity of 91–95% and a specificity of 86–97% in the detection of carotid occlusions and stenoses causing more than 40–50% diameter reduction (39, 45). This level of accuracy surpasses that of conventional duplex scanning, with the added advantage of a significantly shorter examination time. Also, the sensitivity of CDS markedly surpasses that of transvenous digital subtraction angiography (DSA) (11). In the grading of stenoses, CDS and intra-arterial DSA have shown agreement in 90% of cases (46). These results provide a strong rationale for using CDS as an alternative to intravenous DSA, which is obsolete in extracranial cerebrovascular examinations. CDS is the primary screening method in patients with suspected carotid obstructive disease.

The widely used techniques of CW Doppler sonography (19) can provide a satisfactory, nonimaging evaluation of the carotid arteries, yielding comparatively good results in the detection of higher-grade stenoses. Accuracy rates of over 90% are reported (32). However, the differentiation of subtotal stenosis from occlusion and the detection of low-grade stenoses are more difficult with CW Doppler than with available CDS, which yields better information in these cases by virtue of its high sensitivity (45). In a kinked or coiled internal carotid artery, CW Doppler findings can be confusing and misleading due to the measurement of varying Doppler angles and varying Doppler frequency shifts within a small volume.

Intra-arterial contrast angiography is decidedly superior to all Doppler techniques for the detection of stenoses located near the aortic arch, near the skull base, or within the cranial cavity. If an obstructive lesion is suspected at these sites, an angiographic study is indicated. This is also true in cases where ultrasound imaging is seriously hampered by extensive vascular calcifications, a high carotid bifurcation, or patient obesity, when there is urgent clinical suspicion of a stenosis, and surgery is being considered. Transcranial Doppler sonography (1, 36) continues to be an important noninvasive method for evaluating intracranial cerebrovascular disease, but its role in selecting patients for carotid surgery remains unclear.

CDS can significantly improve the results of conventional duplex scanning in the detection of vertebral stenoses and occlusions (44). But while CDS shows a specificity of 88–93% compared with angiography, it has shown only a moderate sensitivity of 65–77% (45), based largely on an inability to demonstrate all parts of the vertebral arteries. Angiography, then, is still superior for the detection of obstructive lesions in the vertebral system. Experience to date indicates, however, that CDS is ideal for the diagnosis of subclavian steal syndrome (44).

5.6 References

1 Becker, G., J. Winkler, U. Bogdahn: Die transkranielle farbkodierte Real-Time-Sonographie des Erwachsenen. Ultraschall in Med. 12 (1991) 74–79

2 Bendick, P. J., J. L. Glover, R. S. Dilley: Transcutaneous detection of subcritical arterial stenoses by Doppler signal spectrum analysis. J. Ultrasound Med. 2 (1983) 445–449

3 Blackshear, W. M., D. J. Phillips, P. M. Chikos, J. D. Harley, B. L. Thiele, D. E. Strandness: Carotid artery velocity patterns in normal and stenotic vessels. Stroke 11 (1980) 67–71

4 Brown, P. M., K. W. Johnston, M. Kassam, R. S. C. Cobold: A critical study of ultrasound Doppler spectral analysis for detecting carotid disease. Ultrasound Med. Biol. 8 (1982) 515–523

5 Bruno, A., H. P. Adams, J. Biller, K. Rezai, S. Cornell, C. Aschenbrenner: Cerebral infarction due to Moyamoya disease in young adults. Stroke 19 (1988) 826–833

6 Busuttil, R. W., J. D. Baker, R. K. Davidson, H. I. Machleder. Carotid artery stenosis – hemodynamic significance and clinical course. J. Amer. med. Ass. 245 (1981) 1438–1441

7 Dobkin, B. H.: Orthostatic hypotension as a risk factor for symptomatic occlusive cerebrovascular disease. Neurology 38 (1989) 30–34

8 Fisher, M., A. M. Blumenfeld, T. W. Smith. The importance of carotid plaque disruption and hemorrhage. Arch. Neurol. 44 (1987) 1086–1089

9 Garraway, W. M., J. P. Whisnant, I. Drury: the continuing decline in the incidence of stroke. Mayo Clin. Proc. 58 (1983) 520–523

10 Garth, K. E., B. A. Carroll, F. G. Sommer, D. A. Oppenheimer: Duplex ultrasound scanning of the carotid arteries with velocity spectrum analysis. Radiology 147 (1983) 823–827

11 Gmelin, E., I. P. Arlart: Digitale Subtraktionsangiographie, Thieme, Stuttgart (1987) 59

12 Gross-Fengels, W., W. Steinbrich, H. Erasmi, K. F. R. Neufang, H. Lanfermann, F. E. Zanella: Die perkutane transluminale Angioplastie (PTA) der A. subclavia: Technik, Ergebnisse, Risiken. Röntgen-Bl. 43 (1990) 203–212

13 Hallam, M. J., J. M. Reid, P. L. Copperberg: Color-flow Doppler and conventional Duplex scanning of the carotid bifurcation: Prospective, double-blind, correlative study. Amer. J. Roentgenol. 152 (1989) 1101–1105

14 Hamann, H., S. Cyba-Altunbay, H. Schäfer, J. F. Vollmar: Asymptomatic carotid artery stenosis Surgery versus medical treatment (Casanova-Study). In Maurer, P. C., H. M. Becker, H. Heidrich, G. Hoffmann, A. Kriessmann, H. Müller-Wiefel (eds.): What is new in Angiology? Zuckschwerdt, München 1986 (305 ff)

15 Howard, R., P. Trend, R. W. Russel: Clinical features of ischemia in cerebral arterial border zones after periods of reduced cerebral blood flow. Arch. Neurol. 44 (1987) 934–940

16 Imperato, A. M., T. S. Riles, F. G. Baumann: The importance of hemorrhage in the relationship between gross morphologic characteristics and cerebral symptoms in 376 carotid artery plaques. Ann. Surg. 197 (1983) 195–203

17 Kappert, A.: Lehrbuch und Atlas der Angiologie. Hans Huber, Bern 1987 (73)

18 Katz, M. L., M. Johnson, M. J. Pomajzl, A. J. Comerota, D. Ahrensfield, L. Mandel, W. Hayden, T. Fogarty: The sensitivity of real-time B-mode carotid imaging in the detection of ulcerated plaques. Bruit 8 (1983) 13–16

19 Keller, H. M.: Doppler Sonographie (kontinuierliche Emission) bei extrakraniellen Arterienkrankheiten. In Kriessmann, A., A. Bollinger, H. M. Keller (Hrsg.): Praxis der Doppler-Sonographie, 2. Aufl. Thieme, Stuttgart 1990 (161–263)

20 Klag, M. J., P. K. Whelton, A. J. Seidler: Decline in US stroke mortality. Demographic trends and antihypertensive treatment. Stroke 20 (1989) 14–21

21 Krayenbühl, H., M. G. Yasargil: Zerebrale Angiographie für Klinik und Praxis, 3. Aufl. Thieme, Stuttgart 1979

22 Kriessmann, A., A. Bollinger, H. M. Keller: Praxis der Doppler-Sonographie. Thieme, Stuttgart 1990

23 Lattera, J., S. Gebarski, J. C. Sackellares: Transient amnesia resulting from vertebral artery dissection. Stroke 19 (1988) 98–101

24 Leonberg, S. C., F. A. Elliot: Prevention of recurrent stroke. Stroke 12 (1981) 731–735

25 Loftus, C. M., J. Biller, M. N. Hart: Management of radiation-induced accelerated carotid atherosclerosis. Arch. Neurol. 44 (1987) 711–714

26 Lüscher, T. F., J. T. Lie, A. W. Stanson, O. W. Houser, L. H. Hollier, S. G. Sheps: Arterial fibromuscular dysplasia. Mayo Clin. Proc. 62 (1987) 931–952

27 Lippert, H., R. Pabst: Arterial variations in man. Classifications and frequency. Bergmann, München 1985 (3–9)

28 Mathias, K.: Katheterbehandlung der arteriellen Verschlußkrankheit supraaortaler Gefäße. Radiologe 27 (1987) 547–554

29 May, A. G., L. Van de Berg, J. A. De Weese, G. G. Rob: Critical arterial stenosis. Surgery 70 (1963) 250

30 Middleton, W. D., W. D. Foley, T. L. Lawson: Color-flow Doppler imaging of carotid artery abnormalities. Amer. J. Roentgenol. 150 (1988) 419–425

31 Middleton, W. D., W. D. Foley, T. L. Lawson: Flow reversal in the normal carotid bifurcation: Color Doppler flow imaging analysis. Radiology 167 (1988) 207–210

32 Neuerburg-Heusler, D.: Dopplersonographische Diagnostik der extrakraniellen Verschlußkrankheit. Vasa Suppl. 12 (1984) 59–70

33 Neufang, K. F. R., D. Dolars, W. Gross-Fengels: Einfluß der Geometrie arteriosklerotischer Karotisläsionen auf deren angiographische Darstellbarkeit – eine arteriographische Studie. Röntgen-Bl. 43 (1990) 11–15

34 Petro, G. R., G. A. Witwer, E. D. Cacayorin, C. J. Hodge, C. E. Bredenberg, M. S. Jastremski, S. A. Kieffer: Spontaneous dissection of the cervical internal carotid artery: Correlation of angiography, CT and pathology. Amer. J. Neuroradiol. 7 (1986) 1053–1058

35 Prendes, J. L., W. M. McKinney, F. S. Buonanno, A. M. Jones: Anatomic variations of the carotid bifurcation affecting Doppler scan interpretation. J. clin. Ultrasound 8 (1980) 147–150

36 Rosenkranz, K., R. Langer, M. Cordes, R. Felix: Transkranielle Doppler-Sonographie bei zerebrovaskulären Erkrankungen. Fortschr. Röntgenstr 155 (1991) 72–79

37 Ruff, R. F., W. T. Talman, F. Petito: Transient ischemic attacks associated with hypotension in hypertensive patients with carotid artery stenosis. Stroke 12 (1981) 353–355

38 Sillesen, H., K. Bitsch, H. J. Steenberg, T. Schroeder, L. Hansen, H. J. B. Hansen: The clinical use of objective quantification of flow disturbance in carotid artery disease: correlation between spectral broadening index and arteriography. Ultrasound Med. Biol. 13 (1987) 519–525

39 Steinke, W., C. Kloetzsch, M. Hennerici: Carotid artery disease assessed by color Doppler flow imaging: Correlation with standard Doppler sonography and angiography. Amer. J. Roentgenol. 154 (1990) 1061–1068

40 Trattnig, S., P. Hübsch, P. Barton, F. Karnel, Th. Sautner, B. Schwaighofer, G. Kretschmer: Durchgängigkeit der Carotis externa und interna bei Patienten mit Carotis-communis-Okklusion: Nachweis in der farbkodierten Doppler-Sonographie. Fortschr. Röntgenstr. 154 (1991) 44–48

41 Trattnig, S., P. Hübsch, H. Schuster, D. Pötzleitner: Color-coded Doppler imaging of normal vertebral arteries. Stroke 21 (1990) 1222-1225

42 Trattnig, S., P. Hübsch, B. Schwaighofer, F. Karnel, M. Eilenberger: Vaskuläre Raumforderungen der Arteria carotis - Nachweis mit der farbkodierten Dopplersonographie. Ultraschall in Med. 12 (1991) 70–73

43 Trattnig, S., D. Pötzleitner, P. Hübsch, K. Daha, Ch. Matula, H. Magometschnigg: Nicht-invasive Verlaufskontrolle mittels farbkodierter Doppler-Sonographie nach operativen Eingriffen an den extrakraniellen hirnversorgenden Arterien. Fortschr. Röntgenstr. 156 (1992) 224–227

44 Trattnig, S., B. Schwaighofer, P. Hübsch, M. Schwarz, F. Kainberger: Color-coded Doppler sonography of vertebral arteries. J. Ultrasound Med. 10 (1991) 221–226

45 Tschammler, A., P. Landwehr, M. Höhmann, R. Moll, G. Wittenberg, K. Lackner: Farbkodierte Duplexsonographie der extrakraniellen hirnversorgenden Arterien: diagnostische Aussagekraft und Fehlerquellen im Vergleich zur i.a.DSA. Fortschr. Röntgenstr. 155 (1991) 452–459

46 Wiebers, D. O., J. P. Whisnant, W. M. O'Fallon: Reversible ischemic neurologic deficit (RIND) in a community: Rochester/Minnesota, 1955–1974. Neurology 32 (1982) 459–465

47 Williams, P. L., R. Warwick, M. Dyson, L. H. Bannister: Grays Anatomy. 37th ed. Churchill Livingstone, Edinburgh 1989

48 Wolf, P. A., T. R. Dawber, W. B. Kannel: Heart disease as a precursor of stroke. In: B. S. Schoenberg (ed.): Advances in Neurology 19. Raven, New York 1978 (567–576)

49 Zwiebel, W. J.: Spectrum analysis in carotid Doppler sonography. Ultrasound Med. Biol. 13 (1987) 625–636

50 (European Carotid Surgery Trialists Collaborative Group) MRC European Carotid Surgery Trial: interim results for symptomatic patients with severe (70–99%) or with mild (0–29%) carotid stenosis. Lancet 337 (1991) 1235–1243

51 (North American Symptomatic Carotid Endarterectomy Trial Collaborators) Beneficial effect of carotid endarterectomy in symptomatic patients with high-grade carotid stenosis. New Engl. J. Med. 325 (1991) 445–453

6 Extremity Arteries

P. Landwehr

6.1 General

The life expectancy of a patient with peripheral arterial occlusive disease (pAOD) of the extremities is shortened by approximately 10 years relative to comparable patients without pAOD (37). The findings of the Basel Study and more recent investigations (25) indicate that this is due chiefly to the high rate of concomitant obstructive lesions of the coronary and carotid arteries (e. g., approximately 50% of patients with symptomatic pAOD have significant coronary artery stenosis). The 5-year incidence of new occlusive disease is 3.2–13.9% in the asymptomatic stage and 1–4.6% in the symptomatic stage, depending on age (36). Classic risk factors for the development of pAOD are smoking, diabetes mellitus, arterial hypertension, and hyperlipidemia. As the number of risk factors increases, so does the incidence of pAOD.

As operative and nonoperative treatment options have expanded in recent years, there has been an increasing need for noninvasive arterial imaging techniques that can provide an efficient, low-risk primary workup and can objectively monitor the efficacy of various therapeutic measures and their potential complications. This chapter deals with the capabilities and limitations of CDS in the evaluation of extremity arterial disease.

6.2 Normal Anatomy, Common Variants, and Examination Technique

6.2.1 Preliminary Remarks

The arterial anatomy of the extremities differs from that of the cerebral circulation in that there is only one main artery supplying blood to a particular segment of the extremity. At the same time, occlusive lesions of more gradual onset can lead to the development of a potentially extensive collateral circulation that can do much to compensate for the circulatory impairment, even during strenuous exercise. Consequently, the stenosis or occlusion of a single artery is not necessarily an indication for interventional therapy.

Another distinctive feature of the extremity arteries, especially when compared with the intra-abdominal arteries, is their exposure to mechanical stresses. This particularly applies to the arteries of the lower extremity. Also, peculiarities in the course of an artery (e. g., the superficial femoral artery in the adductor canal, atypical position of the popliteal artery in entrapment syndrome) can predispose to the development of vessel wall lesions.

6.2.2 Arteries of the Lower Extremity

The pelvis and lower extremities derive their blood supply from the abdominal aorta in the retroperitoneum. The inferior mesenteric artery and the paired lumbar arteries arise from the infrarenal segment of the abdominal aorta, and the middle sacral artery arises from the distal end of the aorta, where the great vessel bifurcates into the two common iliac arteries (usually at the level of L4). Since the abdominal aorta is slightly to the left of the midline, the right common iliac artery is usually somewhat longer than the left. The length of the common iliac arteries ranges from 3.5 to 7.5 cm but is subject to marked variations, and the external iliac artery may even spring directly from the aorta (8). The common iliac artery divides at the level of the sacroiliac joint into the internal iliac artery, which supplies the pelvic viscera, pelvic wall, buttocks and perineum, and the external iliac artery, which does not give off any significant branches until just before passing behind the inguinal ligament. The external iliac artery runs along the medial side of the iliopsoas muscle in the pelvis to the inguinal ligament, giving off two branches just before reaching the ligament: the inferior epigastric artery (to the anterior abdominal wall) and the deep circumflex iliac artery (38).

As the external iliac artery passes behind the inguinal ligament through the lacuna vasorum (medial to the lacuna musculorum), it becomes the femoral artery (Fig. 6.**1**), which runs lateral to the femoral vein and anterior to the hip joint. The femoral artery proximal to the origin of the profunda femoris artery is frequently termed the common femoral artery in clinical parlance (analogous to the common femoral vein, see Chapter 8). The profunda femoris artery (deep femoral artery) passes posterolaterally from the common femoral artery to supply the thigh. The profunda femoris generally arises 2–5 cm below the inguinal ligament, though it has been observed to arise at more proximal levels and even as high as the ligament itself.

Past the origin of the profunda femoris, the trunk of the femoral artery is known in clinical parlance as the superficial femoral artery. It first runs anteromedially, then courses medially along the thigh, its middle and distal portions closely approaching the femoral shaft from the medial side. It relates posteriorly to the accompanying superficial femoral vein. At the junction of the middle and distal thirds of the thigh, the superficial femoral artery enters the adductor canal (the Hunter canal) with the accompanying vein and saphenous nerve, then turns posteriorly. The adductor canal is bounded by an anterior aponeurosis made up of fibers of the adductor longus and magnus muscles (vastoadductor membrane) and by the posterior portions of these muscles. The superficial femoral artery gives off small branches in its course and re-emerges from the distal end of the adductor canal in the adductor (tendinous) hiatus as the popliteal artery.

The popliteal artery traverses the popliteal fossa to the tendinous arch of the soleus muscle, coursing medial to its accompanying vein. It mainly gives off branches to the articular network about the knee. The branches of the popliteal artery show a highly variable pattern. Normally the artery divides distal to the knee joint into the anterior and posterior tibial arteries, the latter giving rise to the peroneal artery as its first branch; the segment between the origins of the anterior tibial artery and peroneal artery is also known as the tibioperoneal trunk. But the popliteal artery may bifurcate proximal to the tendinous arch of the soleus muscle and may even divide at the level of the knee joint. In other cases the anterior tibial artery and peroneal artery may arise directly from the popliteal artery, with absence or hypoplasia of the posterior tibial artery.

Ordinarily there are three main arteries in the lower leg, and all can vary markedly in their diameters. The anterior tibial artery pierces the interosseous membrane at the inferior border of the popliteus muscle and runs in the extensor muscles to the dorsum of the foot, where it passes below the cruciform ligament to become the dorsal pedal artery. In one variant the anterior tibial artery courses on the fibula in the distal third of the lower leg. The posterior tibial artery normally has a larger caliber than the anterior tibial artery and runs behind the tibia between the superficial and deep flexor muscles and behind the medial malleolus at the ankle before continuing to the sole of the foot as the plantar artery. The peroneal artery descends on the back of the fibula to the lateral malleolus, traversing a canal formed by the fibula, flexor hallucis longus muscle, and posterior tibialis muscle.

The anterior and posterior tibial arteries can show varying degrees of hypoplasia or may be absent. In such cases the arterial supply is maintained by the other tibial artery or by the peroneal artery, which is less commonly hypoplastic.

At the level of the ankle joint, the tibioperoneal arteries form an anastomotic network that ensures an adequate collateral supply in the event that one or two vessels are incapacitated due to hypoplasia, aplasia, or acquired disease.

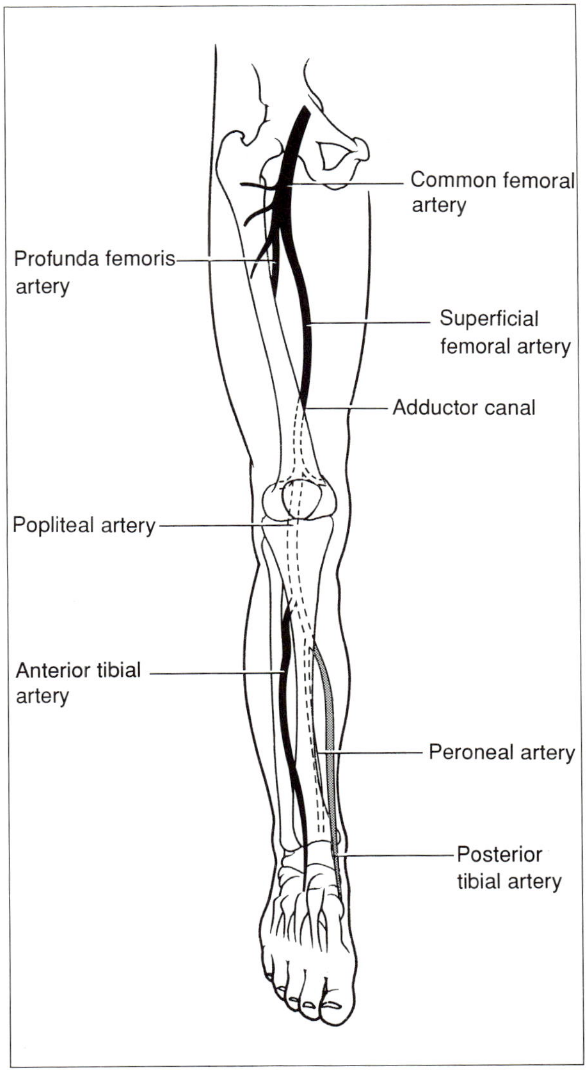

Fig. 6.**1** Arterial anatomy of the lower extremity

The foot is supplied by the dorsalis pedis artery (from the anterior tibial) and the medial and lateral plantar arteries (from the posterior tibial). The latter arteries form the plantar arch, which anastomoses with the deep plantar branch (from the arcuate artery of the dorsalis pedis). The dorsalis pedis system supplies the dorsal metatarsal and digital arteries, while the plantar metatarsal and digital arteries arise from the posterior tibial system (plantar arteries). As at the malleolar level, multiple arterial anastomoses are present in the foot to ensure good collateralization (38).

6.2.3 Arteries of the Upper Extremity

The upper extremity arteries arise from the main supra-aortic trunks on both sides, the right subclavian artery generally arising from the brachiocephalic artery behind the sternoclavicular joint while the left subclavian artery springs directly from the aortic arch. The origins of these vessels are subject to considerable variation (see section 5.2).

The subclavian artery arches over the pleural dome and passes with the brachial plexus through the "scalenus gap" formed by the anterior and medial scalene muscles. It then runs over the first rib to the retroclavicular area, passing in front of the scapula and behind the pectoralis minor muscle before entering the axilla. The subclavian artery becomes the axillary artery at the lateral margin of the first rib. The main branches of the subclavian artery are the vertebral artery (see Chapter 5), the thyrocervical trunk, and the internal thoracic (mammary) artery.

The branches of the axillary artery, which may have extensive collateral connections with branches of the subclavian artery, supply the region of the shoulder girdle. The axillary artery becomes the brachial artery after crossing the inferior border of the pectoralis major muscle.

The brachial artery runs in the medial bicipital groove to the elbow and divides into the radial and ulnar arteries at the level of the joint space. Besides muscular branches, the brachial artery gives origin to the deep brachial artery in the proximal upper arm as well as the superior and inferior ulnar collateral arteries. These branches of the brachial artery join with proximal branches of the radial and ulnar arteries to form an anastomotic network about the elbow, which can usually provide adequate collateral flow to the forearm and hand in response to a distal brachial occlusion. A common variation of the brachial artery is a high division into the radial and ulnar arteries, the radial artery showing an atypically high origin more frequently than the ulnar artery (1 of 8 cases versus 1 of 13 cases) (8). The remaining trunk then gives off the interosseous artery in the proximal forearm, which generally arises from the ulnar artery.

The radial artery continues the course of the brachial artery along the radial side of the forearm, passes through the snuff box at the wrist, and unites with the deep branch of the ulnar artery to form the deep palmar arch. This arch gives rise to the palmar metacarpal arteries, which anastomose with the common palmar digital arteries.

From its origin, the ulnar artery passes obliquely deep to pronator teres and between the superficial and deep flexors to the medial side of the forearm. In the proximal forearm it gives off the common interosseous artery and continues along the flexor carpi ulnaris to the wrist. It forms the major portion of the superficial palmar arch and gives off the three common palmar digital arteries, each of which divides into two proper palmar digital arteries (to the second through fourth fingers). The thumb receives its blood supply directly from the deep palmar arch, and the fifth finger from the superficial palmar arch. The blood supply of the fingers is basically derived from four digital arteries; besides the palmar vessels noted above, dorsal digital arteries arise from the dorsal carpal branch of the radial artery (38).

6.2.4 Examination Technique

6.2.4.1 Preliminary Examinations

The preliminary clinical workup of suspected peripheral AOD should include the history (which covers risk factors, claudication, rest pain, location of ischemia, gangrene, prior therapy, arterial diseases in other regions) and the clinical examination (e. g., quality of peripheral pulses, trophic skin changes, presence of bruits) (14). Peripheral pulse palpation and blood pressure measurements during various provocative maneuvers are helpful in the diagnosis of thoracic outlet syndromes. To assess the severity of lower-extremity pAOD, standardized stress testing with a treadmill ergometer, or accompanied walking on level ground at a designated pace, is preferable to having the patient estimate his or her maximum walking distance (although the latter is helpful for assessing subjective disability).

The Doppler measurement of systolic blood pressures is an essential preliminary study in every pAOD patient. A minimum protocol is the comparative measurement of systolic pressures in both arms and in a pedal artery of the affected limb at rest to determine the Doppler blood pressure ratios (ankle–arm index) [23]). If a CW Doppler unit is not available, this can be accomplished with a CDS instrument. After the blood pressure cuff has been applied, the dorsalis pedis artery or posterior tibial artery is visualized and observed for resumption of arterial flow during cuff deflation to ascertain the systolic pressure (low PRF and wall filter settings should be used to increase sensitivity). The values determined are compared with those measured in the brachial artery. By obtaining segmental blood pressure ratios at various levels and taking postexercise measurements, either pAOD can be excluded with reasonable confidence or, in positive cases, provide a semiquantitative assessment of the severity and approximate location of the disease (2, 13, 20). This noninvasive protocol is easily learned and can be widely implemented at low cost.

6.2.4.2 Instrumentation

The basic instrument requirements for CDS are described in Chapter 4. A 5-MHz linear-array transducer is generally recommended for examination of the lower extremity arteries. A 7.5-MHz transducer may provide enhanced definition, depending on the thickness of the soft-tissue envelope, and is the transducer of choice for most examinations of the upper-extremity arteries. When imaging the pelvic arteries, the examiner should first check to see whether the 5-MHz transducer provides sufficient depth of penetration; otherwise a 3.5-MHz convex transducer should be used.

The color duplex mode should be activated right away in examinations of the extremity arteries. This facilitates the anatomic survey and the localization of abnormalities. Following optimum adjustment of the gray-scale image, the color encoding is adjusted by setting the PRF, wall filter, and sensitivity to eliminate aliasing in healthy vascular segments (see Chapter 4) and to fill the vessel completely with color pixels without producing extravascular color artifacts.

6.2.4.3 Position of the Patient and Examiner

Examinations of the pelvic and lower-extremity arteries are basically performed in the recumbent position. If possible, a patient with suspected pAOD should lie down and rest for 15 min prior to the examination so that any prolonged reactive hyperemia following the walk to the examination room will have time to clear. This is often difficult for logistic reasons but is very important for the optimum evaluation of Doppler blood pressure ratios and Doppler spectra.

For imaging of the pelvic and lower-extremity arteries, the patient lies comfortably in a supine position with the upper body slightly elevated if desired. In some cases the patient may have to be turned to a lateral or prone position to demonstrate the popliteal artery or arteries in the posterior lower leg (for details see below). The supine position is also recommended for examination of the upper-extremity arteries, or the upper body may be tilted up while the arm rests on the table surface.

6.2.4.4 Protocol for Examination of the Lower Extremity

A complete, bilateral CDS examination of the pelvic and lower-extremity arteries by an experienced examiner, with documentation, takes about 25–35 min or perhaps longer if complex pathology is encountered. The examiner should follow an efficient protocol whose scope is oriented toward the clinical inquiry. Often it is unnecessary to examine all the vessels in their entirety. In a patient evaluated for a puncture-related false aneurysm in the groin, for example, CDS may be limited to the region of interest on the affected side (5–10 min) unless there are additional questions that must be addressed (such as embolization from the aneurysm). However, in cases where pAOD is more severe on one side than the other, the less severely affected side should always be examined as well.

The search for pAOD in the lower extremity begins with Doppler spectral sampling (in the color-encoded flow image) at the following sites: the distal anterior tibial artery just above the ankle joint, the distal posterior tibial artery behind the medial malleolus, the external iliac artery, the proximal superficial femoral artery, the profunda femoris, and the popliteal artery. If flow sampling at these sites shows normal-appearing biphasic or triphasic spectra with a steep systolic upslope, and if the Doppler pressure ratio is normal (> 0.9), it is reasonable to exclude therapeutically relevant occlusive disease of the larger arteries. Usually there is no need to proceed with a CDS survey of the entire arterial tree.

If abnormal Doppler spectra are recorded, the proximal-to-distal change in the spectral waveform should indicate the approximate location of the lesion. In this case all portions of the arterial tree from the iliac bifurcation to the distal tibial arteries should be evaluated by CDS imaging if possible. An effort is made to obtain complete longitudinal images of the arteries and search for abnormal flow patterns. The main criteria for evaluating arterial status with CDS are the width of the perfused vascular lumen, the presence of lumen-reducing plaques, increased flow velocities within stenoses, and poststenotic turbulence and vorticity. If definite pathology is found on the basis of CDS criteria, there is generally no need to perform a Doppler frequency analysis at the site of the lesion (Figs. 6.**2**, 6.**3a–d**, 6.**4**, 6.**5a**, **b**, 6.**6a**, **b**, 6.**7a**, **b**). If the stenosis needs to be graded, this can usually be done satisfactorily from the color flow image. If direct color-encoded flow imaging is not possible in certain areas (obesity, bowel gas, wall calcifications), the comparison of Doppler spectra recorded proximal and distal to the inaccessible area pro-

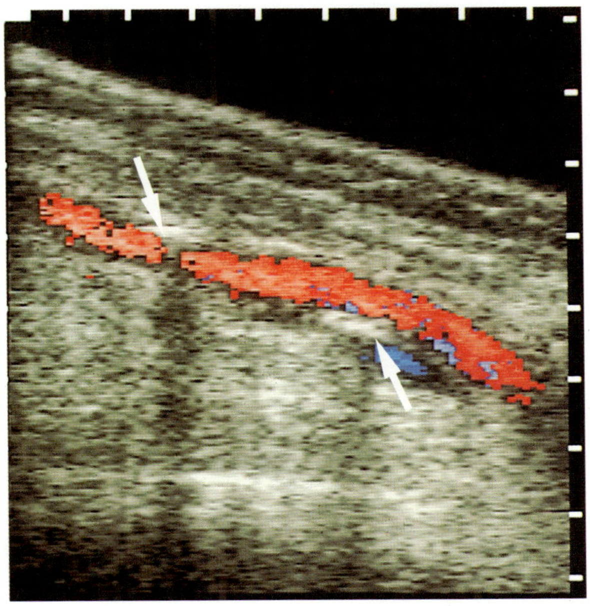

Fig. 6.**2** Calcified wall plaques (arrows) in the superficial femoral artery. Acoustic shadow behind the calcifications, minimal change in the proximal and distal color-encoded flow patterns, indicating no significant stenosis caused by the calcification

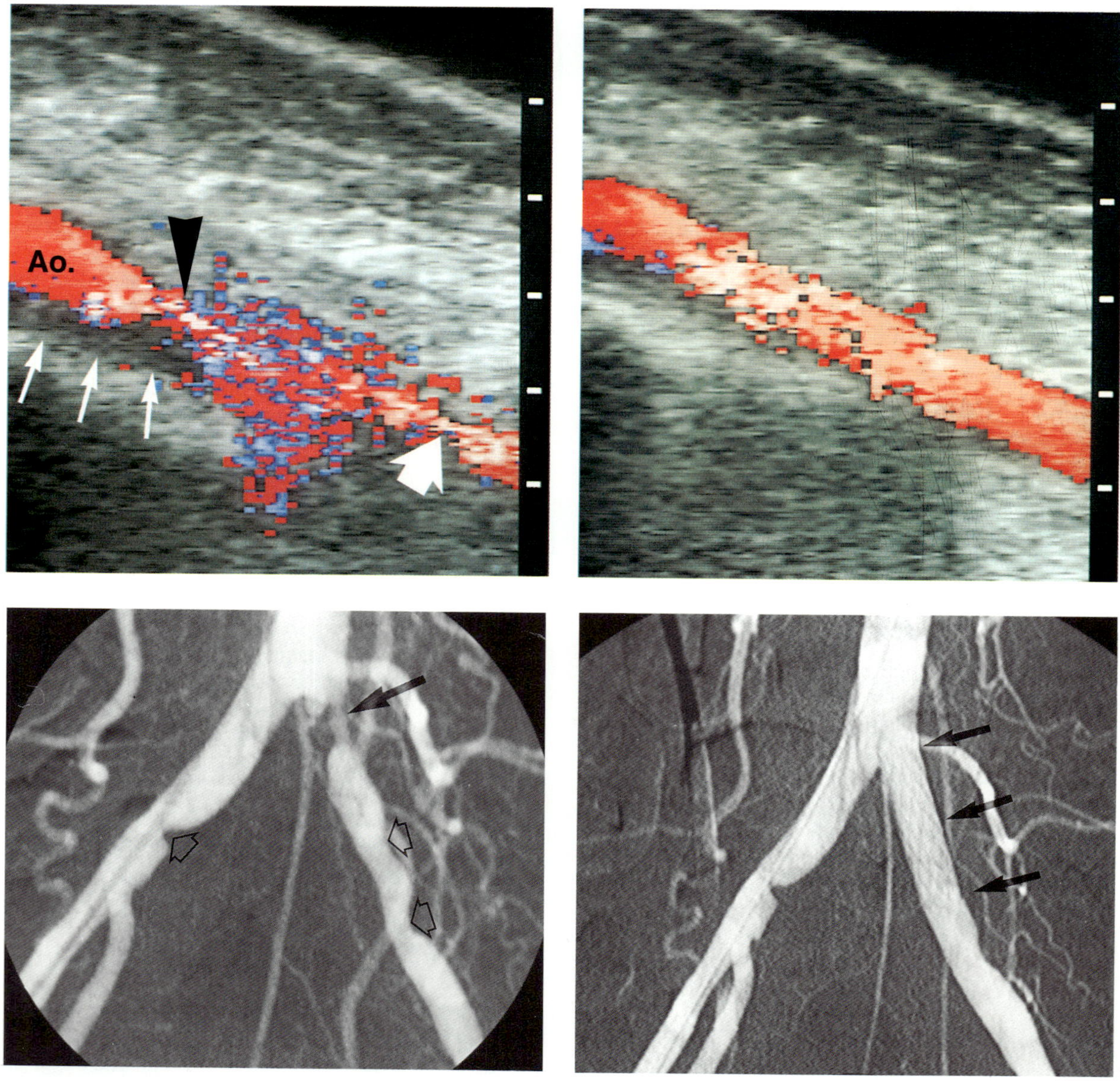

Fig. 6.**3a–d** High-grade proximal stenosis of the left common iliac artery before and after PTA with stent insertion

a CDS demonstrates atherosclerotic wall plaques (white arrows) causing severe luminal narrowing (arrowhead), indicated by the very light color of the high-velocity flow. Marked perivascular tissue vibration artifacts (red and blue "color cloud") appear within and distal to the stenosis. A second stenosis is visible distally (short white arrow). Ao. = Aorta

b Intra-arterial DSA demonstrates a high-grade stenosis in the proximal common iliac artery (solid arrow), two additional stenoses in the distal vascular segment, and a stenosis in the right common iliac artery (open arrows)

c CDS after PTA and stent placement shows a fully patent lumen with laminar flow and absence of vibrational artifacts. The stent casts a faint acoustic shadow that does not hamper evaluation of the vessel lumen

d Angiogram after PTA and stent insertion (Palmaz stent) demonstrates bridging of the proximal stenoses by the stent (arrows) with a normal-size lumen

Fig. 6.**4** Diffuse, dilatative atherosclerosis of the superficial femoral artery. Pronounced, circumferential wall thickening presents a mixed hypoechoic and hyperechoic pattern (arrows = outer boundary of the vessel wall). Irregularities on the inner wall of the vessel give rise to turbulence (manifested by blue speckling). There is a circumscribed stenosis (S) with increased flow velocity (pale red)

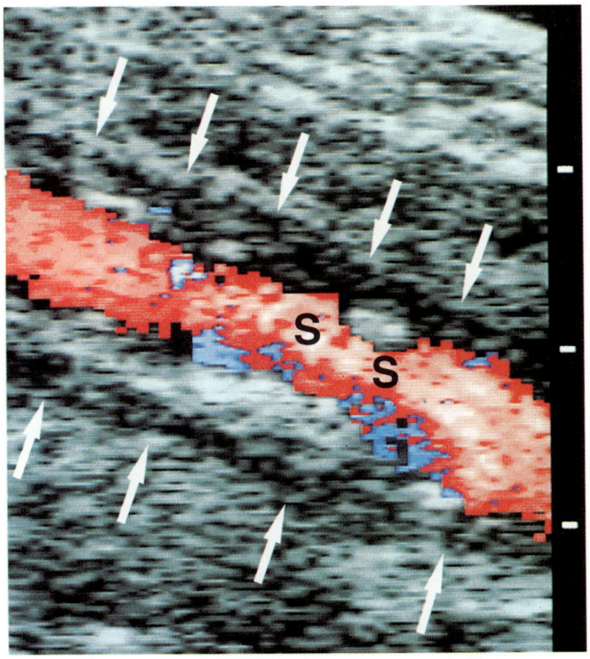

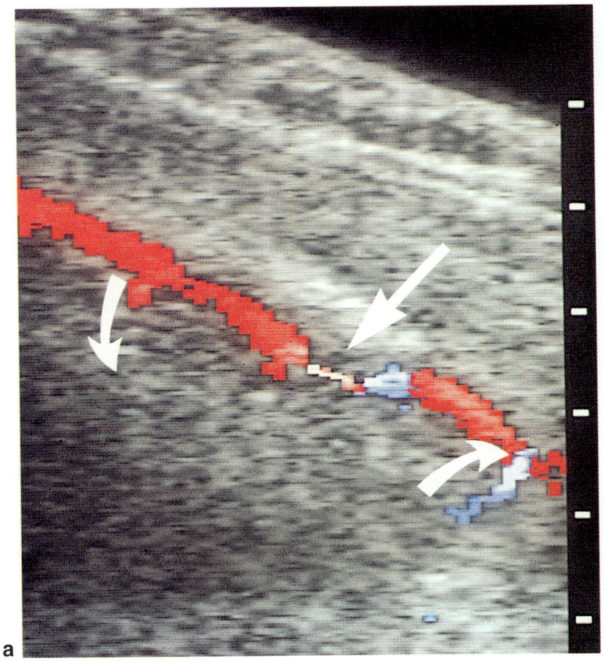

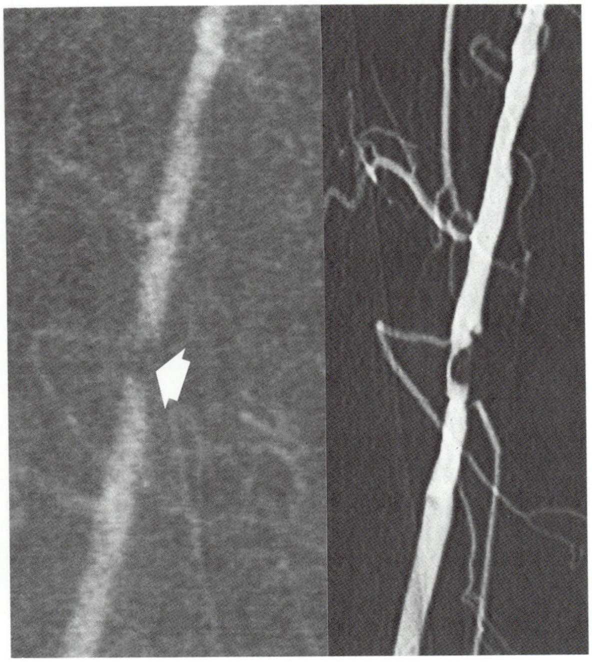

Fig. 6.**5a, b** Short, eccentric stenosis of the superficial femoral artery

a CDS demonstrates severe, eccentric luminal narrowing. The white encoding in the stenosis (straight arrow) indicates a very high frequency shift. The stenosis is circumvented by collaterals whose proximal origin (left curved arrow) and distal site of entry (right curved arrow) can be seen

b Intravenous DSA (left) and intra-arterial DSA (right). The lesion mimics an occlusion on the intravenous DSA (arrow). The arterial study confirms the CDS finding of a high-grade stenosis. The CDS image demonstrates the morphology of the stenosis better than intravenous DSA

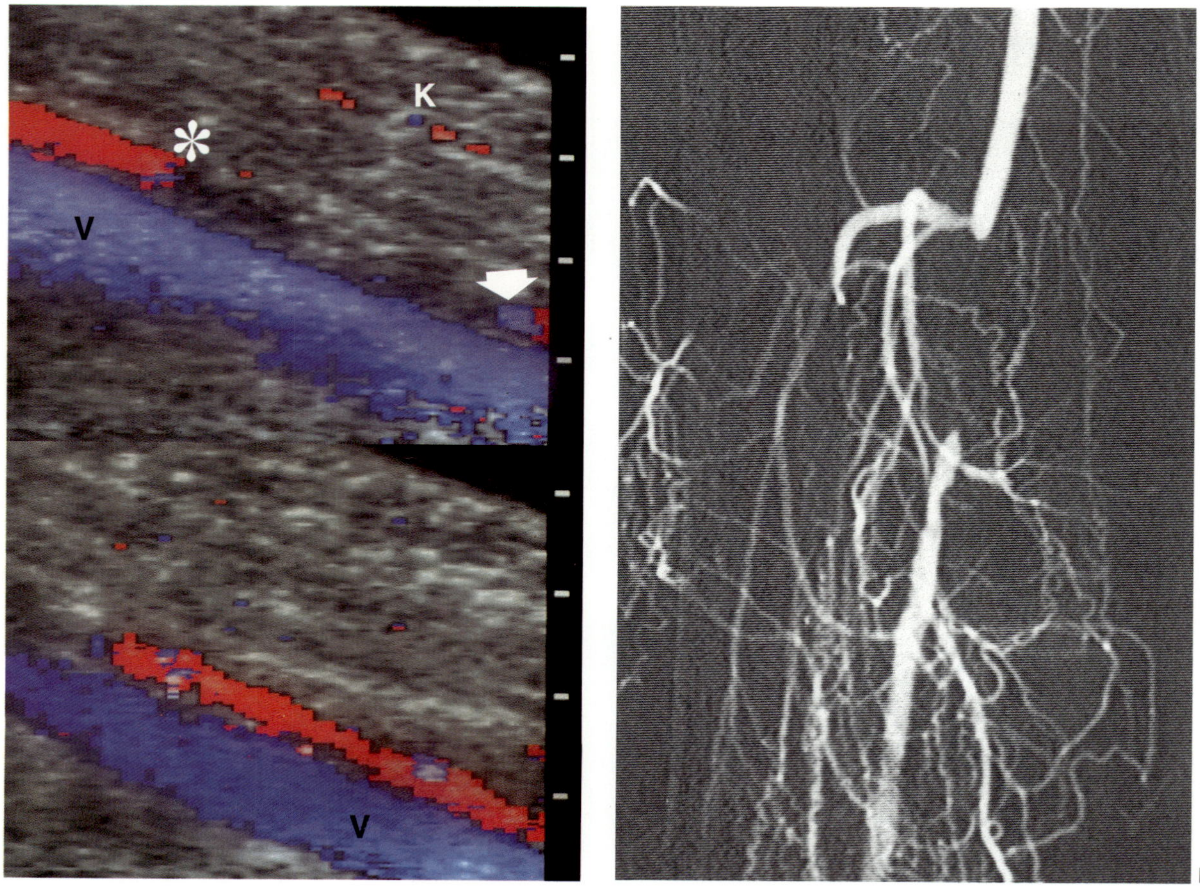

a b

Fig. 6.**6 a, b** Short segmental occlusion of the superficial femoral artery
a CDS: The asterisk in the upper image marks the proximal point of occlusion, and the arrow marks the site where flow is reconstituted distally (also shown in the lower image). The lumen of the occluded vascular segment is nonhomogeneously hypoechoic. Subcutaneous collaterals (K) are visible. The blue-encoded signals are from the superficial femoral vein (V)
b Intra-arterial DSA shows the segmental occlusion and prominent collaterals. The angiogram demonstrates the collateral circulation with greater clarity and completeness

vides a means of detecting or excluding significant occlusive disease.

Ultrasound imaging at the pelvic level is hampered by the retroperitoneal position of the arteries, since the abdominal wall and bowel loops cause marked scattering and attenuation of the sound. Thus, the aortoiliac examination, like normal abdominal sonography, should be performed after adequate patient preparation (special diet 2–3 days before the examination, use of antiflatulents or mild laxatives). Gentle pressure can be applied with the transducer to shorten the distance to the imaged vessel, and often this will displace bowel loops out of the sound field. It may be necessary to locate the best acoustic window by angling the transducer past undisplaced bowel loops or by scanning through the distended urinary bladder.

The distal external iliac artery, the common femoral artery, the main trunk of the profunda femoris, and the proximal portion of the superficial femoral artery are easily examined from an anterior approach owing to the relative proximity of the vessels to the skin. The primary longitudinal scan may have to be supplemented by additional transverse scans to demonstrate eccentric vascular stenoses and aneurysms. In all cases the femoral bifurcation should be imaged transversely to supplement the longitudinal view. Approximately 2–4 cm of the main trunk of the profunda femoris can usually be visualized. From there the course of the superficial femoral artery is followed, always keeping the shortest possible distance between the transducer and the vessel. In most cases the femoral artery can be imaged as far as the adductor canal in the supine patient by moving the transducer to a more posteromedial position. Because of the strong sound absorption by muscle and fascia in the area, the instrument settings usually have to be adjusted (gain, color sensitivity). Also, the distance to the vessel can often be reduced by applying controlled pressure with the transducer on one side and with the

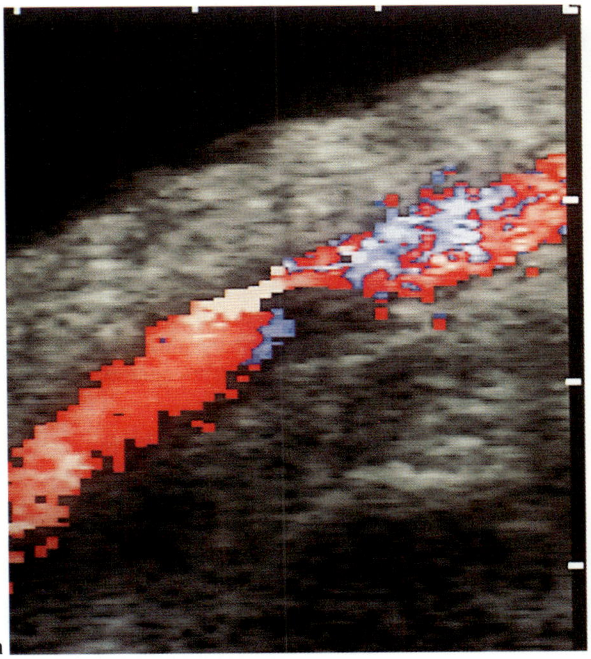

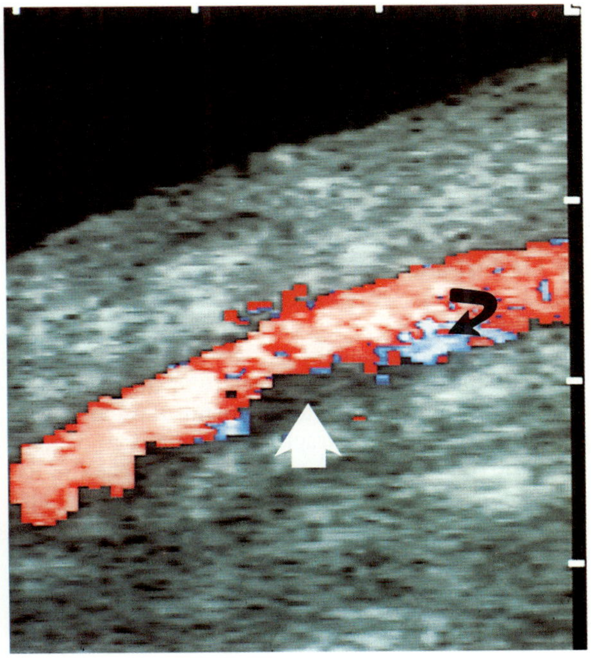

Fig. 6.**7a, b** Stenosis in the common femoral artery before and after percutaneous transluminal angioplasty (PTA)
a CDS before PTA shows a high-grade eccentric stenosis with a high intrastenotic velocity (pale red) and poststenotic turbulence (mixture of red and blue)
b CDS after PTA still shows residual eccentric stenosis by plaque on the posterior vessel wall (white arrow) and a slight persistence of poststenotic flow reversal (curved black arrow)

hand on the other side (see Fig. 8.**6**). The transducer position must be adjusted for the increasing posterior course of the vessel; this can be done either by abducting and externally rotating the hip and flexing the knee slightly or by turning the patient to the prone or lateral position. The popliteal artery will be readily accessible in one of these positions.

Besides the pelvic vessels, the tibioperoneal trifurcation in the lower leg is the most difficult region of the lower-extremity arteries to examine with CDS. Due to the complex spatial arrangement of the main vessels arising from the popliteal artery, it generally is not possible to demonstrate all three origins in one sectional image. The trifurcation region, and especially the origins of the peroneal and posterior tibial arteries, are best surveyed either from the posterior aspect (in the prone position) by scanning distally along the popliteal artery or from the posteromedial aspect by scanning between the posterior tibial border and the medial head of the gastrocnemius muscle (abduction, external rotation, knee flexion, supine position). Because the anterior tibial artery runs anterolaterally from its origin to pierce the interosseous membrane, the proximal segment of this vessel must be evaluated both from the transducer position described above and from an anterolateral approach (lateral to the anterior tibial border). If the tibioperoneal arteries are not hypoplastic, they often can be imaged longitudinally as far as the ankle joint in nonobese patients: the posterior tibial and peroneal arteries are scanned from the back, the anterior tibial artery from the front. Because the complete visualization of all three arteries is very time-consuming, however, the selective sampling of proximal and distal spectra from the tibioperoneal arteries is generally sufficient for the detection of hemodynamically significant disease. In the foot, at least the main trunks of the dorsalis pedis and plantar arteries can be demonstrated. CDS cannot provide reproducible, continuous imaging of the more distal arteries, although segments of individual digital arteries can be seen.

When imaging aneurysmal lesions, the examiner should direct attention to the walls of the lesion so that mural thrombi are not missed. Arteriovenous fistulae can be defined more clearly by slightly compressing the inflow vessel to decrease the flow and reduce typical perivascular tissue vibration artifacts. The hemodynamic significance of the fistula can be estimated by quantifying the flow rates in the artery proximal and distal to the fistula.

6.2.4.5 Protocol for Examination of the Upper Extremity

The basic considerations previously discussed for examinations of the lower extremity arteries apply equally to the arteries of the upper extremity. The examination should start with a search for arterial stenoses and occlusions with comparative Doppler spectral sampling in the axillary artery, the midportion of the brachial artery, and the proximal and distal portions of the ulnar artery and radial artery. CDS imaging of the vessels proceeds in a proximal to distal direction, first scanning the axillary artery from the axilla (with the arm slightly abducted) or from the anterior side (through the pectoralis major muscle). From there the vessel can be tracked proximally to demonstrate the sonographically accessible lateral half of the subclavian artery. Then the axillary artery and brachial artery are imaged longitudinally from the medial side with the arm supinated and are followed distally. The radial and ulnar arteries are observed best from the volar aspect with the arm supinated. As in the foot, the sectional ultrasound images cannot provide a global view of the palmar and metacarpal arteries, although the digital arteries can be reproducibly defined with a high-frequency transducer and their Doppler spectra recorded. The competence of the palmar arch can be assessed by a simple compression test. If manual compression of the proximal radial artery evokes flow reversal in the distal part of the artery, it may be concluded that the palmar arch is functionally competent. This is also evidenced by the persistence of pulsatile flow in the radial thumb artery when the distal radial artery is compressed.

If a thoracic outlet syndrome is suspected, Doppler spectra should be sampled from the axillary or brachial artery with the arm in the neutral position and during a provocative maneuver (e. g., elevation of the arm plus head rotation to the opposite side).

With a suspected obstruction of the subclavian or brachiocephalic artery, the vertebral arteries should also be examined to exclude subclavian steal phenomenon. This assessment can be aided if necessary by the induction of postischemic reactive hyperemia (see Chapter 5).

6.2.4.6 Documentation

The documentation of color duplex findings is geared basically toward the problem of demonstrability. This is far more difficult than with contrast angiography, given the inherent confinement of the duplex image plane to a very small part of the vascular system and the absence of definite anatomic landmarks (such as bones in angiography). The ability to review CDS findings can be enhanced by the videotape documentation of representative sequences and by obtaining hard-copy images of individual frames. Findings must be labeled by means of captions or special symbols.

Minimum CDS documentation of a lower-extremity examination should include the following:

- A longitudinal image and spectrum of the external iliac artery
- A longitudinal image of the femoral bifurcation, the profunda femoris, the proximal and distal superficial femoral and artery
- A longitudinal image and spectrum of the popliteal artery
- A longitudinal image and spectrum of the distal anterior tibial artery and distal posterior tibial artery (the distal peroneal artery should be documented if one or both tibial arteries cannot be visualized)

An examination of the upper extremity arteries should be documented by:

- A longitudinal image and spectrum of the axillary artery, of the distal brachial artery, of the distal radial artery, and of the distal brachial ulnar artery

Pathologic findings should be documented with a longitudinal scan that, in the case of aneurysms, a–v fistulae, and eccentric intravascular and extravascular lesions, is supplemented by transverse views. If stenotic flow abnormalities are poorly depicted on the color flow image (e. g., due to vessel wall calcifications), they should be documented with an additional Doppler spectrum. Written documentation may be freely formulated or recorded on a standard report form.

6.3 Normal Findings

Flow in the extremity arteries is normally very pulsatile due to the high peripheral vascular resistance (see Chapter 3; biphasic or triphasic pattern). This pattern is equally apparent in the color-encoded image and Doppler spectrum, and either mode will demonstrate the diastolic reverse flow component when proper instrument settings are used. Diastolic reverse flow is highly variable even under physiologic conditions and may be abolished by a high ambient temperature or emotional stress (peripheral vasodilation). It is not unusual to observe a marked fluctuation of spectral morphology during the course of an examination. Thus diastolic flow reversal may be initially absent during the examination and may appear later, especially if the patient was not adequately rested before the examination, so the spectrum initially recorded may not signify a true proximal flow obstruction. The individual fluctuations of peripheral vascular resistance that are detectable by Doppler spectral analysis are usually more pronounced in the upper extremities than in the legs.

Various factors determine whether the pelvic and lower extremity arteries can be directly visualized with CDS: the distance from the skin surface to the vessel, overlying bowel loops and bowel gas (in the pelvis), the nature of the intervening soft tissues (10), the wall characteristics of the artery (calcifications, etc.), the average blood flow velocity at the site of interest, and the instrument settings. One study has shown that 89% of the arterial segments from the aortic bifurcation to the ankle joint can be imaged in healthy subjects (22). Most accessible to CDS imaging (demonstrable in 97.5% of subjects) were the common femoral artery, the profunda femoris, the proximal and middle portions of the superficial femoral artery, the popliteal artery, and the anterior and posterior tibial arteries. In this same study 70% of the vascular segments at the pelvic level could be directly visualized, and 60% of the segments in the distal thigh. The peroneal arterial segments were visible in only 78% of subjects, although angiography was not used in this study to check for anatomic variants. It should be noted, however, that poor direct visualization of the pelvic vessels and the superficial femoral artery in the adductor canal can be compensated by obtaining the Doppler spectra proximal and distal to sites that cannot be directly evaluated.

The pelvic arteries have a transverse diameter of 8–10 mm, and the superficial femoral artery measures approximately 5–7 mm. The more distal arterial diameters continue to taper from 4–6 mm in the popliteal artery to 2–4 mm in the tibial arteries. Absolute flow velocities are of little value in the diagnosis of lower-extremity arterial disease. The peak systolic velocity is approximately 100 cm/s at the pelvic and thigh level and approximately 50 cm/s in the popliteal and tibioperoneal arteries (22). The normal range of variation is quite large, however (> 50% of the mean value). This is partly due to the highly variable peripheral resistance, the pulsatility index ranging from 3 to more than 30 under physiologic conditions.

No systematic studies have been done on the accessibility of the upper-extremity arteries to CDS imaging (Fig. 6.**8**). Owing to the relatively thin soft-tissue envelope, however, the upper-extremity arteries can generally be imaged without difficulty from the lateral part of the subclavian artery to the wrist. Often this can be accomplished with a 7.5-MHz transducer alone. As explained in section 6.2.4.5, CDS is very limited in its ability to portray the complex three-dimensional anatomy of the palmar arch, but simple compression tests can be used to assess the function of the radial and ulnar arterial connections in the palmar region. CDS can usually demonstrate one digital artery on each side of the finger, and a Doppler spectrum can be recorded from each vessel. It should be noted that the digital arteries are subject to marked fluctuations of peripheral vascular resistance, producing corresponding changes in the spectral waveform. The steepness of the systolic upslope provides the main criterion for the detection of proximal obstructive lesions.

The sonographically accessible arteries of the upper extremity diminish in caliber from 6–8 mm at the subclavian level to 2–3 mm in the forearm. What was previously said regarding the value of normal velocity data in the lower-extremity arteries applies equally to the arteries of the upper limb.

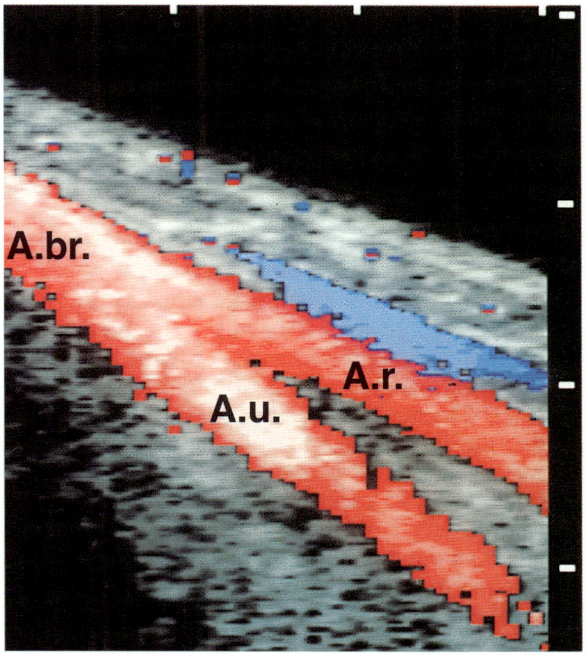

Fig. 6.**8** Normal bifurcation of the brachial artery with homogeneous color encoding, darker shades of red at the vessel wall and a much lighter shade (almost white) at the center, indicating the higher frequency shift. A venous segment ventral to the artery is encoded in blue. A. br. = Brachial arterty, A. u. = ulnar artery, A. r. = radial artery

6.4 Pathologic Findings

6.4.1 Preliminary Remarks

The great majority of patients referred for a peripheral arterial examination suffer from arterial occlusive disease. A basic distinction is drawn between acute and chronic pAOD. Thromboembolism or acute local thrombosis in a previously stenotic artery is responsible for more than 90% of acute arterial occlusions in the extremities. Chronic pAOD is generally due to atherosclerosis, with rare cases resulting from vasculitis, compression syndromes, or other disorders. Transition forms can occur, as illustrated by an acute thrombotic occlusion supervening on stenotic atherosclerotic disease. Once clinical findings and CW Doppler examination have raised suspicion of pAOD, it is the task of diagnostic imaging to localize the lesion and define its extent so that appropriate treatment can be planned.

6.4.2 Clinical Manifestations of Arterial Occlusive Disease

The location and extent of the obstructive disease, its compensation by collateral vessels, and the demands of oxygen-consuming organs (mainly the skin and muscles) determine the timing, location, and severity of clinical manifestations. The staging of extremity AOD distinguishes between ischemic symptoms that occur with exercise and are asymptomatic at rest (intermittent claudication), rest pain, and gangrene. In the staging of pAOD, it must be considered that coexisting coronary or pulmonary disease may limit the patient's general physical stress tolerance to such a degree that he may experience few or no symptoms from the extremity occlusive disease.

Pain is the cardinal symptom of extremity AOD. Other possible symptoms include paresthesias, cold sensitivity, fatigability, changes in skin color, and trophic disturbances ranging from ulceration to gangrene. The location of the symptoms is useful for assessing the approximate location of the disease (e.g., exercise-induced calf pain due to a stenosis in the superficial femoral artery). Steal-type symptoms can also arise (e.g., subclavian steal syndrome, contralateral pain in the gluteal region with an ipsilateral obstruction of the common iliac artery, and collateral flow through the opposite internal iliac artery).

The extent of the collateral circulation depends on the duration of the pAOD and influences the clinical severity. Thus, an acute thromboembolic occlusion tends to produce much more severe symptoms than a progressive thrombosis that occludes a stenosis of long standing.

6.4.3 Ischemia Due to Nonembolic Atherosclerotic Obstruction

6.4.3.1 Preliminary Remarks

The thigh is the most common level of atherosclerotic disease in the lower extremity, accounting for approximately 40% of cases (14). The next most common sites are the external iliac artery (about 20%) and the common iliac artery (about 10%). The tibial vessels are involved in about 20% of cases. Involvement of the distal abdominal aorta or aortic bifurcation is relatively uncommon (5%). Some 20% of patients already have multiple stenoses at the time of diagnosis. Multilevel obstructive disease is most commonly encountered in the thigh and lower leg (about 26%) and in the pelvis and thigh (about 15%). Bilateral disease is present in about 70% of patients and may involve one side more severely than the other. These data indicate that a color duplex examination in a patient with a suspected diagnosis of pAOD should not be limited to one side or one level of involvement.

6.4.3.2 Stenoses and Occlusions of the Pelvic and Lower-Extremity Arteries

Isolated low-grade stenoses (< 50% area reduction) generally produce only local flow changes (Figs. 6.7**b**, 6.9**b**), most notably an increase in the intrastenotic flow velocity (see Chapter 3). A significant reduction in arterial blood pressure may be absent or may occur only with exercise. Doppler spectra recorded proximal and distal to the lesion show no abnormal features.

As the degree of stenosis becomes more severe, the intrastenotic flow velocity increases, and vorticity and turbulence develop distal to the lesion (Figs. 6.5**a**, 6.7**a**, 6.9**a**) (see also Chapter 3). If the stenotic area can be directly visualized, the degree of stenosis can be determined using the method recommended in Chapter 3. As a general rule, stenoses of less than 50% area reduction cause an intrastenotic velocity increase (< 100%) but do not significantly alter the spectral waveform. Standard morphologic criteria for spectral analysis such as a reduction in diastolic reverse flow, widening of the systolic peak, and spectral broadening generally do not appear until the stenosis exceeds 75% in area reduction (> 50% diameter reduction, Fig. 6.**10 a**, **b**). High-grade stenoses (> 90% area reduction) cause a massive intrastenotic velocity increase (possibly with aliasing), significantly reduce the cyclic flow pattern, abolish the diastolic reverse flow component, and cause complete fill-in of the spectral window. Reverse flow elements appear in the distal part of the stenosis and the immediate poststenotic segment, especially in systole, corresponding to turbulent flow in the sample volume. In some cases the high intrastenotic flow velocity can produce vibration artifacts involving the vessel wall and surrounding soft tissues (see section 7.4.2) (25).

A stenotic area that cannot be directly visualized (approximately 20% of cases [19]) can still be evaluated from the proximal and distal spectra. The spectral findings can exclude a hemodynamically significant lesion with considerable confidence (normal-appearing Doppler spectra proximal and distal of the concerned area), or they can provide presumptive evidence of a significant stenosis (reduced systolic amplitude distal to the lesion, absence of diastolic reverse flow) or a high-grade stenosis or occlusion (distal spectrum: flattening of the systolic peak, diastolic plateau of antegrade flow, greatly reduced flow velocity, spectral broadening that persists far distal to the lesion; proximal spectrum: high pulsatility, reduced flow velocity).

The color-encoded flow image demonstrates an occlusion as an intraluminal segment devoid of flow signals (Figs. 6.6**a**, **b**, 6.**11**, 6.**12**). Generally the proximal and distal points of occlusion can be localized, especially in the thigh (Fig. 6.6**a**, **b**). Knowledge of this distance is essential for the selection of optimal treatment (PTA or surgery). Occlusions are frequently marked by collateral arteries arising just proximal to the occlusion, and at least the initial part of the collateral can be visualized by CDS imaging. The presence of increasing collateral branches noted while imaging distally along an artery should direct suspicion toward a more peripheral high-grade stenosis or occlusion ("signal collaterals"). If instrument settings are not optimal, CDS may suggest that the distal site of flow reconstruction is located too far distally due to the very low flow velocities. These cases require a

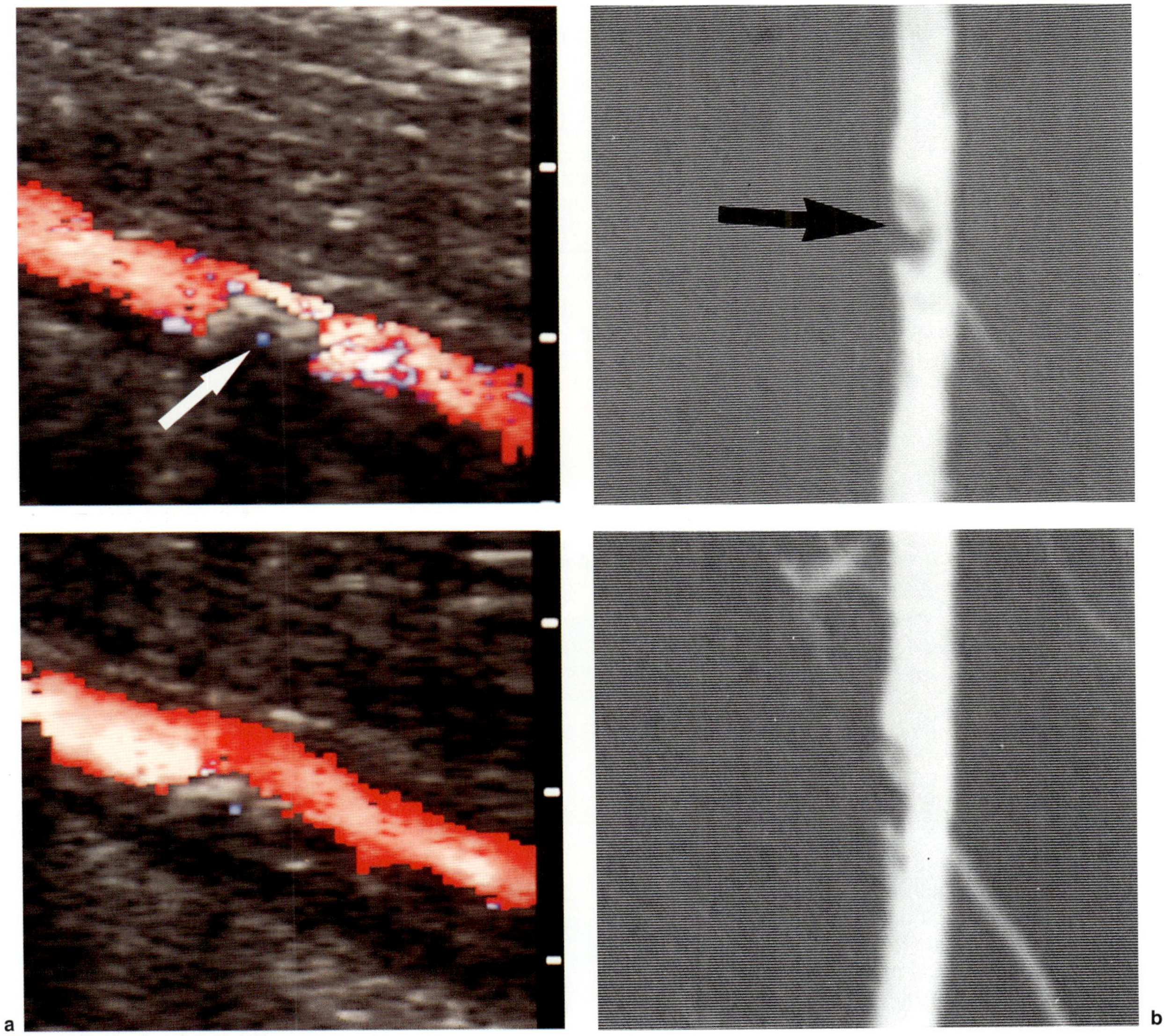

Fig. 6.**9 a, b** Calcified eccentric stenosis of the superficial femoral artery before and after PTA
a The pre-PTA CDS image *(top)* shows eccentric luminal narrowing by a calcified plaque (arrow) with posterior acoustic shadowing and poststenotic turbulence (red and blue). The post-PTA image (bottom) shows slight residual stenosis but no poststenotic flow abnormalities (absence of blue pixels in the red-encoded flow)
b Arterial angiogram confirms the CDS findings of an eccentric stenosis before PTA (*top*, arrow) and residual stenosis after PTA *(bottom)*

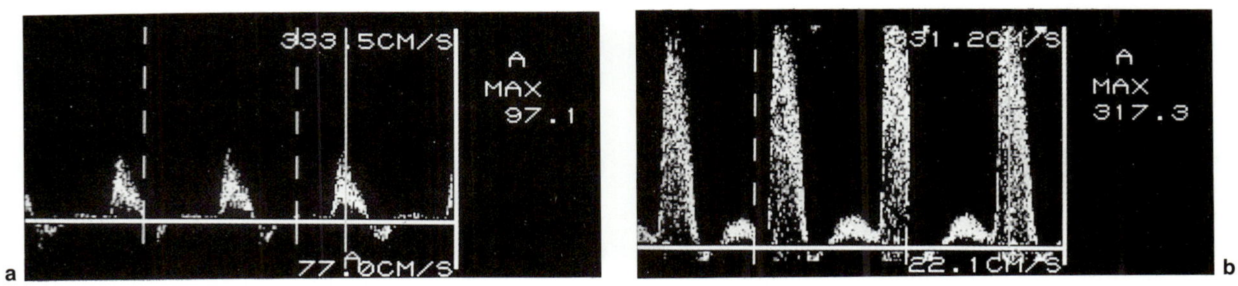

Fig. 6.**10 a, b** Frequency analysis (spectrum) of a stenosis in the iliac artery (50–75% diameter reduction)
a Prestenotic spectrum exhibits a normal triphasic waveform
b Intrastenotic spectrum shows a marked velocity increase (approximately threefold) with marked spectral broadening and an increased antegrade diastolic component. The waveform retains its pulsatile character

Table 6.**1** Classification of the severity of peripheral arterial stenoses. Degree of stenosis is defined as the percentage reduction in cross-sectional area. The classification is not valid for lesions located at vascular bifurcations. Due to the complex dependence of stenosis hemodynamics on numerous factors, there are no firm dividing lines between the different categories (see Chapter 3). The method of calculating degree of stenosis is described in sections 3.4.2 and 3.4.6

Area reduction (degree of stenosis)	Color-encoding/ Doppler spectrum in the stenosis	Color-encoding/ Doppler spectrum just distal to the stenosis	Doppler spectrum far distal to the stenosis	Doppler spectrum proximal to stenosis
0–50%	Increase in V_{max} (by <100%)	Possible flow reversal	Same as prestenotic	Normal
51–75%	Increase in V_{max} (> 100%), slight reduction in pulsatility	Flow reversal, possible slight turbulence, moderate spectral broadening, closure of the spectral window	Normal or slightly reduced pulsatility	Normal
76–90%	Marked increase in V_{max} (> 250%), aliasing, significant reduction in pulsatility	Significant turbulence, marked spectral broadening closure of the spectral window	Increased systolic acceleration time, reduced pulsatility	Amplitude normal or slightly reduced (compare with other side!)
> 90%	Almost no pulsatility (no cyclic changes)	Severe turbulence, marked spectral broadening closure of the spectral window	Flattened systolic peak, significant reduction in pulsatility	Amplitude reduced pulsatility increased
Occlusion	No flow signal	Slow flow (via collaterals)	Very flat and broad complex, low pulsatility	Low amplitude, small complex with relatively high negative component

very diligent examination using maximum instrument sensitivity. The position of the occlusion as determined by CDS should be marked on the skin and the length of the occlusion measured.

Visualization of the main trunk of the profunda femoris is particularly important, because this artery provides the major collateral flow to the distal leg when superficial femoral arterial occlusive disease is present (Fig. 6.**12**). Obstructive disease of the superficial femoral artery involves the profunda femoris in about one-third of cases, jeopardizing the collateral supply to the entire lower leg. The availability of a relatively simple and effective operative treatment for profunda artery stenosis (35) underscores the importance of demonstrating this vascular region, particularly since it is a difficult angiographic site that requires additional oblique projections for reliable evaluation of the proximal profunda segment.

One problem with using CDS for the diagnosis of stenoses and occlusions lies in the detection of multilevel disease. Spectral changes are of very limited value for quantifying a stenosis that is located downstream from more proximal lesions. Additionally, the flow rate past multilevel obstructions may be so greatly reduced that it is below the threshold detectable even by sensitive Doppler instruments. Transpulmonary ultrasound contrast agents could be useful in these cases, as they can significantly enhance the Doppler signal and enable the detection of very slow flow even under unfavorable conditions (see Chapter 16).

6.4.3.3 Stenoses and Occlusions of the Upper-Extremity Arteries

On the whole, the arteries of the upper extremity are less commonly affected by pAOD than the arteries of the pelvis and lower extremity. The most clinically important lesions are proximal stenoses of the subclavian and brachiocephalic artery, which can lead to cerebral ischemia (see Chapter 5) as well as brachial or antebrachial claudication. Often, however, a stenosis or occlusion of the subclavian artery is an incidental finding based on pulse and blood pressure asymmetries.

6.4.4 Nonatherosclerotic Arterial Obstructive Disease

6.4.4.1 Arterial Compression Syndromes

Arterial compression occuring under physiologic conditions, usually during exercise, is generally due to congenital anomalies. Besides the acute peripheral

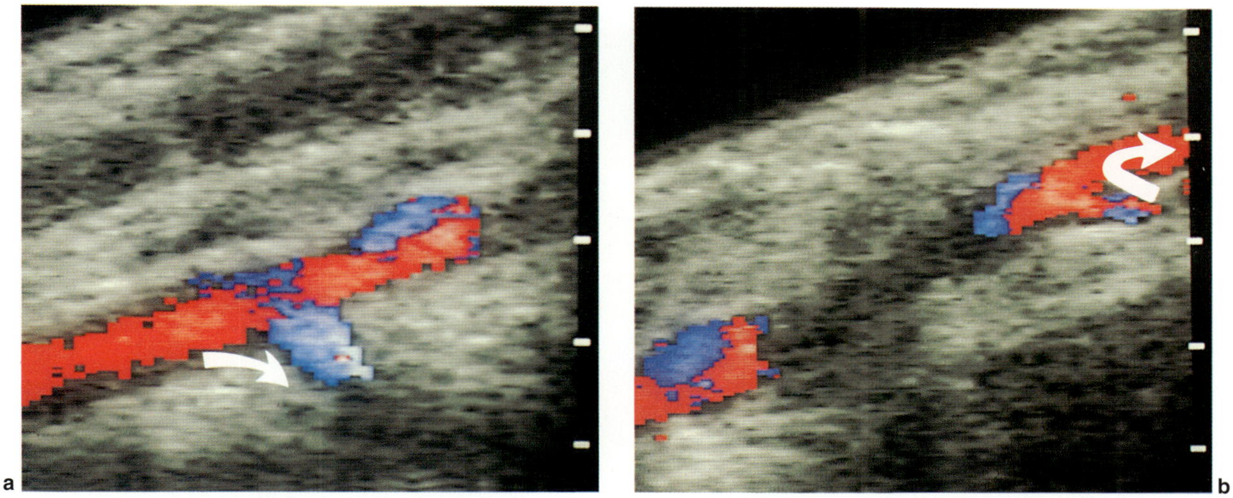

Fig. 6.**11** Short, complete occlusion of the axillary artery circumvented by collaterals

a Longitudinal CDS image shows a large collateral with blue-encoded flow (arrow) arising a short distance proximal to the axillary occlusion (right side of image)

b Section of the vessel distal to **a** with demonstration of the entire occluded segment and the distal reentry of flow (arrow) via a collateral vessel

perfusion deficit caused by the compression itself, the chronic vascular trauma can lead to intimal lesions with stenosis, acute arterial occlusion, aneurysm formation distal to the compression site, and arterioarterial embolization to more distal vessels. Arterial compression syndromes frequently remain asymptomatic until adulthood.

The "thoracic outlet syndromes" usually involve the compression of neural structures (especially the brachial plexus), occasionally accompanied by constrictions in the course of the subclavian artery or subclavian vein. This group of syndromes includes the scalenus anticus syndrome (vascular compression in the interscalene triangle), cervical rib (vascular compression between a cervical rib or associated ligamentous band and the first rib), and the costoclavicular syndrome (vascular compression between the clavicle and first rib) (14). Often the affected vascular segment (usually the brachiocephalic artery or proximal subclavian artery) is not directly accessible to CDS imaging due to overlying lung and bone. But provocative maneuvers (abduction, elevation) make it possible to detect the reversible vascular obstruction and thus differentiate it from a fixed atherosclerotic or inflammatory stenosis (21).

The most common compression syndrome involving the lower-extremity arteries is the popliteal entrapment syndrome. It is based on an atypical course of the artery or an anomaly in the medial head of the gastrocnemius muscle (33). Various types of entrapment syndrome have been described, all involving an atypical medial course of the popliteal artery in relation to the medial head of the gastrocnemius. The symptoms commonly affect young, athletic males and consist of exercise-induced ischemia in the lower leg and possibly an acute occlusion of the popliteal artery and/or the tibial arteries. As in the shoulder girdle region, true aneurysms may develop distal to the compression site. Bilateral occurrence is not unusual (33). CDS can demonstrate the atypical medial course of the popliteal artery as well as any stenoses, occlusions, aneurysms, or distal emboli. A suspected entrapment syndrome can be confirmed by a provocative test. With the patient in the prone position, the knee is

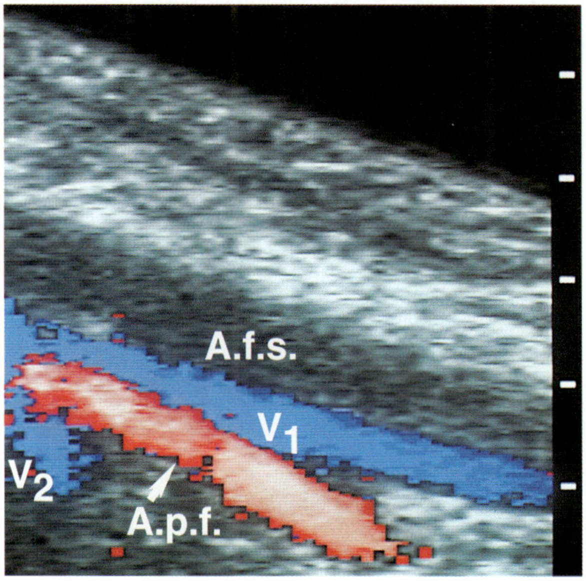

Fig. 6.**12** Complete occlusion of the superficial femoral artery developing 3 days after PTA. The area within the occluded segment (A. f. s.) is uniformly hypoechoic with no evidence of flow. The profunda femoris artery (A. p. f.) is normally perfused by red-encoded flow. Note the blue encoding of the superficial femoral vein (V_1) and profunda femoris vein (V_2)

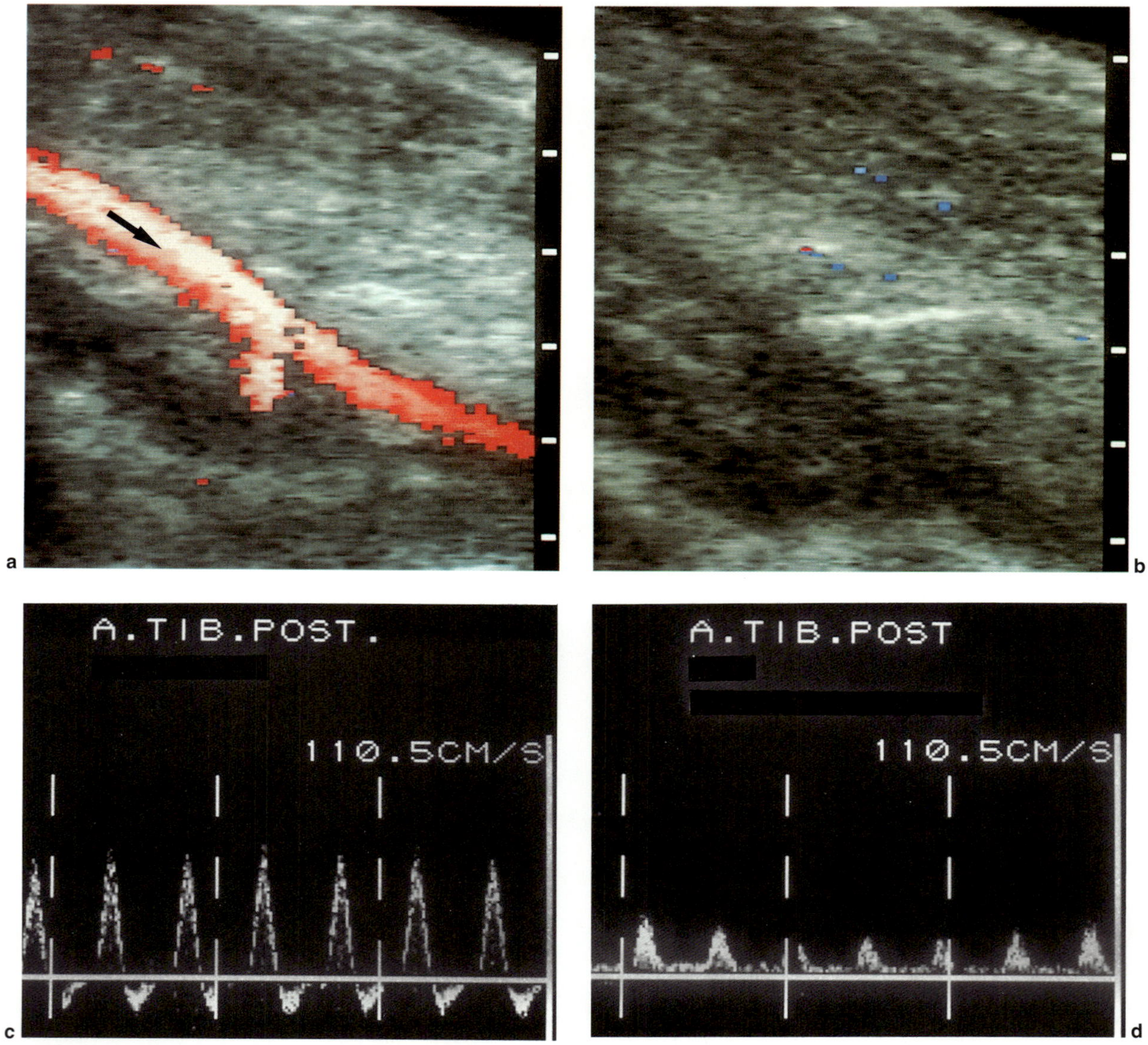

Fig. 6.**13 a–d** Popliteal entrapment syndrome
a Imaging at rest demonstrates normal flow in the proximal popliteal artery (arrow)
b Maximum extension of the knee and active plantar flexion against a resistance evokes a complete cessation of flow in the popliteal artery
c A normal Doppler spectrum is recorded in the distal posterior tibial artery at rest
d The spectrum during provocative testing (see **b**) shows minimal, collateral-derived flow in the distal posterior tibial artery

maximally extended, and the foot is actively and maximally plantar flexed against a resistance. In a positive test, flow in the popliteal artery ceases during effort, and Doppler spectrum sampling of the tibial arteries yields a low-amplitude postocclusive curve (Fig. 6.**13 a–d**). After completion of the maneuver, there is resumption of popliteal artery perfusion with reactive hyperemia in the lower leg.

6.4.4.2 Cystic Adventitial Degeneration

This is an etiologically obscure condition characterized by cyst formation in the adventitia of the vessel wall chiefly affecting the popliteal artery and occasionally involving other vessels (external iliac artery, femoral artery, radial artery, ulnar artery). There may be parallels with the development of articular ganglia (33). The variable state of filling of the cysts can produce luminal distortion ranging from a smoothly marginated, hemodynamically significant vascular obstruction to complete occlusion. The disease predominantly affects middle-aged men (average age 42 years, range 11–70 years) (5). The stenosis can be localized by CDS imaging, and the isolated, eccentric nature of the lesion and the patient's age should suggest a diagnosis of adventitial cyst. The efficacy of CDS in delineating these cysts and making a specific diagnosis is unclear at present due to a lack of personal experience and published reports.

6.4.4.3 Inflammatory Vascular Diseases

Only about 5% of arterial diseases are inflammatory in nature. A complete discussion of these conditions is beyond our present scope, and we refer interested readers to the literature (14). CDS, like other imaging procedures, does not provide a specific diagnosis. But when sonographic findings are interpreted in the light of clinical findings and the pattern of involvement, it may be possible to recognize the nature of the disease. For example, the detection of stenoses or occlusions in multiple supra-aortic arteries in young women would be consistent with Takayasu arteritis, whereas the detection of predominantly distal, rapidly progressive lesions of the upper- or lower-extremity arteries in young smokers would suggest thromboangiitis obliterans. On the whole, symmetric luminal narrowing that involves a long vessel segment and is unassociated with wall calcifications suggests an inflammatory cause. The involvement of small arteries in the setting of arteritis might be presumed from color duplex findings if a very high peripheral resistance or reduced flow velocity is detected in the large arteries accessible to examination.

6.4.4.4 Other Stenosing Disorders

Arterial stenoses and occlusions can have numerous causes besides atherosclerosis and inflammatory disease, and CDS is useful for localizing the lesion and assessing its severity. For example, the detection of symmetrical poststenotic spectra in the pelvic arteries with normal-appearing spectra in the upper extremity arteries is consistent with coarctation of the aorta. Stenoses caused by tumor compression, radiotherapy, trauma, or burns can be demonstrated in accessible vascular segments with the same accuracy as atherosclerotic lesions, whereas an acute traumatic arterial occlusion, with or without hemorrhage, is generally an indication for primary arteriography. The lesions of ergotism affect muscular arteries exclusively and present as long segmental vasospasms that may lead to occlusion in long-standing cases. CDS imaging, like angiography, can provide only indirect evidence of diabetic microangiopathy in cases where clinical signs are suggestive of diabetes mellitus (e. g., diabetic necrosis) and the larger demonstrable arteries are fully patent or show only minor changes that alone cannot account for the clinical symptoms. Often, however, noninvasive procedures are unrewarding in this population because the potentially extreme media sclerosis causes poor visualization of the arteries in the B-mode image and prevents accurate Doppler pressure measurements (noncompressible tibial vessels yield falsely elevated pressures). CDS in these cases can provide only a gross assessment based on comparative Doppler frequency analyses at sites where less calcified vessel wall segments can serve as an acoustic window. Angiography is often the only procedure that can establish a diagnosis in these cases.

6.4.5 Ischemia Due to Arterial Embolism

Acute arterial occlusion by thromboembolism can produce a more dramatic clinical picture than gradual thrombotic occlusion superimposed on preexisting stenosis, since sufficient collateral channels are generally unavailable in a healthy vascular system that is suddenly occluded by an embolus. From 80–90% of arterial emboli originate in the heart. The rest are arterioarterial emboli arising from an aneurysm or an atherosclerotic lesion. Arterial thromboemboli tend to lodge at sites where vessels divide (aortic bifurcation, femoral bifurcation, tibial trifurcation, brachial bifurcation) (Fig. 6.**14**), where they can create a nidus for the formation of proximal and distal appositional thrombi.

CDS imaging can detect the typical changes associated with a subtotal (Fig. 6.**15a**, **b**) or total vascular occlusion (Figs. 6.**11**, 6.**14**). If there is still residual

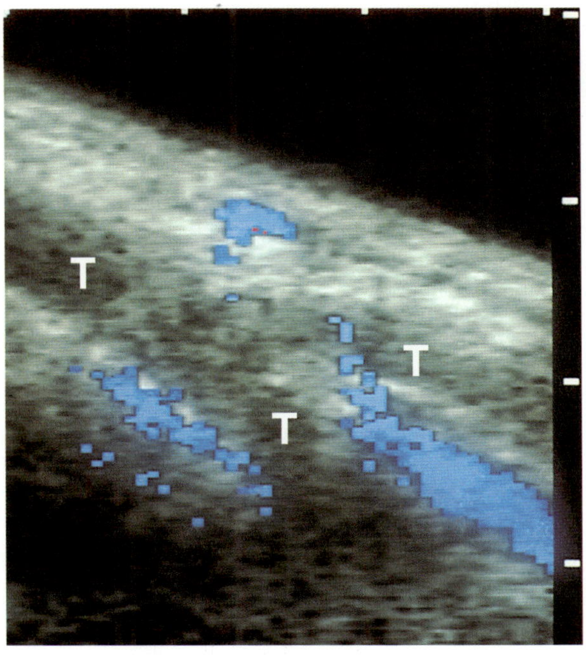

Fig. 6.**14** Complete thromboembolic occlusion of the brachial artery and its bifurcation. The lumina are occluded by hypoechoic thrombi (T) with no evidence of flow. The flow in adjacent veins is encoded blue (after manual compression of the distal forearm muscles)

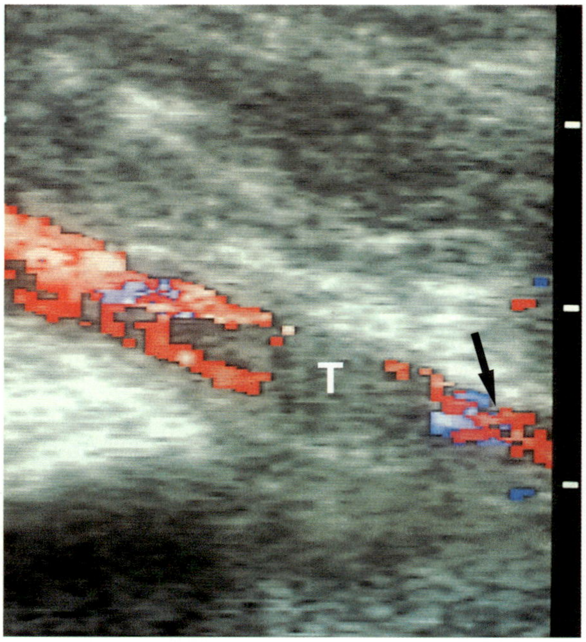

a

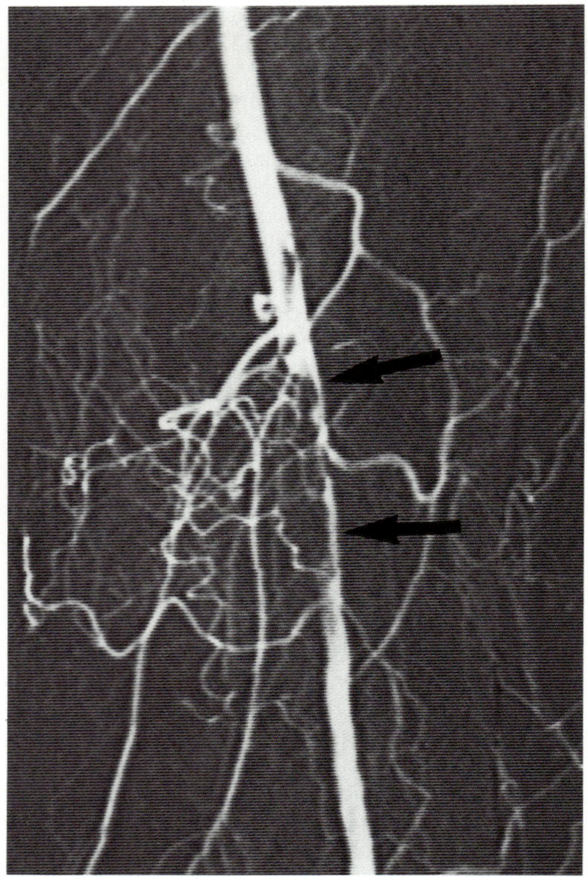

b

Fig. 6.**15a, b** Subtotal embolic occlusion of the superficial femoral artery
a CDS demonstrates the thrombus material (T), slight residual flow, and turbulence distal to the lesion (arrow)
b Intra-arterial DSA confirms subtotal occlusion of the superficial femoral artery by an embolus (arrows)

flow past the thromboembolus, ultrasound will demonstrate a hypoechoic mass in the vessel lumen with flow signals confined to the wall (Fig. 6.**15a**, **b**). With a complete embolic occlusion, it is often difficult to define the distal end of the occluded segment because of the extremely low flow velocities that prevail distally due to inadequate collateralization. Besides localizing the embolic occlusion, CDS is used to search for the source of the embolus in accessible vascular segments (aneurysm? stenosis?).

The most common sites of embolic arterial occlusion in the upper extremity are the distal axillary artery at its junction with the brachial artery and the bifurcation of the brachial artery into the radial and ulnar arteries. These occlusions are easily demonstrated with CDS, which can provide the foundation for planning an embolectomy (Figs. 6.**11**, 6.**14**). An absence of detectable digital artery flow in a patient with acute onset of symptoms and a history of predisposing disease is sufficient for the presumptive diagnosis of an embolic occlusion of the digital arteries.

6.4.6 Follow-up after PTA and Vascular Surgery

CDS also provides a noninvasive method for evaluating the efficacy of percutaneous transluminal angioplasty (PTA) (19) or vascular surgery (6). This pertains both to the outcome of the procedure and to potential complications relating to the procedure.

The goal of the PTA of a stenosis or occlusion is to reestablish a lumen that can deliver adequate flow to the peripheral vessels. This goal can be accomplished only by fragmentation of the atherosclerotic plaque, which tends to cause disruption of the intima or media (1). Besides enlarging the vessel lumen, this procedure often leaves marked surface irregularities that can be thrombogenic. This is transitory, however, and the irregular surface becomes smooth with passage of time. Restenosis can develop as a result of elastic rebound forces, wall dissection, fresh thrombus formation, intimal hyperplasia, or progression of atherosclerotic disease. Intra-arterial thrombolytic therapy (11) aims at dissolution of the thrombus by the combined action of administered plasmin activators and endogenous thrombolytic factors. Atherosclerotic stenosis remaining after the therapy is managed by transluminal dilatation. Other widely used PTA procedures are atherectomy (24) and stent implantation (9, 15, 34).

CDS imaging can demonstrate the vascular segments treated by an interventional procedure, even immediately after PTA (Figs. 6.**7**, 6.**9a** , **b**). The degree of residual stenosis can be described, recognizing,

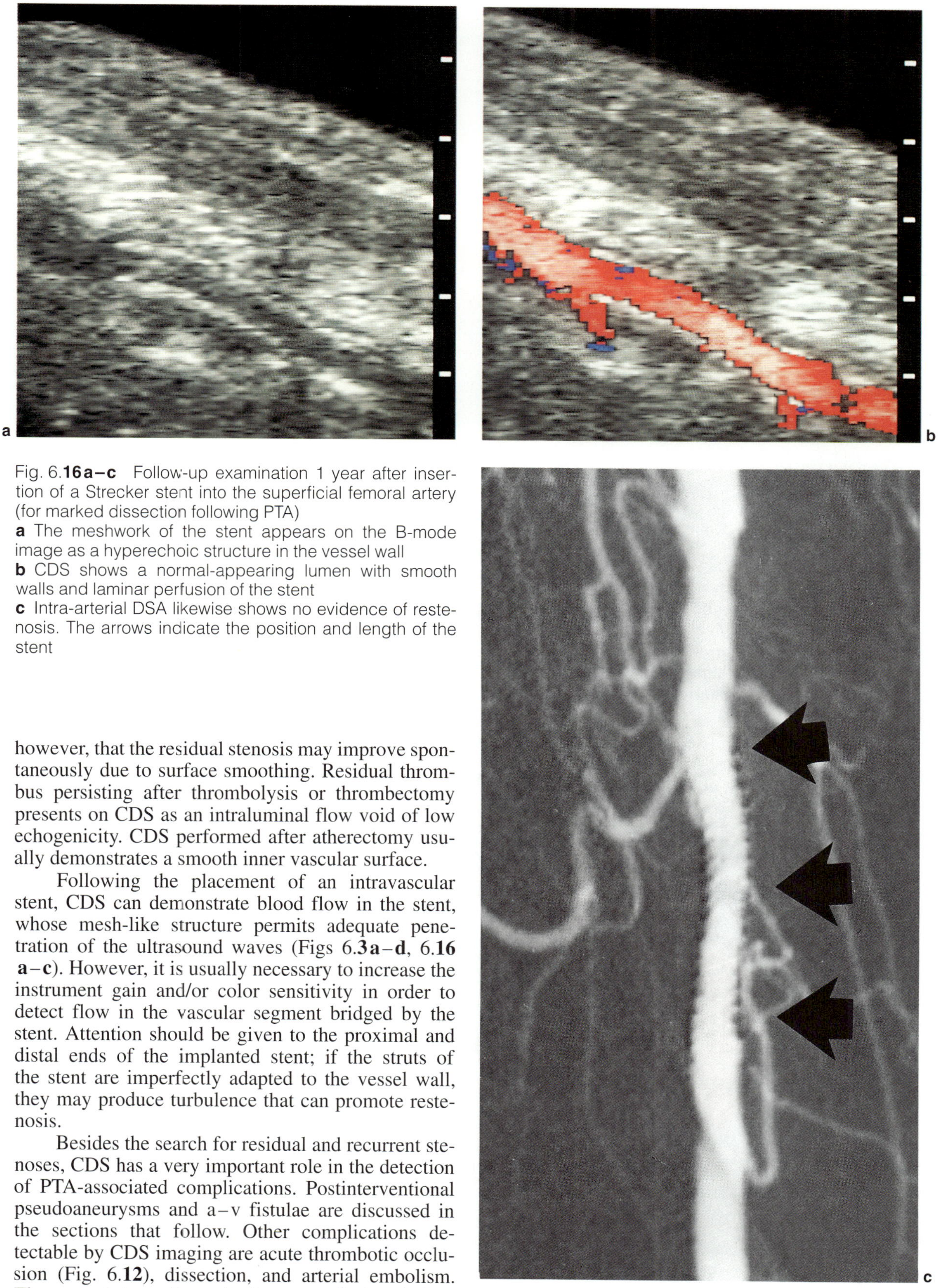

Fig. 6.**16 a–c** Follow-up examination 1 year after insertion of a Strecker stent into the superficial femoral artery (for marked dissection following PTA)
a The meshwork of the stent appears on the B-mode image as a hyperechoic structure in the vessel wall
b CDS shows a normal-appearing lumen with smooth walls and laminar perfusion of the stent
c Intra-arterial DSA likewise shows no evidence of restenosis. The arrows indicate the position and length of the stent

however, that the residual stenosis may improve spontaneously due to surface smoothing. Residual thrombus persisting after thrombolysis or thrombectomy presents on CDS as an intraluminal flow void of low echogenicity. CDS performed after atherectomy usually demonstrates a smooth inner vascular surface.

Following the placement of an intravascular stent, CDS can demonstrate blood flow in the stent, whose mesh-like structure permits adequate penetration of the ultrasound waves (Figs 6.**3a–d**, 6.**16 a–c**). However, it is usually necessary to increase the instrument gain and/or color sensitivity in order to detect flow in the vascular segment bridged by the stent. Attention should be given to the proximal and distal ends of the implanted stent; if the struts of the stent are imperfectly adapted to the vessel wall, they may produce turbulence that can promote restenosis.

Besides the search for residual and recurrent stenoses, CDS has a very important role in the detection of PTA-associated complications. Postinterventional pseudoaneurysms and a–v fistulae are discussed in the sections that follow. Other complications detectable by CDS imaging are acute thrombotic occlusion (Fig. 6.**12**), dissection, and arterial embolism. The same interpretive criteria are applied as before treatment.

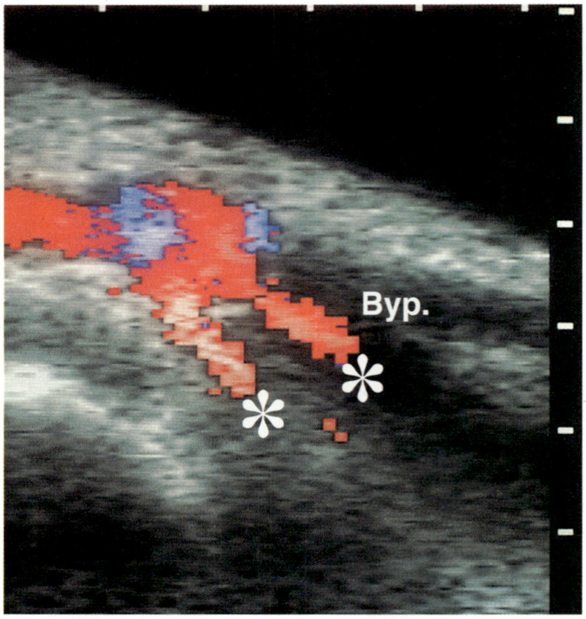

Fig. 6.**17** Complete occlusion of a femoropopliteal venous bypass. Aneurysmal luminal dilatation is evident at the proximal anastomosis. The bypass lumen (Byp.) is uniformly hypoechoic and devoid of flow signals. The asterisks indicate the perfused branches of the profunda femoris artery

After open vascular surgery (Fig. 6.**17**), it is as easy to confirm the patency of an autologous or prosthetic bypass with CDS as it is to demonstrate an artificial a–v fistula (7). At the distal anastomosis of an end-to-side femoropopliteal bypass, retrograde flow is commonly observed in the still-patent arterial segment proximal to the anastomosis. There may be some difficulty in evaluating the sites most commonly responsible for recurrence (intimal hyperplasia)—the anastomotic sites and their connections with the peripheral vessels (6)—due to increased ultrasound wave attenuation caused by surrounding scar tissue. Ultrasound can also demonstrate the status of vessels following endarterectomy, with or without a patch graft. Complications such as false aneurysms (Fig. 6.**18**) can occur after open vascular surgery as well as after PTA. A rare but important complication is prosthetic infection, recognized in the B-mode image by a hypoechoic fluid rim surrounding the prosthesis.

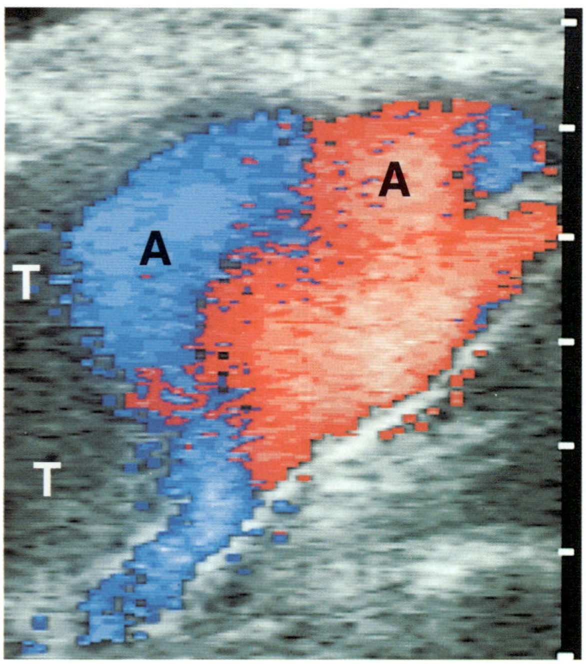

Fig. 6.**18** CDS image at the distal anastomosis of an iliofemoral bypass demonstrates a large false aneurysm (A) with areas of thrombosis (T) in its cranial portion

6.4.7 Dilatative Atherosclerosis, Aneurysms

Besides stenotic changes, atherosclerotic disease may lead to a diffuse or more circumscribed dilatation of arterial segments. The diffuse form of dilatative atherosclerosis leads to a marked slowing of blood flow in the ectatic segment, with risk of thrombotic occlusion. Aneurysms may affect not just the abdominal aorta but also the lower-extremity vessels, especially the iliac, femoral and popliteal arteries.

Other causes of aneurysms besides atherosclerosis include the various forms of arteritis and arterial compression syndromes. The clinical significance of these circumscribed dilatations, besides changes relating to the underlying disease, is based on the potential for rupture, incomplete thrombosis with risk of embolism, and complete vascular occlusion. CDS can quickly demonstrate both diffuse and circumscribed vascular dilatations, and the color-encoded flow image can delineate thrombosed elements (Fig. 6.**18**). Attention is also given to possible compression of surrounding vessels by the aneurysm (especially accom-

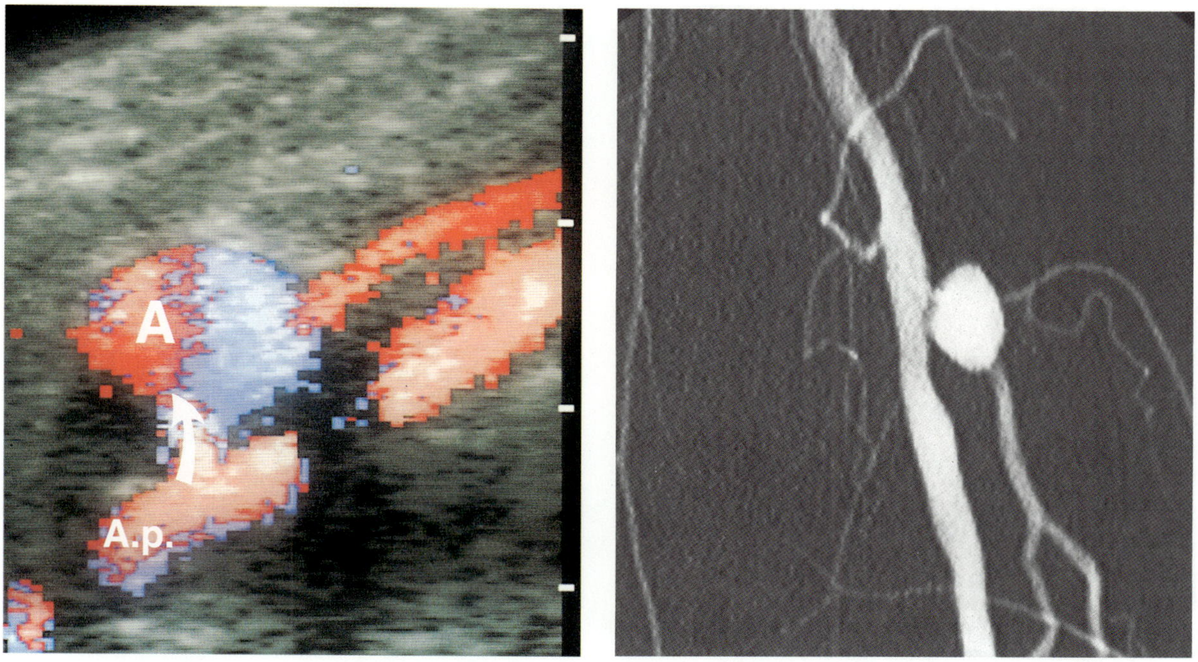

a b

Fig. 6.**19a, b** False aneurysm at the origin of a popliteal arterial branch supplying the anastomotic network of the knee. The lesion formed after a Simpson atherectomy of a popliteal artery stenosis
a CDS demonstrates the popliteal artery (A. p.), the neck of the aneurysm, the absence of mural thrombus in the aneurysm cavity (A), and a distal runoff artery. A short calcified wall segment just distal to the neck of the aneurysm casts an acoustic shadow but does not cause significant lumen reduction (absence of distal turbulence)
b Intra-arterial DSA confirms the CDS findings

panying veins) and to embolic complications. Aneurysms in the upper extremity region most commonly affect the subclavian artery.

6.4.8 False Aneurysms

A false aneurysm (pseudoaneurysm) develops when blood extravasates through a defect in the vessel wall (e. g., following an arterial puncture) and is contained by a pseudocapsule (Fig. 6.**19a**, **b**). The extravasation may stop spontaneously, allowing the aneurysm to resolve by thrombosis. If extravasation into the tissue persists, a pseudoaneurysm will develop that may go undetected for months. The danger of a false aneurysm lies in its potential for rupture, its ability to compress the vessel or origin and adjacent neurovascular structures, and embolization to peripheral vessels.

A false aneurysm develops in up to 4% of patients who undergo PTA or diagnostic cardiac catheterization (27). The typical presentation on CDS images is a pulsating, juxta-arterial mass containing a variable degree of turbulent flow that tends to enter the lesion in systole and exit in diastole. The neck of the aneurysm can usually be defined. For the planning of surgical treatment, it is important to identify the origin of the false aneurysm (in most cases the common femoral artery, profunda femoris, or superficial femoral artery). Mural thrombi appear as hypoechoic areas devoid of flow. Generally the displacement or compression of adjacent vessels is easily visible. Particular attention should be given to the concomitant presence of an a–v fistula.

Postcatheterization pseudoaneurysms have a high propensity for spontaneous thrombosis (approximately 60%). Due to the danger of rupture, which occurs in about 6% of cases, the patient should be closely followed while the lesion is active, and the degree of filling of the pseudoaneurysm cavity should be regularly assessed by CDS. The classic treatment for false aneurysm is surgical repair. It was found in a recent study (4) that definitive repair could be effected nonoperatively in 90% of patients by applying pressure with the transducer for several minutes until flow through the neck of the pseudoaneurysm was eliminated. The aneurysms that develop after vascular operations present basically the same imaging criteria; most form at anastomotic sites (Fig. 6. **18**) and after endarterectomies.

6.4.9 Arteriovenous Fistulae

Arteriovenous (a–v) fistulae can result from iatrogenic or other injury (Fig. 6.**20**) or may represent a congenital abnormality. The pathologic discharge of arterial blood into the venous system (low-pressure system) causes an increase of flow in the artery supplying the fistula. Often this feature alone can direct atten-

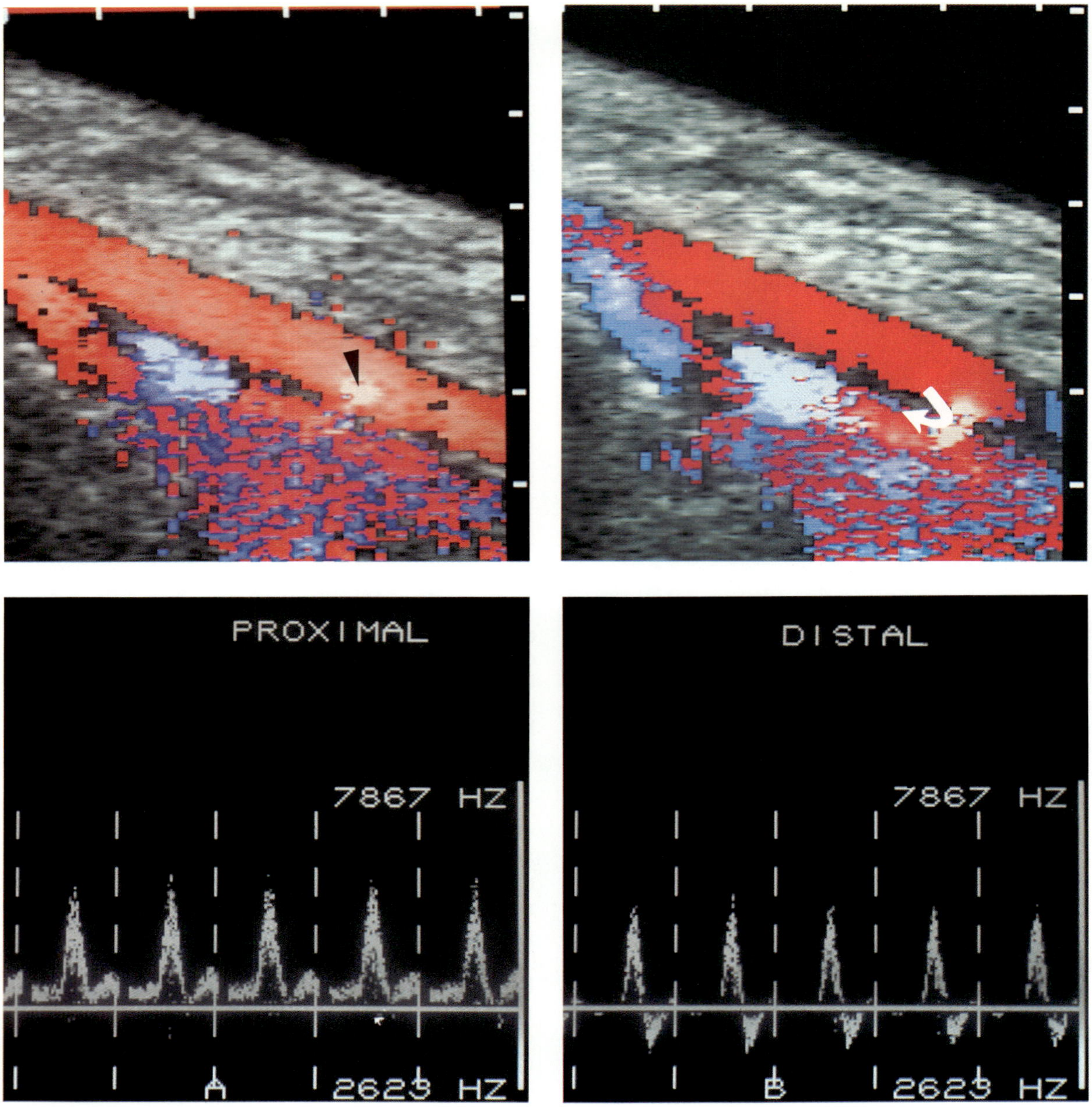

Fig. 6.**20 a–d** Arteriovenous fistula from the superficial femoral artery (SFA) following left heart catheterization. CDS measurement indicated an integral volume flow in the fistula of 130 mL/min (flow in SFA_{prox} – flow in SFA_{distal})
a Image in systole shows locally increased flow velocities (arrow) at the posterior wall of the SFA 3 cm distal to the origin (puncture site), where fast-moving blood is entering the adjacent superficial femoral vein. The high flow velocities cause marked vibration of the venous wall and perivascular soft tissues ("color cloud")
b Image in diastole shows persistence of antegrade flow in the proximal SFA due to the locally decreased peripheral vascular resistance (see **c**). Diastolic reverse flow is observed in the profunda femoris and in the SFA distal to the a–v fistula (high peripheral resistance, see **d**)
c Doppler spectrum from the SFA 1 cm proximal to the a–v fistula confirms the diastolic antegrade flow as a sign of decreased vascular resistance
d A normal waveform is recorded from the SFA 1 cm distal to the a–v fistula

tion to the presence of a fistula (Figs. 6.**20**, 4.7**a**, **b**). The main criterion for a CDS diagnosis of a–v fistula is the detection of perivascular tissue vibrations (25) caused by the high flow velocities in the fistula. The perivascular, cloud-like mosaic of red and blue signals can completely obscure the lesion, but gentle compression of the feeding artery may be able to slow the flow and reduce the mosaic artifact. This is particularly important for the precise localization of the fistula. The volume flow through the a–v fistula can be quantified by making comparative flow determinations in the segments proximal and distal to the fistula.

6.4.10 Common Pitfalls

Besides operator errors and faulty settings (e. g., threshold too low leading to false-positive diagnosis of occlusion, inadequate color encoding due to an unfavorable angle between the transducer and flow direction or a large distance between the transducer and vessel), certain patterns of disease such as multilevel stenoses or occlusions can lead to misinterpretation. This is especially true if the flow distal to one or more stenoses or occlusions is so slow that it is below the instrument's threshold of detection. Therefore, before an occlusion is diagnosed a final attempt should be made to detect blood flow by adjusting the instrument settings (higher sensitivity) and decreasing the Doppler angle.

Short occlusions are occasionally misdiagnosed, especially if the occluded area is bypassed by a large collateral that roughly follows the course of the occluded artery. In this case the collateral can simulate vascular continuity and lead to the false diagnosis of a long stenosis.

In examinations of the distal portion of the anterior tibial artery, excessive plantar flexion of the foot at the ankle joint should be avoided, as this can cause stretching, compression, and functional occlusion of the dorsalis pedis artery.

PTA as well as vascular operations are followed by a period of peripheral arterial dilatation, sometimes lasting days, that results in decreased pulsatility of the arterial flow. The Doppler spectra obtained in this situation should not be misinterpreted as indicating stenotic disease. If necessary, the entire course of the vessel should be surveyed in the color-encoded image to exclude a stenosis as the cause of the spectral changes.

6.5 Diagnostic Value of Color Duplex Sonography in Relation to Other Diagnostic Procedures

CW Doppler blood pressure measurements continue to be a mainstay in screening examinations for arterial occlusive disease (2, 13, 20). They cannot and should not be replaced by the significantly more costly and complex procedure of CDS. But CW Doppler ultrasound does not supply morphologic information, so imaging procedures are necessary for the planning of invasive therapy.

Arterial angiography is the gold standard by which new imaging procedures must be judged (18). Evaluations of CDS in comparison with arterial angiography have consistently documented the high accuracy of CDS in the detection of stenoses and occlusions (Table 6.**2**). Problems exist, however, in the quantification of lesions distal to a significant proximal lesion in patients with multilevel disease. The examiner is apt to overinterpret a high-grade stenosis as an occlusion, or mistake an occlusion for a severe stenosis in cases of this kind. This particularly applies to lesions in the adductor canal, where it may not be possible to demonstrate the finding accurately, and the diagnosis must rely on the analysis of proximal and distal spectra.

In the gross classification of stenoses, it has been found that CDS can correctly classify the severity of a lesion as a low-grade stenosis, high-grade stenosis, or occlusion in 81–87% of cases (Table 6.**2**), although only a subjective classification of angiographic findings was made in these studies. The proximal point of an occlusion can almost always be accurately defined with CDS. The length of the occlusion may be overestimated due to the very slow flow that often prevails distal to the occluded site.

Disadvantages of CDS compared with arterial angiography relate to the physical barriers posed by obesity and intervening bowel gas. This can lead to diagnostic uncertainty, especially in the pelvis, although many doubts can be resolved by analysis of the Doppler spectrum distal to the nonvisualized vessel section. A significant advantage of angiography over CDS lies in its ability to provide a broad, continuous survey of the arterial tree, making the findings eas-

Table 6.**2** Results of CDS in the diagnosis of lower extremity AOD in comparison with arteriography (* = tibial arteries also evaluated)

Authors	n (patients)	Sensitivity	Specificity	Accuracy	Correct grading of severity
Koennecke (16)	53*	97%	97%	97%	81%
Landwehr (19)	52*	92%	99%	96%	87%
Polak (32)	17	88%	95%	93%	–

ier to demonstrate and review. This places particularly high demands on the CDS examiner.

CDS can achieve markedly better results than conventional duplex scanning, especially with regard to sensitivity (which is about 80% with conventional duplex [12]). Moreover, CDS is much more rapid and efficient since the flow dynamics can be appreciated at once from the color-encoded image.

The diagnostic accuracy of CDS in the detection of aneurysms and a–v fistulae is very high and generally obviates the need for angiography (26, 27, 31).

Given the importance of conservative treatment options, an invasive diagnostic procedure should be performed only if invasive therapy appears promising and is consented to by the patient. Thus CDS has a place in the diagnostic evaluation of pAOD whenever the clinical findings and Doppler pressure measurements are suggestive of pAOD, and a decision has to be made with regard to further invasive procedures. If CDS demonstrates a lesion that is probably accessible to a PTA procedure (e. g., isolated stenosis or short-to-moderate arterial occlusion in the pelvis or thigh), then PTA may be planned without having to perform diagnostic and therapeutic angiography in separate sittings (3, 19). Diagnostic arterial angiography should be performed only if the CDS findings are equivocal. Generally there are no valid indications for intravenous DSA (Fig. 6.**5**). At present, CDS alone is not believed to provide an adequate workup prior to reconstructive vascular surgical procedures, because arterial angiography can provide the surgeon with a significantly broader and more detailed vascular survey than is obtainable with CDS. As this still relatively new procedure gains wider acceptance, however, it is reasonable to speculate that certain reconstructive vascular procedures (e. g., profundaplasty, endarterectomy of short stenoses in the common femoral artery, revision of stenotic bypass anastomoses) will increasingly be performed without angiography (17). In cases where a major bypass procedure is proposed, global angiographic views of the vascular anatomy and pathology probably cannot be replaced by CDS scanning. On the other hand, even today the detection of certain postinterventional and postoperative complications by CDS, such as aneurysms and a–v fistulae, is entirely sufficient in most cases for the planning of corrective surgery.

If the results of CDS imaging and/or general factors contraindicate an invasive therapy, further diagnostic investigations are not required.

In evaluating the results of PTA (19) and vascular operations (7), CDS generally leads to a definitive diagnosis without the need for angiography. The patency of a bypass graft following a revascularization procedure can be reliably assessed (6, 30). Even stenoses and a–v fistulae can be detected or excluded with high accuracy in comparison with angiography, though in some cases it can be difficult to evaluate the connecting vessels distal to the bypass (6).

Magnetic resonance angiography is currently undergoing clinical testing (29). It remains to be seen how this noninvasive procedure will compare with CDS in terms of reliability, cost effectiveness and required examination time in the evaluation of vascular disease.

6.6 References

1 Becker, G.J., B.T. Katzen: Noncoronary angioplasty. Radiology 170 (1989) 921–940

2 Bernstein, F.F., A. Fronek: Current status of noninvasive tests in the diagnosis of peripheral arterial disease. Surg. Clin. N. Amer. 62 (1982) 473 –487

3 Davies, A. H., T. R. Magee, R. Parry, J. Hayward, P. Murphy, S. E. A. Cole, R. N. Baird, M. Horrocks: Duplex ultrasonography and pulse-generated run-off in selecting claudicants for femoropopliteal angioplasty. Br. J. Surg. 79 (1992) 894–896

4 Fellmeth, B.D., A.C. Roberts, J.J. Bookstein, J.A. Freischlag, J.R. Forsythe, N.K. Buckner, R.J. Hye: Postangiographic femoral artery injuries: nonsurgical repair with US-guided compression. Radiology 178 (1991) 671–675

5 Flanigan, D.P., S.J. Burnham, J.J. Goodreau et al.: Summary of cases of adventitial cystic disease of the popliteal artery. Ann. Surg. 189 (1979) 165

6 Fürst, G., F.-P. Kuhn, R.-P. Trappe, H.-W. Kniemeyer, U. Mödder: Bildgebende Diagnostik nach rekonstruktiver Arterienchirurgie der unteren Extremitäten. Fortschr. Röntgenstr. 151 (1989) 666–673

7 deGier, P., S. Sommeling, E. van Dulken, E. Truyen, J. Buth: Stenosis development at the distal anastomosis of prosthetic bypasses for aortoiliac occlusive disease. Incidence and accuracy of colour flow duplex in the diagnosis. Eur. J. Vasc. Surg. 7 (1993) 237–244

8 Gray, H., C.M. Goss: Anatomy of the human body. Lea & Febiger, Philadelphia (1973)

9 Günther, R.W., D. Vorwerk, K. Bohndorf, I. Peters, A. El-Din, B. Messmer: Iliac and femoral artery stenoses and occlusions: treatment with intravascular stents. Radiology 172 (1989) 725–730

10 Hendrickx, Ph., U. Roth, F. Brassel, K. Taubert, C. Ranke, H.H. Wagner: Phantomuntersuchungen zur Wertigkeit der farbkodierten Doppler-Sonographie bei der arteriellen Verschlußkrankheit der Extremitäten. Fortschr. Röntgenstr. 152 (1990) 1–5

11 Hess, H., A. Mietaschk, R. Brückl: Peripheral arterial occlusions: a 6-year experience with local low-dose thrombolytic therapy. Radiology 163 (1987) 753–758

12 Jäger, K.A., D.J. Phillips, R.L. Martin, C. Hanson, G.O. Roederer, Y.E. Langlois, H.J. Ricketts, D.E. Strandness jr.: Noninvasive mapping of lower limb arterial lesions. Ultrasound. Med. Biol. 11 (1985) 515–521

13 Johnston, K.W., M.Y. Hosang, D.F. Andrews: Reproducibility of noninvasive vascular laboratory measurements of the peripheral circulation. J. vasc. Surg. 6 (1987) 147–151

14 Kappert, A.: Lehrbuch und Atlas der Angiologie. H. Huber, Bern (1987)

15 Kauffmann, G.W., G.M. Richter, G. Nöldge, Th. Roeren, P. Landwehr, K. Lackner: Vier Jahre Erfahrung mit der ballonexpandierbaren Endoprothese. Radiologe 31 (1991) 202–209

16 Koennecke, H.-C., F. Fobbe, M.M. Hamed, K.-J. Wolf: Diagnostik arterieller Gefäßerkrankungen der unteren Extremitäten mit der farbkodierten Duplexsonographie. Fortschr. Röntgenstr. 151 (1989) 42–46

17 Kohler, T.R., G. Andros, J.M. Porter, A. Clowes, J. Goldstone, K. Johansen, E. Raker, D.R. Nance: Can duplex scanning replace arteriography for lower extremity arterial disease? Ann. vasc. Surg. 4 (1990) 280–287

18 Lackner, K., Th. Harder, M. Herter, N. Leipner: Vergleich der intraarteriellen digitalen Subtraktionsangiographie mit der konventionellen Angiographie. Fortschr. Röntgenstr. 141 (1984) 616–624

19 Landwehr, P., K. Lackner: Farbkodierte Duplexsonographie vor und nach PTA der Arterien der unteren Extremität. Fortschr. Röntgenstr. 152 (1990) 35–41

20 Lepäntalo, M., O. Lindfors, P. Pekkola: The ankle/arm systolic blood pressure ratio as a screening test for arterial insufficiency in the lower limb. Ann. Chir. Gynaecol. 72 (1983) 57–62

21 Longley, D. G., J. W. Yedlicka, E. J. Molina, S. Schwabacher, D. W. Hunter, J. G. Letourneau: Thoracic outlet syndrome: evaluation of the subclavian vessels by color duplex sonography. Amer. J. Roentgenol. 158 (1992) 623–630
22 Luska, G., U. Risch, M. Pellengahr, H. v. Boetticher: Farbcodierte doppler-sonographische Untersuchungen zur Morphologie und Hämodynamik der Arterien des Beckens und der Beine bei gesunden Probanden. Fortschr. Röntgenstr. 153 (1990) 246–251
23 Mahler, F.: Systolische Blutdruckmessung. In Kriessmann, A., A. Bollinger, H. Keller: Praxis der Doppler-Sonographie, 2. Aufl. Thieme, Stuttgart (1990) 21–32
24 Maynar, M., R. Reyes, V. Cabrera, M. Roman, J.M. Pulido, F. Castaneda, J.G. Letourneau, W.R. Castaneda-Zuniga: Percutaneous atherectomy as an alternative treatment for postangioplasty obstructive intimal flaps. Radiology 170 (1989) 1029–1031
25 Middleton, W.D., S. Erickson, G.L. Melson: Perivascular color artifact: pathologic significance and appearence on US color Doppler images. Radiology 171 (1989) 647–652
26 Mitchell, D.G., L. Needleman, M. Bezzi, B.B. Goldberg, A.B. Kurtz, R.G. Pennell, M.D. Rifkin, M. Vilaro, O.H. Baltarowich: Femoral artery pseudoaneurysm: Diagnosis with conventional duplex and color Doppler US. Radiology 165 (1987) 687–690
27 Moll, R., W. Habscheid, P. Landwehr: Häufigkeit des Aneurysma spurium der Arteria femoralis nach Herzkatheteruntersuchung und PTA. Fortschr. Röntgenstr. 154 (1991) 23–27
28 Müller-Bühl, U., C. Diehm, U. Sieben et al.: Prävalenz und Risikofaktoren von peripherer arterieller Verschlußkrankheit und koronarer Herzkrankheit. Vasa 16 (Suppl.) 4 (1987)
29 Mulligan, S.A., T. Matsuda, P. Lanzer, G.M. Gross, W.D. Routh, F.S. Keller, D.B. Koslin, L.L. Berland, M.D. Fields, M. Doyle, G.B. Cranney, J.Y. Lee, G.H. Pohost: Peripheral arterial occlusive disease: prospective comparison of MR angiography and color duplex US with conventional angiography. Radiology 178 (1991) 695–700
30 Polak, J.F., M.C. Donaldson, G.R. Dobkin, J.A. Mannick, D.H. O'Leary: Early detection of saphenous vein arterial bypass graft stenosis by color-assisted duplex sonography. Amer. J. Roentgenol. 154 (1990) 857–861
31 Polak, J.F., M.C. Donaldson, A.D. Whittemore, J.A. Mannick, D.H. O'Leary: Pulsatile masses surrounding vascular prostheses: real-time US color flow imaging. Radiology 170 (1989) 363–366
32 Polak, J.F., M.I. Mitchell, J.A. Mannick, D.H. O'Leary, M.C. Donaldson, A.D. Whittemore: Determination of the extent of lower-extremity peripheral arterial disease with color-assisted duplex sonography. Amer. J. Roentgenol. 155 (1990) 1085–1089
33 Rich, N.: Popliteal entrapment and adventitial cystic disease. Surg. Clin. N. Amer. 62 (1982) 449–465
34 Strecker, E.-P., D. Liermann, K.H. Barth, H.R.D. Wolf, N. Freudenberg, G. Berg, M. Westphal, P. Tsikuras, M. Savin, B. Schneider: Expandable tubular stent for treatment of arterial occlusive diseases: experimental and clinical results. Radiology 175 (1990) 97–102
35 Towne, J.B., D.L. Rollins: Profundaplasty: its role in limb salvage. Surg. Clin. N. Amer. 66 (1986) 403–414
36 Widmer, L.K., A. Da Silva, G. Madar: Epidemiologie der Gefäßkrankheiten. In Kappert, A.: Lehrbuch und Atlas der Angiologie. Huber, Bern (1987) 312–318
37 Widmer, L.K., H.B. Stähelin, C. Nissen, A. Da Silva: Venen-, Arterien-Krankheiten, koronare Herzkrankheit bei Berufstätigen. Huber, Bern (1981)
38 Williams, P. L., R. Warwick, M. Dyson, L. H. Bannister: Grays Anatomy, 37th ed, Churchill Livingstone, Edinburgh 1989

7 Hemodialysis Shunt

P. Landwehr

7.1 General Remarks

The surgical creation of an arteriovenous (a–v) fistula for hemodialysis access has become a standard procedure in the treatment of chronic end-stage renal failure. Percutaneously or surgically implanted central venous catheter systems are only suitable for short-term vascular access prior to the construction of an a–v fistula, in patients with reversible renal failure, or as a fallback procedure for creating access under unfavorable conditions (5, 14, 27). For all the patients with renal failure who either wait for a donor kidney or have contraindications for renal transplantation or peritoneal dialysis, the only option is long-term hemodialysis. The survival and quality of life of dialysis patients in this situation are critically influenced by the functional competence of the a–v fistula.

The use of a dialysis fistula requires frequent venipunctures (several per week using one or two needles) that inflict chronic trauma on the access vein, which is already traumatized by the unphysiologically high flow rates through the fistula. Published reports on the patency rates of Brescia–Cimino (BC) fistulas and prosthetic grafts vary depending on patient selection, study criteria, surgical technique, and experience. Recent findings indicate that 80–90% of BC fistulas are still functioning well at 1 year, 63–87% at 2 years, and approximately 65% at 4 years. The corresponding rates for synthetic grafts are 62–90% at 1 year, 50–79% at 2 years, and about 40% at 4 years (1, 16, 17, 23, 25, 26, 28). With passage of time, then, functional problems arise in a substantial percentage of hemodialysis fistulas.

The frequency of recurring access problems requires a method of examination that is accurate, noninvasive, and can be repeated as often as needed to evaluate the morphology and function of the fistula. Clinical examination of the fistula by palpation and auscultation and the assessment of fistula function during dialysis by estimating the maximum attainable flow rate, measuring blood pressure in the venous outflow tract, and determining serum parameters of retention are useful for assessing the nature and extent of access failure. But an accurate evaluation of the pathologic changes and optimum therapeutic solution (modifying the puncture technique, moving the access site, percutaneous transluminal angioplasty [PTA], surgical revision) must rely on imaging procedures. CDS has established itself in recent years as the procedure of first choice for the evaluation of hemodialysis access problems (18, 21, 29).

7.2 Types of Vascular Access and Examination Technique

7.2.1 Preliminary Remarks

A basic distinction is drawn between native internal arteriovenous fistulas and synthetic graft fistulas. The most commonly used internal fistula involves the surgical creation of an anastomosis between a subcutaneous vein and an artery. The low resistance in the venous system leads to a substantial increase of blood flow in the artery and thus in the communicating vein. The unphysiologically high venous flow leads to dilatation of the vein and thickening of its wall, providing a vascular access segment that can be punctured several times weekly with a large-gauge needle for performing hemodialysis at a flow rate of 200–300 mL/min. If adequate venous segments are not available for the development of an access vein, a synthetic bridge graft can be used to establish the necessary arteriovenous fistula.

The potential need for reintervention must be considered during creation of the fistula. The first principle is to place the fistula as far distally as the condition of the vessels will permit. The first fistula is constructed near the wrist, therefore. The internal arteriovenous anastomosis is usually performed using an end-of-vein-to-side-of-artery technique (13) so that the arterial segment distal to the anastomosis will remain patent even if the anastomosis or vein becomes occluded. If the anastomosis or perianastomotic vein develops a stenosis that cannot be corrected by PTA, the access vein can be reanastomosed to the artery at a site several centimeters proximal to the original a–v fistula.

A second principle of vascular access surgery is that it is better to place the fistula in the upper extremity than in the leg. This is advantageous in terms of care of the access site. Also, the arterial supply of the leg is more frequently involved by peripheral arterial occlusive disease (pAOD), which can jeopardize the function of the fistula and exacerbate AOD-related complaints.

A third principle of access surgery is that it is better to use a native internal a–v fistula than a synthetic graft, since the patency rates of internal fistulas are superior to those of bypass grafts (see section 7.1), and synthetic materials are more susceptible to infection than endogenous veins.

Despite the general validity of these principles, recurring access problems or a lack of suitable peripheral vessels may make it necessary to deviate from these principles during the course of long-term dialysis. In evaluating access problems, the user of color duplex sonography is confronted with a variety of fistula designs, some incorporating synthetic materials and some involving the use of "atypical" vessels. Often, therefore, the examiner must work jointly with the vascular surgeon and nephrologist to elucidate the morphology of complicated fistulas. The most common types of vascular access are described in the sections below.

7.2.2 Brescia–Cimino Fistula

This type of a–v fistula, first described in the 1960s (4), is still the procedure of choice for the initial construction of a dialysis fistula. The classic Brescia–Cimino (BC) fistula involves the creation of a distal anastomosis between the radial artery and cephalic vein (forearm fistula). An end-of-vein-to-side-of-artery anastomosis is currently favored over the original side-to-side technique (see Section 7.2.1) (Fig. 7.**1a**, **b**). In the event of perianastomotic access problems, the basic access design can be maintained by progressive "proximalization" of the fistula, which may be done at the time of revision. As an alternative to the radiocephalic fistula, anastomosing the ulnar artery to the basilic vein can also provide an effective forearm fistula. The brachiocephalic or brachiobasilic fistula replicates the basic BC fistula design in the upper arm (Figs. 7.**1b**, 7.**2**). Occasionally the proposed access vessel (e. g., the basilic vein) can be translocated to a subcutaneous position to provide a longer venous segment for dialysis.

The primary BC fistula is usually not ready for immediate use, because time is needed for the vein to undergo sufficient dilatation and wall thickening. An average of 3–4 weeks is needed for maturation of the primary a–v fistula. If an initially functioning fistula must be moved to a more proximal site due to perianastomotic stenosis, it is usually possible to use part of the former access segment, so the fistula can be utilized for dialysis immediately after the revision.

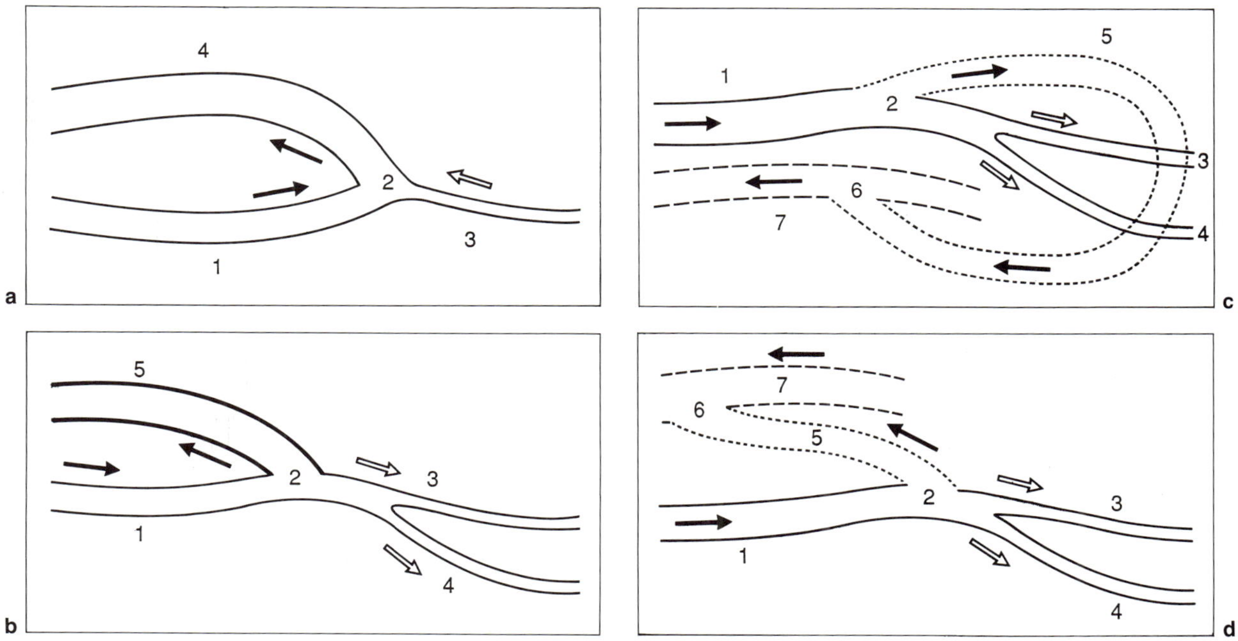

Fig. 7.**1a–d** Most common types of surgically constructed a–v fistulas for hemodialysis (arrows = direction of blood flow)

a Forearm fistula (Brescia–Cimino). 1 = Afferent artery (usually the radial artery), 2 = side-to-end a–v anastomosis, 3 = radial artery distal to the anastomosis, usually carries retrograde flow with a competent palmar arch, 4 = arterialized access vein

b Upper arm fistula (Brescia–Cimino). 1 = Afferent artery (brachial artery), 2 = side-to-end a–v anastomosis, 3 = radial artery, 4 = ulnar artery, 5 = access vein

c Synthetic loop graft in the forearm. The anastomoses (2 = arterial, 6 = venous) are usually placed in the distal upper arm. 1 = Afferent artery (brachial artery), 3 = radial artery, 4 = ulnar artery, 5 = loop synthetic graft (access segment), 7 = outflow vein

d Synthetic interposition graft in the upper arm. 1 = Afferent artery (brachial artery), 2 = arterial anastomosis, 3 = radial artery, 4 = ulnar artery, 5 = interposition graft (access segment), 6 = venous anastomosis, 7 = outflow vein

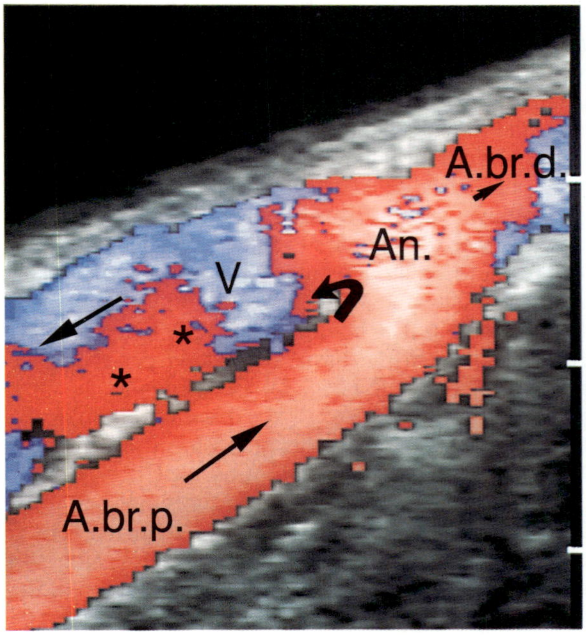

Fig. 7.**2** CDS appearance of a normally functioning Brescia–Cimino dialysis fistula in the upper arm. Most of the inflow is diverted proximally into the access vein, while some continues on toward the periphery. The scan demonstrates normal zones of flow reversal at the wall of the access vein (asterisks). A. br. p. = Brachial artery proximal to the anastomosis, A. br. d. = brachial artery distal to the anastomosis, An. = anastomosis, V = access vein, arrows = direction of blood flow

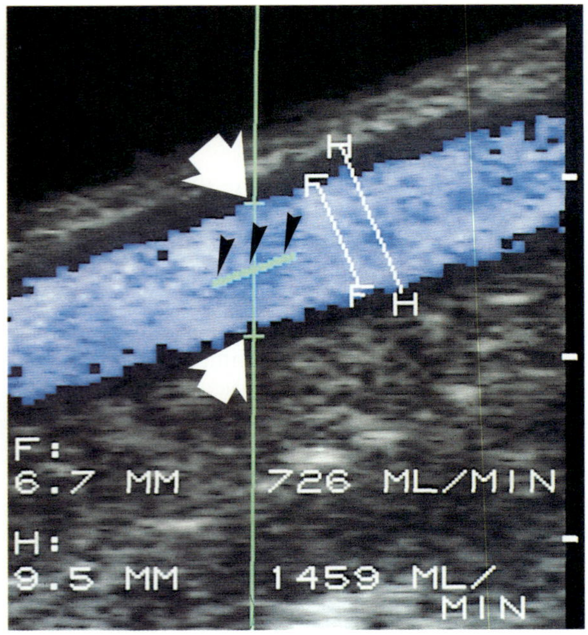

Fig. 7.**3** Normal PTFE bridge graft after several years' use. CDS image demonstrates normal blood flow in the graft with uniform, hypoechoic thickening of all portions of the graft wall. Color encoding of the perfused lumen makes it easier to determine the vessel diameter (*F*) and position the boundary markers (arrows) for determining volume flow. Without color-encoded flow, there would be a tendency to overestimate the vessel diameter (*H*) and thus the volume flow. Arrowheads indicate the angle-correction cursor

7.2.3 PTFE Graft

If there is a lack of usable forearm vessels, either primarily or as a result of previous access prodedures, synthetic grafts can be implanted to replace the function of the access vein. Polytetrafluoroethylene (PTFE) has proved to be an excellent graft material. This material has a mesh-like texture that is receptive to the formation of a neointima.

Two basic types of PTFE graft design are commonly used for graft fistulas in the upper extremity. In both types the distal brachial artery functions as the inflow vessel (end-of-graft-to-side-of-artery), since its larger diameter affords more favorable conditions for anastomosis to synthetic material than the more distal arteries. The graft itself may be placed as a subcutaneous U-shaped loop in the forearm and anastomosed to the basilic or brachial vein (forearm PTFE loop graft), or it may be interposed as a straight graft between the brachial artery and the basilic, cephalic, brachial, or axillary vein (upper arm PTFE interposition graft) (Fig. 7.**1 c**,**d**). Loop grafts can also be placed in the upper arm if the arterial and venous anastomoses are at a more proximal level (e. g., axillary artery and vein).

Occasionally, when there is a lack of usable vessels in both arms, a leg shunt can be constructed by anastomosing a PTFE loop graft end-to-side to the proximal superficial femoral artery and to the great saphenous vein or femoral vein.

In principle, functioning PTFE jump grafts require no maturation delay and can be used for dialysis immediately after surgery. The standard diameter of a PTFE tube graft is about 6 mm. A tapered graft (e. g., 4 mm at the anastomotic site and 6 mm in the access segment) can be used to reduce the flow rate through the fistula. This may be done, for example, to avoid a steal syndrome in patients with preexisting pAOD or to avoid exacerbation of preexisting cardiac failure by excessive fistula flow.

7.2.4 Other Grafts and Shunts

If a sufficiently long access segment is not available for dialysis in a BC fistula with a functioning a–v anastomosis, the fistula can be salvaged by resecting the affected venous segment and interposing a PTFE graft in end-to-end fashion (venovenous PTFE interposition graft). Short arteriovenous PTFE interposition grafts also can be used in patients with anastomotic stenoses.

Autologous saphenous vein interposition grafts or bovine carotid artery heterografts can be used in principle, but these materials are not recommended because of their markedly poorer long-term results .

In the Scribner extracorporeal shunt, a length of external silicone tubing connected between an arterial and venous cannula is used for insertion of dialysis needles (24). Rarely used today, this shunt has been largely superseded by central venous dialysis catheters for short-term vascular access.

7.2.5 Examination Technique

7.2.5.1 Preliminary Remarks

If possible, the CDS examination of a dialysis fistula should be performed either prior to dialysis or on a day when dialysis is not scheduled, to avoid examination-related infection or postprocedural bleeding from the last puncture site. If acute problems arise that may require prompt intervention (especially if there is suspicion of acute thrombosis), the fistula may be examined with the dialysis needle in place, with the dressing in place, or after careful removal of the dressing. In the latter case an antiseptic spray or sterile ultrasound gel should be used as a coupling medium.

7.2.5.2 History and Preliminary Studies

Before the fistula is examined by CDS, a specific vascular access history is taken, giving particular attention to how many fistulae have been constructed, the age of the present fistula (since its construction, PTA, or surgical revision), previous access-related infections, underlying diseases that might affect the vessels, the puncture technique (single-needle or two-needle system), and the nature of the dialysis problem (poor arterial flow, increased venous pressure, difficulties with needle placement, development of collateral veins, underdialysis despite an adequate flow rate, postdialysis bleeding or hematoma, pain in the access extremity, swelling of the extremity, progressive cardiac failure with suspicion of excessive fistula flow, suspected access infection). Quantitative data should be obtained on the maximum possible flow rate during dialysis and on the venous outflow pressure for a given flow rate. The examiner should palpate the fistula himself to gain an impression of its configuration.

7.2.5.3 Instrumentation

Because the fistula is almost always located near the skin surface, and to achieve the highest possible spatial resolution, a transducer with a high operating frequency (7.5 MHz) should be used for examination of the fistula. A 5-MHz transducer should also be available for examining the afferent arteries and the veins in the upper arm and axilla, especially in obese patients. A linear transducer with a wedge-shaped standoff pad or electronic beam steering is preferred (see Chapter 4). If a transducer with beam steering is used, it may be helpful to attach a standoff pad to the transducer, depending on the quality of the image in the near field. The instrument gain setting and color sensitivity usually have to be reduced due to the proximity of the fistula to the transducer.

7.2.5.4 Position of the Patient and Examiner

The fistula may be examined with the patient sitting or supine, depending on available space and the patient's clinical condition. Ambulatory patients can sit on a low chair or stool next to the examination table with the slightly flexed arm resting on the side of the table. The examiner then sits opposite the patient. The advantage of the sitting position is that the dialysis patient can watch the monitor more easily than from a supine position. Involving the patient in the examination and explaining the most important findings is of great psychological benefit in the examination of dialysis fistulas, because most dialysis patients ascribe a vital, central importance to the fistula, whose function dictates the patient's state of health. Also, most dialysis patients are so familiar with their fistula that they can occasionally contribute important information to the ultrasound examination (e. g., location of failed puncture attempts, puncture sites that yield a poor arterial flow, etc.).

7.2.5.5 Examination Protocol

The examination should always include visualization of the afferent arteries, the anastomosis, the access vein (that is cannulated for dialysis), and the runoff veins. It may also be necessary to examine the arteries distal to the anastomosis, depending on the clinical inquiry (e. g., suspected steal syndrome).

Visualization of the arterial limb of the fistula in the upper extremity begins in the axilla. Generally it is sufficient to demonstrate the axillary artery in longitudinal section and follow it distally, then do the same for the brachial artery and the afferent artery in the forearm. As in all CDS arterial studies, the vessels are evaluated for luminal size and flow pattern. When these criteria are applied, stenoses and occlusions are easily and quickly identified. When the flow rate through the fistula is high, a relatively high pulse repetition frequency should be used because of the markedly increased flow velocity in the proximal arterial segment. If that segment cannot be continuously defined in its proximal to distal course, or if it is uncertain which forearm artery is supplying the fistula, it may be helpful to identify the arterial inflow segment at the anastomosis and follow it proximally.

In the examination of a native fistula, once the anastomosis has been defined the transducer should be applied with very light pressure to avoid false-positive findings caused by compression of the veins. This should also be done when examining the venous side of the fistula. At this stage the transducer should be steadied by bracing several fingers or the edge of the hand against the extremity. The transducer should not be placed directly on the vein; rather, the maximum transducer pressure should be directed slightly past the apex of the vein wall. The maximum vessel diameter is than imaged in longitudinal section by slight angulation of the transducer. Copious ultrasound gel should be used to improve coupling. This technique avoids significant vascular compression by the transducer, even when there is a low perfusion pressure in the outflow vein. PTFE bypass grafts are less compressible, regardless of the intravascular pressure.

The region of the arteriovenous anastomosis is now examined in transverse section to evaluate its course and luminal size. This is followed by a longitudinal scan that should demonstrate the inflow artery, the perianastomotic portion of the outflow vein, and possibly the distal arterial segment. The surgical design of the fistula (e. g., end-to-side) can generally be appreciated from this biplane examination of the anastomosis.

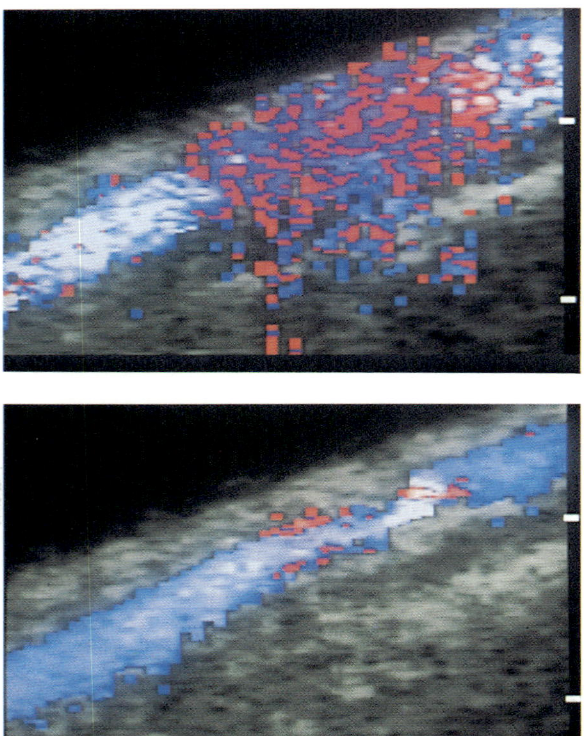

a

b

Fig. 7.**4** Visualization of a stenosis of the shunt vein improved by controlled compression of the afferent artery. Perivascular tissue vibrations (color cloud) in the area of the stenosis (upper image) obscure pathologic findings. Controlled compression of the artery supplying the fistula eliminates the artifacts, and the stenosis is well defined (lower image)

Next the transducer is moved up the extremity, defining the entire course of the access vein or graft in transverse and longitudinal views. Attention is given to any circumscribed or diffuse areas of wall thickening, luminal narrowing or expansion, venous branches, perivascular masses (hematoma, abscess), and the depth of the access vein in relation to the skin surface. Access vein tortuosity and venous collaterals are appreciated better on transverse images than in longitudinal views. If collateral veins are numerous (more than two) or present a relatively large lumen (diameter more than one-third that of the primary access vein), they should be tracked individually with the scanner to identify the principal runoff vein.

The need to evaluate the more proximal veins depends on the fistula design and the clinical problem. If the fistula incorporates a synthetic graft, it is essential to demonstrate the venous anastomosis and the adjacent native venous segments, as these are sites of predilection for stenosis. If there is clinical evidence of a proximal venous outflow obstruction (arm swelling, pain, high venous pressure), attention should be given to the basilic or cephalic vein, brachial vein, axillary vein, or subclavian vein depending on the fistula design. The medial portions of the subclavian vein and the brachiocephalic vein generally are difficult to demonstrate with ultrasound. However, observation of blood flow in the ipsilateral internal jugular vein gives indirect evidence of an obstructive lesion of the brachiocephalic vein.

Normal dialysis fistulas and especially stenoses can generate high flow velocities that cause vessel-wall and perivascular tissue vibrations that are most pronounced in the region of the anastomosis and outflow vein. These vibrations, which produce an audible bruit and palpable thrill, cause prominent cloud-like artifacts in the CDS image that transcend the lumen and hamper evaluation of the vessel (20). Usually this artifact can be eliminated by controlled manual compression of the feeding artery or the shunt vein; this reduces the flow through the fistula and provides clear definition of the vascular segment (Fig. 7.**4**). The degree of compression should be sufficient to eliminate the artifact while still allowing adequate perfusion for color flow imaging.

The CDS image, with its directional color encoding, usually permits a straightforward orientation even in complex fistulas. Doppler frequency analysis is unnecessary for evaluation of the venous part of the fistula, but spectra recorded from the artery can be useful for identifying a higher-grade obstruction (Fig. 7.**5 a,b**). A Doppler spectrum is routinely sampled and documented in the artery supplying the fistula. In forearm fistulas, a spectrum should also be recorded in the nonfistula artery to detect the shunting of blood from, say, the ulnar artery to a radial artery fistula via the palmar arch.

Basically the same examination technique is applied to evaluating a fistula in the lower extremity. If

Fig. 7.**5 a, b** Doppler spectrum before and after PTA of a shunt venous stenosis
a Spectrum from the radial artery with a high-grade stenosis of the perianastomotic access vein (fistula flow = 55 mL/min) exhibits a narrow systolic peak and slight diastolic flow reversal, characteristic of a high peripheral vascular resistance
b Spectrum after successful PTA of the stenosis shows high diastolic antegrade flow in the afferent artery based on the lower peripheral resistance (fistula flow = 410 mL/min)

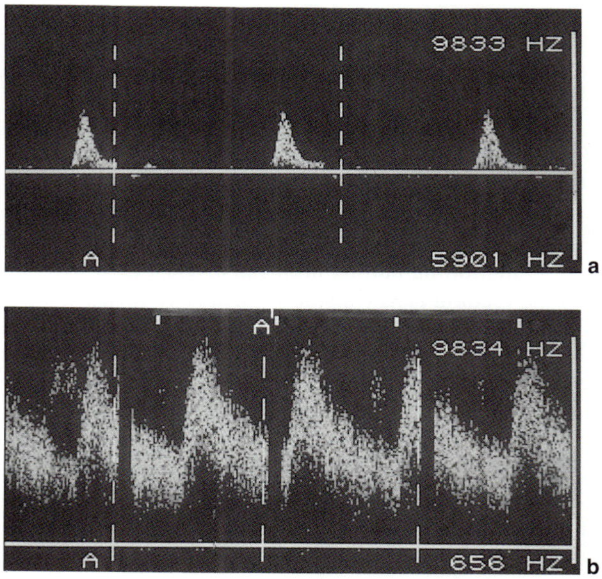

the problem relates to arterial occlusive disease in an access arm, the entire arterial system of the lower extremity should also be examined (see Chapter 6).

If there is clinical suspicion of a steal syndrome (signs of ischemia distal to the anastomosis), it may be necessary to sample Doppler spectra at various sites in the distal artery or in a digital artery, with and without maximum manual compression of the access vein, to detect an increase in peripheral flow.

7.2.5.6 Measurement of Fistula Flow Rate

The hemodynamic significance of pathologic changes in the dialysis fistula is most accurately assessed by measuring the flow rate at designated points in the fistula. If possible, the flow rate should first be measured in the access segment. The measurement should be performed in a straight segment that is free of turbulent flow (see Chapter 3; Fig. 7.**3**). As stated above, the transducer must not cause venous compression. After the mean flow velocity integrated over the vessel cross section has been determined, the transverse diameter of the vessel is measured, and the volume flow rate is calculated in ml/min (see section 3.5). Velocity and diameter measurements should be repeated three times and averaged.

If accurate measurement cannot be made in the access segment due to an unfavorable course of the vessel or turbulent flow, alternative sites can be used in the afferent artery or outflow vein. With a proximal venous measurement, one must be certain that there are no collateral veins branching distal to the site of measurement. If a perianastomotic branching is present, the total fistula flow can still be determined (disregarding the relatively low flow at rest to supply the peripheral arteries) by measuring the arterial flow and the partial flow rates in the outflow tract by taking individual measurements in the constituent veins.

7.2.6 Documentation

The condition of the anastomosis, the anastomotic vessels, and in some cases the extra-anatomic vessels, should be reproducibly documented in examinations of dialysis fistulas. Representative imaging sequences should be recorded on videotape and clearly labeled. Also, a video printer or photo unit should be used to document representative frames, including:

- a longitudinal image and spectrum of the artery supplying the fistula
- a longitudinal and transverse image of the anastomotic region
- a longitudinal image of the access vein showing the transverse diameter of the vessel, the mean integral flow velocity, and the calculated flow rate
- a longitudinal image (and possibly a transverse view) of pathologic findings

Every examination should include a written description of the findings and a drawing showing the condition of the fistula. This may be done freehand or on a preprinted diagram that shows the principal arteries. The drawing should indicate the anatomy of the fistula, the involved vessels, stenoses, occlusions, aneurysms, and large collaterals, and the measured fistula flow rate should be entered at the appropriate site.

If special problems arise that require modification of the access site, it may be necessary to trace the course of the fistula on the skin with a waterproof marker, indicating regions that would make good access sites as well as regions to be avoided. Occasionally the person who inserts the dialysis needle may need to attend the examination and note the details of the fistula anatomy. The length of the examination is approximately 10–20 min.

7.3 Normal Findings

Due to the low peripheral resistance in the venous system, the blood flow in the arterial and venous limbs of the fistula shows an almost continuous pattern that is only slightly modulated by pulsatile systolic peaks. The physiologic biphasic or triphasic arterial Doppler spectrum is replaced by a monophasic waveform (Fig. 7.**5b**). The low resistance in the fistula in the presence of a functioning palmar arch can cause a flow reversal in the feeding artery distal to the anastomoses. This is manifested by spectral changes in the nonfistula artery (loss of biphasic or triphasic waveform) and by retrograde flow in the distal segment of the fistula artery.

The increased blood flow induces a gradual dilatation not only of the access vein but also of the artery supplying the fistula (Fig. 7.**6**). Not infrequently, sites of relative luminal narrowing or expansion compared with the more proximal arterial segment are observed at the anastomosis, especially in Brescia–Cimino fistulas. In most cases, these sites lack hemodynamic significance. In almost all fistulas, some degree of turbulence can be observed at the anastomosis and for several centimeters along the outflow tract due to the frequently rapid alternating flow direction and exit effects in that region (see Chapter 3) (Fig. 7.**2**). As the venous flow moves proximally, it tends to assume an almost continuous pattern which differs from that of ordinary veins in the decreased respiratory modulation of the venous perfusion. This finding is characteristic of a functioning fistula.

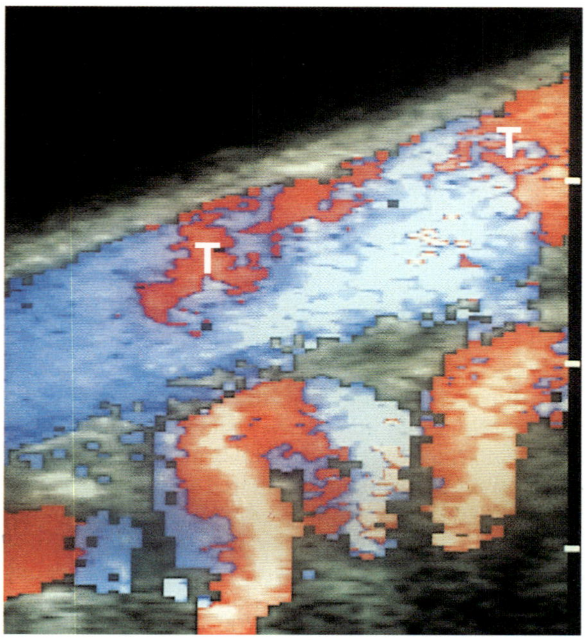

Fig. 7.**6** CDS image of a distal forearm fistula shows marked tortuosity of the radial artery (dorsal) secondary to prolonged high fistula flow (650 mL/min). Zones of physiologic turbulence (T) are visible in the perianastomotic shunt vein (ventral)

PTFE grafts are as accessible to CDS examination as venous fistulas (Fig. 7.**3**). The wall of the graft is clearly displayed as a straight, sharply defined line, and flow within the graft (except for the perianastomotic section) is nonturbulent owing to the uniform wall diameter. The graft material leads to greater absorption of the sound waves than veins, causing moderate acoustic shadowing behind the graft.

The outflow vein of a Brescia–Cimino fistula dilates to approximately 6–10 mm depending on the age of the fistula, the condition of the vein, and the flow rate through the fistula (2, 3, 22). Larger venous diameters are compatible with good fistula function, but significantly smaller diameters can cause difficult needle placement with an increased risk of wall injury and stenosis.

According to reports in the literature, the mean flow rates range from 500 to 1000 mL/min in both native and graft fistulas (2, 3, 11, 22). Thus, there is no true "normal value" for fistula flow, although a flow rate of at least 200–300 mL/min is necessary for adequate hemodialysis. Flow rates less than 200 mL/min at duplex scanning almost always lead to underdialysis, and flow rates of 200–300 mL/min can lead to dialysis problems if there are concomitant, minor disruptive factors such as venous branches or a fall of blood pressure during dialysis. Significant problems should not arise at flow rates above 300 mL/min with correct needle placement in a normally configured fistula. The "normal range" for fistula flow, then, may vary intraindividually with no compromise of dialysis efficiency. Whether very high fistula flows (> 1000 mL/min) may be considered normal in an individual case depends mainly on the primary cardiac status of the patient.

7.4 Pathologic Findings

7.4.1 Preliminary Remarks

Pathologic changes most commonly involve the venous limb of the fistula and the anastomotic sites. Various clinical access problems that can arise in hemodialysis patients are listed in Table 7.**1** and are correlated with the most common morphologic and functional causes. The morphologic findings are far less important than their functional effects, which determine the selection of patients for intervention (fistula PTA, fistula revision, creation of new fistula, closure of the fistula, collateral vein ligation, aneurysm resection, etc.). The CDS examination, then, should always cover the morphology and the function of the fistula (flow measurement, flow changes in other vascular regions) so that the clinical significance of fistula abnormalities can be appreciated.

Table 7.**1** The most important clinical dialysis access problems and their most frequent causes

Clinical problem	Possible cause
1. Inadequate flow during dialysis (< 200–300 mL/min), but dialysis may still be possible	– Stenosis of the artery – Stenosis of the anastomosis – Stenosis of the access vein – Venipuncture misses main access vein (enters tributary) – Puncture technique
2. Recurring difficult needle placement, possibly with wall entrapment by the needle	– Same as 1, or occlusion – Deeply situated access vein
3. Little (< 100 mL/ min) or no flow during dialysis	– Same as 1, or occlusion
4. Difficulty or inability to palpate and auscultate the access vein	– Same as 1, or occlusion
5. Increased venous outflow pressure (> 150 mm Hg at maximum blood flow rate)	– Venous stenosis or occlusion proximal to the puncture site
6. Cardiac failure and/or steal syndrome	– Excessive fistula flow
7. Local swelling, possible redness	– Hematoma – Aneurysm – Abscess
8. Diffuse swelling	– Same as 5 – Relative proximal stenosis due to excessive fistula flow – Infection
9. Redness, fever, pain	– Infection
10. Ischemia distal to the fistula	– Arterial occlusive disease – Excessive fistula flow
11. Inadequate dialysis despite good flow	– Proximal stenosis with circulation of partially dialyzed blood into peripheral veins

There are five basic pathologic situations in which abnormal fistula flow rates may occur:

1. Decreased flow rates on both the arterial and venous sides of the fistula due to stenoses or an occlusion in the artery, anastomosis, or vein
2. Decreased flow rate on the venous side of the fistula due to venous branches
3. Increased flow rate with signs of venous outflow obstruction
4. Increased flow rate with signs of cardiac failure
5. Increased flow rate with signs of a steal syndrome

7.4.2 Stenosis and Occlusion

The development of stenotic changes depends on the surgical technique., the preoperative condition of the vascular segments used in constructing the fistula, the degree of dilatation of the arterialized access vein, and the quality of the puncture technique.

Even before the first dialysis fistula is created, venous stenoses may be induced by venipuncture procedures (blood sampling, indwelling venous cannula, central venous catheter). This applies equally to peripheral and central veins. Excessive intraoperative traumatization of the vessels in the anastomotic region can induce intimal lesions that predispose to subsequent stenosis. Arterial occlusive disease that is preexisting or develops over time can lead to stenotic changes in the artery supplying the fistula. Each needle puncture of the access vein inflicts vessel-wall trauma that ideally resolves by thrombic occlusion of the needle tract with subsequent thrombus organization and intimal repair. If a large thrombus forms at the puncture site, it may obstruct flow immediately or after the thrombus has organized. Intimal hyperplasia can lead to stenosis as readily as a puncture-related dissection of the vessel wall. The chronically high blood flow can incite intimal hyperplasia in the area of venous valves, with thickening of the valve leaflets and consequent stenosis. The same mechanism can underlie the transformation of primarily nonsignificant, puncture-related sites of venous wall thickening to hyperplastic, hemodynamically significant lesions through the action of the constant high flow. Venous thoracic outlet syndromes can also lead

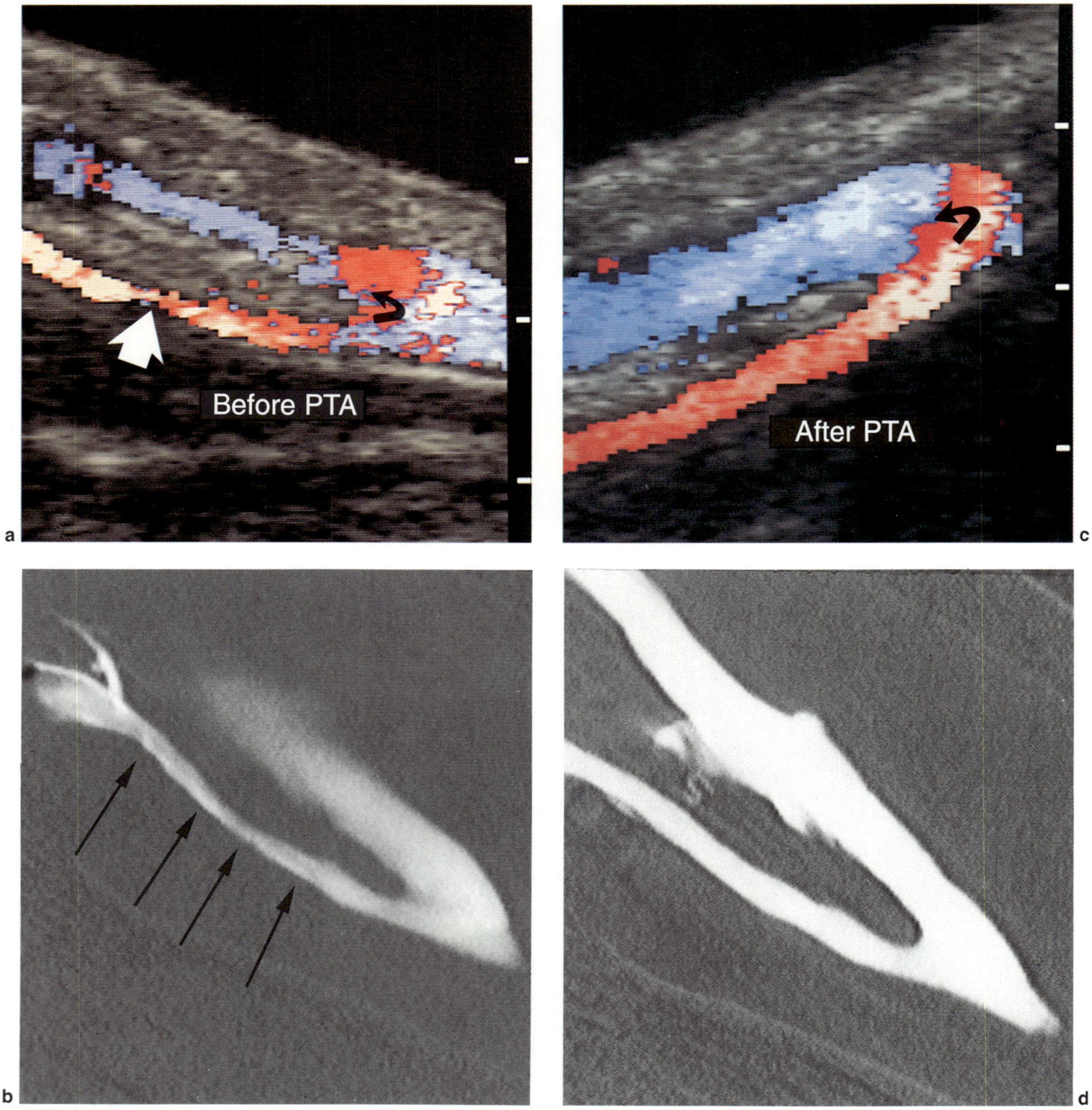

Fig. 7.**7a–d** Long stenosis of the perianastomotic radial artery before and after PTA

a CDS shows a long, circumscribed, high-grade stenosis in the proximal artery (arrow) with deficient perfusion of the access vein. Flow rate = 135 mL/min

b DSA following antegrade puncture of the brachial artery and selective catheterization of the radial artery. Black arrows indicates the sites of stenosis

c CDS after PTA demonstrates a normal lumen of the radial artery with good perfusion of the access vein. Flow rate = 380 mL/min

d DSA after PTA confirms the CDS findings

to stenoses, which normally are hemodynamically irrelevant but may become significant in dialysis patients due to the unphysiologically high flow. Ipsilateral pacemaker cables can also cause intimal lesions that predispose to stenosis.

From a hemodynamic standpoint, obstructive lesions of the inflow artery (Fig. 7.**7a–d**), the anastomosis (Fig. 7.**9a**, **b**), and the perianastomotic venous segments (Fig. 7.**9a**, **b**) can produce the same clinical symptom: a reduction of flow during dialysis. The sonographic features of a stenosis in a dialysis fistula are basically the same as those of an arterial stenosis (see Chapters 5 and 6). They can be difficult to detect in curved vascular segments, however. Turbulence is

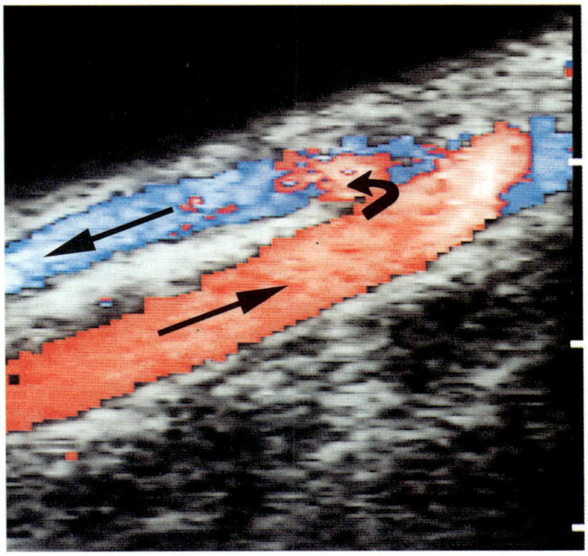

a

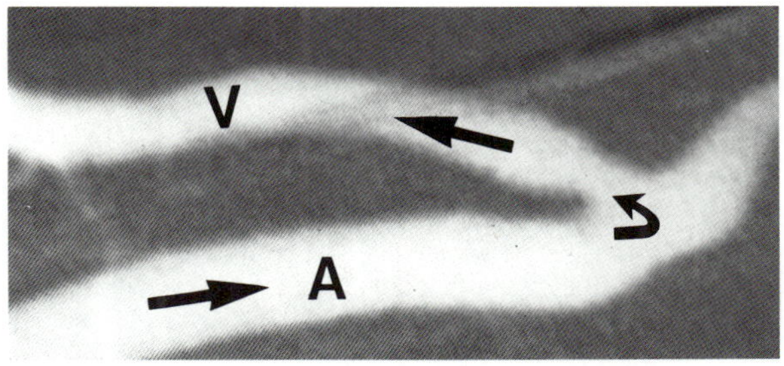

b

Fig. 7.**8a, b** Moderate narrowing of the perianastomotic access vein in a well-functioning BC fistula in the distal forearm
a CDS shows slight luminal narrowing on the venous side of the anastomosis (venous diameter less than arterial diameter) with turbulence. Measured fistula flow = 390 mL/min, arrows = direction of flow
b Intra-arterial DSA (puncture of the brachial artery) confirms the findings. A = Artery, V = shunt vein

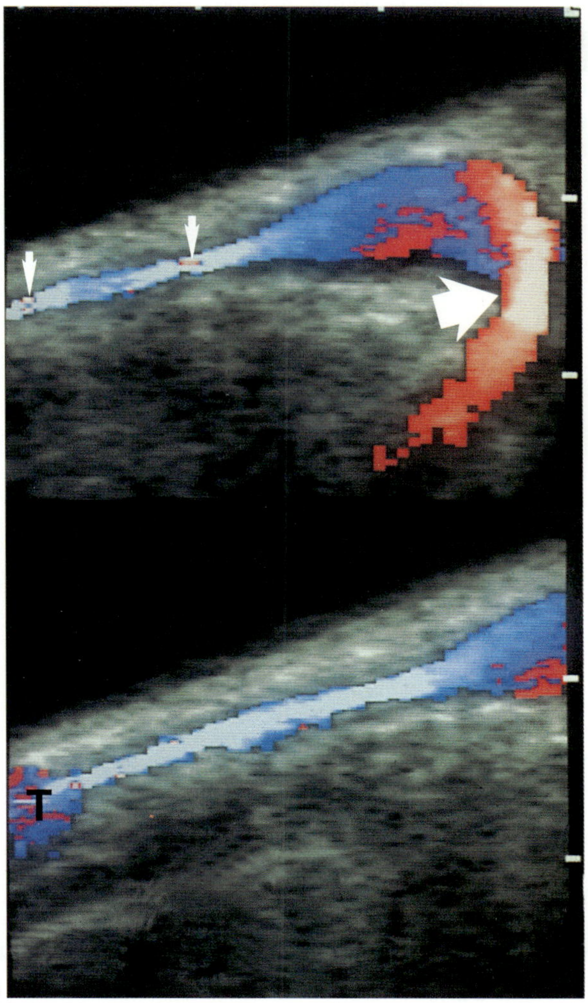

a

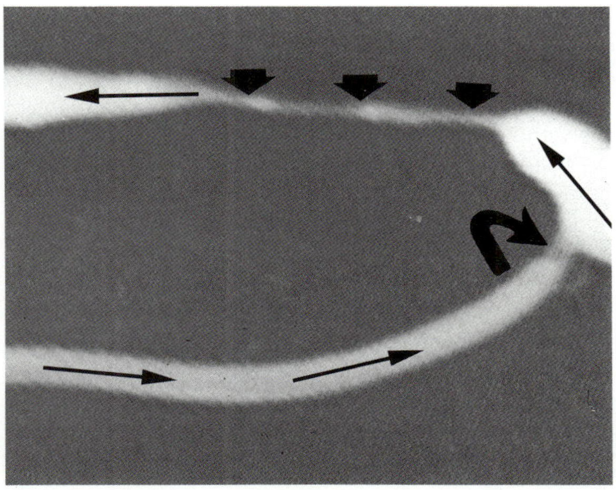

b

Fig. 7.**9a, b** Long, high-grade stenosis of the access vein in a distal radial fistula with mild anastomotic stenosis, leading to decreased arterial flow and inadequate dialysis
a CDS shows concentric luminal narrowing of the shunt vein starting 1 cm proximal to the anastomosis and involving about a 2.5-cm segment of the vein. Increased color saturation toward pale blue indicates high flow velocities in the stenosis with some aliasing (thin arrows) and post-stenotic turbulence (T, lower image). Low-grade anastomotic stenosis is also present (short wide arrow). Flow rate = 165 mL/min
b Intra-arterial DSA confirms a long, high-grade stenosis in the shunt vein (wide arrows) and a mild anastomotic stenosis (curved arrow). Long thin arrows = direction of blood flow

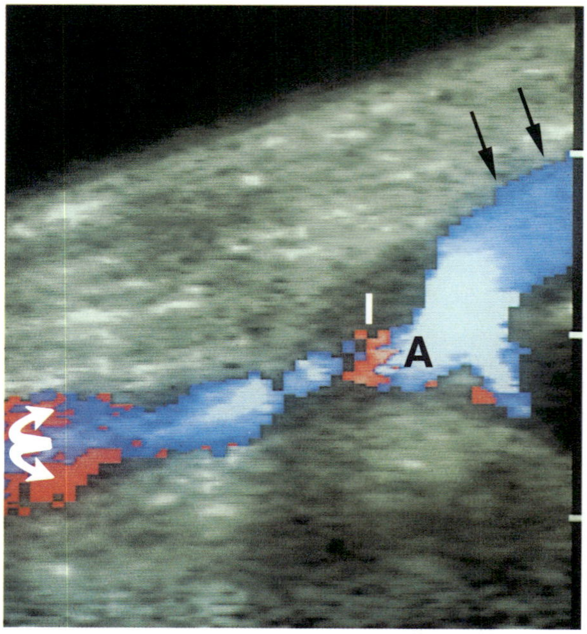

Fig. 7.**10** Stenosis at the venous (proximal) anastomosis (A) of a PTFE jump graft (arrows). Flow direction is from right to left. The image shows wall thickening (I) in the anastomosis caused by intimal hyperplasia, also zones of poststenotic flow reversal in the outflow vein (curved arrows) cranial to the stenosis

more pronounced in the intrastenotic and especially the poststenotic segments, because the prestenotic flow velocity is often higher than with an non-dialysis shunt extremity artery stenosis, and because most dialysis patients have a markedly reduced hematocrit with a decrease in blood viscosity. Aliasing is common within the stenosis due to the high flow rate, so the intrastenotic flow velocity usually cannot be quantified. As noted in section 7.2.5.5, even a nonstenosed access vein can produce significant perivascular vibrations leading to prominent color artifacts. These artifacts are especially pronounced when there is a stenosis in the access vein, so the typical perivascular color cloud should direct attention to the stenotic lesion and prompt closer scrutiny of the area using the described compression technique.

An access vein stenosis may be eccentric or concentric, depending on the etiology, and the lesion may be circumscribed or involve a long segment of the vein. Thickening of the venous wall may be substantial and often is well demonstrated by ultrasound (Fig. 7.**10**). A special circumscribed form is membranous stenosis, which probably develops from a hypertrophied venous valve. While these stenoses can be difficult to detect on angiograms, their appearance on CDS images is far more impressive due to the extensive poststenotic flow abnormalities. Stenoses can also result from partial thrombosis of the access vein (Fig. 7.**11 a**, **b**). Proximal stenoses, which usually are manifested by symptoms of venous congestion, can be demonstrated as far as the middle part of the subclavian vein by CDS.

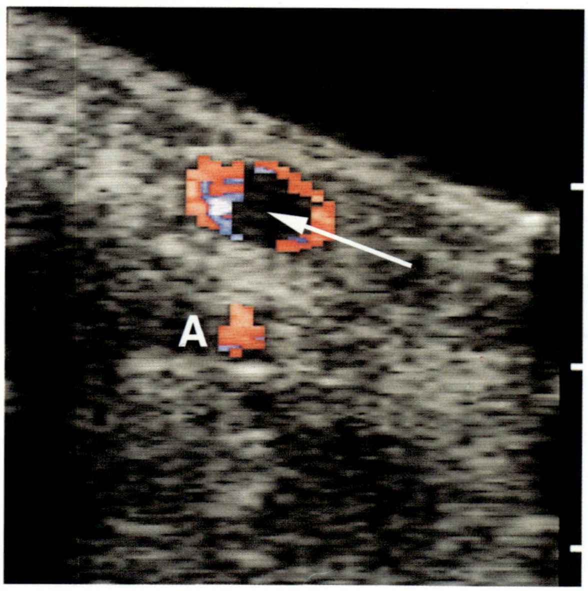

a

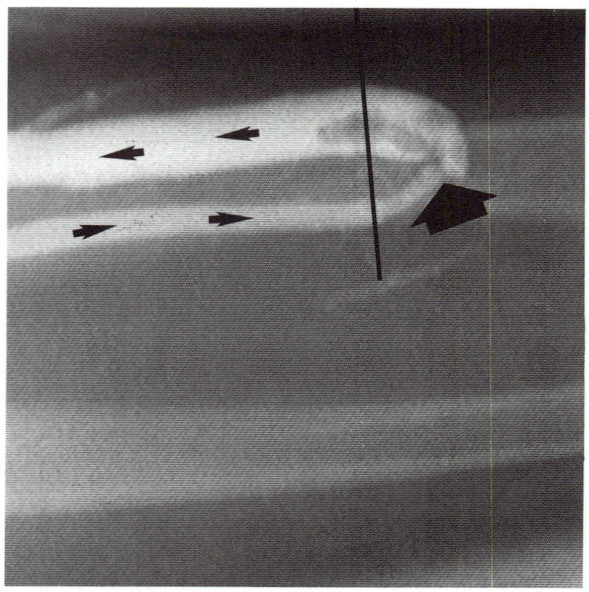
b

Fig. 7.**11 a, b** Partial thrombosis of the shunt vein with an anastomotic stenosis (forearm BC fistula)
a Transverse CDS image just above the anastomosis demonstrates a nonocclusive thrombus (arrow) in the access vein. A = Radial artery

b Arterial DSA shows a high-grade anastomotic stenosis (arrow) and a nonocclusive thrombus extending proximally from the stenosis into the vein. The solid line indicates the image plane in **a**

It should again be emphasized that the examination of a dialysis fistula includes visualization of the arterial limb starting from the axillary artery. Dialysis patients suffer a high incidence of chronic arterial occlusive disease, which also may involve the upper extremity. Arterial stenoses, which generally are readily accessible to balloon dilatation (PTA) should not be overlooked as a cause of access failure—particularly since their extent can be important in predicting the success of additional fistulas in the same extremity.

Stenotic lesions in a dialysis fistula are almost always detectable by CDS. Doppler spectral analysis is seldom necessary for this purpose, although spectra recorded during examination of the arterial limb of the dialysis fistula may indicate significant obstructions distal to the sampling site if the spectral waveform resembles that of a normal extremity artery (Fig. 7.**5a,b**). This is attributable to a stenosis-induced increase in the peripheral vascular resistance, which normally is very low in the fistula region. A high-resistance spectrum recorded in a fistula artery or in the perianastomotic portion of the access vein is pathognomonic for a significant obstructive lesion downstream. Antegrade flow in the arterial segment distal to the anastomosis is another sign of a high-grade obstruction of the access vein or an a–v anastomosis in a peripheral BC fistula (19).

The quantification of a stenosis in a dialysis fistula is based largely on the measurement of its functional effects, regardless of the site of occurrence (artery, anastomosis, access vein, far proximal vein). The essential functional parameters in this regard are:

1. The fistula flow rate available for dialysis, and
2. The intravenous blood pressure

While the fistula flow rate can be quantified by CDS, the venous pressure cannot. Because the most common fistula problem is insufficient arterial flow due to obstructive lesions in the artery, anastomosis, or vein, morphologic assessment of the fistula must be followed by flowmetry to quantify the extent of the lesions. This makes allowance for the frequently multifocal distribution of fistula stenoses, since the hemodynamic effects of multiple stenoses are additive, and for the fact that the effect of a stenosis on fistula flow depends partly on the cardiac output for a given local degree of stenosis. Thus, in contrast to carotid artery examinations, it is usually unnecessary to determine the degree of stenosis as a relative reduction in cross-sectional area or diameter, since the demonstration of a stenosis that reduces fistula flow serves to prove its hemodynamic significance.

Even so, it is occasionally necessary to state the degree of severity of a vascular stenosis. This is the case, for example, when multiple lesions are present whose cumulative effect is a flow reduction that hampers dialysis, but which for technical reasons cannot all be treated in the same sitting (by PTA or surgery). In this situation it is useful to determine the relative diameter reduction in relation to the feeding artery. The local grading of an access vein stenosis in relation to an adjacent segment is unrewarding because of normally occurring variations in the caliber of the vessel.

Some proximal venous stenoses that do not initially cause a significant flow reduction are manifested clinically by frequent, painful swelling in the arm (19). During dialysis an increased venous outflow pressure is often recorded in these cases. CDS can detect proximal stenoses only as far as the middle part of the subclavian vein; the more central venous segments are difficult or impossible to examine with ultrasound. Nevertheless, if CDS shows no fistula abnormalities in a patient with swelling of the access arm, there is a high probability of a central stenosis, and angiographic evaluation should be performed. Occasionally the detection of retrograde flow in the ipsilateral internal jugular vein will suggest a significant obstruction in the brachiocephalic vein, leading to flow reversal in the jugular vein and diversion of the returning blood to the opposite side through cervical collaterals (19).

Occlusions may result from inadequate surgical technique, preexisting stenoses, or as a complication of dialysis (wall dissection or hematoma with luminal obstruction). Factors that predispose to fistula thrombosis are hypotensive episodes, hypovolemia, fistula infection, overcompression of the fistula site after dialysis, unfavorable positioning of the access arm, treatment with erythropoietin, and renal transplantation. Anastomotic thrombosis generally involves the adjacent venous segment as well, while the fistula artery always remains patent if the distal arterial segment is still perfused (with an end-of-vein-to-side-of-artery anastomosis).

A complete, fresh venous thrombosis is easily recognized by the absence of an intraluminal flow signal (Fig. 7.**12a**, **b**) and the incompressibility of the vein. The flow in the afferent artery again shows marked pulsatility, and a biphasic or triphasic spectral waveform reappears. If the anastomosis is still patent, CDS can also demonstrate segmental occlusions of the access vein that are bridged by collateral veins. These sites are best observed in the transverse view. Old venous occlusions, associated with collaterals of varying competence, may appear only as a thin scar-tissue band or an abrupt direction change in the course of the fistula (former collateral origin).

7.4.3 Aneurysms

In dialysis fistulas as in other vascular systems, a distinction is drawn between true aneurysms and false aneurysms (pseudoaneurysms). Aneurysms can develop at virtually any site in a dialysis fistula. Most occur in the access vein (Figs. 7.**13**, 7.**14**), but arterial aneurysms can also form (e. g., after inadvertent puncture of the feeding artery with a large dialysis needle).

A true aneurysm represents a more or less circumscribed dilatation of the entire vessel involving all the layers of the vessel wall (Fig. 7.**13**). This type

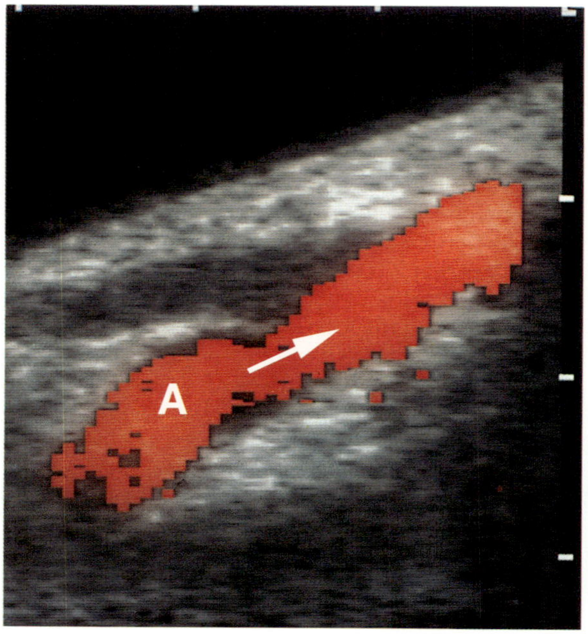

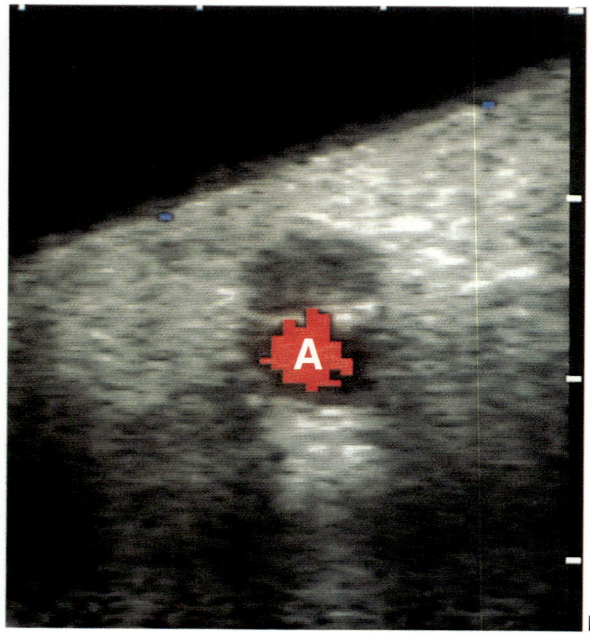

Fig. 7.**12 a, b** Complete, fresh occlusion of the shunt vein
a Longitudinal scan of the anastomotic region shows a patent radial artery (A) and an occluded, homogeneously hypoechoic access vein devoid of flow signals (ventral of the artery). Arrow = direction of blood flow
b Transverse image of the same region. Radial artery (A)

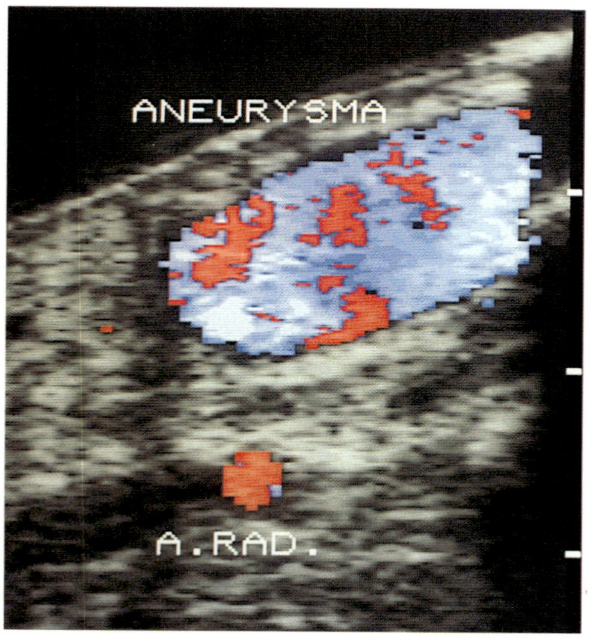

Fig. 7.**13** Transverse image demonstrates a prominent aneurysm of the access vein. A. RAD. = Radial artery

of aneurysmal dilatation occurs almost exclusively in native fistulas and may be caused by excessive dilatation of the access vein during arterialization or by perianastomotic turbulence. The dividing line between venous dilatation and an aneurysm depends on the absolute diameter of the vessel and the local change in caliber. If the transverse diameter of a native access vein exceeds 15 mm or there is a circumscribed diameter increase of 50% or more, an aneurysm is said to be present.

Pseudoaneurysm may occur as a complication of a vascular suture or needle puncture in which a small vascular leak gives rise to a contained hemorrhage that persists due to absent or inadequate hemostasis and thus maintains the perfusion of the newly formed cavity. Pseudoaneurysms can develop in all types of vascular access. It is not uncommon for an aneurysm of the access vein to coexist with a circumscribed stenosis at the inlet or outlet of the aneurysmal sac.

Not all aneurysms are clinically significant. Aneurysms may cause problems due to:

1. Compression of adjacent structures (vessels, nerves)
2. Restriction of the accessable segment of the fistula (puncture of the aneurysm is avoided)
3. Thrombosis (though a limited thrombosis may be desirable for the resolution of a pseudoaneurysm)
4. Rupture, hemorrhage
5. Flow reduction due to an adjacent stenosis

Aneurysms are easily detected in access fistulas by CDS. Besides vascular dilatation, there is typically a suspension of the regular, almost laminar flow profile with the formation of substantial turbulence (Fig. 7.**14 a**, **b**). An eccentric dilatation most likely represents a pseudoaneurysm, while concentric dilatation is more suggestive of a true aneurysm. Mural thrombi are easily distinguished from the perfused lumen by

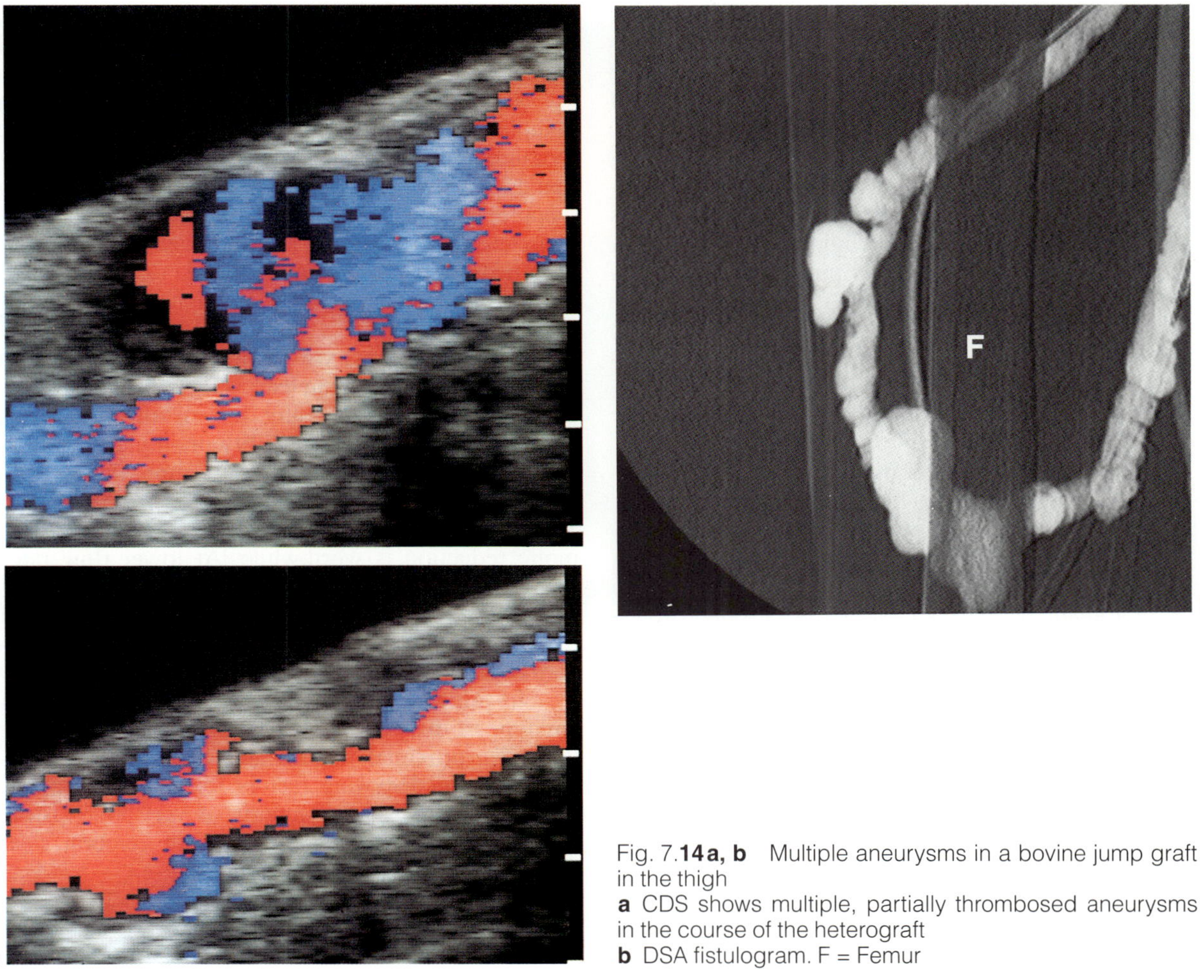

Fig. 7.**14a, b** Multiple aneurysms in a bovine jump graft in the thigh
a CDS shows multiple, partially thrombosed aneurysms in the course of the heterograft
b DSA fistulogram. F = Femur

their lack of flow signals. Long-standing aneurysms may contain wall calcifications, recognized by their high echogenicity and associated acoustic shadow.

7.4.4 Branched or Deeply Situated Access Vein

Despite a good flow rate in the region of the a–v anastomosis, dialysis problems may arise if the access vein branches early so that only a portion of the volume flow is available. This results in difficulties with needle placement and inadequate flow rates for dialysis.

Venous branches are most easily identified in transverse views. Their hemodynamic effect can be quantified by determining the flow rates in the individual tributaries and identifying the vein that is carrying the largest partial volume flow. If adequate dialysis cannot be performed through that vein (marked on the skin), the remaining, unused collateral veins could be ligated.

Puncture problems can also arise if the access vein is not directly subcutaneous but is separated from the skin by a relatively thick layer of subcutaneous fat. Even a large access vein can be very difficult to palpate and puncture in this situation. It may occasionally be necessary to mobilize the vein surgically and transpose it to a more superficial position.

With an abnormally deep position of the outflow veins, marking the most favorable puncture site (after confirming a flow rate adequate for dialysis) and determining the distance from the skin surface to the access vessel is often a simple and effective method of ensuring a reliable venipuncture. If surgical transposition of the access vein is proposed, the course of the fistula should be marked on the skin preoperatively with the aid of CDS imaging.

7.4.5 Pathologically Increased Fistula Flow

A large anastomosis and widely dilated access vein can permit fistula flow rates in excess of 1000 mL/min, especially if the fistula is located in the upper arm. Because dialyzers are limited to a maximum blood flow rate of 500 mL/min, these values cannot be measured during dialysis and can only be determined noninvasively using Doppler ultrasound methods. For this reason, an excessive fistula flow rate is often suspected only when clinical problems, such as cardiac failure, recurrent swelling of the access arm, or steal syndromes (see section 7.4.6) arise. The clinical significance of excessive fistula flow depends chiefly on the patient's cardiac status. In the absence of preexisting cardiac disease, even high fistula flow rates may produce no appreciable clinical symptoms for a long period of time. If there is preexisting heart disease, even a moderately increased fistula flow or flow rates in the high–normal range (800–1000 mL/min) can evoke symptoms of cardiac failure. Thus, an individual correlation should always be established between the flow rate through the fistula and the patient's cardiac status.

Excessive fistula flow may in some cases necessitate surgical reduction of the anastomotic orifice or closure of the anastomosis with creation of a new fistula (8, 11). So far no prospective studies have been done on the tolerance of high fistula flow rates in asymptomatic patients, although it is reasonable to assume a causal relationship between the development of cardiac failure and an increased volume load on the heart. Grosser et al. (11) define 1600 mL/min as the absolute upper limit for fistula flow, above which surgical intervention is indicated.

In patients with proximal venous stenoses, fistula flow is an important factor in the development of venous congestive symptoms. The greater the obstruction of the proximal flow path and the poorer the venous collateralization, the less fistula flow is needed to evoke decompensation of venous outflow in the access arm with congestive phenomena such as edema, pain, and trophic skin changes. In our experience, the average fistula flow in patients with proximal venous stenoses producing congestive symptoms is approximately 860 mL/min. Following successful PTA of the stenosis, the average flow rate increased to 1340 mL/min, but congestive symptoms were eliminated in all patients by reduction of the stenosis.

7.4.6 Steal Syndromes

The low peripheral resistance in the venous system not only causes the arteriovenous shunting of blood through the surgically constructed fistula but frequently leads to the "stealing" of blood from other arterial regions. As noted previously, flow reversal commonly occurs in the distal arterial limb of a radial-cephalic fistula due to the shunting of blood from the ulnar artery via the palmar arch (19, 21). This situation alone normally does not produce clinical symptoms. A true steal syndrome with peripheral ischemia (10) develops only if there is coexisting arterial occlusive disease. Stenoses or occlusions of digital arteries or a more proximal obstruction (e. g., in the ulnar artery) can, in the presence of a radial artery fistula, cause deficient perfusion of the fingers or even the entire hand and in rare cases can lead to gangrene. The main factors influencing steal-related ischemia are the fistula volume flow and the extent of the arterial occlusive disease.

In the case of ischemia in the access arm a complete fistula evaluation including flow-rate measurements and examination of the large arteries that do not supply the fistula is required. By sampling Doppler spectra from a digital artery with and without complete compression of the shunt vein, it can be determined whether reducing the fistula flow (simulated ligation) leads to an increase in peripheral arterial perfusion.

Even in patients with mild occlusive disease, a very high fistula flow can lead to significant ischemia. By using CDS to measure the fistula flow, it is possible to predict the feasibility of surgically reducing the anastomosis as a means of improving peripheral ischemia. If the fistula flow is greater than 500 mL/min, our experience indicates that anastomotic reduction is worthwhile. At lower flow rates there is insufficient reserve down to the critical rate of 250–300 mL/min, because the extent of a surgical fistula reduction cannot be accurately planned with regard to achieving a specific volume flow.

In principle, a steal syndrome can develope in any type of dialysis fistula (Fig. 7.**1a–d**). According to (6, 7), proximal fistulas and side-to-side anastomoses are predisposing factors for steal syndromes. Also, there are isolated reports of very high fistula flows promoting the development of cerebral steal syndromes (11).

7.4.7 Perivascular Lesions

CDS is superior to angiography in its ability to demonstrate not only the perfused vascular lumen but also the vessel wall and surrounding soft tissues. Hematomas, seromas, and abscesses in proximity to a dialysis fistula are clearly defined (Fig. 7.**15**) and are easily distinguished from a pseudoaneurysm by the absence of flow signals. It is a simple matter to distinguish compression-induced narrowing from a true vascular stenosis. A hypoechoic or anechoic rim around a synthetic graft may signify a graft infection.

7.4.8 Findings Before Fistula Construction, after Shunt PTA, and after Surgical Revision

The need for routine vascular imaging prior to the construction of a dialysis access fistula is at present uncertain. In patients with arterial occlusive disease, however, CDS should always be used preoperatively to assess the patency of the arterial system in the access extremity.

CDS is advised for the noninvasive follow-up of dialysis shunt angioplasties (PTA) and fistula revisions (Figs. 7.**5a**, **b**, 7.**7a–d**). It is used after PTA mainly to evaluate for restenoses and complications

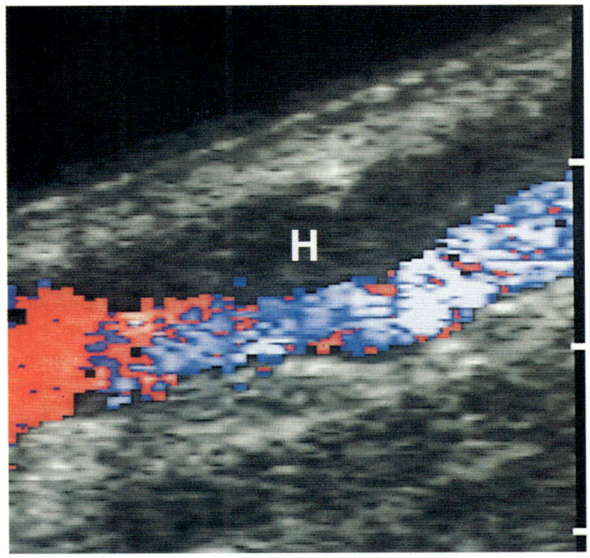

Fig. 7.**15** Perivascular hematoma (H) secondary to faulty needle insertion, with moderate narrowing of the access vein

of balloon dilatation such as dissection and pseudoaneurysm. It can also be used after the implantation of vascular stents in dialysis fistulas, since the mesh construction of the stent permits adequate penetration of ultrasound waves (19). The measurement of fistula flow is of central importance for the functional follow-up of access procedures. The improvement of dialyzability following PTA correlates closely with an increase in volume flow measured by color duplex sonography (18).

7.5 Diagnostic Value of Color Duplex Sonography in Relation to Other Diagnostic Procedures

Clinical examination of the dialysis fistula with attention to the hemodynamic parameters of dialysis (maximum possible dialyzer flow rate, venous outflow pressure, arterial blood pressure) can yield important clues to the nature and location of an access problem. An imaging procedure is needed, however, for the accurate characterization, localization, and quantification of the pathologic changes. The relative strengths and weaknesses of angiography and CDS are summarized in Table 7.**2**.

Angiography has served as the traditional gold standard by which new procedures are appraised. A dialysis fistula can be opacified by fine-needle puncture of the brachial artery or by direct puncture of the access vein. The latter method requires suprasystolic proximal compression of the arm to provide retrograde opacification of the anastomosis and fistula artery. The advantage of DSA over conventional angiography is that it eliminates superimposed bone while using a smaller dose of contrast medium and causing less puncture trauma. Angiography is advantageous in that it provides continuous visualization of the vessels and permits review of the angiographic films. Disadvantages relate to the occasional difficulty of interpreting complex access vein configurations involving numerous superimposed veins (neces-

Table 7.**2** Comparison of the advantages and disadvantages of arteriographic and CDS examination of hemodialysis fistula (based on the literature and the author's own experience). The more "plus" signs are given for an entry, the more favorable the rating of the procedure

Problem	Angiography	CCDS
Peripheral stenosis, occlusion	+++	+++
Central venous stenosis, occlusion	+++	(+)
Entire arterial limb	+++ (invasive)	+++
Aneurysm	++	+++
Branched access vein	+++	+++
Deeply situated vein	+	+++
Perivascular abnormalities	(+)	+++
Steal syndrome	++	+++
Quantification of flow	–	+++
Invasiveness, repeatability	+	+++
Ability to demonstrate examination	++	+++
Ability to review image documentation	+++	+
Examiner dependence	++	+

sitating additional film sequences in different projections), the invasiveness of the procedure, the need for radiographic contrast medium, and radiation exposure.

CDS is at least equal to angiography in its ability to demonstrate stenoses, occlusions, aneurysms, and fistula branching. Compared with conventional duplex scanning (15), CDS permits a much more efficient and straightforward demonstration of the dialysis access fistula. The sensitivity and specificity of CDS compared with DSA are, respectively, 91–100% and 93–95% in the evaluation of the feeding artery, the anastomosis, and the access vein (19). Angiography is markedly superior to CDS only in the demonstration of central venous obstructions (sensitivity of CDS 36%). But the sonographic method offers several important advantages over angiography in its lack of invasiveness, plane-of-section image, and the inclusion of functional information—advantages that are especially valuable in the examination of dialysis fistulas. The noninvasiveness permits the examination to be repeated as often as desired with no risk to the patient. While a transfemoral approach is generally required for angiographic visualization of the more proximal arterial segments (axillary artery, brachial artery), these areas can be routinely covered during the CDS examination. The concomitant demonstration of the perivascular soft tissues is another advantage of sonography over angiography. This is important not only for the detection of hematomas and abscesses but also for investigating problems of needle insertion in deeply placed access veins. While angiography obviously provides a better global view of the vascular tree than CDS, we have found that the demonstrability and acceptance of CDS are very high when the vascular surgeon or dialysis personnel are involved in the examination. When relevant findings are marked on the skin for the purpose of modifying the puncture technique, for preoperative orientation of the surgeon, or for the radiologist planning a PTA, this can be done more easily and accurately with CDS than with angiography. The ability to measure the flow rate through an a–v fistula represents another important advantage of CDS over angiographic methods. Although DSA can be used in principle to quantify flow velocities (9), this cannot be done when the region of interest is obscured by overlying bone or other opacified vessels. Neither the clinical examination nor angiography can routinely answer the question of whether a pathologically high fistula flow rate is present. This can be accomplished only with Doppler ultrasound, and CDS is inherently superior to all other Doppler techniques for the quantitation of flow.

On the whole, the combination of morphologic and functional information supplied by CDS makes it the procedure of first choice for the investigation of dialysis access problems. In most cases a complete diagnosis can be established with CDS, the combined interpretation of clinical data and CDS findings providing a sound basis for therapeutic decision making. Angiography is necessary only for the elucidation of equivocal findings, the search for central venous obstructions, the monitoring of PTA, and for certain preoperative investigations.

7.6 References

1 Ahmad, S., C.R. Blagg, B.H. Scribner: Center and home chronic hemodialysis. In Schrier, R.W., C.W. Gottschalk (Eds.): Diseases of the kidney, 4th ed. Little, Brown, Boston (1988) 3281–3322

2 Bergmann, H., P. Brücke, C. Gross: Nichtinvasive Flowmessung beim Cimino-Shunt mittels Ultraschall. Wien. med. Wschr. 11 (1982) 245–247

3 Bouthier, J.D., J.A. Levenson, A.C. Simon, J.M. Bariety, P.E. Bourquelot, M.E. Safar: A noninvasive determination of fistula blood flow in dialysis patients. Artif. Org. 7 (1983) 404–409

4 Brescia, M.J., J.E. Cimino, K. Appel, B.J. Burwich: Chronic hemodialysis using venipuncture and surgically created arteriovenous fistula. New Engl. J. Med. 275 (1966) 1089–1092

5 Broviac, J.W., J.J. Cole, B.H. Scribner: Silicone rubber atrial catheter for prolonged parenteral nutrition. Surg. Gynecol. Obstet. 136 (1973) 602

6 Bussel, J.A., J.A. Abbott, R.C. Lim: A radial steal syndrome with arteriovenous fistula for hemodialysis. Ann. intern. Med. 75 (1971) 387–394

7 Castro, L.A.: Permanente Gefäßzugänge für die Dauerdialysebehandlung. In Wetzels, E., A. Colombi, P. Dittrich, H.J. Gurland, M. Kessel, H. Klinkmann (Hrsg.): Hämodialyse, Peritonealdialyse, Membranplasmapherese und verwandte Verfahren. Springer, Berlin (1986) 157–183

8 Compty, C.M., F.L. Shapiro: Cardiac complications of regular dialysis therapy. In Drukker, W., F.M. Parsons, J.F. Maher (eds.): Replacement of renal function by dialysis, 2nd ed. Martinus Nijhoff, Boston (1988) 595–610

9 Dölken, W., P. Landwehr, E.F. Frank, K. Lackner: Calculation of flow velocities from the geometrical shape of contrast-induced time-density curves using DSA. Europ. J. Radiol. 8 (1988) 208–213

10 Duncan, H., L. Ferguson, I. Faris: Incidence of the radial steal syndrome in patients with Brescia fistula for hemodialysis: its clinical significance. J. vasc. Surg. 4 (1986) 144–147

11 Grosser, S., G. Kreymann, A. Kühns: Duplex-sonographisch quantifiziertes Shuntvolumen und dessen klinische Relevanz. Angio Archiv 22 (1991) 74–77

12 Haimov, H., F. Giron, J.H. Jacobsen: The expanded polytetrafluoroethylene graft. Three years' experience with 362 grafts. Arch. Surg. 114 (1979) 673–677

13 Haisch, C. E., J. Cerilli: Vascular access procdures for renal dialysis (including peridoneal dialysis). In: Sabiston, D. C. (ed.): Textbook of Surgery 14th ed. Saunders (Philadelphia) (1991) 393–401

14 Hickman, R.O., C.D. Buchner, R.A. Clift, J.E. Sanders, P. Stewart, E.D. Thomas: A modified right atrial catheter for access to the venous system in marrow transplant recipients. Surg. Gynecol. Obstet. 148 (1979) 871

15 Kathrein, H., P. König, S. Weimann, G. Judmaier, P. Dittrich: Nicht-invasive morphologische und funktionelle Beurteilung arteriovenöser Fisteln von Dialysepatienten mit der Duplexsonographie. Ultraschall 10 (1989) 33–40

16 Keller, F., H.J. Loewe, K.J. Bauknecht, A. Schwarz, G. Offermann: Kumulative Funktionsraten von orthotopen Dialysefisteln und Interponaten. Dtsch. med. Wschr. 113 (1988) 332–336

17 Kjellstrand, C.M.: The Achilles' heel of the hemodialysis patient. Arch. intern. Med. 138 (1978) 1063–1064

18 Landwehr, P., K. Lackner: Color Doppler flow imaging of the hemodialysis shunt. Acta Radiol. (Suppl.) 377 (1991) 15–19

19 Landwehr, P., A. Tschammler, R.M. Schaefer, K. Lackner: Wertigkeit der farbkodierten Duplexsonographie des Dialyseshunts. Fortschr. Röntgenstr. 153 (1990) 185–191

20 Middleton, W.D., S. Erickson, G.L. Melson: Perivascular color artifacts: Pathologic significance and appearance on color doppler US images. Radiology 171 (1989) 647–652

21 Middleton, W.D., D.D. Picus, M.V. Marx, G.L. Melson: Color Doppler sonography of hemodialysis vascular access: Comparison with angiography. Amer. J. Roentgenol. 152 (1989) 633–639

22 Moran, M.R., J.M.R. Rodriguez, M.R. Boyero, A.A. Enriquez, A.I. Morin: Flow of dialysis fistulas. Noninvasive study performed with standard Doppler equipment. Nephron 40 (1985) 63–66

23 Munda, R., M.R. First, J.W. Alexander, C.C. Linnemann, J.P. Fidler, D. Kittur: Polytetrafluoroethylene graft survival in hemodialysis. J. Amer. med. Ass. 249 (1983) 219–222

24 Quinton, W., D. Dillard, B.H. Scribner: Cannulation of blood vessels for prolonged hemodialysis. Trans. Amer. Soc. artif. intern. Org. 6 (1960) 104–113

25 Reilly, D.T., R.F.M. Wood, P.R.F. Bell: Prospective study of dialysis fistulas: problem patients and their treatment. Brit. J. Surg. 69 (1982) 549–553

26 Sabanayagam, P., A.B. Schwartz, R.R. Soricelli, P. Lyons, J. Chinitz: A comparative study of 402 bovine heterografts and 225 reinforced expanded PTFE grafts as AVF in the ESRD patient. Trans. Amer. Soc. artif. intern. Org. 26 (1980) 88–91

27 Shaldon, S.L., L. Chiandussi, B. Higgs: Hemodialysis by percutaneous catheterization of the femoral artery and vein with regional heparinization. Lancet II (1961) 857

28 Tellis, V.A., W.I. Kohlberg, D.J. Bhat, B. Driscoll, F.J. Veith: Expanded polytetrafluoroethylene graft fistula for chronic hemodialysis. Ann. Surg. 189 (1979) 101–105

29 Vorwerk, D., R.W. Günther, K. Bohndorf, A. Asgarzadeh, K. Borchers: Farbkodierte Duplexsonographie (Angiodynographie) in der Beurteilung arteriovenöser Shunts. Fortschr. Röntgenstr. 148 (1988) 265–268

8 Peripheral Veins

F. Fobbe

8.1 General Remarks

Diseases of the extremity veins are a common occurrence. Deep venous thrombosis (DVT) is the most clinically significant of these disorders because of its associated morbidity and mortality. In the United States approximately 20 million cases of DVT of the lower extremity are estimated to occur each year and 187 000 patients were treated for DVT in hospitals in 1987 (6, 13, 31). Deep venous thrombosis can lead to pulmonary embolism, postthrombotic syndrome due to venous insufficiency, and recurrent thrombosis. The clinical symptoms of deep venous thrombosis are often nonspecific, and a suspected pulmonary embolism may first direct suspicion toward thrombosis in an extremity. For these reasons, there is need for a diagnostic procedure that is easy to perform, low in cost, reliable, causes no side effects, requires no patient cooperation, and can be performed at bedside. Essentially all of these requirements are satisfied by diagnostic ultrasound.

8.2 Normal Anatomy and Common Variants

8.2.1 Veins of the Pelvis and Lower Extremity

The veins of the lower extremity consist of three anatomically and functionally distinct groups: (1) superficial veins, (2) deep veins, and (3) perforating veins.

1. The **superficial veins,** located directly below the skin, have a relatively thick muscular wall. The main vessels pass through connective-tissue pouches in the superficial fascia. The long (greater) saphenous vein and the short (lesser) saphenous vein are the principal superficial venous trunks of the lower extremity and receive blood from numerous, mostly unnamed tributaries. The long saphenous vein is the longest vein in the human body. It arises at the medial border of the foot, ascends about 2–3 cm anterior to the medial malleolus, crosses to the medial border of the tibia, then runs along the medial side of the leg to its termination at the femoral vein about 3 cm below the inguinal ligament. In many cases the vessel is duplicated, especially below the knee. The short saphenous vein begins behind the lateral malleolus as a continuation of the lateral marginal vein of the foot. From there it ascends along the back of the calf, perforates the deep fascia between the heads of the gastrocnemius muscle, and empties into the popliteal vein 3–8 cm above the level of the knee joint.

2. The **deep veins** of the lower extremity are accompanied by the homonymous arteries. They have a very thin muscular wall compared with the superficial veins. There are three groups of veins in the calf named for their accompanying arteries, each consisting of a variable number of veins.

- The posterior tibial veins originate from the plantar veins behind the medial malleolus. The largest tributaries come from the soleus muscle. They ascend in the postero-medial part of the calf.
- The peroneal veins (Vv. fibulares) receive tributaries from the heel region and soleus muscle. They unite with the posterior tibial veins in the proximal third of the lower leg.
- The anterior tibial veins are the proximal continuations of the dorsal veins of the foot. After ascending in front of the interosseous membrane in the distal two-thirds of the lower leg, they pass through the interosseous membrane in the proximal third and unite dorsally with the posterior tibial veins to form the popliteal vein.
- The popliteal vein ascends in the popliteal fossa, passing between the heads of the gastrocnemius and also bordered laterally by an extension of the biceps femoris and medially by the semitendineus. In the lower half of its course the vein is medial to the popliteal artery; above the knee joint it is posterolateral to it. In the adductor canal the popliteal vein becomes the femoral vein at the adductor hiatus (fissure between the insertions of the adductor magnus muscle).
- The femoral vein is posterior to the femoral artery except for its proximal one-fourth, which courses medial to the artery. It occupies the intermediate compartment of the femoral sheath and is bounded medially by the femoral canal. The fatty tissue in the femoral canal permits considerable expansion on the vein. Besides smaller muscle veins, the profunda femoris vein is the most important tributary, entering the back of the femoral vein 4–12 cm below the inguinal ligament and generally containing a valve just below its termination. The profunda femoris mostly drains the muscles of the thigh.

As in the femoral artery, clinical parlance subdivides the femoral vein into two anatomic segments: the superficial femoral vein below the entry of the profunda femoris, and the common femoral vein above the entry of the profunda femoris vein. The medial and lateral circumflex femoral veins either enter the common femoral vein directly above the profunda femoris vein or terminate at the profunda femoris vein itself. The long saphenous vein enters the common femoral vein anteriorly at the same level. The relatively small-caliber external pudendal vein enters from the medial side, establishing a communication with the internal iliac vein (Fig. 8.**1**).

- The common femoral vein becomes the external iliac vein behind the inguinal ligament. The vein follows the arcuate line upward and terminates in front of the sacroiliac joint by uniting with the internal iliac vein to form the common iliac vein. The inferior epigastric vein and deep circumflex iliac vein enter the external iliac vein anteriorly in its lower portion. These tributaries establish a communication with the superior vena cava. The right and left common iliac veins unite at the L5 level to form the inferior vena cava. Before this junction, the left common iliac vein crosses behind the ipsilateral common iliac artery (where the vein lumen may become compressed between the artery and the vertebral body). Unlike the lower extremity veins, the iliac vein is usually valveless.

3. The **perforating veins** run transversely through the deep fascia to establish connections between the superficial and deep veins. Like the deep veins, they have a very thin muscular wall. The perforating veins in the lower leg are of primary clinical interest. In the American literature, the perforators are divided by their location into three main groups: a posterolateral group, an anterolateral group, and a medial group. Valvular incompetence in the perforating veins is a major factor in the pathogenesis of varicose veins.

Anatomic variations are very common in the venous system. The deep veins generally accompany the corresponding arteries, so variants usually relate not to the course of the veins but to the number of lumina. No hard and fast rule can be stated for the superficial veins. Venographic studies indicate that the superficial femoral vein is duplicated in approximately 20% of individuals and is more than duplicated in 14%; the popliteal vein is duplicated in 20% and tripled in 2%. The number and course of the tibial veins are also subject to considerable variation (22, 35).

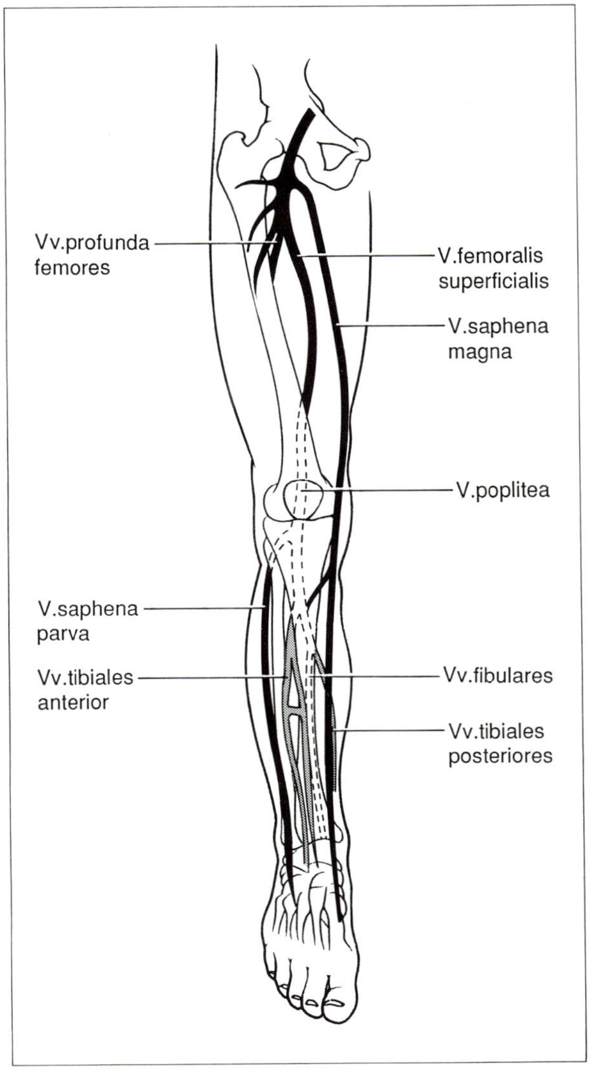

Fig. 8.**1** Venous anatomy of the lower extremity

8.2.2 Veins of the Upper Extremity, Shoulder, and Neck

As in the lower extremity, the veins of the upper extremity can be broadly classified as superficial or deep. Both groups communicate through multiple connections. The superficial veins are subcutaneous, while the deep veins are accompanied by arteries. Venous valves occur in both groups but are more numerous in the deep veins.

1. **Superficial veins.** Besides innumerable unnamed veins, there are two main superficial veins that merit discussion: the cephalic and the basilic vein.

- The cephalic vein arises from the dorsal radial network of the distal forearm and winds obliquely over the palmar side of the forearm to the elbow, receiving multiple side tributaries in its course. At the elbow it gives off the large median cubital vein, which enters the basilic vein. The main trunk then ascends subcutaneously in the groove formed by the brachioradialis muscle laterally and the biceps brachii muscle medially. In the proximal part of the upper arm the vein lies between the medial border of the deltoid muscle and the lateral border of the pectoralis major muscle. It then pierces the

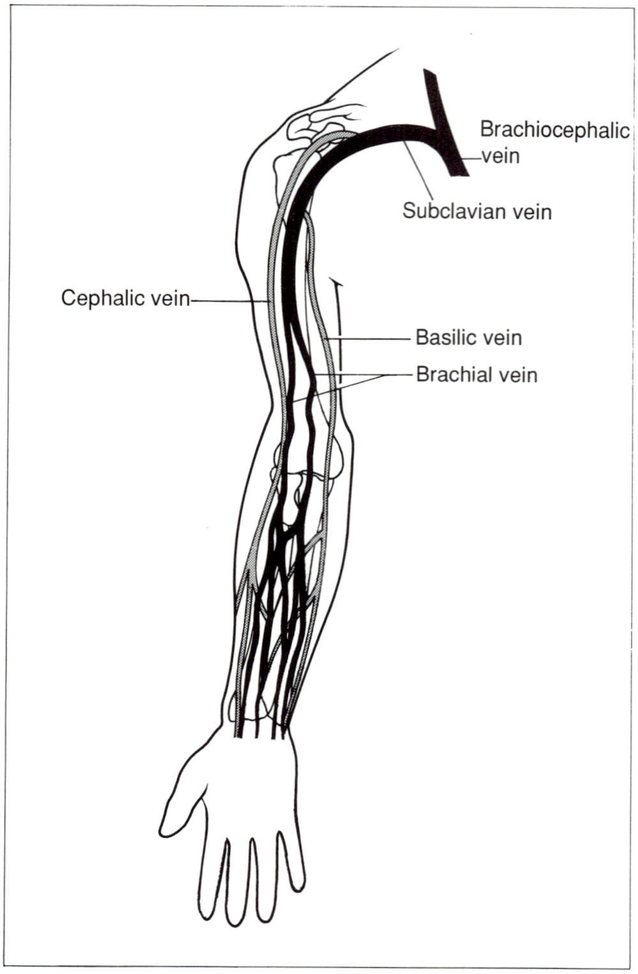

Fig. 8.**2** Venous anatomy of the upper extremity

clavipectoral fascia and enters the axillary vein just below the clavicle.

- The basilic vein begins in the dorsal ulnar network of the distal forearm. It ascends along the ulna before crossing to the palmar side in the proximal forearm. At the elbow it is joined by the medial cubital vein. The vessel continues to ascend in the groove formed by the biceps brachii muscle laterally and the pronator teres muscle medially. It perforates the deep fascia in the middle third of the upper arm, then follows the course of the brachial artery medially. The basilic vein becomes the axillary vein at the lower border of the teres major.

2. The **deep veins** of the upper extremity accompany the corresponding arteries. Occasionally there are several brachial veins in the upper arm that ensheath the brachial artery and empty into the axillary vein. The vessels have various communications with one another and with the superficial veins. The axillary vein begins by definition at the lower border of the teres major as the continuation of the basilic vein. It follows the course of the axillary artery and becomes the subclavian artery at the outer margin of the first rib. The subclavian vein relates anteriorly with the clavicle and subclavius muscle and behind and above with the subclavian artery. Inferiorly, the vein rests upon the first rib and the pleural dome. The medial third of the subclavian vein is separated from the artery by the scalenus anterior and the phrenic nerve. The subclavian vein unites with the internal jugular vein in front of the scalenus anterior to form the brachiocephalic vein (Fig. 8.**2**). The internal jugular vein is the downward continuation of the sigmoid sinus. It is related laterally to the internal and common carotid arteries. The brachiocephalic vein begins at the medial end of the clavicle, both brachiocephalic veins uniting behind the manubrium sterni to form the superior vena cava (35).

8.3 Examination Technique and Normal Findings

8.3.1 Lower-Extremity Veins

For examination of the proximal venous segments, the patient is placed in a supine position with the head as flat as possible. Particularly in obese patients, this gives better access to the groin and does not compromise venous return to the heart. In patients with dyspnea, the head may be elevated on a pillow. The legs should be extended with slight external rotation. The popliteal and lower leg regions are best examined in a supine position with the knee flexed to about 20°; this relaxes the soft-tissue structures in the popliteal fossa and makes it easier to apply compression. The lateral decibitus position also may be used. If the patient's condition prohibits this, an assistant can raise the leg so that the transducer can be applied from below. In all cases the patient should be positioned as comfortably as possible. Soft-tissue compression is much easier to apply when the patient is relaxed, especially in the area of the adductor canal. Due to the high acoustic absorption by structures in this region, compression is often necessary to obtain satisfactory grayscale imaging.

A 5-MHz transducer is best for examination of the deep veins. Though some authors advocate higher frequencies to improve spatial resolution, this is obtained at the cost of depth penetration. The vessels in the adductor canal and lower leg, for example, may be poorly defined by a higher-frequency transducer, especially in obese patients. In any case, the spatial resolution achieved with a 5-MHz transducer is adequate for the evaluation of the veins and the detection of thrombosis.

The velocity scale should be adjusted so that the relatively slow venous blood flow generates color-encoded flow signals without interference from the "fast" signals in adjacent arteries. Also, the movement of the transducer on the skin should produce as few artifacts as possible. Color encoding above a

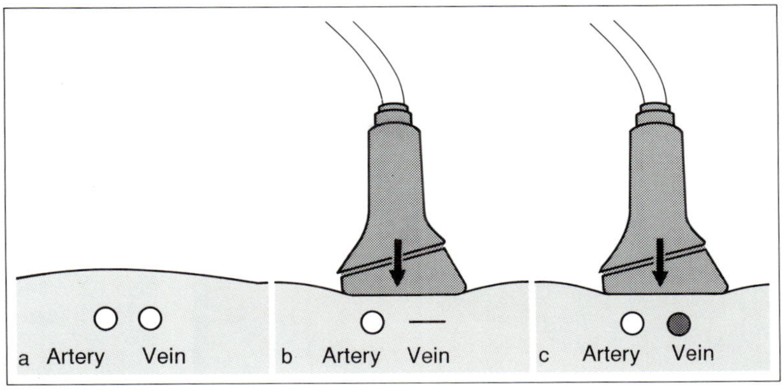

Fig. 8.**3** Principle of compression sonography (modified from [15]): Gentle pressure from the transducer can completely obliterate a normal vein (**b**), but transducer pressure does not alter the cross section of a thrombosed vein (**c**)

frequency shift of 50–100 Hz is satisfactory when a 5-MHz transducer is used (see Chapter 4).

The time required for a CDS examination of the lower-extremity veins depends on the examiner's experience. But a suitably trained and experienced sonographer should require no more than 10 min of pure examination time per leg.

The lumen of a normal vein, unlike an artery lumen, can be completely compressed and occluded by gentle pressure with the transducer. When completely compressed, the apposed venous walls are in most cases not distinguishable from the surrounding fatty tissue on the gray-scale image (Figs. 8.**3**, 8.**4a**, **b**). The complete compression of the venous lumen excludes venous thrombosis with a high degree of confidence. Pathologic changes are marked either by an inability to fully compress the vein lumen or by thickening of the vein wall. These are the basic criteria used in the venous examination. The vessel should be imaged transversely to ensure that the entire lumen is visualized. Longitudinal scanning (Fig. 8.**5**) is useful only as an adjunct to the transverse views. Both lower extremities should be examined routinely, because asymptomatic contralateral involvement may be found in patients with unilateral complaints, and findings are easier to interpret by comparison

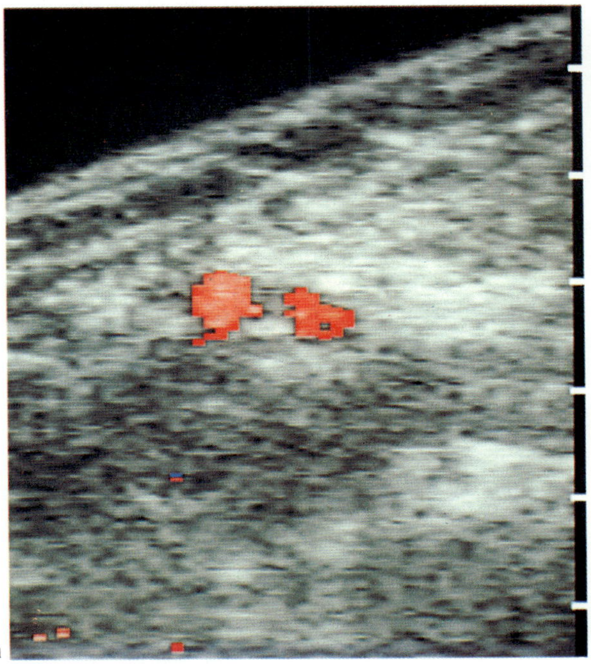

a

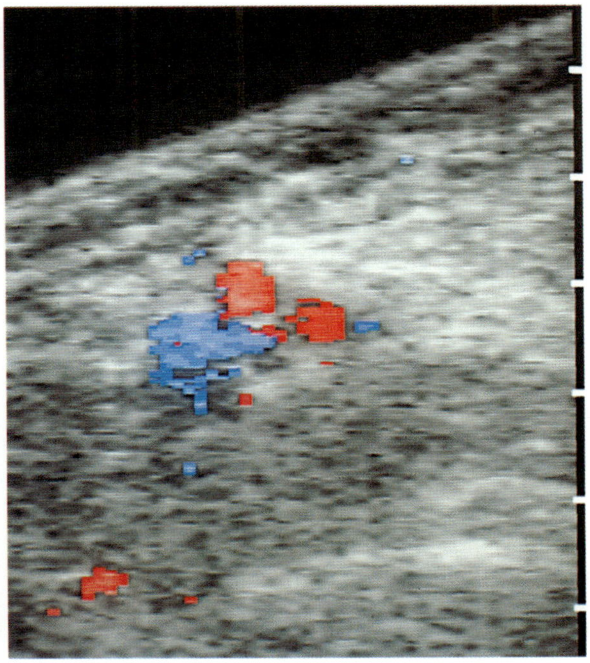

b

Fig. 8.**4a, b** Transverse scan through the upper thigh just above the division of the common femoral artery into the superficial femoral artery *(left)* and the profunda femoris artery *(right)*

a When pressure is applied with the transducer, flow signals are obtained from the arteries (red), but the walls of the veins are not clearly defined

b On release of the pressure, the venous lumen reopens, and there is an immediate resumption of increased venous flow (blue)

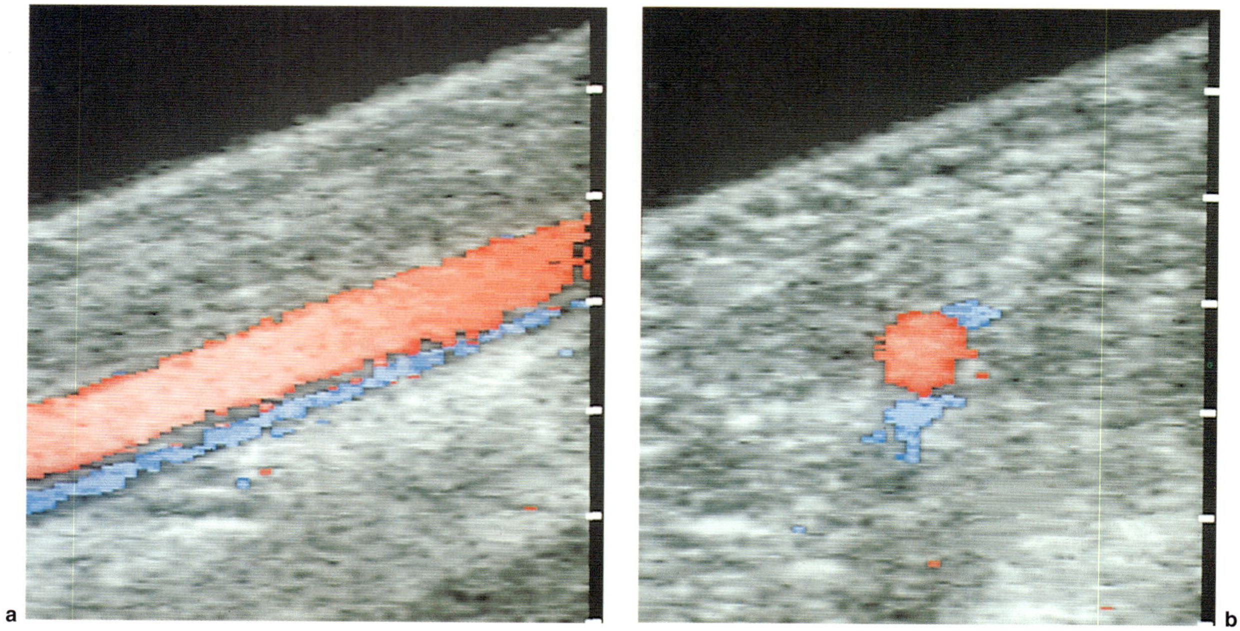

Fig. 8.**5a, b** Normal superficial femoral artery and vein
a Longitudinal image shows almost complete collapse of the vein in response to transducer pressure (venous flow is encoded in blue, arterial flow in red)
b Transverse image demonstrates the duplicated vein (blue)

with the opposite side. A side-to-side comparison is necessary in any case for the indirect evaluation of the pelvic veins.

The examination begins in the proximal thigh. The transducer is applied just below the inguinal ligament and oriented transversely so that the vein appears at the center of the image. The color-encoded signals from the accompanying artery permit rapid identification of the vessels. The artery and vein are easily differentiated in transverse view by color encoding, even when compression is not applied. While a rhythmic alteration of signals is noted in the arterial lumen, the venous flow is unidirectional and shows only phasic changes in response to respiration. A markedly obese patient is instructed to hold the abdomen cephalad with both hands. The vessels in this region are relatively superficial even in very obese patients and are easily assessed. Gentle pressure is applied with the transducer to compress the venous lumen. Just enough pressure is applied to occlude the vein without altering the shape of the artery (Fig. 8.**3**). From this position the transducer can be moved cephalad on the skin to define the distal portion of the external iliac vein. The rest of the pelvic veins can be indirectly evaluated by placing the transducer lightly on the skin (compression only with the weight of the transducer) and, maintaining the transverse orientation, angling the transducer slightly cephalad (beam angle $\neq 90°$) and instructing the patient to perform a Valsalva maneuver. If the pelvic veins are fully patent, deep inspiration will first produce a cessation of venous flow and an increase in the vascular diameter. Further straining will then induce a variable degree of venous reflux into the vessels of the thigh. Because the Valsalva response varies greatly among different individuals, comparison with the opposite side is imperative.

Maintaining a transverse orientation, the examiner moves the transducer several centimeters distally while applying compression, then stops and releases the pressure until the vein opens. He then reinitiates compression and moves the transducer farther distally. The examination proceeds distally in this fashion—moving the transducer with compression, then pausing and releasing the pressure—down to the adductor channel. Starting from the common femoral artery, first the profunda femoris artery and then the superficial femoral artery are identified, and the accompanying veins are examined. At each step the examiner makes certain to identify the signals from the accompanying artery. If the superficial femoral artery is occluded, the acoustic shadowing from arterial wall calcifications provides an obvious landmark in the gray-scale image.

The release of compression from patent veins is followed by an increase in venous blood flow due to the occlusive effect of the compression. In some patients, however, little or no evidence of blood flow will be seen on release of transducer pressure even if the venous system is fully patent. This can be remedied by carefully compressing the soft tissues distal to the examination site while maintaining a very light transducer pressure. This distal compression should augment the venous flow and make it detectable on the color-encoded flow image.

Adequate compression in the adductor canal can be achieved by manually pushing the soft tissues toward the transducer from the posteromedial aspect of the thigh (Fig. 8.6). Examination of the popliteal vein is assisted by appropriate repositioning (see above). Again, this segment is examined in transverse planes by moving the transducer distally with compression and pausing while the compression is released.

The deep veins of the proximal lower leg are easily identified as the distal continuations of the popliteal vein. The entry of larger gastrocnemius veins can also be identified. Positive identification of the short saphenous vein is rarely possible, however, due to its variable junction with the popliteal vein. Due to the great variability of venous anatomy below the knee, no attempt is made to identify all the vessels individually (in contrast to the examination technique in the thigh and knee). Rather, the transverse examination proceeds distally along the calf using the same technique as in the thigh, watching for rounded structures of low echogenicity. Because an isolated muscle fiber can appear as a rounded hypoechoic structure in the transverse image, comparison with the opposite side is again warranted. It is important to examine all segments of the lower leg. One can start by using one of the tibial arteries as a landmark and then proceeding with examination of the intervening areas. In very obese patients it may also be necessary to additionally examine the calf in the supine position. It is helpful in this situation to demonstrate the anterior tibial veins from an anterolateral approach between the tibia and fibula (the vessels are in front of the interosseous membrane!).

In the recumbent patient, the veins of the lower leg are in a collapsed state, and gray-scale image quality is compromised by the numerous myofascial planes. In many cases, therefore, the examiner will be unable to define the venous wall. One possible solution is to examine the patient in a sitting position with the lower leg unsupported. In this position the veins are filled and easier to visualize. But all the deep veins cannot be seen even with this technique, and examination in the supine position, as described above, is adequate for the detection or exclusion of thrombosis. Longitudinal venous examination is necessary only as an adjunct. For example, a longitudinal scan may provide a better view of blood flowing past a partially occlusive thrombosis. By itself, however, a longitudinal venous examination can be misleading, because any lateral deviation of the transducer during compression would yield a false-negative result.

Among the superficial veins, the long saphenous vein should be visualized in the proximal thigh. The rest of the superficial veins are collapsed in the supine patient. Due to the lack of a useful sonographic landmark for these veins, they can be identified only at their site of entry into a deep vein and in the thigh while the patient performs a Valsalva maneuver. In contrast, in patients with varicose veins, the dilated superficial vessels can be traced and followed when the patient is in an upright position. In some cases, even incompetent perforating veins can be identified by the display of retrograde venous flow.

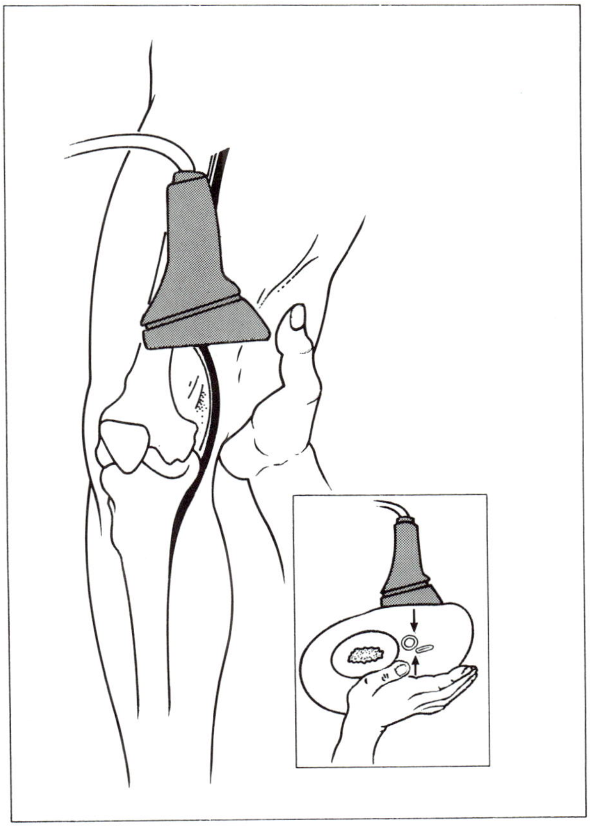

Fig. 8.**6** Examination of the vessels in the adductor canal. Because the vessels wind behind the femur from the medial side, manual pressure is applied posteromedially to displace the soft tissues toward the transducer

8.3.2 Veins of the Upper Extremity, Shoulder, and Neck

The examination technique for the upper extremity is similar to that for the lower extremity. The patient is positioned supine with the head as flat as possible. The arms are extended and slightly abducted with the forearms supinated. The axillary vessels are examined most easily in the elevated arm. The subclavian vein can be identified only in its lateral portion before it passes behind the clavicle. As in the lower extremity, the routine comparison of both sides is recommended.

The examination begins at the neck with identification of the internal jugular vein. The common carotid artery is imaged in transverse section. The jugular vein is collapsed in the supine patient and during quiet respiration, and it opens in response to deep inspiration and straining. Vessel-wall pulsations transmitted from the heart are occasionally observed. The vessel is tracked inferiorly to a point slightly above its junction with the subclavian vein. The brachiocephalic vein can be evaluated only indirectly by the change in the venous signals during respiration. The transducer is then placed on the chest wall, parallel to the long axis of the body, and moved laterally until the subclavian artery and vein are identified behind the clavicle. The vein courses slightly anteroinferior to the artery in this region. They are further differentiated by their distinctive color-encoded flow signals (continuous flow in the vein versus rhythmic flow in the artery). The quality of the flow signals can be improved by slight angulation of the transducer. If pathologic changes are present, a frequency analysis may also be required to differentiate the vessels. After the subclavian vein has been identified, the patient is instructed to perform a Valsalva maneuver. If the vein is fully patent, the maneuver will evoke an abrupt cessation or reversal of the venous flow.

The examination is continued in the axilla, proceeding with transverse views of the artery and vein and evaluating the proximal segments indirectly by the response of the flow signals to forced respiration. The rest of the examination proceeds as in the lower-extremity veins. The vein is transversely compressed by light transducer pressure on the soft tissues, and the transducer is moved distally. The deep veins and accompanying arteries in the upper arm should be comprehensively surveyed. In the forearm as in the lower leg, the examination is limited to a search for pathologic changes; no attempt is made to demonstrate all the veins in their entirety. The superficial veins are identifiable only at their site of entry into a deep vein or if they are thrombosed.

8.3.3 Documentation

The documentation of pathology should specify the exact location of the lesion, its extent, its relation to other structures, and the nature of the abnormality (e. g., partial or complete thrombosis, fresh or old thrombus). Given the limited scope of the ultrasound scan, the exact location of a lesion often cannot be determined from the image itself, so a detailed description must be provided. This description can be supplemented by recording the location and extent of the lesion on a standardized schematic diagram (like that in Fig. 8.**1**). For follow-up purposes, it is also helpful to mark the extent of the pathology on the skin with a waterproof marker. Venous thrombosis should be documented by a transverse image depicting the greatest diameter of the thrombus and by images at its proximal and distal ends. The description should indicate the composition of the thrombus and its relation to the vein wall. An older, partially occlusive thrombus in the popliteal vein, for example, might be described in these terms: venous lumen incompletely compressible, with a nonhomogeneously hypoechoic intraluminal echogenicity; maximum vein diameter on compression is 1.4 times that of the adjacent artery; flow signals detected near the vessel wall after manual compression of the calf; distal limit of thrombus at the entry of the anterior tibial vein, proximal limit at the level of the inferior patellar border.

8.4 Pathologic Findings

8.4.1 Lower-Extremity Veins

Venous disorders are a very common clinical problem. Relatively few disease entities are causative, however, with thrombosis and varicosity accounting for more than 90% of cases. The rest are based on rare vascular malformations, which may occur alone or in association with complex anomalies (e. g., Klippel–Trenaunay–Weber syndrome).

Venous stasis is the most important contributory factor to venous thrombosis. Accidental or surgical trauma and hypercoagulability also have causal importance. Thrombosis is thought to originate most commonly in the sinuses between the valve cusps and vein wall, from which point the thrombus propagates proxiesedfmally or distally through the aggregation of blood constituents. With passage of time the vein may recanalize (spontaneously or as a result of therapy) or remain occluded. In any case the inflammation accompanying the thrombosis damages the functional competence of the venous valves, leading to varicosity (postphlebitic syndrom). This differs from "primary varicose veins" occurring in the absence of detectable preexisting disease. Genetic and environmental influences have been implicated in the pathogenesis of primary varicose veins. Varicosity is characterized by a dilated vessel lumen, tortuosity, and a thin, fragile venous wall. Because of the luminal dilatation, even venous valves that are initially functional are rendered incompetent.

The most reliable criterion for the sonographic diagnosis of venous thrombosis is lack of compressibility of the vein lumen. Whereas a normal vein is easily obliterated by light transducer pressure, a thrombosed vessel shows little or no collapse in response to compression. A partially occluded vein may show elliptical distortion by pressure from the transducer.

A completely thrombosed deep vein appears in the gray-scale image as a hypoechoic structure, devoid of flow signals, located directly adjacent to the artery (Figs. 8.**7a–c**, 8.**8a**, **b**). Careful compression of the soft tissues distal to the examination site does not elicit flow. Both the transducer pressure and the manual soft-tissue compression should be applied gently and carefully to avoid at least the theoretical possibility of dislodging a thrombus and causing pulmonary embolism. It is unclear how real this danger is in practice. During the clinical examination of the lower extremities, the examiner may, for example, check for pain in response to calf compression or for

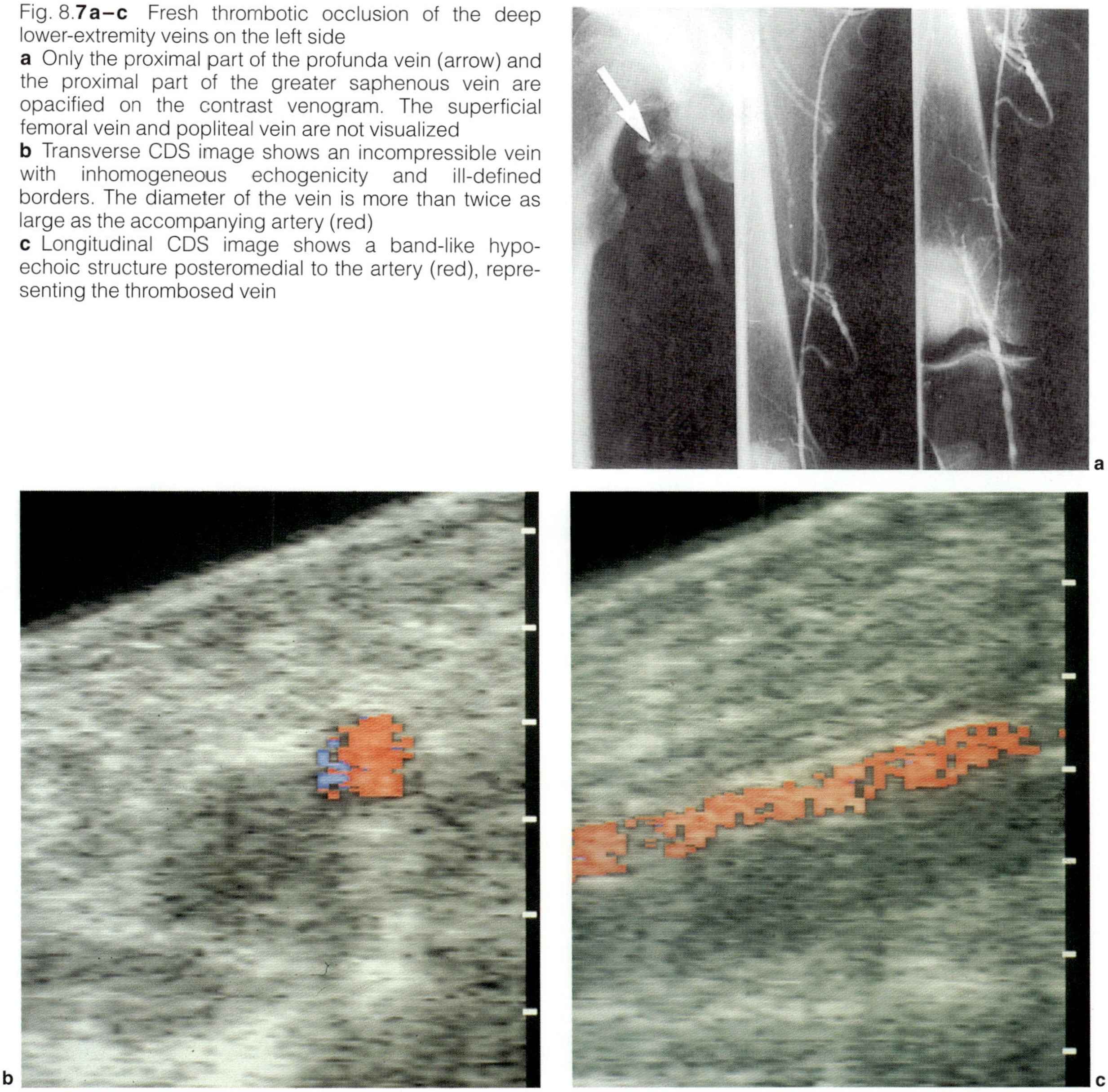

Fig. 8.**7a–c** Fresh thrombotic occlusion of the deep lower-extremity veins on the left side
a Only the proximal part of the profunda vein (arrow) and the proximal part of the greater saphenous vein are opacified on the contrast venogram. The superficial femoral vein and popliteal vein are not visualized
b Transverse CDS image shows an incompressible vein with inhomogeneous echogenicity and ill-defined borders. The diameter of the vein is more than twice as large as the accompanying artery (red)
c Longitudinal CDS image shows a band-like hypoechoic structure posteromedial to the artery (red), representing the thrombosed vein

calf pain evoked by compression of the thigh. There are no reported instances of pulmonary embolism provoked by the clinical examination. We have performed this examination in more than 7000 patients in the past 6 years and have seen no evidence of compression-induced embolization. The literature contains two reported case of a thrombus embolizing to the lung from the femoral vein during compression sonography of the lower extremity (27, 36). One of our patients suffered a pulmonary embolism after performing a Valsalva maneuver. But this maneuver is necessary for the maintenance of physiologic processes, and the embolism might easily have occurred at any other time. Nevertheless, the potential for an examiner-induced pulmonary embolism should be kept in mind and should prompt the examiner to proceed carefully (e.g., by gradually increasing the transducer pressure when applying compression).

With a complete venous thrombosis, color-encoded flow signals are detected only in the accompanying artery. With a partially occlusive thrombosis, compression may alter the vessel lumen depending on the diameter of the thrombus. The CDS image is particularly helpful in these cases and can differentiate thrombus-related flow voids from areas of residual perfusion (Fig. 8.**9a**, **b**). Longitudinal examination is a helpful adjunct to transverse scans for demonstrating slow blood flow without having to adjust the transducer angle. Spontaneous flow may not be apparent in the supine position, especially if the thrombus oc-

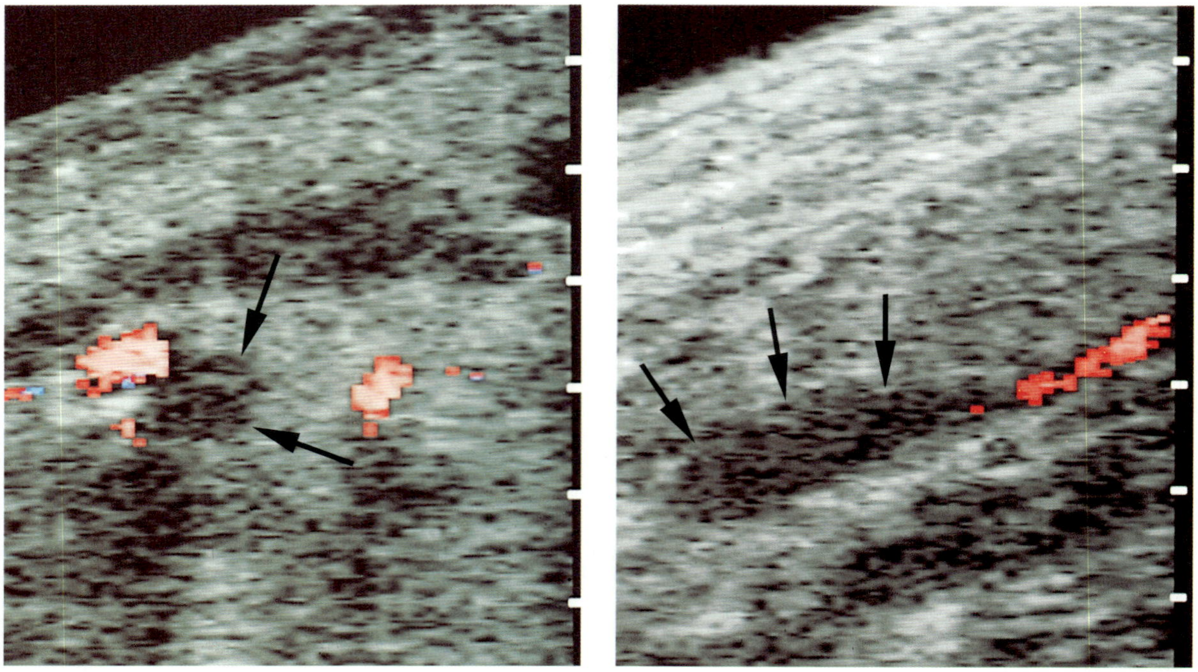

Fig. 8.**8a, b** Thrombotic occlusion of a calf vein (peroneal group)
a Transverse image shows a rounded, well-defined hypoechoic structure (arrows) directly adjacent to the artery (red). The structure contains no flow signals and has an echogenicity similar to that of adjacent muscle
b Longitudinal image shows a well-defined, fusiform, uniformly hypoechoic area with no flow signals (arrows) adjacent to the artery

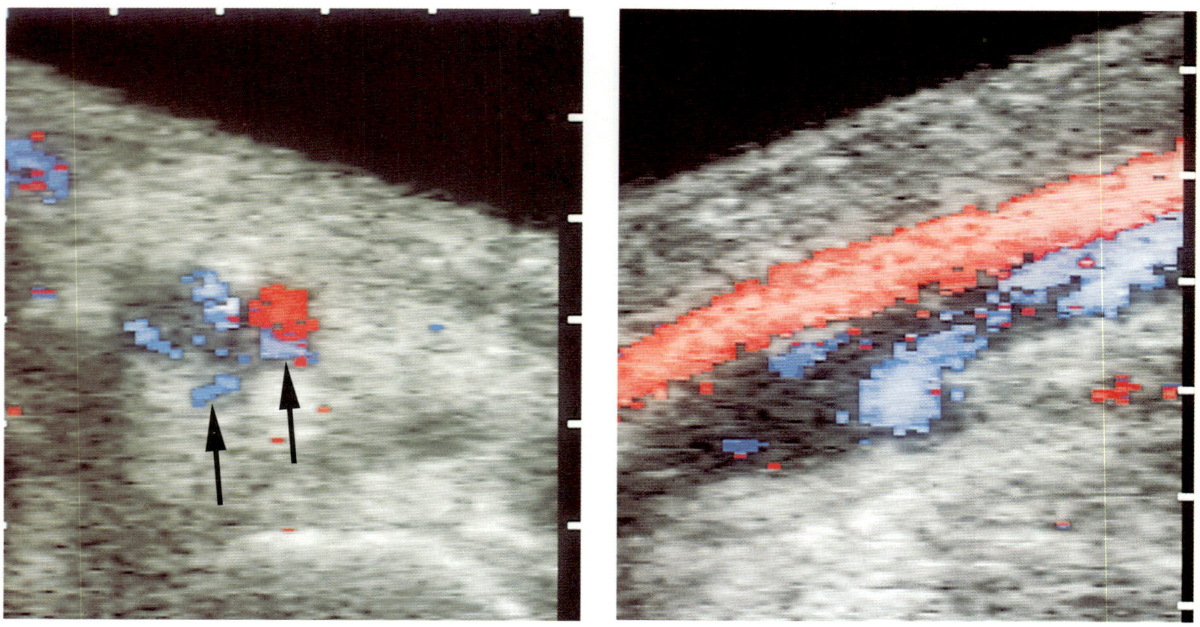

Fig. 8.**9a, b** Old, partially occlusive thrombus in the left superficial femoral vein
a Transverse image shows an incompletely compressible, sharply demarcated vein with a hypoechoic texture medial to the accompanying artery (red). The diameter of the vein is about 50% greater than that of the artery. Venous (blue) flow signals are registered at the posteromedial and anterolateral borders of the vessel. Two profunda veins (arrows) enter the vessel posterolaterally. A superficial vein (= greater saphenous vein) appears at upper left
b Longitudinal image shows a well-defined, hypoechoic band-like structure posteromedial to the artery (red) containing residual areas of venous flow (blue)

cludes almost all of the lumen, so the extent of the residual flow channels should always be evaluated separately. This is done by defining the thrombus in the gray-scale image and then carefully compressing the soft tissues distal to the transducer with the hand. This augments the venous outflow so that residual perfusion channels are clearly defined (Figs. 8.**9a**, **b**, 8.**10a**, **b**). Generally the Valsalva maneuver is not useful for demonstrating a partially occlusive thrombus in the upper leg.

If the compression with the transducer leads to deformation of the accompanying artery, too much pressure is being applied, and it is reasonable to assume the presence of pathologic changes. This finding is typical, for example, of a complete proximal occlusion of the common iliac vein with patency of the external iliac vein and thigh veins. The outflow obstruction causes stasis in the veins distal to the occlusion, with consequent dilatation of the vessels. With a fresh occlusion, the intraluminal pressure is often so high that the vein can be compressed only by applying sufficient force to deform the accompanying artery. The diagnosis can be made more easily with CDS: when the shape of the vein is altered (by transducer pressure), blood will move within the venous lumen even if severe stasis is present. These color-encoded flow signals reliably differentiate a thrombotically distended vessel from a vessel that is dilated due to proximal outflow obstruction. In the case of a partially occluded proximal pelvic vein, a side-to-side comparison may show dilatation of the common femoral vein or distal external iliac vein on the uninvolved side at rest, or a right–left discrepancy may be noted in response to the Valsalva maneuver.

The boundaries of the thrombosed vein may be sharp or ill-defined, and its internal structure may be homogeneous or nonhomogeneous. These criteria are unreliable for estimating thrombus age. Relatively few authors have dealt with the problem of determining the age of venous thrombi using ultrasound. In vitro experiments, for example, have involved the sonographic study of fresh blood allowed to clot in plastic tubes (1, 5). These experiments showed that freshly clotted blood has a high echogenicity that diminishes over time. These findings probably cannot be applied to the venous system in a patient. On the one hand, filling the tubes with blood causes air to mix with the blood, and the trapped air will increase the echogenicity of the clot. The decreasing echogenicity could result from a gradual escape of the air over time. Moreover, thrombus formation in vivo cannot be compared to the clotting of blood in a plastic tube. Even the examination of alcohol-sclerosed superficial varices (24) is of limited value due to the entirely different mechanism of the vascular occlusion.

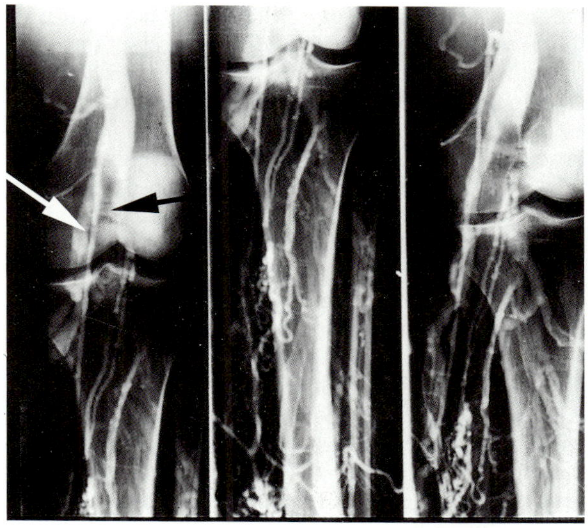
a

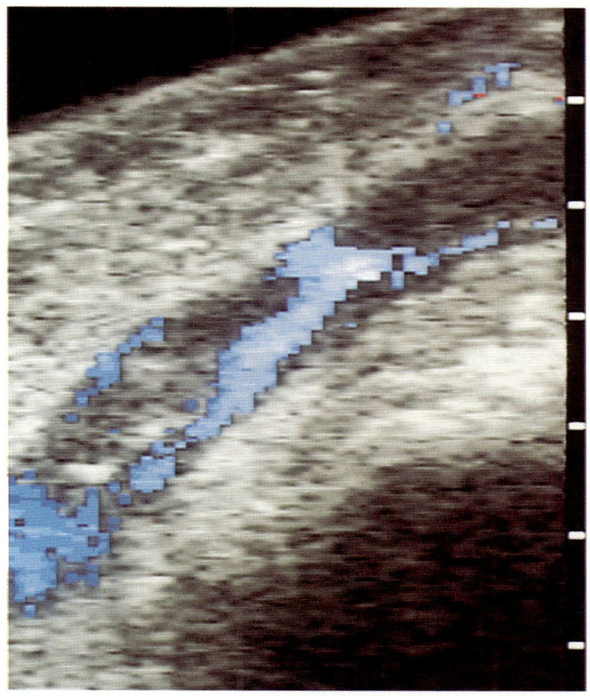
b

Fig. 8.**10a, b** Partially occlusive thrombus in the popliteal vein accompanied by venous thrombi in the lower leg
a Venograms demonstrate partial occlusion of the deep veins of the lower leg with flow of contrast medium past a thrombus (arrows) in the popliteal vein
b Longitudinal CDS image shows a noncompressible popliteal vein with a nonhomogeneous echogenicity and venous flow signals (blue) near the vessel wall representing areas of residual blood flow past the thrombus

Regardless of the results of experimental studies, there are problems with using echogenicity or the definition of the venous wall as a criterion. A major difficulty is that the characterization of echogenicity as "homogeneous" (uniform) or "nonhomogeneous" (nonuniform, heterogeneous) depends on the examiner, the instrument settings, and the constitution of the patient. The gray-scale image gain can be adjusted to produce either a homogeneous or heterogeneous echo pattern. In obese patients the increased absorption and scatter of sound waves tends to impart a heterogeneous echo pattern to the vessel lumen. For the same reasons, the definition of the boundaries of the vessel wall are not useful for the assessment of thrombus age.

In our experience the only useful criterion for estimating thrombus age is the diameter of the thrombosed vein. Acute thrombosis leads to venous distention, and the diameter of the vein can be determined sonographically with reasonable accuracy. To allow for individual differences, it is advisable to take the ratio of the greatest diameter of the thrombosed vein (under compression) to the greatest diameter of the accompanying artery. A ratio of 2 or more suggests very strongly that the thrombosis is less than 10 days old (12). If the ratio is less than 2, the thrombosis is more than 10 days old (Figs. 8.**7a–c**, 8.**9a**, **b**). This method will yield a reliable assessment of thrombus age in the majority of cases, although equivocal or misleading results are possible. Thus the question of thrombus age should always be considered within the context of all the available clinical data.

While it is possible to differentiate an acute thrombosis (up to 10 days old) from an older thrombosis by measuring the venous diameter, older thrombotic changes cannot be further differentiated. A thrombosed vessel may undergo spontaneous recanalization, or it may remain occluded. At present there is no reliable way to determine whether recanalization will occur in a particular vessel or patient in response to a particular treatment. When a thrombosed vein is detected whose diameter approximates that of the accompanying artery, the thrombus may be 2 weeks old or 6 months old (12, 15). A further differentiation cannot be accomplished with imaging procedures. The ultrasound appearance of an intravenous thrombus may remain unchanged for months after the acute inflammation. The thrombus may undergo lysis, which can culminate in recanalization or occlusion of the vessel. In the latter case ultrasound may fail to demonstrate the vein in its expected position next to the artery, or it may demonstrate only short, partially recanalized venous segments. With CDS, however, a varying degrees of venous collaterals in proximity to the original vein will be demonstrated. These collateral veins, which are not present in a healthy venous system, frequently have small lumina (Fig. 8.**11**) and are detectable only by the presence of color-encoded flow signals (especially after soft-tissue compression distal to the examination site). Following recanalization of the vessel lumen, the vein may present a completely normal sonographic appearance, or it may show a variable degree of wall thickening (Fig. 8.**12**). These wall changes are best appreciated during luminal compression. Longitudinal examination of the vein shows a disappearance of normal laminar flow and the appearance of conspicuous turbulent zones (red–blue alternation) caused by the wall irregularities (Table 8.**1**). Even if a vein appears normal sonographically, postthrombotic changes may still be present. This is due to

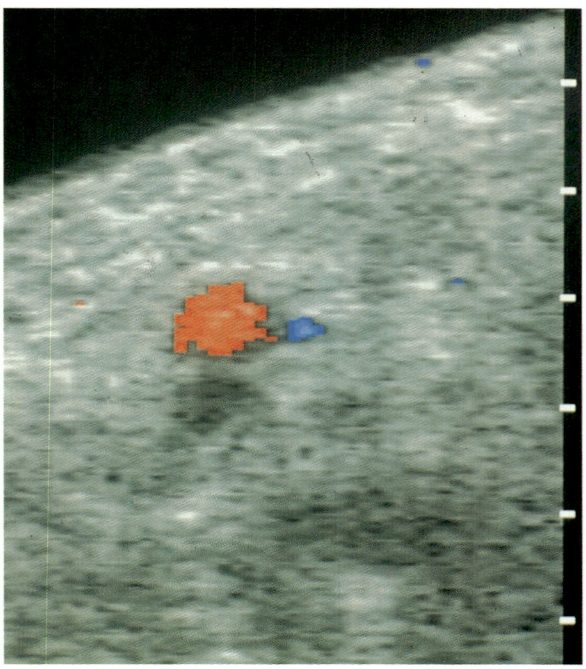

Fig. 8.**11** Transverse image of an old thrombotic occlusion of the left superficial femoral vein. Dorsal to the artery (red) is a well-defined rounded area of uniformly low echogenicity (smaller diameter than the artery) containing no flow signals. The blue-encoded area lateral to the artery represents a small-caliber collateral vein

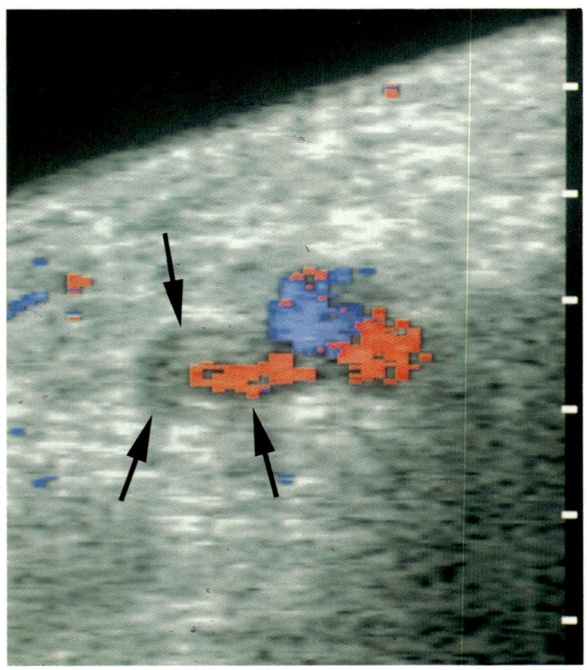

Fig. 8.**12** Postphlebitic changes in the left superficial femoral vein. Transverse image demonstrates flow signals in the lumen (here encoded red) with marked thickening of the venous wall (arrows). A profunda vein (red) of normal wall thickness enters posterolateral to the artery (blue)

Table 8.1 Summary of CDS findings in the lower-extremity veins

Normal	Vein completely compressible, thin venous wall, flow response to respiration and distal soft-tissue compression are equal on both sides
Fresh thrombosis (< 10 days old)	Vein incompressible, lumen diameter two or more times larger than that of the accompanying artery, possible residual flow near the vessel wall
Older thrombosis (> 10 days)	– Occlusion: vein incompressible, lumen diameter less than twice that of the accompanying artery, no flow signals – Partial occlusion: vein partially compressible, lumen diameter less than twice that of the accompanying artery, some residual flow at the vessel wall
Postthrombotic changes	Thickened venous wall, turbulent flow, short or longer segmental venous occlusion, collateral vessels

postinflammatory changes of the venous valves, whose function are difficult to assess even with CDS.

One problem of differential diagnosis relates to the detection of recurrent thrombosis in a postthrombotic vein. Due to the scarred, thickened condition of the vein wall, recurrent thrombosis does not produce as much vascular distention as a fresh thrombus does in a normal vessel. Because all segments of a vessel usually do not show the same degree of inflammatory change, the fresh thrombus may be detected in a segment where only minimal wall changes are present. This again underscores the importance of routinely examining the veins in all portions of the lower extremity.

Venous thrombosis may be followed by a "postphlebitic syndrome" caused by postinflammatory valvular incompetence and/or persistent deep venous occlusion. The role of CDS is limited to detection of the postinflammatory changes in the deep venous system. Primary and secondary varicose veins cannot be differentiated on the basis of sonographic findings. In particular, CDS is rarely successful in the detection of perforator vein incompetence. It is true that venous valves can be defined with ultrasound, and their motion and changes in blood flow direction (e. g., during a Valsalva maneuver) can be demonstrated by CDS imaging. But this is possible only in certain venous valves that are readily accessible to CDS examination (e. g., the terminal valve of the great saphenous vein). The function of the venous system is a complex process that cannot be evaluated sufficiently by local examination. Moreover, the results of a CDS examination depend partly on the patient's position and muscle tonus and therefore are difficult to standardize. Functional evaluation of the venous system is still the province of the clinical examination, supplemented by intravenous pressure measurements (4) and contrast venography to demonstrate the incompetent perforating veins. CDS is only used as a supportive diagnostic procedure.

Perivenous changes can induce clinical changes similar to that of DVT. The most commonly encountered lesions are a (ruptured) Baker cyst, hematoma, or an aneurysm of the accompanying artery. The color-encoded flow signals permit the rapid differentiation of aneurysm from other pathologic fluid collections (see Chapters 5 and 6).

Vascular malformations and tumors of the venous system are rare. Klippel–Trenaunay–Weber syndrome (partial angiectatic gigantism) is marked by ectasia of the extremity veins. The deep and/or superficial veins may be affected in varying degrees. The vessels, which may be grotesquely enlarged, can be emptied by pressure from the transducer, and the connections among the individual venous segments can be demonstrated with CDS. Hemodynamically significant congenital a–v fistulae are extremely rare. Arteriovenous communications are most commonly the result of arterial needle puncture or other trauma. Superficial angiomas usually show very little perfusion on CDS images. CDS can differentiate these lesions from glomus tumor, which typically has a copious blood supply (see Chapters 5 and 6).

8.4.2 Veins of the Upper Extremity, Shoulder, and Neck

Venous lesions in the neck and upper extremity have the same sonographic features as in the lower extremity. A common cause of upper extremity venous thrombosis is central venous catheterization. The Paget–Schroetter syndrome (axillary vein thrombosis, effort thrombosis) is characterized by a sudden swelling of the arm that usually is preceded by physical exertion. The cause is a thrombotic occlusion of the subclavian vein, often without involvement of the axillary vein. Examination reveals marked distention of the axillary vein relative to the opposite side and lack of flow response to respiration. Scanning of the accessible (lateral) portions of the subclavian vein shows venous distention with no evidence of blood movement. Isolated occlusion of the brachiocephalic vein leads to distention of the distal veins and a pathologic Valsalva response.

8.5 Diagnostic Value of Color Duplex Sonography in Relation to Other Diagnostic Procedures

The value of a diagnostic procedure is measured in relation to other methods of examination. A diagnostic procedure may be classified as direct or indirect. Indirect procedures for examining the venous system include radionuclide imaging, thermography, plethysmography, and CW Doppler sonography. The main disadvantage of these modalities is that they do not demonstrate the vein itself but only the changes produced by thrombosis. Thus thrombosis is detected with a relatively high sensitivity but poor specificity, and a positive study warrants further investigation by direct imaging procedures. The indirect procedures, moreover, can cover only portions of the extremity veins. Radionuclide scanning can reliably detect only thromboses below the knee, while CW Doppler is limited to thromboses in the thigh and pelvic veins (3, 10, 17, 30, 38). These procedures cannot be meaningfully compared with CDS, therefore. Additionally, these noninvasive studies have declined in relative importance with the development of ultrasound techniques and probably will continue to do so.

The standard by which every venous examination procedure must be judged is contrast venography. This modality provides direct visualization of venous lumina opacified by contrast medium. It permits direct evaluation of changes in the venous wall and valves and the indirect evaluation of perivascular processes. Venography has been used as the decisive reference standard for many years. While there is no question as to the diagnostic value of venography, it is important to note that the modality has never been truly validated, and that attempts to provide this validation have been inadequate. Two studies illustrate this point: Lund et al. (23) demonstrated the lower-extremity veins in fresh cadavers by intraosseous venography and compared the results with autopsy findings obtained immediately after the contrast study. It is unclear, however, whether such a study can be validly applied to living patients. Hull et al. (18) used serial examinations in patients with clinical signs of lower-extremity venous thrombosis and a negative venogram to test the reliability of the method. Clinical manifestations increased in 1.3% of their subjects during the first 5 days after venography, prompting repeat venograms that demonstrated obvious thrombosis. This study, too, may be called into question because repeat venography was performed only because of clinical progression, so any resolving thrombi that may have been missed on initial examination went undetected. Serial venographic examinations are not very feasible because of their cost and potential side effects. The inadequate validation of venography as a reliable modality is due ultimately to a lack of available reference methods.

Table 8.**2** Sensitivity and specificity of ultrasound in the detection of thrombotic changes in the deep lower-extremity veins compared with venography. (B) = Examination with B-mode sonography, (CDS) = examination with color duplex sonography

	Sensitivity (%)	Specificity (%)
Lensing et al., 1989 (B) (220 legs) (21)	91	99
Krings et al., 1990 (B) (235 legs) (20)	93	96
Fobbe et al., 1989 (CDS) (129 legs) (11)	96	97
Rose et al., 1990 (CDS) (75 legs) (32)	*96	*100

In a study from Picolet et al. (28) venograms from a multicenter study were evaluated by two independent radiologists. Three months after the first evaluation the same radiologists performed a new reading: 35% of the readings had at least one difference and 15% the discrepancies were due to the presence of a thrombosis. This emphasizes that even venography is a subjective method and differences may be based on the divergent technique and/or evaluating (2, 26, 28).

Every new method is judged by traditional procedures. When the results of sonography and venography are compared in terms of detecting lower-extremity venous thrombosis, sonography is found to provide a high sensitivity (91–96%). The four studies cited in Table 8.**2** are representative of the many that have been published in recent years. However, in a recent study of asymptomatic patients Davidson et al. (7) found a sensitivity of only 38% for the detection of proximal leg thrombosis. The authors suggested that fresh thrombi may be fully compressible and therefore are not detectable by compression ultrasound. This explanation is questionable, however: even a fresh thrombus will lead to a small residual vessel lumen on compression and therefore should be detected with careful examination technique. The examinations in this study were done in different centers, by different technicians and physicians, with no proper information given about the examination protocol, the adjustment of the ultrasound machine, or the criteria for a thrombosis. At least this study emphasizes the dependence of the method on the examiner and the importance of a proper technique: In all cases the veins of the entire leg have to be scanned, and the result must be compared with the contralateral side. In our opinion, there is no reason to examine only parts of the veins (as described in [16]) because the time saved is minimal and small thrombi can be missed.

The importance of venography and CDS in evaluating the veins of the calf is controversial. Until a few years ago, it was widely believed that the number and variability of the veins in the calf prohibited a comprehensive sonographic evaluation, so that thrombosis could not be excluded by that method (11, 29). In all symptomatic patients who have patent veins in the thigh and about the knee, lack of information about the below-knee veins inevitably leads to a demand for a supplementary venogram. But this policy seriously limits the value of sonography. A breakthrough came when it was discovered that it is unnecessary to demonstrate all the normal deep veins of the lower leg, and that the examination can be limited to a search for thrombosed veins (15). Working from this premise, even an isolated venous thrombosis in the lower leg can be detected with acceptable confidence in comparison with venography (Table 8.**3**). It should be added that even venography cannot define all the deep veins in the lower leg. In particular, thrombi in smaller veins that completely occlude the vessel may be missed due to the absence of an obvious filling defect (Table 8.**4**). In our experience, the majority of thromboses of the deep veins of the pelvis and lower extremity can be detected with sufficient confidence by CDS.

Besides the detection of thrombosis, thrombus age is a key factor in the planning of optimum treatment. The history and clinical presentation are of limited value in this regard. In venography, the degree of collateralization and the appearance of the thrombus itself can be used in estimating thrombus age (25). But these changes are not very reliable, especially in cases of recurrent thrombosis. The diameter of the thrombosed vein is easily determined sonographically and, when correlated with the history and clinical findings, usually permits a reliable assessment of thrombus age (12). This applies to all veins proximal to and including the popliteal vein. It is not yet known whether vessel diameter is also useful for estimating the age of venous thrombi in the calf.

Sonography is of limited value in patients with significant edema, hematomas, soft-tissue calcifications, and/or a deficient acoustic window due to a recent surgical wound or cutaneous defect. Even so, CDS can always be tried since it is well tolerated, can be performed quickly and economically, and does not require a cooperative patient. If this attempt is unsuccessful, one can always proceed with contrast venography if necessary.

Two serious drawbacks of CDS compared with venography are its examiner-dependence and the difficulty of a complete documentation of findings. Venography customarily provides a straightforward global view of relevant vascular anatomy that is superior to the cross-sectional or short segmental sonographic views, which make it difficult to relate findings to a specific location. Additionally, the quality of the ultrasound examination cannot be assessed by reviewing the documentation. One solution to this problem is close cooperation among the involved disciplines. In doubtful cases the examination can be repeated as often as desired, even in bed-confined patients.

Essentially all the foregoing points apply with equal validity to venous examinations in the upper extremity and neck. Although few comparative studies have been done due to the low incidence of thrombosis in these veins (14, 19), the results of these studies are fully consistent with experience in the vessels of the lower extremity.

Because sonography portrays the vascular system and its surroundings differently from venography, it is reasonable to expect a divergence of findings among different authors. The strengths and weaknesses of both procedures are also different and are not adequately described by statistical terms such as sensitivity and specificity. In Table 8.**5**, therefore, we use a three-point rating system in an attempt to objectify these differences. This assessment is based on the author's many years of experience with both modalities and on current reports in the literature. In several of the points listed in Table 8.**5**, venography and CDS are given the same or similar ratings. Significant differences are noted, for example, in examinations of the pelvic veins. While CDS permits only an indirect evaluation of this region, venography can

Table 8.**3** Sensitivity and specificity of ultrasound in the detection of isolated thrombotic changes in the veins of the calf compared with venography

	Sensitivity 5%	Specificity 5%
Elias et al., 1987 (92 legs) (8)	91	96
Habscheid et al., 1990 (37 legs) (15)	89	99
Yucel et al., 1991 (45 legs) (37)	88	
Vanninen et al., 1993 (51 legs) (34)	77	93

Table 8.**4** Comparison of venography and CDS in the detection of isolated thrombotic changes in the veins of the calf leg in asymptomatic and symptomatic patients (our investigation)

		Venography	
	Ultrasound	Normal	Thrombotic
Asymptomatic (n = 70)	Normal	64	–
	Thrombotic	–	6
Symptomatic (n = 47)	Normal	21	3
	Thrombotic	5	18

Table 8.**5** Relative value of venography and CDS in various aspects of lower-extremity venous examinations. The more "plus" signs given for an entry, the more favorable the rating of the procedure

	Venography	CDS
Pelvic veins	++	+
Femoral vein	+++	+++
Profunda veins	+	+++
Popliteal vein	+++	+++
Below-knee veins	++	++
Superficial veins	+++	+
Patency	+++	+++
Wall changes	++	+++
Complete/partial occlusion	++	+++
Extent of thrombosis	++	+++
Thrombus age determination	+	+++
Collaterals	+++	++
Perivascular structures	+	+++
Venous valves	+++	+
Edema/hematoma, cutaneous defect/postoperative	+++	+
Soft-tissue calcifications	++	+
Documentation	+++	+
Examiner dependence	++	+
Patient cooperation	+	+++
Side effects	+	+++
Cost	+	+++
Technical complexity of procedure	+	+++
Examination time	+	+++

demonstrate the proximal extent of the thrombosis, at least in the case of older and partially occlusive thrombi. With a fresh, complete occlusion of the pelvic veins, neither modality can provide a meaningful assessment. Computed tomography (CT) with contrast enhancement is the modality of choice for ascertaining the cause of venous thrombosis in the pelvis. Sonography and CT are better than venography for detecting the extension of thrombus into the vena cava (see Chapter 11). The profunda femoris veins require retrograde contrast perfusion in order to be evaluated on venograms, but valvular competence and muscular tension often prevent this retrograde opacification. The proximal portions of the profunda veins, however, can be evaluated by CDS with the same reliability as the other veins of the thigh.

An important point in this discussion relates to the advantages of CDS over (conventional) gray-scale ultrasound. This point is especially important when one considers that gray-scale instruments are widely available, whereas CDS instruments are less so due to their high procurement cost. The criterion of venous compressibility can be applied with a conventional B-mode scanner, thus permitting the detection of thrombosis and eliminating the need for venography in many cases. CDS offers the added capability of indirect evaluation of the pelvic veins and of vascular segments that are obscured by overlying structures. Only color-encoded flow imaging permits an accurate description of residual blood flow in case of a partially occlusive thrombus and the reliable detection of postphlebitic changes. Also, the flow signals from the accompanying artery provide a very useful landmark for identifying and tracking the vein.

Conventional duplex scanning, which permits the assessment of blood flow only at a single point, is similar in its capabilities to pure B-mode sonography. It is advantageous over B-mode ultrasound only in its ability to evaluate blood flow in the pelvic veins.

The extremity veins can also be demonstrated with CT and MRI. CT provides only cross-sectional images of the vessels, and contrast medium must be administered to exclude pathologic changes. This procedure is indicated for pelvic venous examination in the presence of a complete thrombotic occlusion and in cases of suspected extrinsic venous compression. MRI can define thrombotic changes even without contrast medium (9, 33). It remains to be seen whether this modality will acquire a significant role in peripheral venous examinations.

Sonography and especially CDS imaging are reliable procedures for evaluation of the peripheral veins. This method can replace venography in most cases. If CDS is to become established clinically, however, the examiner must know the advantages and the limitations of the method and the adjunctive studies that are appropriate for each individual case.

8.6 References

1 Alanen, A., M. Kormano: Correlation of the echogenicity and structure of clotted blood. J. Ultrasound Med. 4 (1985) 421–425
2 Borris, L.C., M.R. Lassen: Venography in deep venous thrombosis: postoperative screening of patients in prophylaxis studies. Haemostasis 23 (Suppl.) (1993) 80–84
3 Browse, N.L., W.F. Claphan, N.N. Croft: Diagnosis of established deep vein thrombosis with J 125 fibrinogen uptake test. Brit. med. J. 4 (1971) 325–328
4 Burnham, S.J.: Operative treatment of varicose veins. In Rutherford, R.B. (Ed.): Vascular Surgery. Saunders (1984) 1348–1353
5 Coelho, J.C.U., B. Sigel, J.C. Ryva, J. Machi, S.A. Renigers: B-mode sonography of blood clots. J. clin. Ultrasound 10 (1982) 323–327
6 Cronan, J.J.: Venous thromboembolic disease: the role of US. Radiology 186 (1993) 619–630
7 Davidson, B.L., C.G. Elliot, A.W.A. Lensing: Low accuracy of color Doppler ultrasound in the detection of proximal leg vein thrombosis in asymptomatic high-risk patients. Ann. intern. Med. 117 (1992) 735–738
8 Elias, A., G. Le Corff, J.L. Bouvier, M. Benichou, A. Serradimigni: Value of real-time-B-mode ultrasound imaging in the diagnosis of deep vein thrombosis of the lower limbs. Int. Angiol. 6 (1987) 175–182
9 Erdman, WA., H.T. Jayson, H.C. Redman, G.L. Miller, R.W. Parkey, R.W. Peshock: Deep venous thrombosis of extremities: role of MR imaging in the diagnosis. Radiology 174 (1990) 425–431
10 Fobbe, F., D. Felsenberg, C. Laaß, Sörensen, R.: Tele-Thermographie bei der Diagnostik tiefer Beinvenenthrombosen. Fortschr. Röntgenstr. 149 (1988) 31–34
11 Fobbe, F., H.-C. Koennecke, M. El Bedewi, P. Heidt, J. Boese-Landgraf, K.-J. Wolf: Diagnostik der tiefen Beinvenenthrombose mit der farbkodierten Duplexsonographie. Fortschr. Röntgenstr. 151 (1989) 569–573

12 Fobbe, F., M. Ruhnke-Trautmann, D. v. Gemmeren, C.A. Hartmann, U. Kania, K.-J. Wolf: Altersbestimmung venöser Thromben im Ultraschall. Fortschr. Röntgenstr. 155 (1991) 344–348
13 Gillum, R.F.: Pulmonary embolism and thrombophlebitis in the United States. 1970–1985. Amer. Heart J. 114 (1987) 1262–1264
14 Grassi, C.J., J.F. Polak: Axillary and subclavian venous thrombosis: follow-up evaluation with color doppler flow US ans venography. Radiology 175 (1990) 651–654
15 Habscheid, W., M. Höhman, St. Klein: Kompressionssonographie als Verfahren zur Diagnostik der akuten tiefen Beinvenenthrombose. Med. Klin. 85 (1990) 6–12
16 Hejboer, H., H.R. Büller, A.W.A. Lensing, A.g.G. Turpie, L.P. Colly, J.W. Ten Cate: A comparison of real-time compression ultrasonography with impedance plethysmography for the diagnosis of deep-vein thrombosis in symptomatic outpatiens. New Engl. J. Med. 329 (1993) 1365–1369
17 Huisman, M., H.R. Büller, J.W. ten Cate, J. Vreeken: Serial impedance plethysmography for suspected deep venous thrombosis in outpatients. New Engl. J. Med. 314 (1986) 823–828, 315 (1986) 765
18 Hull, R., J. Hirsh, D. Sackett, D.W. Taylor, C. Carter, A.G.G. Turpie, P. Powers, M. Gent: Clinical validity of a negative venogramm in patients with clinically suspected venous thrombosis. Circulation 64 (1981) 622–625
19 Knudson, G.J., D.A. Wiedemeyer, S.J. Erickson, T.L. Lawson, M.W. Mewissen, E.O. Lipchik: Color doppler sonographic imaging in the assessment of upper-extremity deep venous thrombosis. Amer. J. Roentgenol. 154 (1990) 399–403
20 Krings, W., J. Adolph, S. Diederich, S. Urhahne, P. Vassallo, P.E. Peters: Diagnostik der tiefen Becken- und Beinvenenthrombose mit hochauflösender real-time and CW-Doppler-Sonographie. Radiologe 30 (1990) 525–531
21 Lensing, A.W.A., P. Prandoni, D. Brandjes, P.M. Huisman, M. Vigo, G. Tomasella, J. Krekt, J.W. ten Cate, M.V. Huisman, H.R. Büller: Detection of deep-vein thrombosis by real-time B-mode ultrasound. New Engl. J. Med. 320 (1989) 342–345
22 Ludbrook, J., G.G. Jamieson: Disorders of veins. In Sabiston, D.C. (Ed.): Textbook of Surgery, 12th ed. Saunders, Philadelphia (1981) 1808–1827
23 Lund, F., L. Diener, L.E. Ericsson: Postmortem intraosseous phlebography as aid in studies of venous thromboembolism. Angiology 20 (1969) 155–176
24 Marshall, M.: Sklerosierungsreaktion großer Varizen im hochauflösenden Ultraschallbild. Phlebol. Proktol. 19 (1990) 205–214
25 May, R., R. Nißl: Zur Symptomatik der frischen Thrombose der tiefen Beinvenen. Fortschr. Röntgenstr. 107 (1965) 262–270
26 Nylander, G.: Comments on reason for conflicting results of venography. Haemostasis 23 (Suppl.) (1993) 85–88
27 Perlin, S.J.: Pulmonary embolism during compression US of the lower extremity. Radiology 184 (1992) 165–166
28 Picolet, H., A. Leizorovicz, D. revel, P. Chirossel, M. Amiel, J.P. Boissel: Reliability of phlebography in the assessment of venous thrombosis in a clinical trial. Haemostasis 20 (1990) 362–367
29 Polak, J.F., S.S. Culter, D.H. O'Larry: Deep veins of the calf: assessment with color doppler flow imaging. Radiology 171 (1989) 481–485
30 Ramchandani, P., R.L. Soulen, L.M. Fedullo, V.D. Gaines: Deep vein thrombosis: significant limitations of noninvasive tests. Radiology, 156 (1985) 47–49
31 Roberts, H.J.: Controversies and enigmas in thrombophlebitis and pulmonary embolism: perspectives on alleged overdiagnosis. Angiology 31 (1980) 686–699
32 Rose, S.C., W.J. Zwiebel, B.D. Nelson, D.L. Priest, R.A. Knighton, J.W. Brown, P.F. Lawrence, B.M. Stults, J.C. Reading, F.J. Miller: Symptomatic lower extremity deep venous thrombosis: accuracy, limitations, and role of color duplex flow imaging in diagnosis. Radiology 175 (1990) 639–644
33 Spritzer, C.E., H.D. Sostman, D.C. Wilkens, R.E. Coleman: Deep venous thrombosis: experience with gradient-echo MR imaging in 66 patients. Radiology 177 (1993) 235–241
34 Vanninen, R., H. Manninen, S. Soimakallio, T. Katila, O. Suomalainen: Asymptomatic deep venous thrombosis in the calf: accuracy and limitations of ultrasonography as a screening test after total knee arthroplasty. Brit. J. Radiol. 66 (1993) 199–202
35 Williams, P.L., R. Warwick, M. Dyson, L.H. Bannister: Gray's Anatomy, 37th ed. Churchill Livingstone, Edinburgh (1989)
36 Yedlicka, J.W., D.W. Hunter, J.G. Letourneau: Pulmonary embolism after femoral vein compression during sonography: case report. Semin. intervent. Radiol. 7 (1990) 24–26
37 Yucel, E.K., J.S. Fisher, T.K. Egglin, S.C. Geller, A.C. Waltman: Isolated calf venous thrombosis: diagnosis with compression. US. Radiology 179 (1991) 443–446
38 Zwiebel, W.J.: Introduction to vascular ultrasonography. Grune & Stratton, Orlando (1986) 333–349

9 Aorta and its Symmetrical Branches

R. Kubale

9.1 General Remarks

For a long time intra-abdominal vessels have been used only as landmarks in ultrasonography. But with improvements in instrumentation and the advent of duplex and CDS, the capabilities of sonography have gone beyond the diagnosis of aortic aneurysms to the detection of other disorders of the smaller intra-abdominal vessels, particularly stenoses, occlusions, thromboses, variants, and collateral vessels. Just as these diseases are detected from qualitative flow information, analysis of the Doppler spectrum can be used to yield additional information on functional and regulatory processes.

This chapter deals with the technique of examining the aorta and its symmetrical branches by CDS and the principal disorders that can be recognized. The splanchnic arteries and intra-abdominal veins are discussed in Chapters 10 and 11.

9.2 Normal Anatomy and Examination Technique

9.2.1 Normal Anatomy and Variants

9.2.1.1 Abdominal Aorta

The aorta pierces the diaphragm, accompanied by the thoracic duct, at the level of T12–L1. It descends directly in front of or slightly to the left of the vertebral column, dividing into the common iliac arteries at the level of the fourth lumbar vertebra.

The diameter of the aorta below the diaphragm averages 24.4 mm in men and 21.3 mm in women. The aorta tapers from the diaphragm to the bifurcation, where its diameter is only 19.3 mm (men) and 17.2 mm (women). Enlargement up to 30 mm is described as dilatation. Aortic aneurysm is characterized by a relatively abrupt caliber increase to more than one and a half times the diameter of the proximal, normal vascular segment.

Anatomic variants are uncommon: most occur in the setting of situs inversus visceral transposition or secondary to kyphosis, retroaortic hematomas, or neoplasms. A slender aorta is frequently seen in asthenic patients but may also result from aortitis or may signify a coarctation of the thoracic aorta. Hypoplasia, atresia and duplication are rare.

9.2.1.2 Symmetrical Branches Including the Renal Arteries

Except for the splanchnic arteries (see Chapter 10), most of the branches of the abdominal aorta are paired. The inferior phrenic arteries branch from the aorta just below the diaphragm, followed distally by the suprarenal arteries and the first pair of lumbar arteries. In most patients, the testicular or ovarian arteries arise from the anterior or anterolateral aspect of the infrarenal aorta. Generally, however, they can be detected sonographically only in the area of the testis or ovary (see Chapter 13).

The renal arteries arise in 75% of cases at the level of the L1–L2 intervertebral disk from the lateral or anterolateral aspect of the aorta. Usually their origin is slightly below the origin of the superior mesenteric artery.

The right renal artery curves behind the vena cava and courses obliquely downward to the right renal hilum. The left renal artery runs posterolaterally behind the body of the pancreas and renal vein to the left renal hilum. The arteries may give off several branches in their extrarenal course. Smaller branches supply the pararenal tissue, pelvis, and proximal ureters. Other possible branches are the inferior suprarenal arteries, an atypical origin of the testicular or ovarian arteries, and especially the inferior phrenic artery.

Both renal arteries divide within or just before the hilum into an anterior and a smaller posterior branch, which in turn split into segmental, lobar, and interlobar arteries in accordance with the renal anatomy. The anterior branch supplies the apical, superior, middle, and inferior renal segments, while the posterior branch supplies only the posterior segment.

The interlobar arteries supply the renal pyramids and pass between the pyramids to the corticomedullary junction, where they divide into the arcuate arteries that supply the glomerula by way of the interlobular arteries and vasa afferentia. Individual interlobular arteries run to the surface of the kidney, where they anastomose with capsular arteries (superior, middle, and inferior capsular arteries). The inferior phrenic arteries, lumbar arteries, suprarenal arteries, and testicular arteries can in cases of occlusion provide additional collateral pathways.

The complex embryologic development in this region can confront the examiner with numerous variations in vascular positions and branching patterns. Anatomic variants such as supernumerary kidneys, ectopia, malrotation, and horseshoe kidneys are associated with atypical patterns of blood supply. The difficulty of the examination can be further compounded by aberrant polar veins and vessels arising from iliac or visceral branches of the aorta, which often are only definable by angiography. The renal artery is duplicated in 24–25% of the population, and three or more renal arteries are present in up to 3%.

9.2.2 Examination Technique and Documentation

The abdominal examination begins with analysis of the gray-scale image. Optimum B-mode image adjustment should be the basis for every examination. A linear or curved-array transducer with an operating frequency of 2–4 MHz is recommended for adults; a 5-MHz transducer can be used in thin patients and children. The acoustic power level and TGC are first set in a subcostal oblique scan of the liver. Then the aorta is imaged longitudinally, and the TGC, focus, and gain are finely adjusted so that the aortic lumen and the origins of the celiac trunc, superior mesenteric artery, and renal arteries are as free of echoes as possible.

With the patient supine, the first scan is carried out through the acoustic window of the liver during inspiration to define the proximal aorta and the origins of the celiac trunk and superior mesenteric artery. The transducer is then moved caudad, and the distal aorta is imaged as far as the bifurcation in two planes. As the transducer is moved, pressure is applied mainly with the superior end of the transducer; this maneuver, plus imaging during maximum expiration, should give clear definition of the entire abdominal aorta even if the abdomen is markedly distended by gas. After the aorta has been defined with gray-scale from the diaphragm to the bifurcation, a normal-appearing vascular site is identified, and the color image is switched on and adjusted as described in Chapter 4.

The patient should receive a low-bulk diet and antiflatulents on the day before CDS examination of the renal arteries, and no oral intake should be allowed on the day of the examination. The patient must be cooperative to the extent of suspending respirations on command and lying quietly. The origins of the renal arteries are first identified in transverse sections. This is aided by placing the patient in a relaxed position and having the patient exhale and hold, especially those with obesity or abdominal wall firmness. Using the color-encoded flow image, the sonographer identifies the proximal part of each renal artery and tracks it distally. If the patient has been adequately prepared, the proximal third of both renal arteries can be visualized in 85–90% of cases. In the rest, these segments cannot be seen despite adequate preparation because of obesity, meteorism, or a very firm, incompressible abdominal wall. Rapid identification of the left renal artery is facilitated by first locating the left renal vein; it passes through the nutcracker-like aorticomesenteric angle and generally is conspicuous by its caliber. The left renal artery is found just posterior to the vein. The middle portion of the renal artery can generally be imaged on the right by using the inferior right lobe of the liver as an acoustic window. In contrast this is very rarely possible on the left side. The distal third of both renal arteries is demonstrated best by scanning from a lateral approach. In this technique the renal hilum is visualized through a posterolateral window and from there the large hilar vessels are followed medially. Occasionally it is helpful to distend the stomach with fluid to create a “water path” for scanning. If meteorism is present, the bowel loop overlying the renal artery can be emptied or pushed aside by applying constant pressure with the transducer, taking care that the pressure does not narrow the renal arterial lumen and mimic stenosis. The renal arteries of children and adolescents can also be visualized from a posterior approach. This is not possible in adults due to the marked absorption and scattering of the sound waves by the spinal muscles.

A medium-to-high velocity scale is adequate for examination of the healthy abdominal aorta and its branches. Color gain and threshold should be adjusted to a point that just eliminates color artifacts when the transducer is held quietly. The angle between the vascular segment of interest and Doppler beam should be less than 70°. Curved vascular segments should be insonated from several directions to allow for adequate evaluation. When a vessel is examined in transverse section, the transducer should be angled at least 20° relative to the perpendicular of the vessel axis. This is essential for obtaining an adequate Doppler signal. The range and color window (see Chapter 4) should be set as low as possible to permit the use of a sufficiently high frame rate.

If flow is not detectable, or if color-encoded flow signals occupy only part of the aorta and renal artery, the velocity scale should be reduced before a diagnosis of thrombosis is made. If, for example, the same instrument has been previously used for cardiovascular examinations, cardiologic wall-pulsation filters should be removed and the user should check that the wall filter is set below 400 Hz.

A period of 15–20 min is recommended for examination of the kidneys and renal artery and 10–15 min for the aorta.

The sonographer should document the diameter of the abdominal aorta, its pulsatile characteristics, calcified plaques, and the major vascular origins in two planes. If renovascular hypertension or renal artery occlusion is presumed, the documentation should include the size of the kidneys, the parenchyma-pelvic relation, parenchymal pattern, and the appearance of the medullary pyramids. The renal arteries are imaged in standard planes from an anterior approach, and renal perfusion is documented in longitudinal and transverse planes from the lateral side. Doppler spectra should be sampled from the proximal and distal portions of each renal artery, including

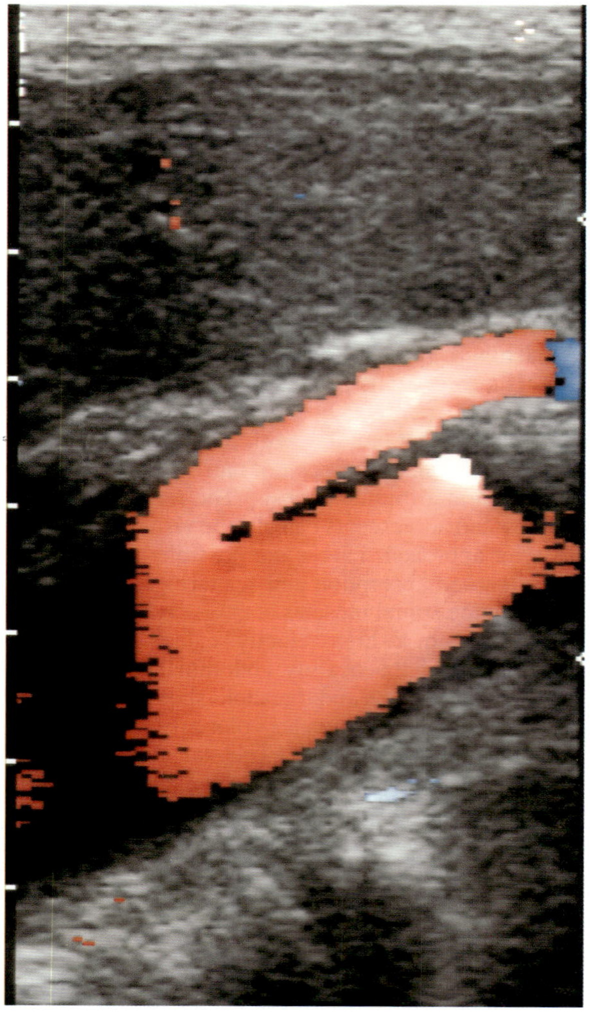

Fig. 9.**1** Longitudinal view of a normal proximal abdominal aorta, showing the normal origin of the superior mesenteric artery. Red pixels uniformly fill the aortic lumen during systole. The color saturation toward white in the superior mesenteric artery represents the higher flow velocity prevailing in that vessel during systole

measurements at the interlobar level. In areas with turbulence or increased flow velocity a spectrum should be acquired from the pathologic area following appropriate angle correction. An aneurysm is documented in its greatest diameter in two planes, and the thrombosed portion of the aneurysm should be determined.

9.3 Normal Findings

9.3.1 Abdominal Aorta

The normal abdominal aorta is completely filled with color-encoded flow signals on the CDS image during systole (Fig. 9.**1**). The flow pattern in diastole depends on the examination site: the aorta proximal to the origin of the celiac trunk and renal arteries shows continuous residual antegrade diastolic flow, especially in younger patients. This antegrade diastolic flow fills at least the center of the vessel with color-endoded signals but may be detectable over its entire cross section.

The infrarenal aorta, like the peripheral arteries, is characterized by a brief reverse-flow component followed by zero flow (Fig. 9.**2a**, **b**). This is probably due to reflections generated by the high impedance in the distal vascular bed (19, 25). These complex flow patterns are physiologic and should not be mistaken for turbulence. The physiologic patterns are modulated by hyperemia in the distal vascular bed and by severe aortic valve regurgitation.

9.3.2 Symmetrical Branches

The only symmetrical branches of the abdominal aorta that are consistently identifiable with ultrasound are the renal arteries and, sometimes, portions of the gonadal vessels. The ovarian and testicular artery are best viewed caudally in the area of the ovary or testis itself, but their origin and course can only occasionally be seen with CDS imaging.

By contrast, the origins of both renal arteries generally can be seen in about 90% of adequately prepared patient (Fig. 9.**3**). The central portion of the renal arteries (lateral to the vertebral margin) is ob-

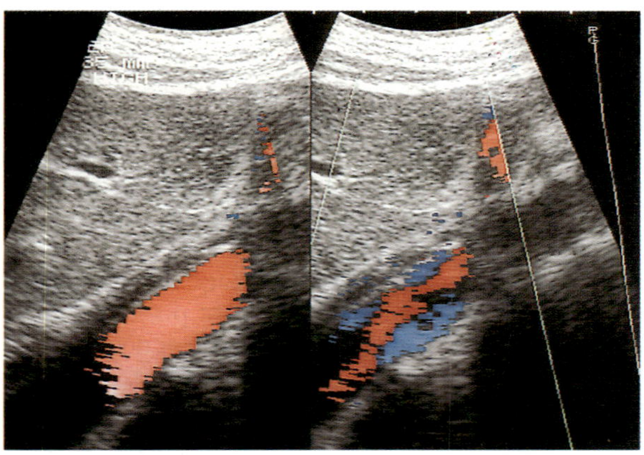

a b

Fig. 9.**2** Longitudinal views of a normal proximal abdominal aorta at different points in the cardiac cycle

a During systole the aortic lumen is uniformly filled with color-encoded signals

b At the beginning of diastole residual antegrade flow (encoded red) persists at the center of the vessel, while reverse flow (encoded blue) is starting to appear along the vessel walls. These complex flow patterns are physiologic and do not signify turbulence scured by overlying bowel gas, and the obstructing bowel loops in this region cannot be adequately compressed even from the anterior side. A diligent, systematic search enables detection of multiple or aberrant renal arteries (Fig. 9.**4a**, **b**). However, accessory renal vessels, the presence of smaller branches, or polar vessels with atypical origins may not be visualized.

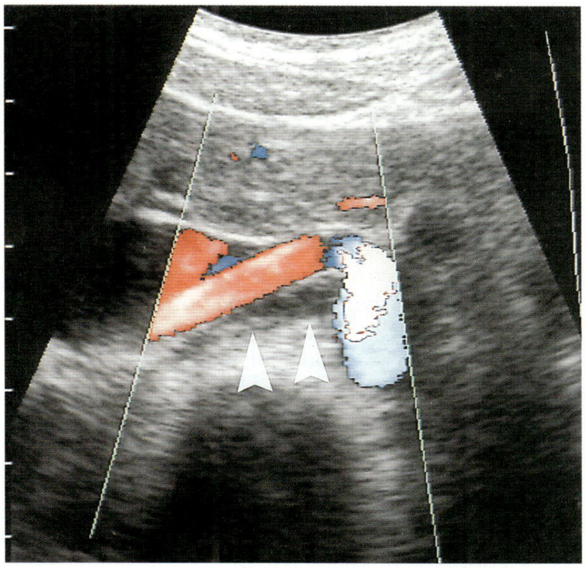

Fig. 9.**3** Origin of the right renal artery from the aorta. The proximal part of the vessel runs sharply anterolaterally and then posterolaterally, resulting in blue-encoded blood flow at the origin and red-encoded flow in the posterolateral course. The aorta is encoded in blue. The hypoechoic band-like structure posterior to the renal artery (arrows) represents the inferior right crus of the diaphragm

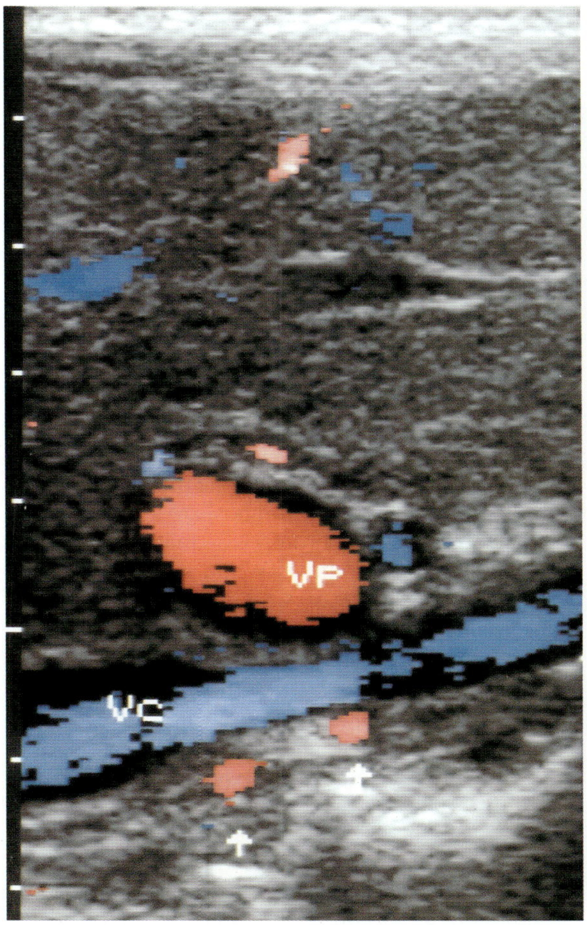

a

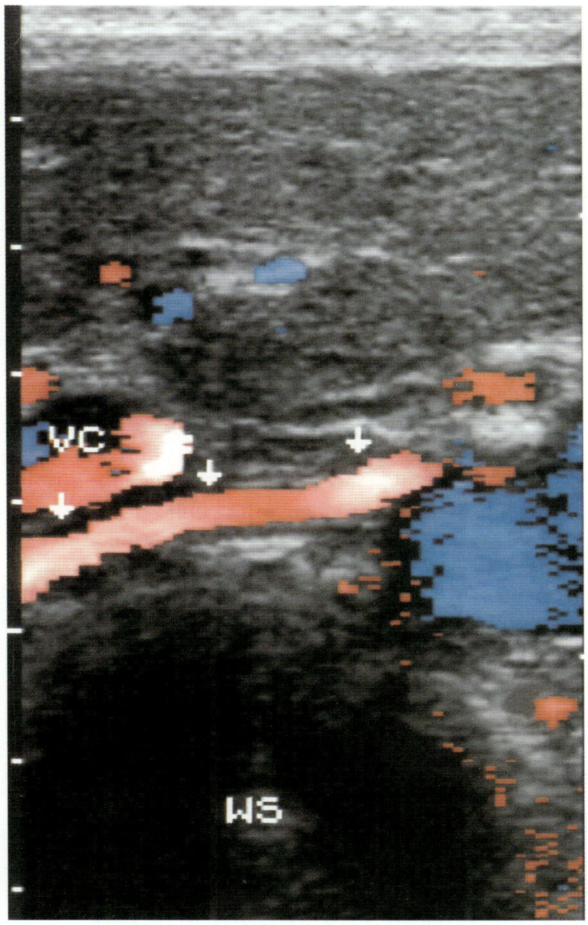

b

Fig. 9.**4a, b** Duplicated right renal artery

a Longitudinal scan through the liver shows the portal vein (VP), cut transversely by the image plane, and the inferior vena cava (VC), which is cut longitudinally. The two renal arteries passing behind the vena cava (arrows) appear as rounded areas with red-encoded blood flow

b Transverse image demonstrates one of the two renal arteries (arrows) to the site where it is crossed by the vena cava. Aortic perfusion is encoded in blue. WS = Spinal column

Normal renal arteries show uniform color saturation on real-time imaging with constant antegrade flow throughout the cardiac cycle due to the low intrarenal resistance (unlike the lower-extremity arteries, for example) (Fig. 9.**3**). Thus, when proper instrument settings are used, any color change (from red to blue) should be interpreted as indicating pathology. The intrarenal arteries of thin patients can be visualized as far as the arcuate or interlobular arteries.

Doppler spectra in healthy patients show a narrow systolic peak with persistence of antegrade flow in diastole. The Pourcelot index is between 0.5 and 0.8. This index is age dependent, increases with the severity of sclerosis (10, 36) and is influenced by physical activity and state of hydration. Hypotension, dehydration, thick fatty and muscle layers, and cutaneous emphysema hamper evaluation of the renal arteries. Renal arterial blood flow is augmented by the infusion or bolus injection of furosemide. This produces a brief but dramatic rise in systolic and diastolic blood flow, allowing clear imaging of even smaller intrarenal branches (35). However, after 30 minutes there is a transient decrease in blood flow, making it more difficult to visualize flow in smaller vessels. This is particularly important in patients with impaired renal function.

9.4 Pathologic Findings

The leading cause of pathologic changes in the aorta and renal arteries is atherosclerosis. Mechanical factors, deposits, degenerative changes, and numerous endogenous and exogenous factors can initiate a complex process involving lipid infiltration and proliferation of the intima and smooth muscle. The precursors of these changes appear as streak-like vessel wall lesions, which initially are still reversible and can be seen after 1 year of age. These "fatty streaks" most commonly involve the ductus arteriosus, the origins of the supra-aortic branches, the celiac trunk, the superior mesenteric artery, and the renal arteries. Further deposits, intramural hemorrhages, ulceration, and intravascular thrombi lead to the formation of plaques, stenoses, and occlusions, whose clinical manifestation vary according to the site of involvement. Changes in the aorta may remain asymptomatic for some time, whereas stenoses of the renal artery quickly induce hypertension, which is an absolute indication for treatment, especially in younger patients (15, 18).

9.4.1 Abdominal Aorta

9.4.1.1 Wall Thickening, Plaque, Stenosis, and Occlusion

Only high-resolution probes can demonstrate wall thickening in its early stage. The normal arterial wall presents a trilaminar structure consisting of two bright lines separated by a hypoechoic zone. The distance between these lines correlates histologically with the thickness of the intima and media. Comparative histologic studies have shown that expansion of the hypoechoic intermediate layer is a very early sign of infiltration and proliferation.

Conventional B-mode imaging can detect only the later stages in which significant wall thickening and plaque formation have developed. Location, size, and echogenicity of the wall should be evaluated. Fibrous plaques are moderately hyperechoic. Calcifications appear as very bright echoes with shadowing. The morphology of the plaques is of prognostic significance: they may dislodge and embolize (3) or incite local thrombosis causing vessel occlusion.

CDS is the only modality that can detect homogeneous, hypoechoic foci and fresh thrombotic deposits, which appear as intraluminal color voids. Continued progression of luminal narrowing leads to stenosis, whose hemodynamic manifestations are like those in the peripheral arteries: spectral broadening, turbulence, flow acceleration, and occasional vibration artifacts (12). The CDS features of stenoses described in Chapter 3 are equally valid for the aorto-iliac region (Figs. 9.**5a**, **b**, 9.**6a**, **b**).

Occlusion of the aorta is not uncommon. It almost invariably results from atherosclerosis and usually extends past the bifurcation to involve the common iliac arteries. Many connections between the celiac trunk, superior mesenteric artery, inferior mesenteric artery, and pelvic arteries can in most cases adequately compensate for an isolated chronic occlusion at rest. Therefore most of these lesions are diagnosed fortuitously or during the investigation of impotence. Other potential causes of aortic occlusion are embolism, trauma, sepsis relating to umbilical artery catheterization, and primary idiopathic hyperlipidemia. An acute occlusion in adults is generally diagnosed from clinical signs and warrants immediate surgical intervention. In neonatology, the use of CDS in septic infants has proven valuable in the early detection of abdominal aortic thrombosis (5).

The occluding thrombotic material remains hypoechoic for some time. While occlusion is suggested by an absence of wall pulsations on the B-mode image, it is proven only by demonstrating the absence of flow. The level of the occlusion, involvement of the renal arteries, and the principal collaterals can be accurately described using CDS.

9.4.1.2 Aneurysms and Retroperitoneal Fibrosis

An aortic aneurysm is a circumscribed concentric or eccentric dilatation of the vessel wall secondary to inflammation, degeneration, trauma, or malformation of the supportive wall elements. Rarefaction or fragmentation of the elastic membranes and atrophy of the medial muscle fibers cause weakening of the vessel wall. Another factor is the hemodynamic load: increased reflections at the splayed bifurcation due to elongation and the asymmetric flow following a uni-

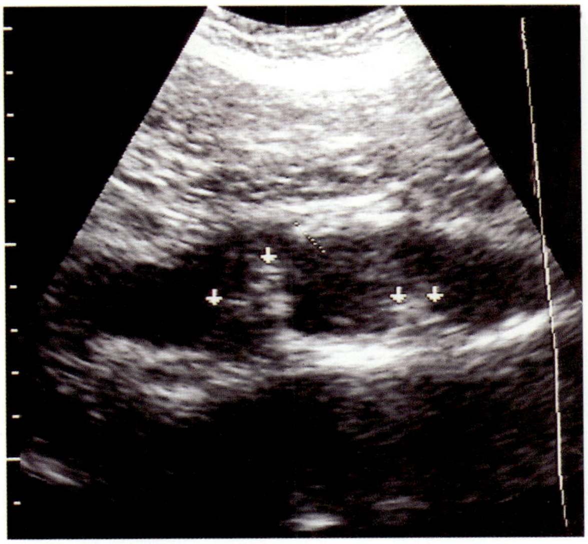

a

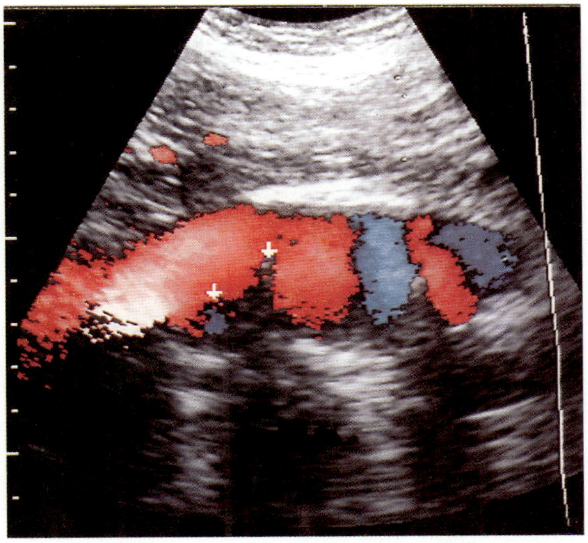

b

Fig. 9.**5a, b** Longitudinal scans demonstrating plaques in the distal abdominal aorta
a The gray-scale image shows nonhomogeneous wall irregularities (arrows) with associated luminal narrowing. At some sites it is difficult to distinguish the irregularities from artifacts due to scattering
b CDS shows that the lumen is still patent. The red-to-blue shifts on the right side of the image are due partly to the diastolic reverse flow component and partly to a change in flow direction relative to the convex transducer face (toward the transducer proximally, away from the transducer distally)

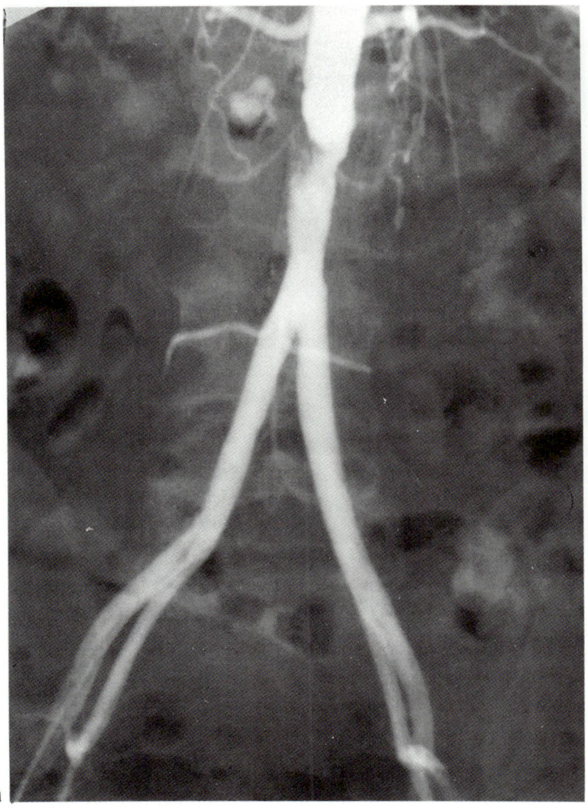

a

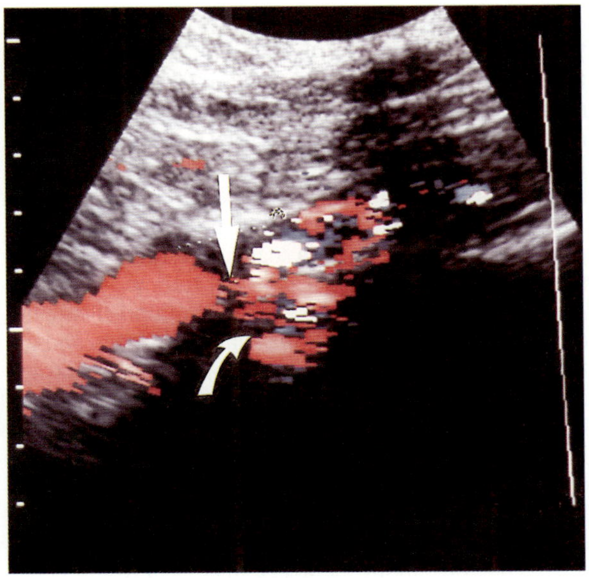

b

Fig. 9.**6a, b** Significant stenosis of the abdominal aorta
a Angiogram shows asymmetric luminal narrowing of the infrarenal aorta by plaque
b Longitudinal CDS image shows asymmetric luminal narrowing (straight arrow) with poststenotic turbulence and vibrational artifacts that transgress the lumen (curved arrow)

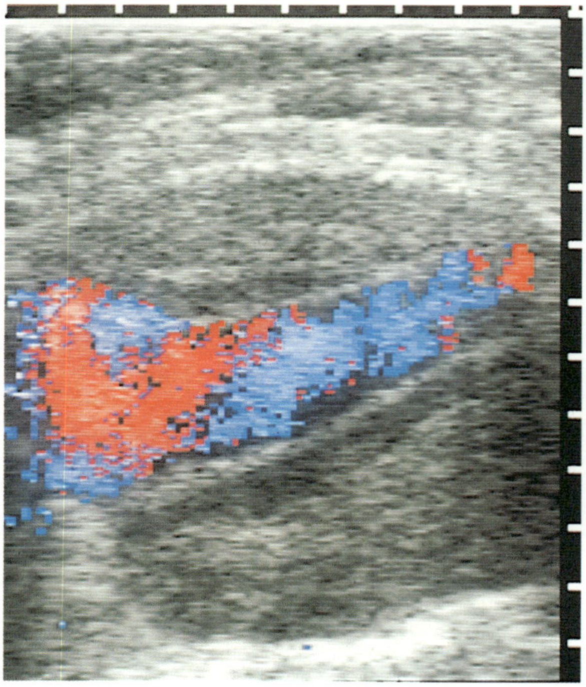

Fig. 9.**7** Aneurysm of the infrarenal aorta with layered mural thrombus and laminar flow (the red-to-blue color change is caused by diastolic reverse flow)

lateral amputation have been implicated as causing local wall stresses that promote aneurysm formation (33). The three main pathoanatomic types of aneurysm are: (1) a true aneurysm involving all three layers of the vessel wall; (2) a dissecting aneurysm; and (3) a false aneurysm (pseudoaneurysm), which is an encapsulated hematoma that communicates with the aortic lumen through a tear in the inner layers of the vessel wall; typically caused by trauma.

True aneurysm, the most common form, is caused by atherosclerosis, is usually fusiform, and affects the infrarenal aorta in 95% of cases. Symptoms result from compression of adjacent structures or perforation. Sonography can demonstrate the outer borders and diameter of the aneurysm and the extent of intraluminal thrombosis. Eccentricity of the perfused lumen, diverticula-like outpouchings, and a diameter greater than 6 cm imply a high risk of rupture. The thrombotic deposits may be layered, may partially separate from the wall, or may reliquefy. All this information can be derived from conventional B-mode ultrasound imaging.

With CDS, two distinct flow patterns can be identified (6). Laminar flow is observed in uncomplicated cases. Some aneurysms are associated with significant turbulence and with blood flow toward the vessel wall (Figs. 9.**7**, 9.**8a**, **b**). This finding may correlate with a higher expansion rate (32) and is independent of the size of the aneurysm. Another advantage of CDS is its ability to analyze the origins and course of the aortic branches and their relation to the aneurysm.

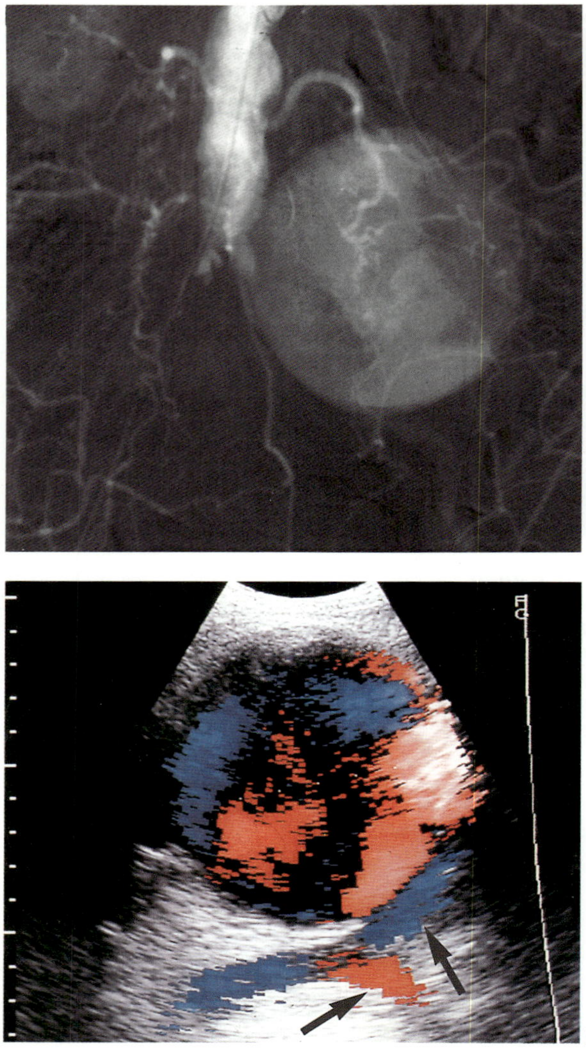

Fig. 9.**8a, b** Giant aneurysm of the distal aorta
a Angiography demonstrates the neck of the aneurysm just proximal to the aortic bifurcation. The aneurysm is compressing the left common iliac artery. The catheter occupies the lumen of the severely stenosed right common iliac artery
b Left paramedian longitudinal scan of the distal aorta (encoded blue) and iliac arteries (arrows). CDS in all flow phases shows lancet-like flow in the aneurysm directed toward the inferior wall, with significant vorticity

A dissecting aneurysm is caused by hemorrhage involving the vasa vasorum with secondary tearing of the intima, allowing blood to enter the wall of the aorta and separate its layers. It may be precipitated by trauma, idiopathic cystic medial necrosis, syphilitic aortitis, medial degeneration in the Marfan syndrome, and especially atherosclerotic disease. Dissection most commonly originates in the ascending thoracic aorta. The lesion may progress through further expansion, thrombosis or rupture. A distal reentry tear limits the condition and leads to sudden improvement in pain, whereas outward rupture of the dissection leads to acute hemorrhage. If the dissection extends into the abdominal aorta, it may acutely obstruct the renal arteries, superior mesenteric artery, and iliac arteries with associated signs of ischemia.

The B-mode diagnosis is established by demonstrating the intimal flap, which typically oscillates in the flow. Problems of differential diagnosis may arise by misinterpretation of the crus of the diaphragm or the connective-tissue isthmus of a horseshoe kidney for a second lumen. CDS can demonstrate blood flow in both lumina (Fig. 9.**9a**, **b**). The reentry point may also be seen under proper conditions (16, 45, 46).

The most feared complication of an infrarenal aneurysm is rupture, which occurs into the retroperitoneum in 88% of cases, into the free abdominal cavity in 7.3%, and into the duodenum or inferior vena cava in 2% each (18). The clinical picture is marked by the classic triad of abdominal pain, a pulsatile mass, and shock. Aneurysmal rupture into the bowel is characterized by severe gastrointestinal hemorrhage, while rupture into the inferior vena cava is marked by acute cardiac failure.

Depending on the site of the hemorrhage, sonography may reveal a distended, nonhomogeneous, usually hypoechoic retroperitoneum, free intraperitoneal fluid, or, with rupture into the gastrointestinal tract, fluid-distended bowel loops and nonspecific wall thickening. CDS does not contribute to the diagnosis of rupture, but it can be helpful in detecting aneurysmal perforation into the vena cava. As in aortocaval fistulas of other etiology, whether traumatic, iatrogenic, or spontaneous (e. g., due to retroaortic renal veins [28]), exceptionally high diastolic flow is noted in the aorta as an indirect sign. The flow signal from the vena cava is pulsatile ("arterialized"). The site of the fistula may be marked by coarse vibrational artifacts and turbulence, depending on the flow rate through the lesion (see Chapter 5).

A chronic rupture, characterized by a small, usually eccentric, annular retroperitoneal hematoma, is difficult to diagnose. The hematoma may escape sonographic detection due to the unfavorable imaging conditions, and even CT may reveal only subtle changes (13).

Mycotic aneurysms, which account for up to 5% of cases, develop in the setting of atherosclerotic disease due to bacterial endocarditis, sepsis, or an abdominal abscess. Sonography usually demonstrates a saccular aneurysm surrounded by a fluid margin (which may show small gaseous inclusions). Mycotic aneurysm requires differentiation from inflammatory aneurysm, a relatively common form accounting for 3–5% of all aneurysms (18, 30). It is characterized by a solid thickening of the aortic wall and perianeurysmal or secondary retroperitoneal fibrosis, the latter producing a uniformly hypoechoic, cuff-like rim surrounding the aortic wall. CT demonstrates a solid structure that enhances with contrast medium.

The same applies to primary retroperitoneal fibrosis, characterized by a proliferation of connective tissue in the retroperitoneal space. This disease is accompanied by varying degrees of cellular infiltration, depending on the cause and stage of the disorder. The cause of primary retroperitoneal fibrosis is unknown. It may relate to a disturbance of fibrinolysis with a proliferation of fibroblasts due to fibrin exudation into the tissue. Secondary forms are caused by drugs, irradiation, adjacent inflammatory conditions, trauma, and chronic hematoma (e. g., blood seepage from aneurysms).

Circumferential encasement of the aorta by uniformly hypoechoic tissue is seen with ultrasound, while CT demonstrates solid, contrast-enhancing structures. Most cases show bilateral ureteral obstruction and congestion of the pelvis of the kidneys. The fibrotic area is usually confined to the region between the renal hilum and promontory.

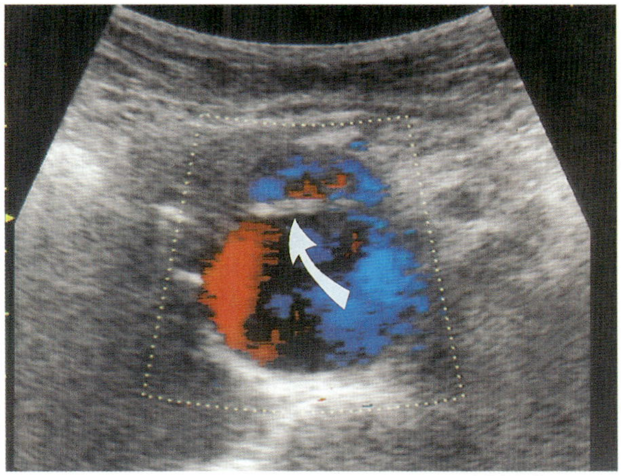

a

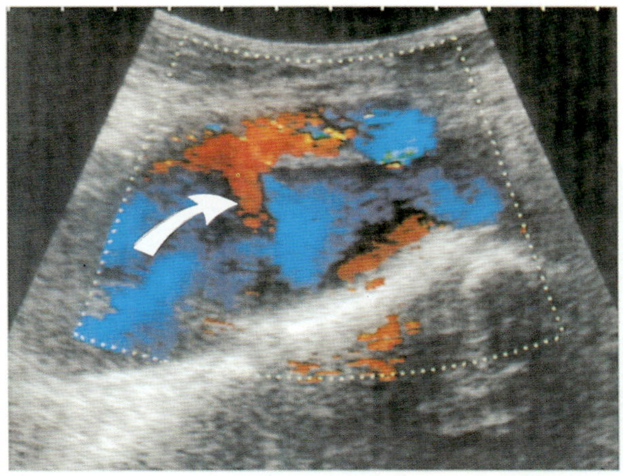

b

Fig. 9.**9a, b** Dissecting aortic aneurysm (iatrogenic)
a Transverse aortic scan demonstrates the oscillating intimal flap (arrow). Blood flow is detected in both lumina
b Longitudinal scan demonstrates the communication between the true and false lumina (arrow). Diastolic reverse flow (encoded blue) is visible in the true lumen

9.4.1.3 Synthetic Grafts and Postinterventional Follow-up

Color duplex sonography is gaining importance in vascular surgery and for interventional radiologic procedures because it provides a noninvasive follow-up method:

- Synthetic vascular grafts generally present smooth, mostly hyperechoic walls enclosing a lumen perfused by laminar flow (Fig. 9.**10a**, **b**). Loss of the wall pulsations in the B-mode image or an absence of flow signals in the CDS image permit an occlusion to be diagnosed in minutes.
- Postoperatively hemorrhage is rare and is due mainly to anastomotic dehiscence. The principal risk factors are blood pressure elevation following anesthesia and excessive anticoagulation. A fresh hematoma is anechoic and easily distinguished from aneurysm by CDS. The echogenicity of the hemorrhage changes over time with its degree of organization, showing patterns ranging from hypoechoic to nonhomogeneously hyperechoic. Even after a period of months, the hemorrhage may be demonstrable as a solid, encapsulated mass.
- Problems of interpretation occasionally arise in patients with atypical extra-anatomic bypass grafts and end-to-side bifurcation grafts. The apparent expansion of the proximal suture site is a summation effect caused by the "piggyback" placement of the aorta upon the graft. Postoperative dilatation of the implanted grafts is common and may be as much as 34% at 6 years (37).

If CDS is supplemented by regular, standardized hemodynamic measurements following bypass grafting, PTA, or thrombolysis, it is possible to predict the risk of occlusion (2): initially the blood flow is elevated as a result of postoperative or postinterventional hyperemia. Flow returns to a normal level by 7–14 days. A fall of the peak systolic velocity to less than 40 cm/s is associated with a high risk of occlusion or recurrent thrombosis and warrants frequent follow-up examinations and anticoagulant therapy. This value of 40 cm/s is based on a transverse vascular diameter of 8–10 mm (2). All flow measurements should be calibrated in a flow phantom, and a normal reference population should be defined. The importance of hemodynamic measurements lies in the monitoring of patient progress. Early detection of anastomotic stenosis and of post-PTA restenosis due to intimal proliferation offers another possibility to improve long-term results.

a
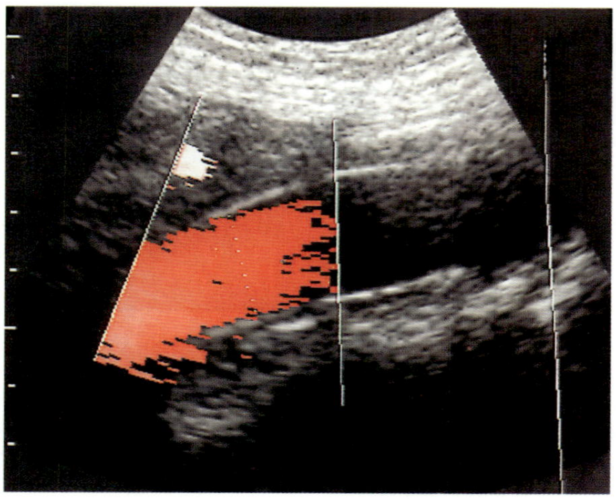

b
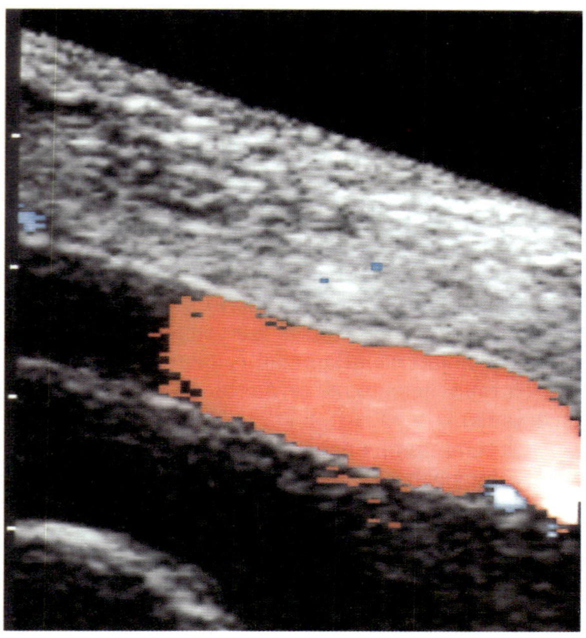

Fig. 9.**10a, b** Aortobifemoral bypass performed for a distal aortic aneurysm involving the iliac arteries
a Longitudinal scan of the distal aorta shows normal laminar flow (homogeneous color encoding). The graft wall appears as a hyperechoic band-like structure. The aneurysmal sac is generally left in place and may still be identifiable years later as a hypoechoic band around the graft wall
b Distal end of an aortobifemoral bypass graft with attachment to the common femoral artery. CDS demonstrates normal graft perfusion. The very light color on the right side of the image represents the higher frequency shift associated with a direction change just proximal to the anastomosis

9.4.2 Symmetrical Branches of the Abdominal Aorta

9.4.2.1 Basic Clinical Considerations

Renal vascular hypertension has been defined as high blood pressure caused by occlusive disease of the main renal artery or its branches. The prevalence of renovascular hypertension is 3–5% in adults, and a renovascular cause can be established in up to 60% of hypertensive children (15).

Renovascular hypertension has numerous potential causes (Table 9.**1**). Sixty percent of cases are caused by atherosclerotic stenoses and occlusions and 35% by fibromuscular dysplasia (15). Atherosclerotic stenosis most commonly involves the proximal part of the renal artery and is most prevalent in older individuals. Fibromuscular dysplasia chiefly affects women in the third and fourth decades of life and frequently involves the central third of the renal artery (15). Intrarenal stenosis can also occur, however, and stenoses of the polar arteries are particularly challenging in terms of diagnosis. The remaining 5% of cases are due to neurofibromatosis, pheochromocytoma, connective tissue bands, arteritis, embolism, thrombosis, neoplasia, aneurysms, and other vascular malformations (21). Early detection allows for definitive interventional or operative treatment.

Table 9.**1** Causes of renovascular hypertension (after [19])

Common causes (90–95%)	Atherosclerosis, fibromuscular dysplasia
Rare causes (5–10%)	Aneurysm, a–v fistula, arteritis, neurofibromatosis, tumors, congenital bands, retroperitoneal inflammatory conditions, coarctation of the aorta (abdominal and thoracic), subcapsular or retroperitoneal hematoma, abscess, fibrosis, etc.
Mass lesions	Juxtaglomerular cell tumor, Wilms tumor, renal cell carcinoma
Inflammatory diseases	Pyelonephritis, radiogenic nephritis, tuberculosis
Congenital anomalies	Hypoplasias, dysplasias, hydronephrosis

9.4.2.2 Wall Thickening, Stenosis, and Occlusion

Early changes such as wall thickening and calcified plaques are only occasionally demonstrable with ultrasound; the latter are sometimes manifested only by posterior acoustic shadowing. Progression of these early lesions leads to stenosis or occlusion, whose site of occurrence depends on the cause: atherosclerotic lesions most commonly involve the ostium and proximal third of the renal artery, while fibromuscular changes occur more peripherally and involve the central or distal third. Concomitant involvement of the segmental arteries is frequent.

In most cases the renal arteries cannot be seen on the gray-scale image due to the inadequate definition of the vessel wall. Further luminal reduction leads to flow disturbances that can be depicted by CDS (Figs. 9.**11**–9.**13**). CDS provides direct visualization of the stenosis and the poststenotic dilatation (Fig. 9.**12**). Local flow acceleration and poststenotic turbulence confirm the hemodynamic significance of the lesion. Coarse vibrational artifacts ("color cloud") signify a high-grade stenosis (Fig. 9.**11**).

Analogous to the criteria used in carotid diagnosis, stenosis is characterized by spectral broadening with a closed spectral window and an increased peak systolic frequency with turbulence. More severe grades of stenosis are associated with a complete loss of the normal cyclic pattern of the spectral waveform. For practical purposes, a classification of the renal artery stenosis into five groups has proven useful (Fig.

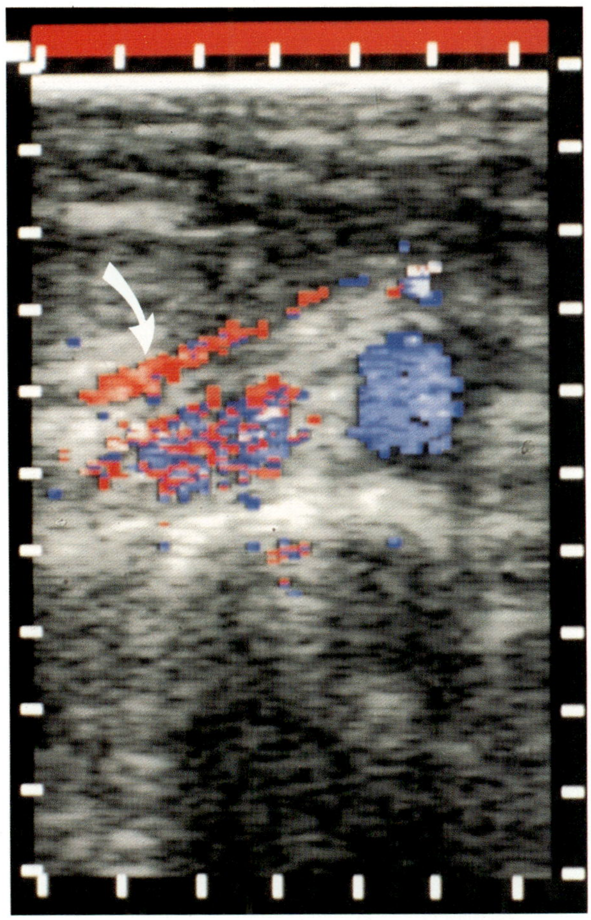

Fig. 9.**11** Transverse scan of the aorta (encoded blue) demonstrating a high-grade stenosis of the right renal artery. The circumscribed "cloud" of mixed red and blue pixels at the intersection of the right renal artery and inferior vena cava reflects the presence of a high-grade stenosis causing vibration of the vessel wall and perivascular structures. The vena cava is encoded in red (arrow)

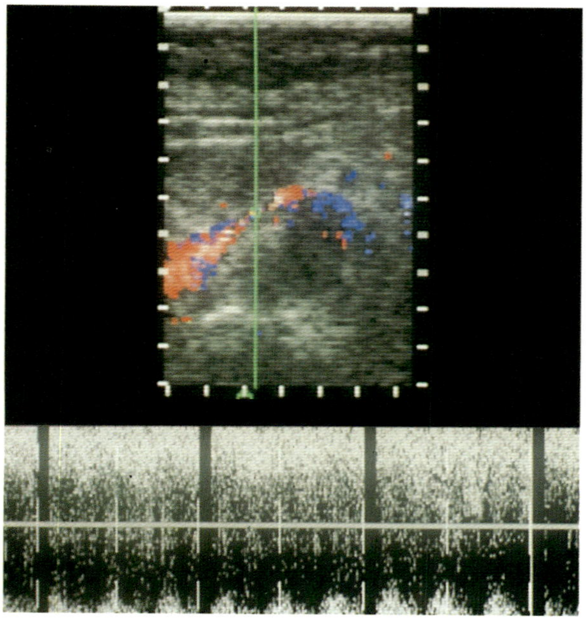

Fig. 9.**12** CDS and Doppler spectrum of a high-grade stenosis of the right renal artery. The renal artery arises from the anterolateral aspect of the aorta (no color-encoded flow in the aortic lumen = end of diastole and start of systole). The very light color saturation signifies a markedly increase frequency shift in the stenosis, while the spectrum (green spot = sampling site) shows an almost complete loss of cyclic variation and a diffuse distribution of the measured frequency shifts

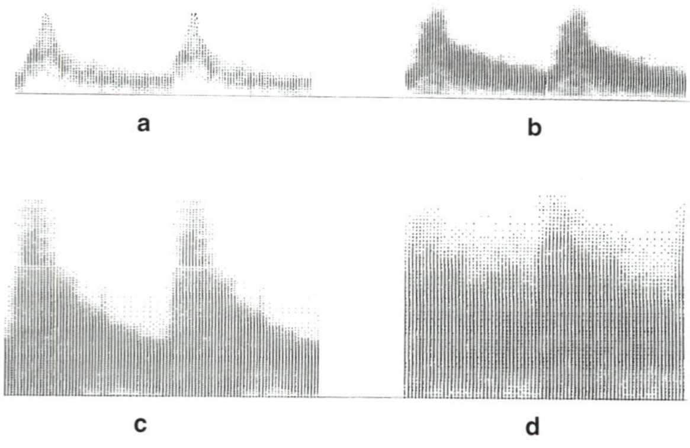

Fig. 9.**13 a, b** Schematic representation of Doppler spectra recorded from renal arteries

a Normal renal artery: narrow systolic peak, constant antegrade diastolic flow (Pourcelot index 0.6–0.8), clear spectral window

b Less than 50% diameter reduction: widening of the systolic peak with fill-in of the spectral window

c Between 50% and 75% diameter reduction: marked increase in systolic velocity (compared with opposite side, after angle correction), spectral fill-in, pronounced post-stenotic flow disturbance

d More than 75% diameter reduction: almost complete loss of cyclic waveform changes (diffuse distribution of points over the spectrum = "spectral noise")

9.**13**): (1) normal renal artery, (2) less than 50% narrowing, (3) 50–75% narrowing, (4) greater than 75% narrowing, and (5) occlusion.

It should be noted in the interpretation of spectra and flow images that a change in the angle of the vessel axis relative to the incident ultrasound beam can cause an apparent acceleration of flow (see Chapter 4; [43]). Therefore using the magnitude of the frequency shift for grading of a stenosis alone is not sufficient. In addition, the measured frequency shift depends on the operating frequency of the transducer. Thus, the grading of a stenosis should always be performed with angle-corrected velocity measurements (1).

Although first reports based on identification of the peak velocity at the stenosis site showed sensitivity and specificity of 69–98% (1, 7, 11, 14, 20, 22, 29), more recent prospective studies have resulted in failure or incomplete CDS examination rates up to 41% (4). Vessel wall calcifications, obesity, and accessory renal artery vessels are the main causes for this failure (43). Discrepancies in specificity are due to different cutoff velocities ranging from 100 cm/s (14) to 180 cm/s (22). It has to be kept in mind that the absolute velocity in a vessel depends largely on the cardiac output and the diameter of the vessel. According to the Hagen–Poiseuille law the velocity depends on the fourth power of the diameter of the vessel. Thus, a generally larger vessel diameter will result in a slower velocity and a smaller increase in case of a stenosis (see Chapters 3 and 4).

These problems may be overcome by using indirect criteria such as the shape of the Doppler frequency spectrum (Fig. 9.**13**). The frequency spectrum is largely independent of the angle, the cardiac output, and the general diameter of the vessel and shows relatively specific changes in cases of a local stenosis. Even in difficult examination conditions, a frequency analysis can be obtained and used for quantification of the stenosis. In our experience, this method is relatively easy to use and permits differentiation between hemodynamically relevant stenosis.

The relation between the maximum systolic frequency shift and the minimal diastolic frequency shift (resistive index = RI) measured in the distal renal artery or in the renal parenchyma itself could also be used. In a recent study (40) a difference of RI left versus right of more than 5% was significant for a hemodynamically significant stenosis. A stenosis of less than 50% did not affect the RI. Some authors recommend the analysis of the shape of the systolic complex of the Doppler frequency spectrum (41). Problems arise in patients with unilateral kidney disease (e. g. infection), bilateral stenosis, and aberrant polar arteries. Additional problems could arise due to different compliance or distensibility of the distal intraparenchymal vessels (8).

Occlusions are caused by thrombosis or embolism precipitated by trauma, aneurysm, inflammatory disease, or emboli from the heart. The extent of renal parenchymal damage and the clinical manifestations are diverse and depend on the site and level of the occlusion. An acute bilateral occlusion leads swiftly to renal failure, while a gradual occlusion can be initially compensated by collateral flow.

The sonographic appearance of the renal parenchyma is still normal in the early stage of an occlusion. Within hours of a segmental occlusion, the infarcted areas become demarcated as zones of low echogenicity. Partial renal distension may be observed depending on the degree of the accompanying edema. Sites of hemorrhage into the parenchyma lead to a nonhomogeneous, sonodense pattern. The volume of the infarcted areas decreases in 2–7 days, and the kidney shows residual scarring or atrophy. Intraluminal material in a distended renal artery and the absence of pulsations can sometimes permit a diagnosis of occlusion from the B-mode image, but proof is provided by flow information: CDS can confirm or exclude a complete occlusion of the main artery in patients with acute renal failure. If the renal artery cannot be directly visualized, it may be helpful to scan from a lateral approach. The detection of flow to the level of the interlobular arteries indirectly excludes a complete occlusion of the main artery. Segmental voids cannot be demonstrated in all cases, however, due to weak signals from the parenchyma and strong absorption and scattering by the skin and abdominal wall. Nonvisualization of the intrarenal vasculature may warrant immediate angiography or at least an isotope scan, depending on the clinical implications. The diagnosis may be improved by the use of ultrasound contrast medium (see Chapter 16) or by new technicall developments (38).

9.4.2.3 Aneurysms and Arteriovenous Malformations

Aneurysms of the renal artery are usually detected as incidental findings. The most common causes besides atherosclerosis and fibromuscular dysplasia are trauma and congenital aneurysms. Most aneurysms due to fibromuscular dysplasia involve the main trunk of the artery. Lesions due to polyarteritis nodosa, necrotizing arteritis, or trauma tend to occur at the intrarenal level, while most atherosclerotic aneurysms involve the main trunk and larger intrarenal branches. Renal artery aneurysms may rupture, embolize to peripheral vessels, or undergo thrombosis. An intrarenal hemorrhage induced by surgery or biopsy has a similar morphology and can lead to massive hematuria.

Sonography demonstrates renal artery aneurysm as a hypoechoic mass, and many atherosclerotic aneurysms exhibit a small calcified shell. The presence of turbulent, still-pulsatile flow in the color-encoded image is pathognomonic for aneurysm, permitting diagnosis and differentiation from parapelvic cysts and ectatic or convoluted veins. The next step is angiography with a check for possible therapeutic embolization.

Arteriovenous malformations are rare, usually congenital lesions that are most commonly located in the medullary region. Other causes are trauma, biopsy, or aneurysmal rupture. Frequent symptoms are hematuria and hypertension. Large-flow a–v fistulae can lead to an increasing cardiac load.

Sonography usually demonstrates cystic structures or a convoluted mass of vessels. A large-caliber artery and dilated runoff veins can suggest a hemodynamically significant a–v shunt, but proof is furnished by direct CDS detection of the fistula based on coarse, mosaic-like vibrational artifacts or modulation of the Doppler signal from the artery and vein as described in Chapter 6 (42). These changes are observed with increasing frequency in renal transplants (see Chapter 12) but can also be diagnosed in native kidneys.

9.4.2.4 Tumors and Tumor Vessels

Accurate information on the extent of tumor thrombi is necessary for the planning of operative treatment. While it is difficult, for example, to demonstrate the terminal portion of the renal vein in arterial DSA, the strength of CDS lies in the evaluation of the renal vein terminations and in the visualization and measurement of the vena cava (see Chapter 10 for details). An additional application is the detection of tumor vessels (10). Although the assessment of tumor vascularity has little importance in terms of differential diagnosis, the efficacy of embolization can be assessed by CDS imaging.

9.4.2.5 Synthetic Grafts and Postinterventional Follow-up

In contrast to an aortic prosthesis or aortobifemoral bypass, the possibility of postoperative follow-up of a renal arterial bypass depends on the type of operation: the more common splenorenal bypasses and aortic reimplantation are often obscured by stomach and colon. They are oriented perpendicular to the anterior plane of examination limiting the detection of flow, so that only flow measurements in the kidney from the lateral aspect can indirectly confirm bypass patency. In contrast, iliacorenal bypasses generally are favorably positioned; at least some segments can be visualized (Fig. 9.**14a–d**) allowing detection of anastomotic stenoses and aneurysms.

9.5 Diagnostic Value of Color Duplex Sonography in Relation to Other Diagnostic Procedures

Diseases of the abdominal aorta were one of the earliest indication for vascular ultrasonography. Despite the usual difficulties of abdominal examination, such as obesity and overlying bowel gas, in most patients ultrasound can demonstrate the full length of the aorta and at least the proximal portions of the renal arteries.

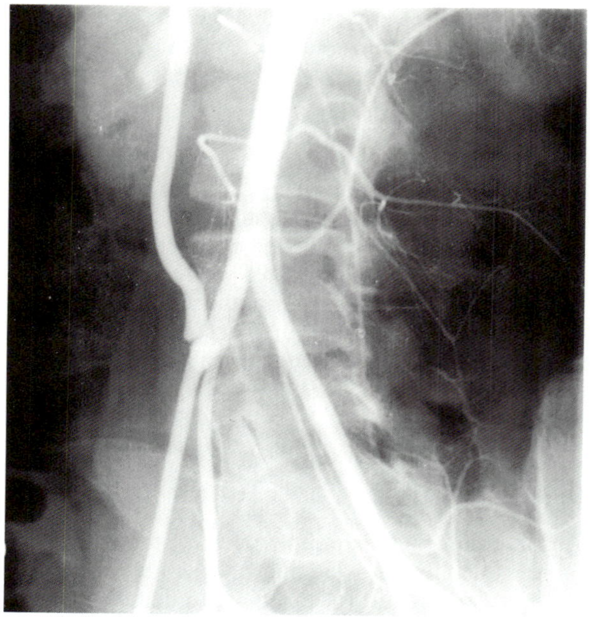

a

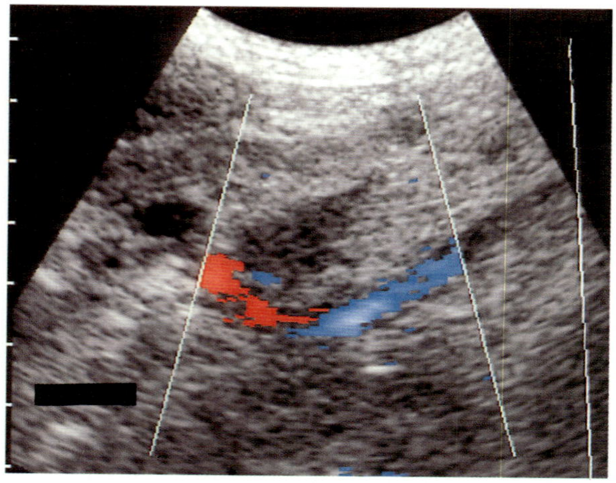

b

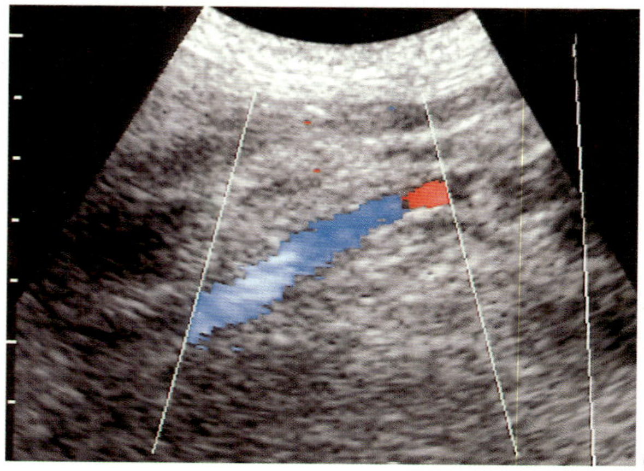

c

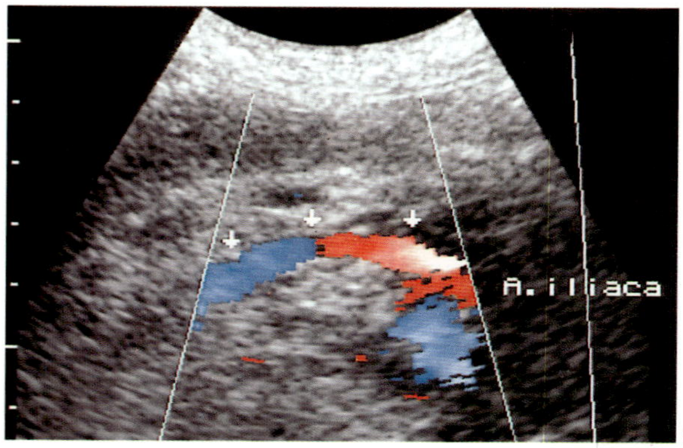

d

Fig. 9.**14a, b** Iliacorenal bypass (angiography and CDS)
a Angiography demonstrates the bypass graft arising from the right common iliac artery and ascending to the right renal hilum
b CDS image of the proximal third of the graft. The anastomosis of the graft with the renal artery is visible on the left side of the image
c Image of the middle third of the graft demonstrates its ascending, distal-to-proximal course
d The distal third of the graft (arrow) and the anastomoses with the common iliac artery (A. iliaca) on the right side of the image

Angiography has been the traditional gold standard for renovascular studies. Other options for vascular diagnosis are CT with selective contrast enhancement, radionuclide scanning for the detection of renal perfusion abnormalities, and more recently MR imaging and MR angiography. Initial studies confirm the value of magnetic resonance for the evaluation of the aorta, pelvic vessels, and renal arteries (23). The value of the different modalities is largely a matter of patient selection and cost effectiveness, however:

1. Sonography is a well-established modality for the screening and follow-up of aortic aneurysms (26). Its sensitivity is 97–100%, depending on examination conditions. Whereas preoperative angiography was once considered indispensable, most surgeons now regard a combination of ultrasound and CT as adequate for the preoperative evaluation of abdominal aneurysms. Both modalities are superior to angiography in their ability to define both the extent and structure of mural thrombi. The advantage of CDS over B-mode ultrasound is that it makes it easier to locate the renal arteries and assess their involvement. Another aspect is the analysis of flow characteristics (6). There is evidence to show that significant tur-

bulence with wall-directed flow peaks is of prognostic importance in the expansion of aneurysms (6, 32).

2. B-mode imaging can offer presumptive evidence of a dissecting aneurysm, but CDS establishes the diagnosis and helps to evaluate flow conditions in the affected abdominal branch vessels. The disadvantage of sonography is that it cannot adequately demonstrate the thoracic aorta. Contrast-enhanced CT, transesophageal sonography, and especially MRI are the procedures of choice in these cases.

3. Although conventional duplex scanning (without color encoding) was once considered promising in the diagnosis of stenoses of the aorta and pelvic arteries, difficulties relating to vessel-wall calcifications in older patients and vessel tortuosity at the pelvic level tended to make a complete examination prohibitive. With the advent of CDS and especially newer instruments providing adequate penetration depth and improved techniques of motion artifact suppression, the examination time could be significantly reduced. Already this has made CDS an established technique for the follow-up of surgical and interventional procedures on the aortic and pelvic arteries. Though the capabilities of MRI are intriguing (23), the more favorable cost–benefit ratio of ultrasound supplemented by color duplex imaging will continue to make it the modality of first choice for diseases of the aorta and pelvic arteries.

4. CDS is still controversial as a screening method for renal arterial stenosis (1, 4, 7, 11, 20, 24, 27, 31, 34, 40, 41, 43). Whereas proximal atherosclerotic stenoses are detected very reliably with CDS, it is difficult to detect narrowing in the central third of the artery—a site of predilection for fibromuscular dysplasia mostly in younger women. Because these stenoses can be successfully treated by PTA, their detection is of major importance. CDS is also limited in its ability to detect stenoses in the polar arteries and within the renal parenchymal. Results in this region might be improved by the use of ultrasound contrast agents (see Chapter 16), but this possibility has not yet been explored in prospective studies. Published reports on the sensitivity and specificity of duplex scanning and CDS in the detection of renal artery stenosis range from 40–98%. The discrepancy results from the use of different criteria for stenoses, different instrumentation, different reference methods (arterial or intravenous angiography), and especially differences in patient populations. It has been our general experience that CDS is equivalent to intravenous DSA. It should be used to resolve suspicion of atherosclerotic renal artery stenosis and especially for the follow-up of PTA.

CDS cannot definitively exclude renal artery stenosis, however, so arterial angiography should be performed whenever negative CDS findings are obtained in a younger patient with suspected fibromuscular dysplasia or intrarenal stenosis.

5. CDS is of much greater value in the detection of renal artery occlusion. If the study clearly defines the segmental and interlobar arteries with peripherally directed flow, occlusion is unlikely. Nonvisualization of the intrarenal vessels may warrant emergency angiography and possible thrombolytic treatment, depending on the clinical situation.

6. Angiography can be omitted for most postinterventional studies and for the follow-up of bypass procedures and thrombolysis in the aorta and pelvic arteries. However, the ability of sonography to demonstrate renal bypass grafts depends strongly on the examination conditions and the location of the bypass. The early detection of malformations and occlusions and the ability to conduct noninvasive follow-up examinations at frequent intervals are helpful and indeed essential for many interventions (14, 39, 42).

References

1 Avasthi, P.S., W.F. Voyles, E.R. Greene: Noninvasive diagnosis of renal artery stenosis by echo-Doppler velocimetry. Kidney int. (N.Y.) 25 (1984) 824–829

2 Bandyk, D.F., G.R. Seabrock, P. Moldenhauer, J. Lavin, J. Edwards, R. Cato, J.B. Towne: Hemodynamics of vein graft stenosis. J vasc. Surg. 8 (1988) 688–695

3 Benvegna, S., I. Cassina, G. Giuntini, F. Rusignuolo, F. Talarico, M. Florena: Atherothrombotic microembolism of the lower extremities (the blue toe syndrome) from atherosclerotic non-aneurysmal aortic plaques. J. cardiovasc. Surg. 31 (1990) 87–91

4 Berland, L.L., D.B. Koslin, W.D. Routh, F.S. Keller: Renal artery stenosis: Prospective evaluation of diagnosis with color duplex US compared with angiography – work in progress. Radiology 174 (1990) 421–423

5 Bhat, R., E. Fisher, U. Doshi, S. Raza, B. Sepehri, P. Flanigan, D. Vidyasagar: Neonatal abdominal aortic thrombosis. Crit. Care Med. 9 (1981) 858–61

6 Bluth, E.I., S.M. Murphey, L.H. Holier, MA Sullivan: Color flow Doppler in the evaluation of aortic aneurysms. Int. Angiol. 9 (1990) 8–10

7 Breitenseher, M., F. Kainberger, P. Huebsch, S. Trattnig, M. Baldt, P. Barton, F. Karnel: Screening von Nierenarterienstenosen. Erste Ergebnisse zur Aussagekraft der Farbdopplersonographie. Fortschr. Röntgenstr. 156 (1992) 228–31

8 Bude, R.O., J.M. Rubin, J.F. Platt, K.P. Fechner, R.S. Adler: Pulsus tardus: its cause and potential limitations in detection of arterial stenosis. Radiology 190 (1994) 779–784

9 Deeg, K.H., B. Nagler, E. Schoenau, H. Ruder: Farbkodierte Doppler-Sonographie der Nierengefaesse im Kindesalter. II. Pathologische Befunde (Color-coded Doppler sonography of the kidney blood vessels in childhood. II. Pathological findings). Mschr. Kinderheilk 138 (1990) 337–348

10 Denys, A., O. Helenon, M. Souissi, E. Attlan, Y. Chretien, B. Dufour, J.F. Moreau: Doppler pulse et couleur des masses renales. Correlation angiographique et anatomo-pathologique. J. Radiol. 72 (1991) 599–608

11 Desberg, A.L., D.M. Paushter, G.K. Lammert, J.C. Hale, R.B. Troy, A.C. Novick, J.R., J.V. Nally, A.M. Weltevreden: Renal artery stenosis: evaluation with color Doppler flow imaging. Radiology 177 (1990) 749–753

12 de Smet, A.A., P.J. Kitslaar: A duplex criterion for aorto-iliac stenosis. Europ. J. vasc. Surg. 4 (1990) 275–278

13 Dore, R., M. Alerci, G. Cornalba, A. DeAgnosti: Unusual CT Features in ruptures of abdominal aortic aneurysms. Fortschr. Roentgenstr. 148 (1988) 127–130

14 Duda, S.H., C.M. Erley, J.P. Wakat, P.E. Huppert, W. Lauchart, T. Risler, C.D. Claussen: Posttransplant renal artery stenosis—outpatient intraarterial DSA versus color aided duplex Doppler sonography. Europ. J. Radiol. 16 (1993) 95–101

15 Franklin, S.: Renovascular hypertension. In Benner, H. (Ed.): Diseases of the Kidney and Urinary Tract. New York (1989)

16 Giyanani, V.L., C.A. Krebs, L.A. Nall, R.L. Eisenberg, H.R. Parvey: Diagnosis of abdominal aortic dissection by image-directed Doppler sonography. J. clin. Ultrasound 17 (1989) 445–448

17 Handa, N., R. Fukunaga, A. Uehara: Echo-Doppler velocimeter in the diagnosis of hypertensive patients: the renal artery Doppler technique. Ultrasound Med. Biol. 12 (1986) 945–952

18 Heberer, G., R.J.A. van Dongen: Kirschnersche Operationslehre. Springer-Verlag, Berlin (1987)

19 Holenstein, R., D.N. Ku: Reverse flow in the major infrarenal vessels–a capacitive phenomenon. Biorheology 25 (1988) 835–842

20 Hudspeth, D.A., K.J. Hansen, S.W. Reavis, S.M. Starr, R.G. Appel; R.H. Dean: Renal duplex sonography after treatment of renovascular disease. J. Vasc. Surg. 18 (1993) 381–8; discussion 389–390

21 Kadir, S.: Diagnostic Angiography. Saunders, New York (1989)

22 Karasch, T., A.L. Strauss, B. Gruen, M. Worringer, D. Neuerburg-Heusler, F.J. Roth, H. Rieger: Farbkodierte Duplexsonographie in der Diagnostik von Nierenarterienstenosen (Color-coded duplex ultrasonography in the diagnosis of renal artery stenosis). Dtsch. med. Wschr. 118 (1993) 1429–1436

23 Kim, D., R.R. Edelman, K.C. Kent, D.H. Porter, J.J. Skillman: Abdominal aorta and renal artery stenosis; evaluation with MR angiography. Radiology 174 (1990) 727–731

24 Kliewer, M.A., R.H. Tupler, B.A. Carroll, S.S. Paine, J.S. Kriegshauser, B.S. Hertzberg, L.P. Svetkey: Renal artery stenosis: analysis of Doppler waveform parameters and tardus–parvus pattern. Radiology 189 (1993) 779–787

25 Kontis, S., R.G. Gosling: On-line Doppler ultrasound measurement of aortic compliance and its repeatability in normal subjects. Clin. Phys. physiol. Measure. 10 (1989) 127–135

26 Kremer, H., B. Weigold, W. Dobrinski, M. Schreiber, N. Zöllner: Sonographische Verlaufsbeobachtungen von Bauchaortenaneurysmen. Klin. Wschr. 62 (1984) 1120–1125

27 Lafortune, M., H. Patriquin, E. Demeule, B.C. Trinn, M.P. Dufresne, L. Legault, J. Raymond: Renal arterial stenosis: slowed systole in the downstream circulation – experimental study in dogs. Radiology 184 (1992) 475–478

28 Mansour, M.A., R.B. Rutherford, R.K. Metcalf, W.H. Pearce: Spontaneous aorto-left renal vein fistula: the "abdominal pain, hematuria, silent left kidney" syndrome. Surgery 109 (1991) 101–106

29 Miralles, M., A. Santiso, A. Gimenez, V. Riambau, A. Saez, J. Daumal, M.A. Cairols: Renal duplex scanning: correlation with angiography and isotopic renography. Europ. J. vasc. Surg. 7 (1993) 188–194

30 Müller-Schwefe, Ch., G. v. Klinggräf, G. Riepe, A. Schröder. Das inflammatorische Bauchaortenaneurysma. Ultraschall in Med. 12 (1991) 158–163

31 Napoli, V., A. Palla, F. Pinto, P. Pavlica, L. Barozzi, C. Vignali, A. Salvetti, C. Bartolozzi: L'eco-Doppler addominale nella diagnosi della malattia reno-vascolare. Studio prospettico in doppio cieco (Abdominal Doppler ultrasonography in the diagnosis of renovascular diseases. Double-blind prospective study). Radiol. med. 86 (1993) 496–502

32 Omlor, G., K. Guindi, P. Walter, B. Koch, K.W. Ecker: Op-Indikation beim Risikopatienten mit asymptomatischem Bauchaortenaneurysma. Vasa (Suppl.) 32 (1990) 499–502

33 Paes, E., J.F. Vollmar, P. Pauschinger, W. Mutschler, W. Wanjura, E. Laboranovic: Blood flow in the large vessels. In Liepsch, D. (Ed.): Biofluid Mechanics. Springer, Berlin 1990 (159–165)

34 Patriquin, H.B., M. Lafortune, J.C. Jequier, S. O'Regan, L. Garel, J. Landriault, A. Fontaine, D. Filiatrault: Stenosis of the renal artery: assessment of slowed systole in the downstream circulation with Doppler sonography. Radiology 184 (1992) 479–485

35 Renowden, S.A., D.L. Cochlin: The effect of frusemide on the Doppler waveform in normal kidneys. J. clin. Ultrasound Med. 11 (1992) 65–68

36 Riehl, J., W. Clasen, H. Schmidt, H. Kierdorf, H.G. Sieberth: Altersabhängige Veränderungen der renalen Hämodynamik: Untersuchungen mittels Duplex-Sonographie. Ultraschall Klin. Prax. (Suppl.) 1 (1989) 129

37 Riepe, G., G. v. Klinggräff, H. Imig: Prothesendilatation nach Aortenersatz. Angio 11 (1989) 153–157

38 Rubin, J.M., R.O. Bude, P.L. Carson, R.L. Bree, R.S. Adler: Power Doppler US: a potentially useful alternative to mean frequency-based color Doppler US. Radiology 190 (1994) 853–856

39 Saitoh, M.: Color Doppler flow imaging in interventional ultrasound of the kidney. Scand. J. Urol. Nephrol. (Suppl.) 137 (1991) 59–64

40 Schwerk, W.B., I.K. Restrepo, M. Steellwaag, K.J. Klose, C. Schade-Brittinger: Renal artery stenosis: Grading with image directed Doppler US. Evaluation of renal resitive index. Radiology 190 (1994) 785–790

41 Stavros, A.T., S.H. Parker, W.F. Yakes, A.E. Chantelois, B.J. Burke, P.R. Meyers, J.J. Schenck: Segmental stenosis of the renal artery: pattern recognition of tardus and parvus abnormalities with duplex sonography. Radiology 184 (1992) 487–492

42 Takebayashi, S., N. Aida, K. Matsui: Arteriovenous malformations of the kidneys: Diagnosis and follow-up with color Doppler sonography in six patients. Amer. J. Roentgenol. 157 (1991) 991–995

43 Seitz, K.H., R. Kubale: Duplexsonographie der abdominellen und retroperitonealen Gefäße. VCH Verlag, Weinheim (1987)

44 Takenaka, K., T. Sakamoto, A. Dabestani, J.M. Gardin, W.L. Henry: Pulsed Doppler echocardiographic detection of regurgitant blood flow in the ascending, descending and abdominal aorta of patients with aortic regurgitation. J. Cardiol. 17 (1987) 301–309

45 Tartarini, G., D. Bertoli, R. Baglini, A. Balbarini, M. Mariani: Diagnosis of aortic dissection by color-coded Doppler. J. nucl. Med. allied Sci. 32 (1988) 127–30

46 Thomas, E.A., P.A. Dubbins: Duplex ultrasound of the abdominal aorta – a neglected tool in aortic dissection. Clin. Radiol. 42 (1990) 330–334

10 Splanchnic Arteries

R. Kubale

10.1 General Remarks

Diseases of the celiac trunk and mesenteric arteries and veins are frequently overlooked. Most of these diseases are caused by atherosclerosis, thrombosis, embolism, as well as tumors and inflammatory processes, which may involve the splanchnic vasculature primarily as in panarteritis nodosa or secondarily by compression or enzymatic erosion in pancreatitis.

The symptoms depend on the degree and acuteness of blood flow impairment. Occlusions of gradual onset may produce no symptoms, while acute obstruction is a life-threatening event. The mesenteric arteries, celiac trunk, and mesenteric veins are regarded as a single pathophysiologic unit.

The traditional procedure of first choice for acute bowel ischemia is angiography, whose early use has lowered the mortality rate from over 90% to 53% (13). Additional indications for angiography are chronic bowel ischemia and the investigation of intestinal hemorrhage that may be treatable by embolization. The use of angiography as a screening study in patients with chronic abdominal pain or equivocal auscultation findings is unrealistic, however. The major intestinal vessels can be evaluated with "conventional" duplex sonography under favorable conditions, but this method has not gained wide acceptance due to the relatively long examination times and the difficulty of identifying specific vessels and Doppler spectral sampling, especially in obese or restless patients. CDS offers significant advantages in this regard: the color encoding of blood flow permits the reliable visualization and identification of specific vessels. This makes CDS useful for screening as well as for examinations of acute disorders.

The present chapter deals with the most important primary and secondary diseases of the splanchnic vessels and their sonographic features. Diseases of the liver and portal hypertension are discussed in Chapter 11.

10.2 Normal Anatomy, Variants, and Examination Technique

10.2.1 Normal Anatomy, Variants, and Collaterals

The blood supply of the abdominal organs and gastrointestinal tract is derived mainly from the three anterior splanchnic branches of the abdominal aorta: the celiac trunk and the superior and inferior mesenteric arteries. They develop from an initially paired, ventral, stepladder-like vascular array through partial fusion and regression of the embryonic segmental arteries (Fig. 10.**1**). Disturbances of this complex developmental process lead to numerous variations in the origin, position, and course of the arteries, which may mislead the examiner. The principal variants are briefly discussed (11, 29).

10.2.1.1 Celiac Trunk and Branches

The celiac trunk is a short arterial trunk arising from the front of the aorta at the level of the twelfth to first lumbar vertebrae just below the aortic aperture of the diaphragm. Its initial portion passes downward or horizontally or may curve cephalad and divides into three branches in up to 75% of cases: the left gastric artery, the common hepatic artery, and the splenic artery (Fig. 10.**2**). In 5–10% of cases the celiac trunk gives off a fourth branch, which may consist of an accessory pancreatic artery or an atypical origin of the posterior pancreatic artery (37).

In rare cases the celiac trunk is absent or arises jointly with the superior mesenteric artery as the gastrohepatosplenomesenteric trunk (11, 19).

- The **left gastric artery** is the first branch of the celiac trunk in 90% of cases. It runs between the layers of the lesser omentum and anastomoses on the lesser curvature aspect with the right gastric artery and with branches of the right gastroepiploic artery and short gastric arteries. In 2.5% of cases it arises directly from the abdominal aorta.
- The **splenic artery,** with a diameter of 6–10 mm, is the largest branch of the celiac trunk. It follows a tortuous course along the superior border of the pancreas to the hilum of the spleen giving off a variable

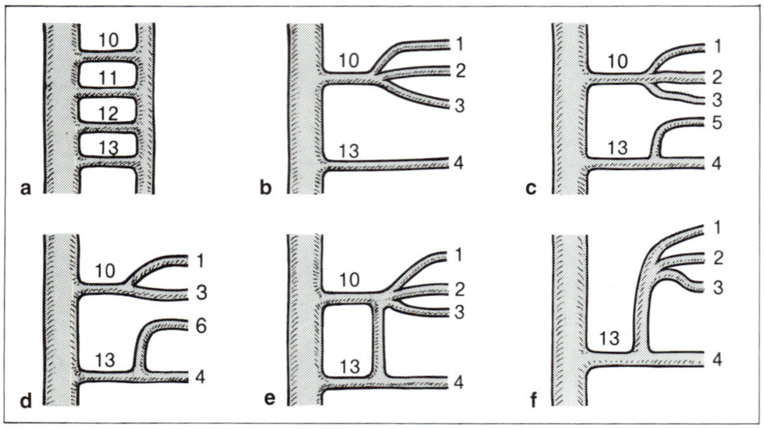

Fig. 10.**1 a–f** Normal and variant embryologic development of the celiac trunk and superior mesenteric artery (after 11). 1 = Left gastric artery, 2 = common hepatic artery, 3 = splenic artery, 4 = superior mesenteric artery, 5 = accessory hepatic artery, 6 = dystopic hepatic artery, 10–13 = embryonic segmental arteries

a The embryonic segmental arteries spring like ladder rungs from the originally symmetrical aorta. They are interconnected initially by a ventral longitudinal anastomotic channel

b After disappearance of the 11th and 12th segmental arteries, the celiac trunk develops from the 10th segmental artery, the superior mesenteric from the 13th segmental artery, and the inferior mesenteric from the 20th or 21st segmental artery. Normally there is complete regression of the ventral anastomosis

c, **d** Partial or complete persistence of the ventral anastomosis leads to an atypical hepatic blood supply from the superior mesenteric artery via an accessory hepatic artery (**c**) or an aberrant right hepatic artery or common hepatic artery (**d**)

e, **f** The longitudinal anastomosis may persist as an anterior collateral vessel (**e** = Bühler anastomosis). In one variant the 10th segmental artery disappears, leaving a common trunk termed the gastromesenteric celiac trunk (**f**)

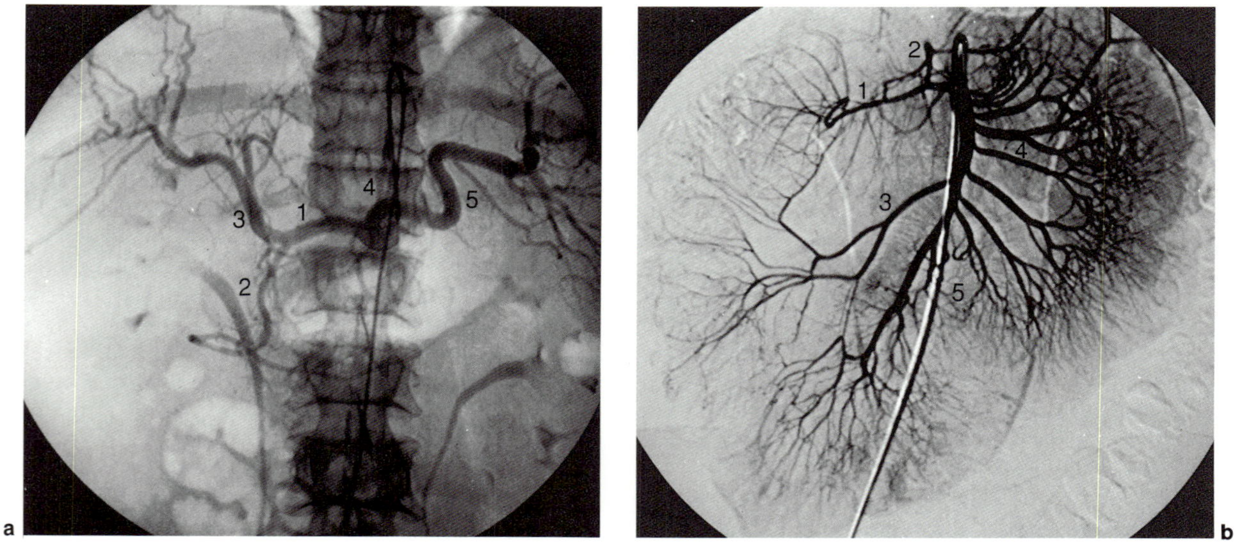

Fig. 10.**2 a, b** Angiographic appearance of the celiac trunk and superior mesenteric artery visualized by selective catheterization

a Celiac trunk with the common hepatic artery (1), gastroduodenal artery (2), hepatic artery proper (3), left gastric artery (4), and splenic artery (5)

b Superior mesenteric artery with right colic artery (1), middle colic artery (2), ileocolic artery (3), jejunal arteries (4), and ileal arteries (5) series of branches to pancreas, stomach and spleen. Its average length is 13 cm. Through the great and dorsal pancreatic arteries and smaller arterial branches, it supplies the body and tail of the pancreas, the greater curvature and fundus of the stomach, and the omentum. It divides at the splenic hilum into an inferior and superior main branch, each of which supplies the splenic parenchyma through four to six segmental arteries.

- From its origin, the **common hepatic artery** runs to the right along the superior border of the pancreas to the hepatoduodenal ligament, where typically it lies on the left of the bile duct and in front of the portal vein. After giving off the gastroduodenal artery, the common hepatic artery passes to the liver as the proper hepatic artery, which divides into the right and left hepatic arteries. In 45% of cases these arteries give off another branch, the middle hepatic artery, which supplies the medial segment of the left hepatic lobe and the quadrate lobe. Variants are numerous. In up to 24% of cases the liver is supplied wholly or in part by the superior mesenteric artery. Numerous accessory arteries arising directly from the celiac trunk or from the left gastric artery or splenic artery as well as crossing branches from the contralateral hepatic lobe can complicate the situation. A collateral supply may exist via the capsule of the liver and through smaller arteries in the hilum (11, 19).
- The **gastroduodenal artery** runs behind the duodenum and in front of the pancreas. It divides further into the right gastroepiploic artery and the superior, anterior, and posterior pancreaticoduodenal arteries, which form arcades that anastomose with the superior mesenteric system. Branches are distributed to the head of the pancreas, the pylorus, portions of the duodenum, and occasionally the jejunum.

10.2.1.2 Superior and Inferior Mesenteric Arteries

The superior mesenteric artery arises 0.5–2.0 cm below the origin of the celiac trunk at the level of the first lumbar vertebra (Fig. 10.**2**). It runs inferiorly, passing behind the body of the pancreas and the splenic artery. After about 4 cm the inferior pancreaticoduodenal artery and the middle and right celiac arteries arise from the right side of the vessel. The jejunum and ileum derive their blood supply from the jejunal and ilial arteries, which interconnect through numerous anastomotic arcades. The iliocolic artery is the terminal branch of the superior mesenteric artery and supplies the cecum, terminal ileum, and appendix.

The inferior mesenteric artery arises from the anterior or left lateral aspect of the aorta about 3 cm above the aortic bifurcation. It first runs downward and divides after 3–6 cm into the left colic artery, the sigmoid arteries, and the hemorrhoidal artery.

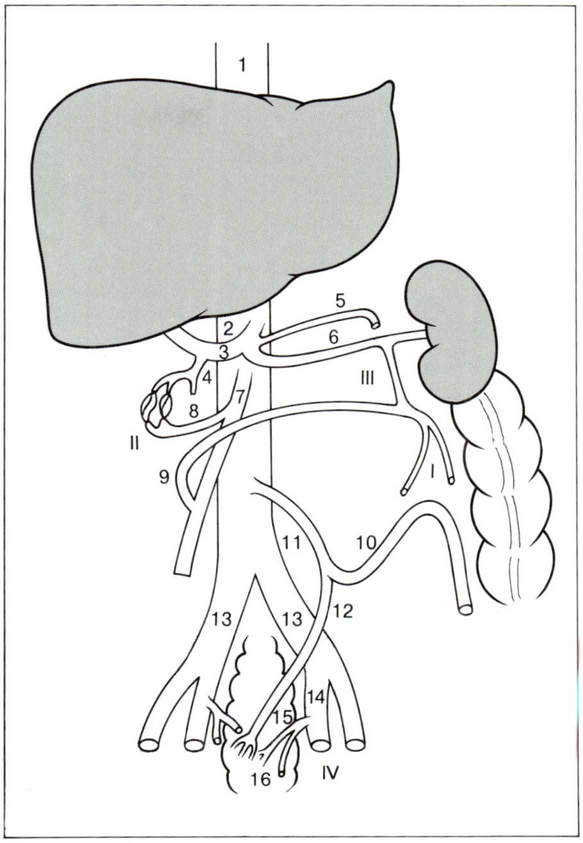

Fig. 10.**3** Existing collateral pathways for the splanchnic arteries (after [20]). The principal cross-connections occur through anastomoses between the middle and left colic arteries (I = Riolan anastomosis), through the superior and inferior pancreaticoduodenal arteries (II = pancreatic arcades), through anastomoses between the middle colic artery and splenic artery (III), and to the territory of the internal iliac artery through the superior and inferior rectal arteries (IV). 1 = Abdominal aorta, 2 = celiac trunk, 3 = common hepatic artery, 4 = gastroduodenal artery, 5 = left gastric artery, 6 = splenic artery, 7 = superior mesenteric artery, 8 = inferior pancreaticoduodenal artery, 9 = middle colic artery, 10 = left colic artery, 11 = inferior mesenteric artery, 12 = superior rectal artery, 13 = common iliac artery, 14 = internal iliac artery, 15 = internal pudendal artery, 16 = inferior rectal artery

10.2.1.3 Preformed Collaterals

Numerous preformed collaterals can supply blood to the intestine in response to a gradual arterial occlusion (Fig. 10.**3**). The most common is the anastomosis of Riolan, which forms a connection between the left colic artery and the first ascending branch of the superior mesenteric, usually the middle colic artery.

Additional cross-links are established through the pancreaticoduodenal arcades (Fig. 10.**1**), and the marginal collaterals that run along the mesenteric side of the colon and are supplied by branches of the middle, right, and left colic arteries. With a complete

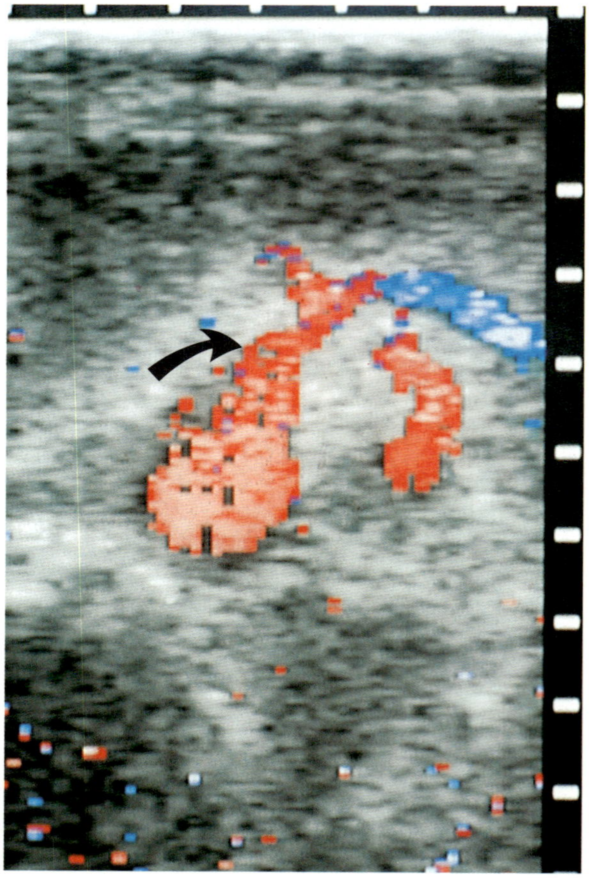

Fig. 10.**4** Transverse view of the celiac trunk (arrow) shows the typical palm-branch division into the splenic artery (right, encoded blue) and common hepatic artery (red). A section of splenic vein (encoded red) is seen posterior to the splenic artery

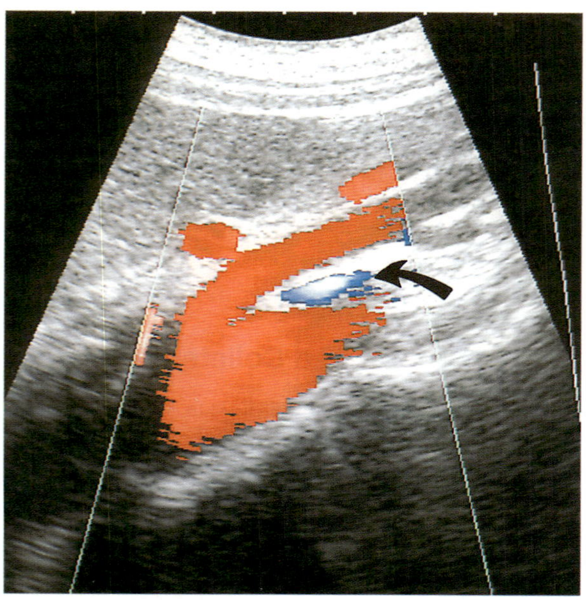

Fig. 10.**5** Longitudinal view of the superior mesenteric artery. After arising from the aorta, the artery crosses in front of the left renal vein (encoded blue, arrow) and usually curves downward along the right side of the aorta

occlusion of all major visceral branches, the intercostal, phrenic, and esophageal arteries can still provide a collateral supply from above. From *below,* blood can reach the inferior mesenteric artery through branches of the internal iliac artery and the inferior and superior hemorrhoidal arteries (20, 37).

10.2.2 Examination Technique

10.2.2.1 Examination Protocol and Vessel Identification

The patient should fast for the examination. Using the settings described in Chapter 9, the examiner first locates the celiac trunk and the origin of the superior mesenteric artery and documents their course in two planes. The examination is performed in the supine or lateral decubitus position, using a 3-MHz transducer or a 5-MHz probe in children and thin patients and applying moderate compression. The celiac trunk and superior mesenteric artery are definable in more than 90% of cases when the liver is used as an acoustic window. After the color encoding is switched on and adjusted, the flow in the celiac trunk is analyzed first (Fig. 10.**4**). The main trunk, common hepatic artery, splenic artery, and if possible the left gastric artery are imaged in longitudinal and transverse views. In 60% of cases at least part of the gastroduodenal artery can be identified anterior to the pancreatic head as a vessel oriented at right angles to the proper hepatic artery. Next the origin of the superior mesenteric artery is identified and traced as far distally as possible in longitudinal views with caudad angulation of the transducer (Fig. 10.**5**).

The inferior mesenteric artery is evaluated by first locating the aortic bifurcation and moving the transducer cephalad with careful compression until the proximal trunk of the inferior mesenteric artery is identified in transverse section about 2–4 cm proximal to the bifurcation. A 2–3 cm segment of the inferior mesenteric artery can usually be defined by rotating the image to a more longitudinal plane (Fig. 10.**6 a–c**).

For an optimum evaluation, the gain and color threshold should be set to a level that just eliminates "color noise." Artifacts induced by peristalsis can be reduced by careful compression of the abdominal wall with the transducer. Some examinations may require temporary gastrointestinal immobilization with an antispasmodic drug (e. g., scopolamine i. v.).

A medium- or high-velocity scale may be needed to obtain adequate flow imaging in the proximal part of the celiac trunk and superior mesenteric artery. Reducing the penetration depth will permit the use of a higher pulse repetition frequency, so that higher flow velocities can be detected without aliasing. Other technical problems can result from echogenic material near the transducer (meteorism, feces, etc.). Vessels that run horizontally can be imaged in transverse section by angling the transducer (see Chapter 4). If the B-mode image demonstrates

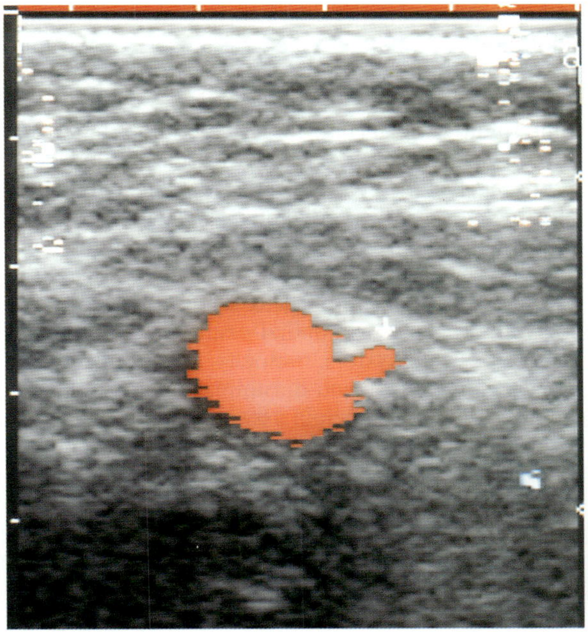
a

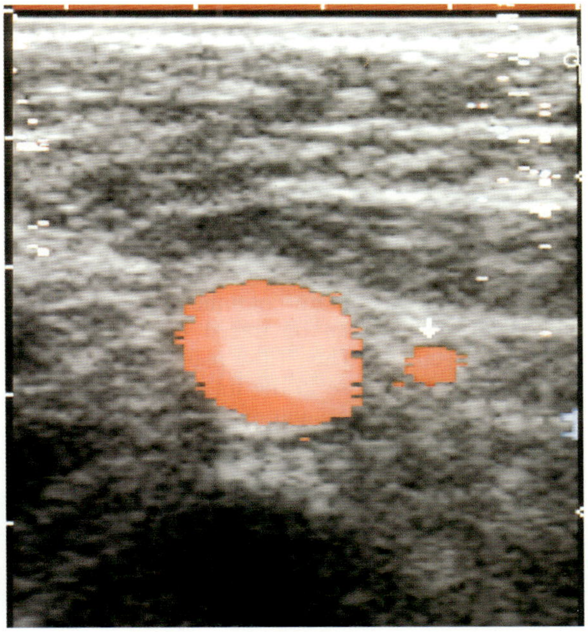
b

Fig. 10.6**a–c** Inferior mesenteric artery
a Transverse scan through the aorta demonstrates the lateral origin of the inferior mesenteric artery (white arrow)
b Scan 1 cm distally shows the cross section of the vessel farther lateral to the aorta (arrow)
c An oblique longitudinal scan demonstrates about a 3-cm segment of the proximal portion of the vessel (blue = section of aorta, red = segment of inferior mesenteric artery

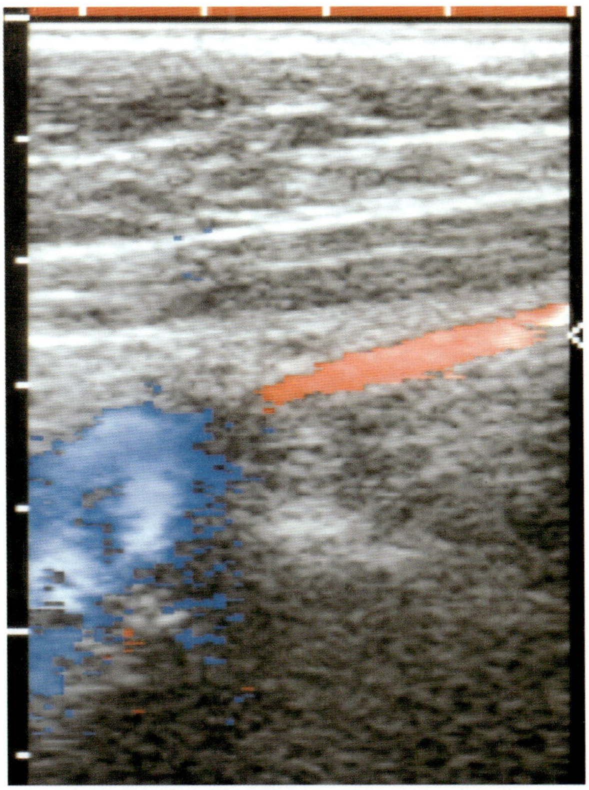
c

plaques, if the color-encoded flow image shows areas of flow acceleration and turbulence, or if the examiner wants to assess drug effects or the regulatory capacity of the mesenteric blood supply, Doppler spectra should be sampled at the origin of the vessels and in suspect areas. The blood flow and the flow direction in the gastroduodenal artery should be visualized to exclude possible steal phenomena (14, 16). In addition, in cases of a stenosis the degree of the stenosis should be assessed in inspiration and in expiration.

The length of the examination depends on the disease. If acute bowel ischemia is suspected, the examiner should allow only a few minutes for the ultrasound examination and quickly proceed to angiography in unequal findings. In patients with a chronic bowel disease, the examiner may take 30 minutes or longer to search for stenosis and, if necessary, proceed with function studies.

10.2.2.2 Documentation

Minimum documentation consists of B-mode and color-encoded flow images of the origins of the celiac trunk and superior mesenteric artery. In cases of suspected chronic bowel ischemia, the trunk of the inferior mesenteric artery should also be imaged.

If CDS demonstrates a local flow acceleration or turbulence, the angle-corrected peak systolic velocity and end-diastolic velocity should be documented in the suspicious area and in two or three additional proximal and distal vascular segments. With a presumed ligamentous stenosis of the celiac trunk, supplementary scans should be obtained in deep inspiration and expiration to assess the extent and persistence of the obstruction. If drug effects or responsiveness to physiologic stimuli are of interest, resistance indices (see Chapter 3) are helpful for further evaluation.

10.3 Normal Findings

The celiac trunk appears as a palm-leaf-shaped structure in the transverse color flow image (Fig. 10.**4**). The common hepatic artery (or hepatic artery proper) and the splenic artery are continuously perfused by pulsatile flow and can be traced to the liver and spleen, respectively. Their flow pattern and Doppler spectrum are like those in the internal carotid artery due to the low distal vascular resistance, which allows persistence of antegrade flow in diastole. Normal values for peak systolic velocity are 60–140 cm/sec. Values up to 250 cm/s are measured in deep expiration in up to 10% of asymptomatic patients.

The left gastric artery can be traced along the inferior surface of the left lobe of the liver in a modified longitudinal scan. Generally only the proximal part of the artery is visualized, though occasionally the vessel may be defined as far as a site of possible anastomosis with the left hepatic artery. Its Doppler spectrum, like that of the gastroduodenal artery, shows greater pulsatility with very little diastolic flow.

The superior mesenteric artery arises from the anterior or anterolateral aspect of the aorta. By watching the monitor and adjusting the transducer position accordingly, the examiner can track the main arterial trunk for up to 8 cm (Fig. 10.**5**). Continuous antegrade flow is observed during systole, with a sharp rise and fall of the systolic peak. In fasted patients a notch occurs in late systolic indicating a brief reverse-flow component that produces a color reversal in the color flow image. Cessation of flow may occur in late diastole. Normal values for peak systolic velocity are 60–180 cm/sec. Postprandial examination shows an increased peak systolic velocity and a disproportionate elevation of end-diastolic velocity reflecting the physiologic hyperemia associated with digestion. Analogous spectral changes occur after the administration of glucagon (10, 15).

Variants, such as a common hepatic artery or right hepatic artery arising from the superior mesenteric artery or the isolated origin of a splenic artery from the aorta, can be seen at once in the color duplex image (Fig. 10.**7a**, **b**).

The inferior mesenteric artery can be visualized in more than 60% of patients by using the examination technique described above. Normally its main trunk is uniformly occupied by color-encoded flow signals during systole. The spectral characteristics re-

a
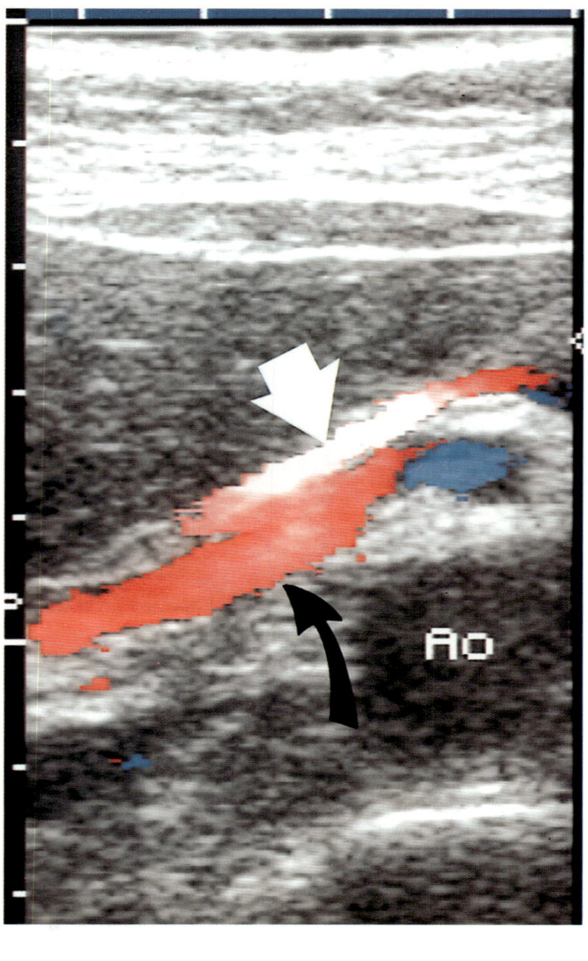

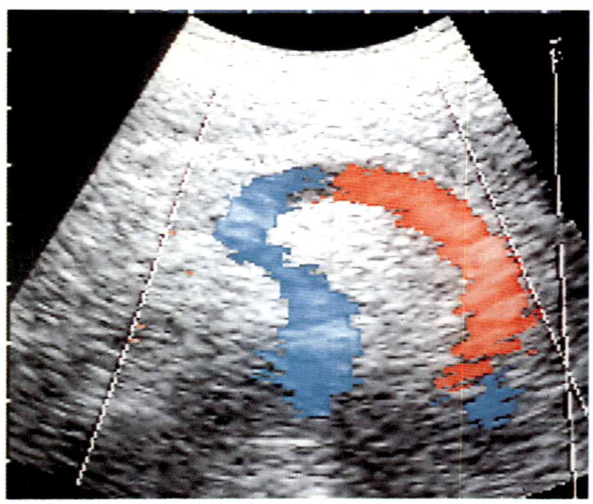
b

Fig. 10.**7a, b** Variants in the origin of splanchnic arteries
a Modified upper abdominal transverse CDS scan shows the aorta (Ao, imaged here at a zero-flow point in the cardiac cycle), the superior mesenteric artery (encoded blue), and a right hepatic artery arising from the superior mesenteric (black arrow). In front of the right hepatic artery, the scan plane cuts the portal vein (white arrow), which is compressed by the transducer, mimicking stenosis (color saturation toward white)
b Origin of the splenic artery from the aorta. Transverse scan demonstrates the tortuous course of the vessel, which first runs anteriorly (blue segment) and then posterolaterally (red segment). Angiography confirmed the isolated origin of the splenic artery from the aorta. The common hepatic artery and superior mesenteric artery form a common trunk

semble those of the superior mesenteric artery: a high velocity in systole and a low velocity or cessation of flow in diastole.

10.4 Pathologic Findings

10.4.1 Preliminary Remarks

Intestinal blood flow is a complex process influenced by mechanical, metabolic, and neurologic factors as well as numerous vasoactive drugs (4). The blood flow increases in accordance with the composition of ingested food and decreases in response to stress and physical activity. Arterial insufficiency can result from stenosis, thrombosis, embolism, tumor compression, volvulus, adhesions, or mesenteric vein thrombosis (see Chapter 11). Lesions of gradual onset can be adequately compensated by collateralization. Acute occlusions, inadequate collateralization, or the involvement of two or more vessels cause ischemic damage to the bowel.

Many of these disorders were formerly misinterpreted as inflammatory bowel disease. But the increasing use of endoscopy, endosonography, histology, and refined angiographic techniques have made it possible to differentiate entities such as ischemic colitis and colitis associated with drug use.

10.4.2 Plaques, Stenoses, and Occlusions

10.4.2.1 Asymptomatic Patients, Atherosclerosis, Arcuate Ligament Compression Syndrome, Fibromuscular Dysplasia, and Vascular Compression by Tumors

The leading cause of stenosis is atherosclerosis. Changes in the splanchnic arteries may be found as early as the third decade of life. Further aging is accompanied by the formation of lumen-reducing plaques or occlusions. Occlusive lesions may involve the proximal part of an artery, the main trunk, first- and second-order branches, or there may be diffuse atherosclerotic involvement of the peripheral branches.

Stenoses caused by calcification and plaque deposits in the aorta are often circumferential. If the stenosis significantly lowers the distal blood pressure, the preformed collaterals will enlarge and supply the territory distal to the stenosis. The main collateral pathway is generally the gastroduodenal artery with the pancreatic arcades (Fig. 10.**3**). If the inferior mesenteric artery is affected, flow is diverted from the superior mesenteric territory via the middle and left colic arteries or from the territory of the internal iliac artery via collaterals.

Atherosclerotic stenosis involving the proximal part of the splanchnic arteries is generally focal and may be circumferential or eccentric. The early stage is often marked only by isolated plaques at the inferior border of the vessel (Fig. 10.**8a**, **b**).

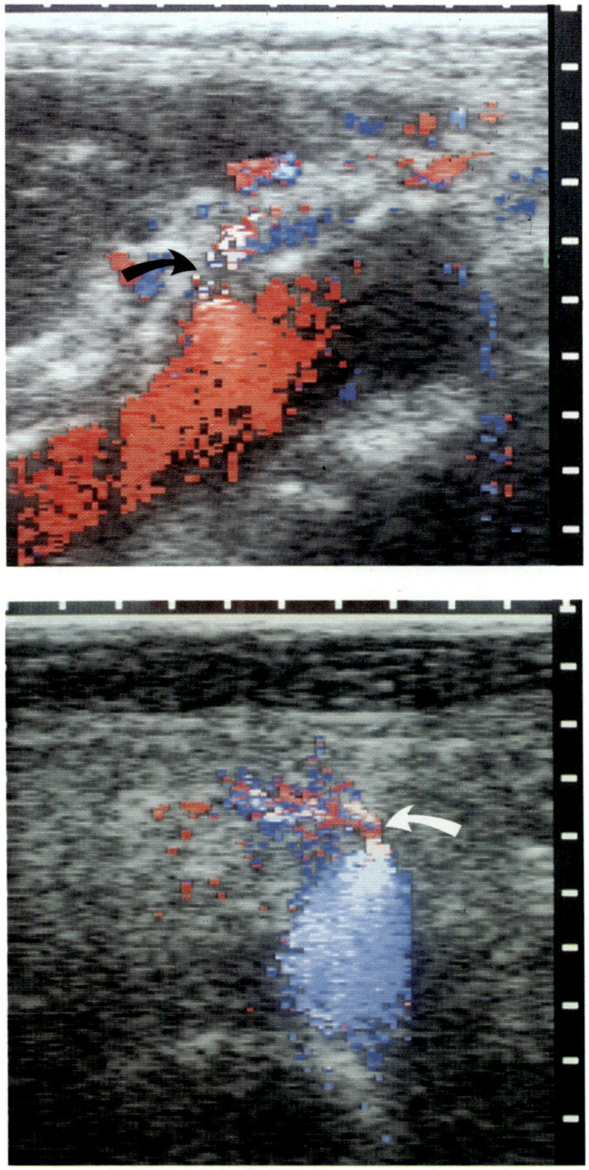

a

b

Fig. 10.**8a, b** Proximal stenosis of the superior mesenteric artery

a Longitudinal view shows a short, high-grade stenosis at the vessel origin (arrow) with poststenotic turbulence (mixed red and blue signals). The stenosed lumen is not defined in the B-mode image due to calcified vessel wall deposits

b Transverse view shows a very high frequency shift (color saturation toward white, arrow) and poststenotic color-encoded artifacts caused by vibration of the vessel wall (diffuse mixture of red and blue pixels). Distal to the stenosis, the vessel turns laterally downward to the right. The aortic lumen is encoded in blue

Diabetics most commonly exhibit a diffuse atherosclerosis with concomitant involvement of the peripheral branches. The vessels appear irregular on angiograms, and collaterals do not develop.

A special entity with controversial clinical implications is arcuate ligament compression syndrome. It is caused by constriction of the celiac trunk at its origin by the medial attachment of the crus of the diaphragm. Angiography demonstrates a characteristic superior, concave indentation at the origin of the celiac trunk from the aorta. The stenosis becomes more severe during expiration, and at maximum inspiration the celiac trunk may appear completely normal (29). Many patients present nonspecific abdominal symptoms. It is unclear whether the symptoms have a primary ischemic cause or result from irritation of the celiac plexus. Some published cases have shown dramatic improvement of complaints following incision of the ligament (34).

Stenosis can also be caused by fibromusular dysplasia—which chiefly affects the renal artery, splenic artery, superior mesenteric artery, and celiac trunk in order of decreasing frequency—and by extrinsic compression from benign or malignant tumors.

Sonography demonstrates calcified plaques as hyperechoic areas that cast a typical acoustic shadow corresponding to plaque size and insonation angle. Luminal narrowing may cause flow acceleration with associated aliasing, turbulence, and dilatation in the poststenotic segment (Fig. 10.**9a**, **b**). High-grade stenosis can produce coarse vibration artifacts that transcend the vessel boundaries (Fig. 10.**8a**, **b**) as described earlier for peripheral vessels and the aorta.

Interpreting the CDS image, one has to consider that the curvature of blood vessels can simulate flow acceleration. The origins of the celiac trunk and superior mesenteric artery, for example, are generally insonated at an optimum Doppler angle of approxi-

a

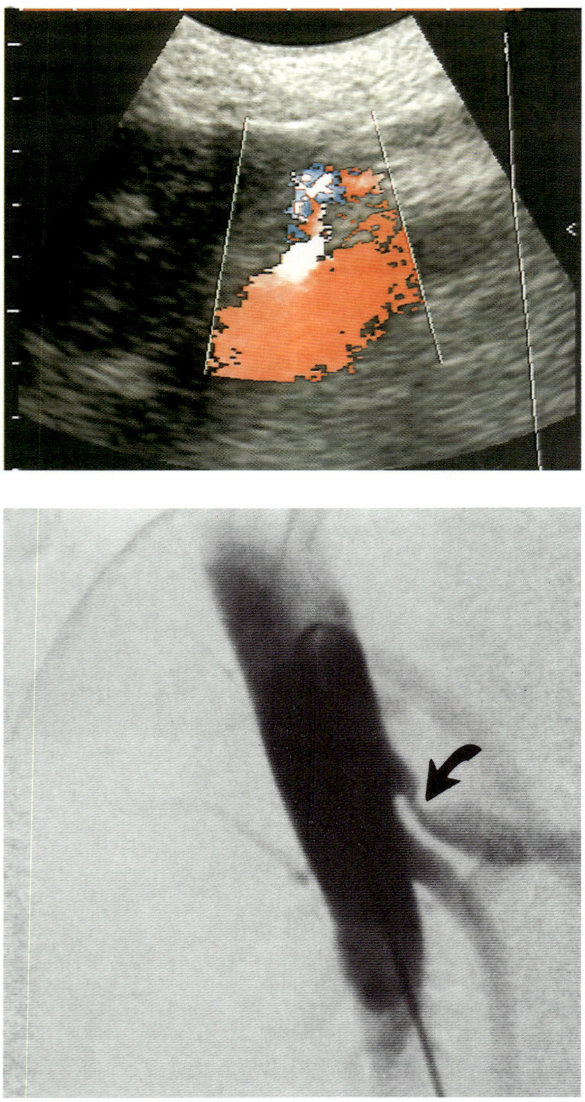

b

Fig. 10.**9a, b** Stenosis of the celiac trunk
a Oblique longitudinal CDS scan shows a markedly elevated frequency shift (color saturation approaching white) at the origin of the celiac trunk and poststenotic turbulence (arrow). The vessel lumen cannot be evaluated in the B-mode image due to wall calcifications
b Corresponding angiogram (DSA) demonstrates more than 50% lumen reduction (arrow)

mately 0° that can mimic accelerated flow. This error can be eliminated by supplementing color-encoded flow data with angle-corrected measurements to confirm or exclude localized flow acceleration with turbulence or vibrational artifacts. While there is no universal criterion for grading celiac and mesenteric stenoses, a rise in the peak systolic velocity of more than 180 cm/s in a fasting patient suggests a hemodynamically sufficient stenosis. A velocity higher than 280 cm/s and/or turbulance indicates a stenosis of more than 75% in the celiac trunk or superior mesenteric artery (9, 15, 16, 21, 23, 24, 32). Higher grades of stenosis are associated with vibration artifacts (see Chapter 3 and 4). One advantage of CDS is that ancillary studies can be performed in various respiratory phases, for example, to evaluate the response of blood flow to inspiration and expiration (Fig. 10.**10**).

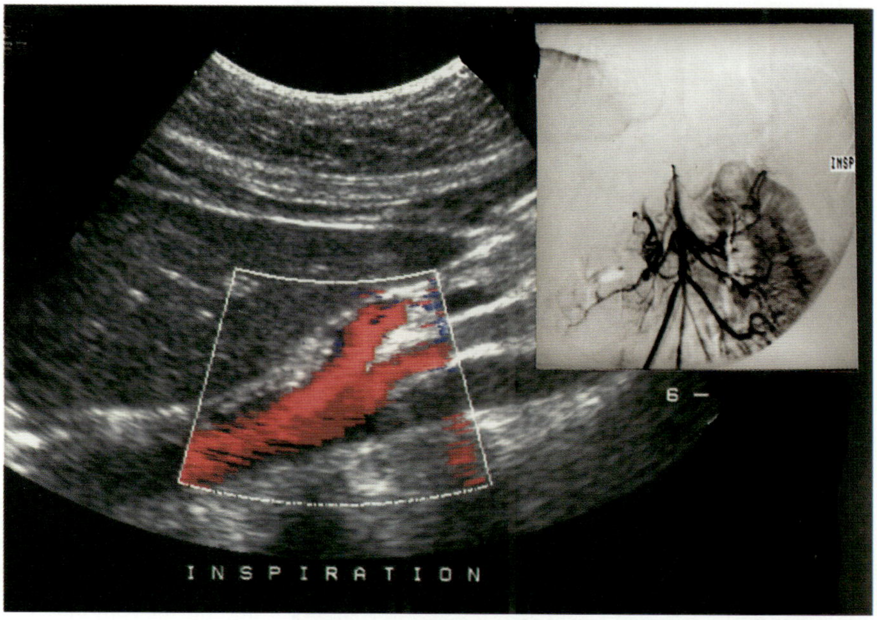

a

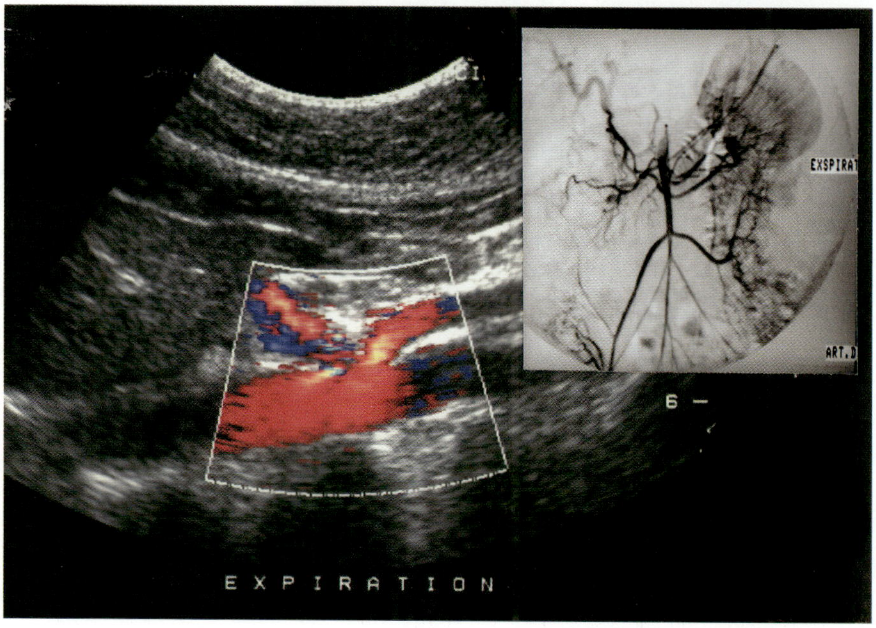

b

Fig. 10.**10 a, b** Functional stenosis of the celiac trunk
a A longitudinal scan with CDS in inspiration shows the normal celiac trunk and the superior mesenteric artery. Selective angiography *(left inset)* of the superior mesenteric artery displays no collaterals with the celiac trunk
b In expiration there is marked turbulence at the origin of the celiac trunk (mixture of red and blue, arrow) and still normal flow in the superior mesenteric artery. The selective angiogram *(left inset)* now shows collaterals with contrast filling of the hepatic artery due to the functional stenosis of the celiac trunk

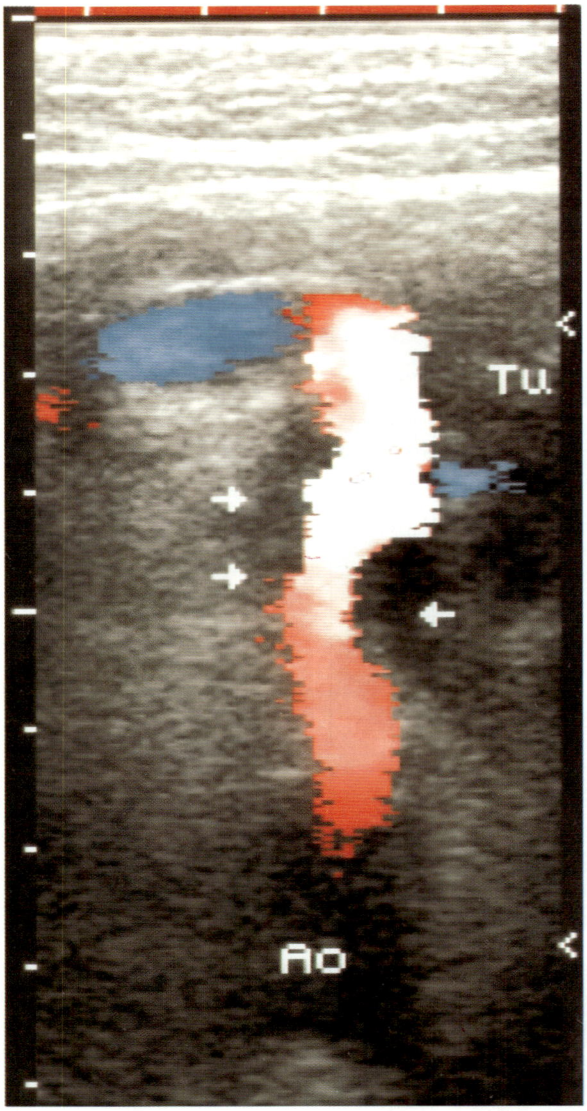

Fig. 10.**11** Carcinoma of the pancreatic head encasing the celiac trunk. Transverse scan shows a nonuniformly hypoechoic mass (Tu, arrows) around the main trunk (encoded red) causing a curved, smoothly marginated pressure defect in the left side of the vessel. The common hepatic artery (encoded blue) branches from the celiac trunk toward the right side. Ao = Aorta

As a rule, tumor compression of splanchnic arteries is easily diagnosed with ultrasound. The main causative lesions are pancreatic carcinoma and lymphoma. While lymphomas spare the blood vessels for some time, other types of malignant tumor tend to produce obvious vascular compression even at an early stage (Fig. 10.**11**).

10.4.2.2 Acute and Chronic Bowel Ischemia, Arterial Embolism, Acute Thrombosis, and "Nonocclusive" Bowel Ischemia

Acute occlusion is a surgical emergency. Its pathogenesis may relate to irregular, thrombogenic plaque, a high-grade stenosis, or embolization. The most common sources of occlusive emboli are the heart, mural thrombi from the aorta, atheromatous wall deposits detached by angiography, or paradoxical emboli from the venous system. The symptoms are varied and often nonspecific. An episode of severe diffuse or colicky pain may be followed initially by an improvement of symptoms. Muscular rigidity and other clinical signs may be absent.

The history is an important key to diagnosis. Particular attention is given to previous embolic events or cardiac disease such as atrial fibrillation, mitral stenosis, or myocardial infarction. A helpful parameter is the serum lactate level, which may show up to a ninefold increase in acute embolism.

Ultrasound imaging in patients with acute bowel ischemia demonstrates increased peristalsis as a nonspecific sign. The rapidly progressive wall edema leads to hypoechoic bull's-eye figures. The further course is marked by a cessation of peristalsis and necrosis of the bowel wall. It is typical to find a relatively normal-appearing abdomen in the plain survey radiograph and continued thickening of the bowel wall with free fluid. In the late stage, the bowel wall and portal vein may contain gas bubbles that produce very bright echoes in the gray-scale ultrasound image. CDS scanning can assist diagnosis in the early stage but generally is of limited value for evaluating the splanchnic vessels in patients with an acute abdomen. If CDS shows an occlusion of the superior mesenteric artery, angiography may be dispensed with, and surgery may be undertaken right away. CDS cannot exclude embolism of the terminal branches, however. If ultrasound shows patency of the major arteries combined with thickened bowel walls in a patient with a nonspecific history and symptoms, immediate angiography is indicated.

An important entity requiring differentiation from acute occlusion is nonocclusive bowel ischemia (NOB). Characterized by severe spasticity in the territory of the mesenteric artery, it predominantly affects patients with multiple morbidity and is managed initially by the intra-arterial infusion of vasodilating agents (33). Precipitating factors are circulatory insufficiency, sepsis, and too rapid digitalization in older patients. Its clinical symptoms are nonspecific in the early stage and are often obscured by underlying disease. Untreated, the condition leads to increasing cellular hypoxia with necrosis and perforation of the bowel wall.

Unlike the plain abdominal radiograph, which is unrewarding in the initial stage, sonography demonstrates increasing hypotony or atony of the small intestine. Initially there is no thickening of the bowel wall. An indirect sonographic sign is a small caliber of the superior mesenteric artery (which may show no flow increase in response to glucagon). CDS is particularly helpful in differentiating NOB from primary mesenteric vein thrombosis (see Chapter 11), which often evokes a reflex arterial constriction that is difficult to distinguish from NOB. Definitive diagnosis and treatment must rely on angiography, however.

10.4.3 Anomalies, Arteriovenous Malformations, and Aneurysms

Arteriovenous malformations are often discovered incidentally during the workup of intestinal hemorrhage. Anomalous differentiation of the embryonic capillary plexus with persistent arteriovenous or arterioportal shunts lead to congenital a–v fistulas of varying morphology (5). The most common form is angiodysplasia, which is most reliably detected by endoscopy and angiography. The same applies to angiomatosis of the colon in patients with the Klippel–Trenaunay–Weber syndrome and Osler disease, in which hepatic involvement is demonstrable with ultrasound. Acquired a–v fistulas may result from atherosclerotic disease, trauma, or surgical procedures.

CDS can detect high-flow fistulas by their associated mosaic-like vibrational artifacts (see Chapter 4). Indirect signs include arterial modulation of the outflow vein or, in arterioportal fistulas, ectasia of the portal vein with turbulent flow (see Chapter 11). A steal effect through the pancreatic arcades or a massive rise in portal venous pressure with reflux into the mesenteric venous system can lead to abdominal angina.

Aneurysms of the splanchnic arteries are considered rare, and most are detected fortuitously. Aneurysms most commonly affect the splenic artery as a result of atherosclerosis, trauma, or enzymatic erosion in pancreatitis. The second most common site of involvement is the hepatic artery, where aneurysms may have an infectious or traumatic etiology. They are observed with increasing frequency following prolonged intravenous catheterization, drug use, valve replacement, or liver transplantation. Only 10% are secondary to trauma or surgical procedures. Eighty percent occur outside the liver, while the rest occur within the liver or porta hepatis. The principal complications are infarction due to the embolization of thrombotic debris and aneurysmal rupture. Far less common sites of occurrence are the cystic artery and the superior mesenteric artery, where aneurysms usually have an infectious etiology (previous *Salmonella* or staphylococcal infection), the gastroduodenal and pancreaticoduodenal arteries, and the celiac trunk.

Ultrasound demonstrates a round or fusiform hypoechoic mass showing color flow evidence of strong and sometimes pulsatile turbulent flow. The B-mode image can define older thrombi, but only CDS can demonstrate all thrombotic material as a flow void.

10.4.4 Inflammatory Changes, Pharmacologic Effects, and Systemic Disease Manifestations

Inflammatory changes may directly involve the vessel wall or, as in pancreatitis, cause secondary erosive changes with hemorrhage, aneurysm formation, or multifocal stenosis syndrome.

Takayasu arteritis predominantly affects the thoracic aorta but may involve the abdominal aorta and visceral branches. The disease progresses episodically, and the underlying cause of this primary arteritis is unknown. Stenosis or occlusion of the superior mesenteric artery and celiac trunk is common. The inferior mesenteric artery is rarely affected and maintains the intestinal blood supply through collateral channels (13).

Panarteritis nodosa is a necrotizing inflammatory vasculitis involving the small and medium-size muscular arteries and caused by the deposition of immune complexes in the vessel wall. The effects of this process in the mesenteric vessels include luminal irregularities, multiple saccular aneurysms of variable size in the medium and small branches, and occasional life-threatening hemorrhage due to rupture. In most cases there is concomitant involvement of the kidneys and liver (13).

While the sonographic features of Takayasu arteritis are indistinguishable from stenoses and occlusions due to other causes, color duplex imaging can in theory provide presumptive evidence of panarteritis nodosa by demonstrating small aneurysms in the terminal branches with a normal-appearing main trunk. The definitive diagnosis is still established by angiography, however.

A more realistic role for sonography is in detecting the marked hyperemia that occurs in florid inflammatory bowel diseases (Crohn disease, ulcerative colitis). While instruments currently available can occasionally demonstrate the hyperemic state of the bowel wall and early venous filling, flow measurements in the inferior mesenteric artery show a relationship between the activity of the inflammatory bowel disease and elevated peak flow velocity and disproportionate diastolic flow increase (12). CDS demonstrates a large-caliber inferior mesenteric artery that is continuously visible in systole and diastole. To diagnose these changes is very helpful in pediatric cases (27) and in patients with necrotizing vasculitis (30). In acute hepatits recent studies showed a significant increase in peak systolic flow of the hepatic artery. Although there is no correlation between enzyme levels and velocity, the interval between the acute phase and the recovery phase did correlate negatively with the peak systolic velocity (36).

Pharmacologic effects on intestinal blood flow can be assessed with CDS (1, 4, 17, 18, 27). Dumping syndrome is manifested by a disproportionately large increase in blood flow, with a potentially marked decrease of flow in response to exercise, depending on the patient's state of training. Blood flow in the superior mesenteric artery is augmented by glucagon and depressed by somatostatin and vasopressin. These effects are well known, but their detectability with ultrasound demonstrates the potential value of CDS for clinical research and pharmacokinetic studies.

10.4.5 Vascular Reconstructions and Postoperative Follow-up

Angiography is still standard for the planning of a vascular surgical procedure owing to its ability to provide a global view of relevant vascular anatomy. The main indication for CDS is in postoperative follow-up, where it provides a noninvasive means of monitoring vascular patency at frequent intervals and permits the early detection of restenosis and other changes. Another indication is the follow-up of organ transplantations (35). The simple and rapid visualization of the portal vein and hepatic artery permits the early detection of anastomotic stenoses and occlusions following liver transplantation. This requires a postoperative baseline examination and frequent follow-up examinations using standard techniques for the delineation and documentation of the portal vein anastomosis and hepatic artery (8). Loss of the typical arterial waveform in the large vessels of the hilum is an indication for immediate angiography to confirm or exclude presence of a thrombosis (35). However, very slow flow caused by massive necrosis or severe systemic hypertension can lead to a false-positive result (31). In contrast to renal and pancreatic transplants, resistance measurements of the hepatic artery have not proven useful for the early detection of liver transplant rejection (22).

By calculating the resistance indices (Pourcelot index) in the artery supplying the pancreatic transplant and taking a value of 0.7 as the threshold, it is possible to differentiate between rejection, pancreatitis, and a normal organ with a reported sensitivity of 76% and specificity of 100% (26). These are preliminary results that must still be validated in larger clinical populations using biopsy confirmation.

10.5 Diagnostic Value of Color Duplex Sonography in Relation to Other Diagnostic Procedures

The traditional first-approach diagnostic procedure for splanchnic arterial disease is angiography with selective catheterization of the celiac trunk, superior mesenteric artery, and inferior mesenteric artery. This method provides clear visualization of the vessels and their branches. By contrast, the results of sonographic vascular examinations are extremely examiner-dependent, may be compromised by overlying bowel gas, and are more difficult to review due to the segmental or plane-of-section imaging format. The advantage of sonography, however, is its lack of invasiveness and the option of repeating the study as often as desired. The importance of newer procedures such as spiral CT with three-dimensional reconstruction of the opacified vascular trunks, MR angiography of the splanchnic arteries, and the radionuclide detection of thrombi using monoclonal antibodies (25) cannot be definitively assessed at the present time.

When first introduced (1986), CDS was used mainly for examinations of the peripheral vessels and superficial organs. Many reports have been published on these applications, and the role of the modality is well established. With the broader introduction of improved scanners, the abdominal region finally became accessible to CDS evaluation. The relative importance and limitations of color duplex imaging in studies of the splanchnic vasculature can be characterized as follows (Table 10.**1**):

1. CDS is of limited importance for the diagnosis of acute intestinal ischemia. Only the main trunk and perhaps the proximal portions of the first-order branches can be visualized. If CDS demonstrates an occlusion, the diagnosis is established and there is no need to proceed with angiography. CDS is of greater value than conventional duplex in this setting, because it can still be used in difficult situations (restless patient, abdominal tenderness) and can be completed in a relatively short time (6, 24). CDS cannot exclude the acute occlusion of a mesenteric vessel, however, so when corresponding clinical signs are present, angiography should be performed without delay. Ultrasound contrast agents may help to demonstrate smaller branches (see Chapter 16), but so far there has been no reported experience in this area.

2. CDS is most valuable as a screening study in patients with chronic intestinal ischemia, nonspecific abdominal complaints, or an unexplained audible bruit. The site of pathology in most of these cases is the proximal part of the vessel, which is accessible to ultrasound imaging. While an experienced sonographer can evaluate the origins of the mesenteric arteries and celiac trunk without benefit of color flow imaging, CDS is essential for locating and tracking collateral vessels and detecting subtle lesions.

3. Although isolated vascular stenoses in asymptomatic patients generally are not clinically significant as a result of good collateral flow, it is recommended that irregular, thrombogenic plaques be closely followed. The detection of collateral flow through pathways such as the colic arcades, splenorenal anastomoses, and especially the pancreatic arcades can be important before major abdominal surgery to avoid postoperative ischemia.

4. Aneurysms are easily detected with CDS. Many lesions that previously were classified as cysts by B-mode imaging can now be rapidly and noninvasively identified using CDS or CT with bolus contrast enhancement (5, 7, 18). Although angiography is still necessary for preoperative planning, the increasing use of ultrasound and CDS permit the early detection

Table 10.**1** Relative value of abdominal plain film, B-mode sonography, duplex sonography, CDS, and angiography in the evaluation of splanchnic vascular disorders (more "plus" signs indicate a more favorable rating; – = no importance, (*) = combination of plain radiography and B-mode imaging, 1 = diagnosis aided by shell-like calcifications)

	Abdomen plain film imaging	B-mode sonography	Duplex sonography	Color duplex sonography	Angiography
Intestinal ischemia					
– Acute (a) initial stage	–	–	+	++	+++
(b) latent stage	(*)+	(*)+	+	++	+++
– Chronic	–	–	++	+++	+++
Tumor compression/ invasion	–	+	++	+++	++
Identification of					
– Variants	–	(+)	+	++	+++
– Collaterals	–	–	+	++	++
– Aneurysms	(+)1	++	++	+++	+++
Postoperative follow-up					
– Vascular reconstruction	–	–	++	+++	+++
– Bypass grafting	–	–	++	+++	+++

even of aneurysms at atypical sites (3) so that elective surgery or embolization can be planned. Color duplex is adequate for monitoring progression and outcome (18).

5. CDS replaces angiography for the postoperative follow-up of stenosis resections and bypass procedures. Frequent follow-up can provide early detection of complications in most cases.

6. The importance of the quantitative assessment of flow velocity and volume flow and the measurement of peripheral resistance in the mesenteric vessels and celiac trunk is not yet fully understood. Experiments in phantoms and laboratory animals have shown good agreement with electromagnetic flow measurements. But the application of these findings to human patients involves much uncertainty. Phantoms always simulate ideal conditions, which do not occur in human patients. The same may be said of animal experiments (see Chapter 4). A more realistic approach employs interindividual measurements of mesenteric blood flow and its response to stimuli, pharmacologic agents, and therapy (1, 6, 14, 17).

10.6 References

1 Aldoori, M.I., M.I. Qamar, A.E. Read, R.C. Williamson: Increased flow in the superior mesenteric artery in dumping syndrome. Brit. J. Surg. 72 (1985) 389–390

2 Alvarez, D., H. Vazquez, J.C. Bai, R. Mastai, D. Flores, L. Boerr: Superior mesenteric artery blood flow in celiac disease. Dig. Dis. Sci. 38 (1993) 1175–1182

3 Barba, C.A., P.M. Bret, E.J. Hinchey: Pseudoaneurysm of the cystic artery: a rare cause of hemobilia. Canad. J. Surg. 37 (1994) 64–66

4 Cooper, A.M., G.D. Braatvedt, M.I. Qamar, H. Brown, D.M. Thomas, M. Halliwell, A.E. Read, R.J. Corrall: Fasting and post-prandial splanchnic blood flow is reduced by a somatostatin analogue (octreotide) in man. Clin. Sci. 81 (1991) 169–175

5 Endress, C., G.A. Kling, B.L. Medrazo: Diagnosis of hepatic artery aneurysm with portal vein fistula using image-directed Doppler ultrasound. J. clin. Ultrasound 17 (1989) 206–208

6 Flinn, W.R., R.J. Rizzo, J.S. Park, G.P. Sandager: Duplex scanning for assessment of mesenteric ischemia. Surg. Clin. N. Amer. 70 (1990) 99–107

7 Fransen, H., R. Kubale, K.D. Wurche, A. Kalaehne: Nicht-invasive Diagnostik von Milzarterienaneurysmata. Fortschr. Röntgenstr. 151 (1989) 532–535

8 Hall, T.R., S.V. McDiarmid, E.G. Grant, M.I. Boechat, R.W. Busuttil: False-negative duplex Doppler studies in children with hepatic artery thrombosis after liver transplantation. Amer. J. Roentgenol. 154 (1990) 573–575

9 Harward, T.R., S. Smith, J.M. Seeger: Detection of celiac axis and superior mesenteric artery occlusive disease with use of abdominal duplex scanning. J. vasc. Surg. (1993) 738–745

10 Jäger, K., A. Bollinger, C. Valli, R. Ammann: Meassurement of mesenteric blood flow by Duplex scanning. J. vasc. Surg. 3 (1986) 462–469

11 Kadir, S.: Atlas of Normal and Variant Angiographic Anatomy. Saunders, Philadelphia (1991)

12 Kathrein, H., A. Dzien, R. Schuhmayer, G. Judmaier, Braunsteiner H: Diagnose von Änderungen des Blutflusses in der Arteria mesenterica inferior bei entzündlichen Darmerkrankungen mit der Duplexsonographie. Vasa (Suppl.) 30 (1990) 129–132

13 Kissane, J.M. (Ed.): Anderson's Pathology, 9th ed. Mosby, St. Louis (1990)

14 Kohler, T.R., H. Debas, M. Crames, J.R. Strandness: Pancreaticoduodenectomy and the celiac artery compression syndrome. Ann. vasc. Surg. 4 (1990) 77–80

15 Kubale, R.: Mesenteriale Gefäße. In Seitz, K.H., R. Kubale (Hrsg.): Duplexsonographie der abdominellen und retroperitonealen Gefäße. VCH, Weinheim (1988)

16 Lampert, V.D., D. Holz, K. Jaeger, J. Landmann: Nouvelle approche therapeutique dans le syndrome de compression du tronc coeliaque (New therapeutic approach in the celiac trunk compression syndrome). Helv. chir. Acta 58 (1991) 169–172

17 Lilly, M.P., T.R. Harward, W.R. Flinn, D.R. Blackburn, P.M. Astleford, J.S. Yao: Duplex ultrasound measurement of changes in mesenteric flow velocity with pharmacologic and physiologic alteration of intestinal blood flow in man. J. vasc. Surg. 9 (1989) 18–25

18 Lim, G.M., R.B. Jeffrey, C.S. Tolentino: Pancreatic pseudoaneurysm. Monitoring the success of transcatheter embolization with duplex sonography. J. Ultrasound Med 8. (1989) 643–646

19 Lippert, H., R. Pabst: Arterial Variations in Man. Bergmann, München (1985)

20 Lusza, G.: Röntgenanatomie des Gefäßsystems. Budapest (1972)

21 Mallek, R., G.H. Mostbeck, R.M. Walter, A. Stuempflen, T. Helbich, D. Tscholakoff: Duplex Doppler sonography of celiac trunk and superior mesenteric artery: comparison with intraarterial angiography. J. ultrasound Med. (1993) 337–342

22 Marder, D.M., G.B. DeMarino, J.H. Sumkin, D.G. Sheahan: Liver transplant rejection: value of the resistive index in Doppler US of hepatic arteries. Radiology 173 (1989) 127–129
23 Moneta, G.L., R.A. Yeager, R. Dalman, R. Antonovic, L.D. Hall, J.M. Porter: Duplex ultrasound criteria for diagnosis of splanchnic artery stenosis or occlusion. J. vasc. Surg. 14 (1991) 511–520
24 Mostbeck, G., R. Mallek, A. Gebauer, D. Tschollakoff: Duplex-Sonographie und farbkodierte Duplex-Sonographie viszeraler Gefäße bei abdominellen Erkrankungen. Wien klin. Wschr. 104 (1992) 227–233
25 Oster, Z.H., P. Som, P.O. Zamora: Mesenteric vascular occlusion: A new diagnostic method using a radiolabeled monoclonal antibody reactive with platelets. Radiology 171 (1989) 653–656
26 Patel, B., M.K. Wolverson, B. Mahanta: Pancreatic transplant rejection: assessment with duplex US. Radiology 173 (1989) 131–135
27 Perko, M.J., S. Just: Duplex ultrasonography of superior mesenteric artery: interobserver variability. J. Ultrasound med. 12 (1993) 259–263
28 Quillin, S.P., M.J. Siegel: Color Doppler US of children with acute lower abdominal pain. Radiographics 13 (1993) 1281–1293; discussion 1294
29 Reuter, S.R., H.C. Redman, J. Ch. Kyung: Gastrointestinal Angiography. Saunders, Philadelphia (1986)
30 Riccabona, M., A. Joannou, U. Maurer, W. Mueller, W. Schwinger: Dopplersonographie bei der nekrotisierenden Enterokolitis. (Doppler ultrasound in necrotizing enterocolitis.) Z. Geburtsh. Perinatol. 197 (1993) 87–89
31 Rollins, N.K., C. Timmons, R.A. Superina, W.S. Andrews: Hepatic artery thrombosis in children with liver transplants: false-positive findings at Doppler sonography and arteriography in four patients. Amer. J. Roentgenol. 160 (1993) 291–294
32 Roobottom, C.A., P.A. Dubbins: Significant disease of the celiac and superior mesenteric arteries in asymptomatic patients: predictive value of Doppler sonography. Amer. J. Roentgenol. 161 (1993) 985–988
33 Schindler, G., H.P. Bruch: Aktueller Stand der Diagnostik und Therapie der nicht okklusiven Darmischämie (NOD). Fortschr. Röntgenstr. 155 (1991) 123–127
34 Schwilden, E.D., M.G.M.H. Barwegen: Zur Problematik des Zöliakiekompressionssyndroms. Angio 4 (1980) 251–258
35 Segel, M.C., A.B. Zajko, A. Bowen, M.L. Skolnick, K.M. Bron, R.J. Penkrot, B.S. Slasky, T.E. Starzl: Doppler ultrasound as a screen for hepatic artery thrombosis after liver transplantation. Transplantation 41 (1986) 539–541
36 Tanaka, K., K. Mitsui, M. Morimoto, K. Numata, S. Inoue, Y. Takamura, M. Masumura: Increased hepatic arterial blood flow in acute viral hepatitis: assessment by color Doppler sonography. Hepatology 18 (1993) 21–27
37 Williams, P.L., R. Warwick, M. Dyson, L.H. Bannister, (Eds.): Gray's Anatomy, 37th ed. Churchill Livingstone, Edinburgh (1989) 1459

11 Abdominal Veins, Portal Venous System, and Liver

R. Kubale

11.1 General Remarks

The main goals in venous examinations of the abdomen and liver are the detection of venous or portal venous thrombosis, the evaluation of portal hypertension, the detection of thrombi in the inferior vena cava and renal and ovarian veins, and the assessment of the vascularization of focal hepatic lesions. Tumor thrombosis in the vena cava can be recognized in the grayscale image, and blood flow can be assessed by conventional duplex scanning. But only CDS imaging makes it possible to evaluate the relevant organs and their perfusion with sufficient accuracy in a reasonable amount of time. The use of duplex scanning, especially CDS, has added new pathophysiologic dimensions to the assessment of portal blood flow. Variants, collaterals, and arteriovenous malformations, once considered extremely rare, are being detected earlier and with increased frequency.

This chapter deals with normal venous anatomy, variants, and the most important sonographic findings in the inferior vena cava, renal and ovarian veins, hepatic veins, and portal venous system along with specific examination techniques for those areas.

11.2 Normal Anatomy and Examination Technique

11.2.1 Normal Anatomy, Common Variants, and Collaterals

Angiogenesis begins in the second half of the third week of embryonic life with two dorsal, longitudinally oriented cellular aggregates that give rise to the aortae, and a capillary plexus, which later forms the heart and primitive venous systems (13, 15). The centerpiece of embryonic venous development is the sinus venosus with the three major embryonic veins:

1. The umbilical veins develop from the chorionic villi and carry oxygen-rich maternal blood to the embryo. The right umbilical vein obliterates whereas the left umbilical vein persists until birth. In postnatal life it remains as an obliterated vessel (the ligamentum teres of the liver).
2. The viteline veins drain the yolk sac. Just before entering the sinus venosus, they form a capillary plexus that is invaded by hepatocytes. This leads to the development of the sinusoidal meshwork of the liver. The portal vein develops from the lower, stepladder-like anastomotic channels between the viteline veins, which form a venous ring encircling the duodenum, through a process of fusion and partial regression. The distal portion of the right vitelline vein becomes the superior mesenteric vein while the proximal portions of both vitelline veins persist as the right and left hepatic veins.
3. The anterior and posterior cardinal veins collect blood from the embryonic body with its primitive kidneys and unite to form a common trunk. The subcardinal veins develop medially as a new venous system; they anastomose between the primitive kidneys and subsequently take over a portion of the venous drainage of the posterior cardinal veins.
4. Last to appear are the supracardinal veins, which anastomose with the subcardinal veins. With further development, the posterior cardinal veins obliterate, and the left inferior supracardinal vein disappears. The right supracardinal vein persists and later becomes the postrenal segment of the inferior vena cava, whose further segments arise from the right subcardinal vein and from anastomoses between the supracardinal and subcardinal veins (13, 15). This complex, multisegmental pattern of embryologic development accounts for the numerous variants and abnormalities that will be discussed below in greater detail.

11.2.1.1 Inferior Vena Cava, Lumbar Veins, and Pelvic Veins

The inferior vena cava, which drains blood from the pelvic viscera and lower extremities, is formed at the L4–L5 level by the junction of the common iliac veins. It ascends initially behind and then to the right of the aorta. In its further course it turns forward at the L2–L3 level and runs a short intrathoracic course before emptying into the right atrium. The caliber of the vena cava varies with its degree of fullness and with respiration. A diameter in excess of 2 cm is not unusual. The size of the lumen decreases with inspiration and may temporarily collapse. It may be physiologically constricted or impressed by the common iliac artery anteriorly by the right renal artery posteriorly, by the liver, and by bony protrusions from the vertebrae.

The lumbar veins and the azygos and hemiazygos venous systems are rarely demonstrable. The vertebral venous plexuses are drained by a stepladder-like network of segmental veins, with some opening into the ascending lumbar vein and others draining directly into the inferior vena cava. The azygos vein originates at the level of the right renal vein as a continuation of the right ascending lumbar vein. It ascends in front of the vertebral column, to the right of the midline, and terminates at the level of the third to fourth thoracic vertebrae in the superior vena cava. The hemiazygos vein runs parallel to the course of the azygos vein on the left side. It crosses to the right at the level of the eighth thoracic vertebrae and enters the back of the azygos vein. Both veins collect blood from the right and left ascending lumbar veins, the posterior intercostal veins, and the subcostal vein. The azygos vein additionally drains bronchial, mediastinal, pericardial, and esophageal veins. These veins assume an important collateral function in portal hypertension and form an important craniocaudal pathway when the superior vena cava is occluded. Other collateral channels exist between the left renal and hemiazygos veins and with the paravertebral veins, which can be demonstrated sonographically in the presence of inferior vena cava occlusion (62).

Variants and anomalies occur in 1.5–4% of the population, and most are detected incidentally. They result from errors in the complex developmental process described above, with disturbances in the transition from the originally bilateral primary embryonic venous system to the predominantly right-sided, asymmetric postnatal system. Chuang (15) recognizes several forms of developmental disturbance (Table 11.**1**), which may pose problems of differential diagnosis: The retrocaval ureter results from a persistent posterior cardinal vein (type A) and can lead to congestion of the right pyelocaliceal system. Mirror-image regression of the supracardinal vein leads to transposition of the inferior vena cava (type C), the persistence of both supracardinal veins to duplication (type BC). Agenesis of the hepatic or prerenal segment presents as an interruption of the inferior vena cava with drainage routed through alternate channels such as the azygos or hemiazygos system.

Other variants occur in the pelvic region at the level of the distal anastomosis of the original posterior cardinal veins. The most important variants in course and termination are duplication of the common iliac vein and internal iliac vein, contralateral anomalous terminations and dysplasia of the left common iliac vein with lumbar collateralization (29, 39).

Table 11.**1** Development and congenital anomalies of the inferior vena cava and renal veins (after 15; see Fig. 11.**11**)

I	**Postrenal segment**	
	Type A	Persistence of right posterior cardinal vein (retro- and circumcaval ureter)
	Type B	Persistence of right supracardinal vein (normal position of inferior vena cava)
	Type C	Persistence of left supracardinal vein (left-sided inferior vena cava)
	Type BC	Persistence of both supracardinal veins (duplicated inferior vena cava)
II	**Renal segment**	
	Persistence of renal venous ring (circumaortic venous ring)	
III	**Prerenal segment**	
	Absence of hepatic segment (azygos or hemiazygos continuation)	

11.2.1.2 Renal Veins and Gonadal Veins

The renal veins develop from anastomoses between the subcardinal and supracardinal veins (see above). A circumaortic venous ring develops that initially receives two veins from each kidney. With further development these vessels normally reduce to a single renal vein per side. The right renal vein is 2–4 cm long and runs obliquely downward to enter the inferior vena cava at the L1 level. The left renal vein is 4–11 cm in length. It follows a more horizontal course and curves anterior to the aorta and posterior to the superior mesenteric artery to enter the vena cava. The intrarenal course of the veins basically follows the arterial distribution pattern: a deep system drains the cortex centrally via the interlobular arteries to the arcuate veins and then to the interlobar veins. Large-caliber draining veins arise from anastomoses at the level of the papillae and calyces, some uniting in front of the renal pelvis and some behind it to form the renal vein. Additionally there is a superficial venous system in which cortical veins collect blood from the renal cortex and carry it to the arcuate veins.

The gonadal veins collect blood from the testes or ovaries. The ovarian veins drain the plexus around the uterus and ovaries, while the spermatic veins are supplied by the pampiniform plexus. Their further retroperitoneal course is the same in both males and females: after crossing over the ureters in the middle third of the iliopsoas, the veins enter the renal vein on the left side and usually open directly into the inferior vena cava on the right side. Portions of these veins can usually be demonstrated sonographically anterior or anterolateral to the psoas muscle.

Variants of the renal veins and gonadal veins are common and have great practical relevance. The most common anomaly is a persistent circumaortic venous ring or a retroaortic left renal vein. Other variants include multiplicity and aberrant terminations that may extend to the common iliac vein. A diligent search for these variants should be conducted during preoperative staging.

The right gonadal vein enters the vena cava just below the right renal vein in 60% of cases and at the same level in 30%. The left gonadal vein opens directly into the inferior vena cava in only 1% of cases. Thirty percent of cases show duplication of the gonadal veins as well as accessory vessels, which are also variable in their mode of termination (29, 39, 62).

11.2.1.3 Portal Venous System, Hepatic Veins, and Segmental Anatomy of the Liver

The portal venous system transports venous blood of the gastrointestinal tract (including the gallbladder, pancreas, and spleen) to the liver via the portal vein. The major tributaries are the splenic vein, the superior and inferior mesenteric veins, the short gastric veins, the left gastroepiploic vein, the pyloric vein, and the gastric coronary veins (Fig. 11.**1**).

The splenic vein is formed by the junction of two to six venous branches in the splenic hilum. It has an average length of 15 cm and courses below and slightly behind the splenic artery (Fig. 11.**2**). The body and tail of the pancreas are anterior to the splenic vein. The inferior mesenteric vein is the largest tributary of the splenic vein, although in 30% of cases it opens into the superior mesenteric vein. It drains blood from the descending colon, sigmoid colon, and rectum. Other branches are the left gastric vein, short gastric veins, and gastroepiploic vein.

The superior mesenteric vein drains blood from the jejunum, ileum, ascending colon, transverse colon, and pancreaticoduodenal arcades (Fig. 11.**1**; 11.**2b**). Intramural veins give rise to the vasa recta and the mesenteric arcades. These in turn form segmental branches that run parallel to the homonymous arteries. The middle colic vein anastomoses with the left colic branch of the inferior mesenteric vein. The veins draining the jejunum and ileum enter from the left side, the veins draining the ascending and transverse colon from the right side. Other nonmesenteric branches are the right gastroepiploic and the pancreaticoduodenal veins, which enter the superior mesenteric vein from the right side.

The cystic veins generally enter the right main branch of the portal vein together and enter the main trunk directly. They unite with the veins of the com-

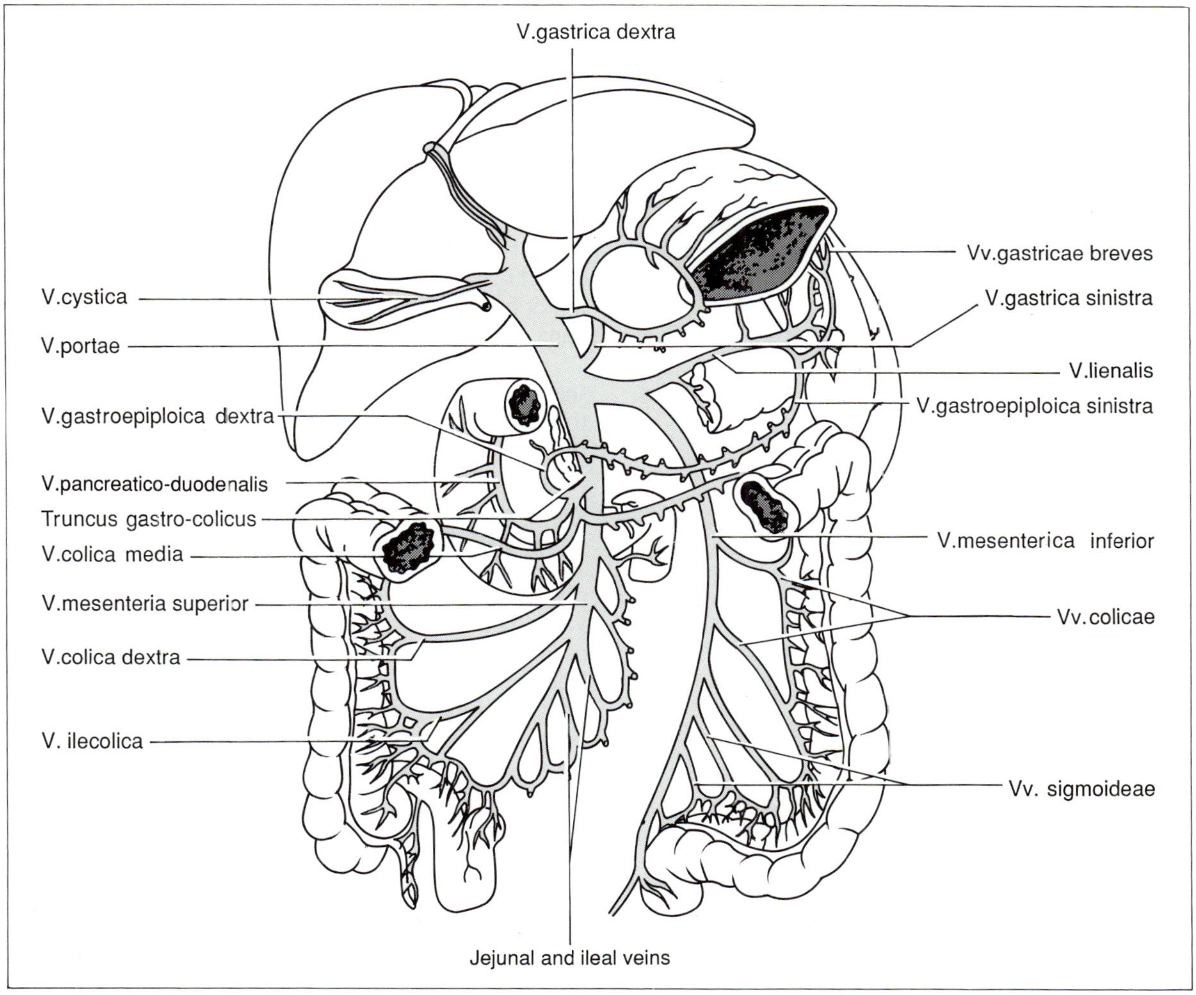

Fig. 11.**1** Tributaries in the portal venous system (after [29])

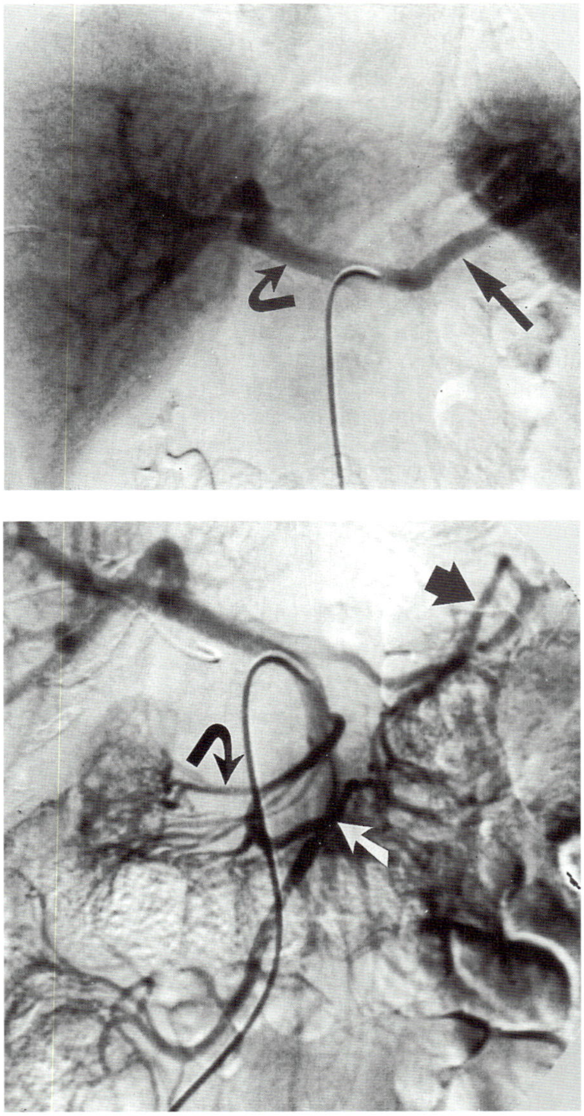

a

b

Fig. 11.**2a, b** Angiographic appearance of the portal venous system
a Indirect splenoportography after injection of contrast medium into the splenic artery demonstrates the splenic vein (straight arrow) and the portal vein (curved arrow) with its intrahepatic branches
b Venous phase after selective catheterization of the superior mesenteric artery. The right and middle colic veins (straight arrow) and the pancreaticoduodenal vein (curved arrow) open into the superior mesenteric vein. Branches from the inferior mesenteric vein (wide arrow) faintly opacify the distal trunk of the splenic vein

mon bile duct and may present as atypical collaterals in the event of portal vein occlusion.

The portal vein begins behind the isthmus of the pancreas at the junction of the splenic and superior mesenteric veins (Fig. 11.**2**). Its extrahepatic portion is 8–10 cm long and ascends obliquely to the porta hepatis, passing between the bile duct and hepatic artery in the hepatoduodenal ligament. The diameter of the portal vein in fasting patients is 8–13 mm. After entering the liver, it divides into branches that accompany the corresponding branches of the hepatic artery and the biliary ducts. It most commonly divides into two main branches: the right branch courses 1–3 cm before dividing into an anterior and a posterior branch, which supply the right lobe of the liver. Each of these branches subsequently divides into a superior and inferior branch. The left main branch of the portal vein courses anterosuperiorly and runs forward and to the right at the boundary of the middle and left lobes.

Variants of intrahepatic branching are common and may consist of early division of the portal vein into three vessels or, rarely, a direct origin of the anterosuperior branch from the main trunk.

Variants in the portal venous trunk are rare. They may arise at various stages of portal vein development. A preduodenal portal vein is generally noted as an incidental finding during surgery. Other anomalies are duplication of the portal vein, strictures, and obstructive valves. Atresia and hypoplasia have traditionally been considered rare and may be associated with a congenital portocaval shunt.

After passing through the preterminal and terminal portal branches, the blood leaves the portal venous system along with blood from the accompanying terminal arterial branches and enters the sinusoids. The sinusoidal anastomoses and the existence of presinusoidal arterial and portal venous sphincters lead to reciprocal influences between the arterial and portal venous hepatopetal pathways (51). The common venous outflow from the liver passes directly from the sinusoids through the central veins of the hepatic lobules and sublobular veins to the segmental veins (Fig. 11.**3**). These vessels normally unite to form three major hepatic veins that open directly into the inferior vena cava with no discernible extrahepatic course.

The principal anatomical variants include absence of the middle hepatic vein, thus eliminating contribution to the drainage of the four central segments. In 30% of cases there are more than three main hepatic veins (34). Other variants relate to variable numbers of accessory veins, which are most common in the area of the diaphragmatic attachment of the liver. The principal accessory veins are the right inferior phrenic veins, posterior hepatic veins, caudate lobe veins, and collaterals to the right suprarenal vein. The caudate lobe veins permit survival in patients with the Budd–Chiari syndrome.

The branching pattern of the portal and hepatic veins is associated with an anatomic segmentation of the liver. Though variable and controversial, this segmentation has proven helpful in the operative treatment of hepatic tumors (5, 18, 28, 33, 34, 62). Each segment is centered on a branch of the portal vein and has a hepatic vein at its periphery. Each lobe of the liver consists of four segments, which are numbered in a clockwise fashion. The horizontal pattern of segmentation is based on the portal venous branches. Segments V and VII, and VI and VII are considered dual segments because of the adjacent positions of their portal segmental hila. Their vertical boundaries are marked by the right and middle hepatic veins (Fig. 11.**4**, Ref. **62**).

11.2.2 Examination Technique and Documentation

11.2.2.1 Examination Technique and Instrument Settings

The examination technique and instrument settings depend on the clinical question. A linear- or curved-array transducer with an operating frequency of 2–5 MHz is recommended for the inferior vena cava and its tributaries. As described in Chapter 4, the gray-scale image should be optimized and analyzed first. This is done by imaging the liver on an oblique subcostal scan and adjusting the gain and TGC so that the parenchyma appears uniformly hyperechoic and the hepatic veins can be traced to the level of their second-order branches. When this has been accomplished, the inferior vena cava is first imaged in longitudinal scans from the front supplemented by coronal scans from a right lateral approach. Its further course can be followed to the pelvic level while careful compression is applied. The common and external iliac veins can be visualized as far as the inguinal ligament at this time by rotating the caudal end of the transducer slightly outward.

The renal veins are best evaluated in transverse views. They are located by moving the transducer caudad from the celiac trunk and superior mesenteric artery. The left renal vein is identified between the aorta and superior mesenteric artery and followed to the inferior vena cava. The right renal vein is visualized by slight caudad rotation of the transducer to the right side. The renal veins can also be examined from a lateral approach using coronal image planes that are angled slightly forward. The full length of the right renal vein can usually be visualized with this technique. In contrast to examination of the inferior vena cave, time is saved by examining the renal veins with color flow right away, rather than starting with a gray-scale survey.

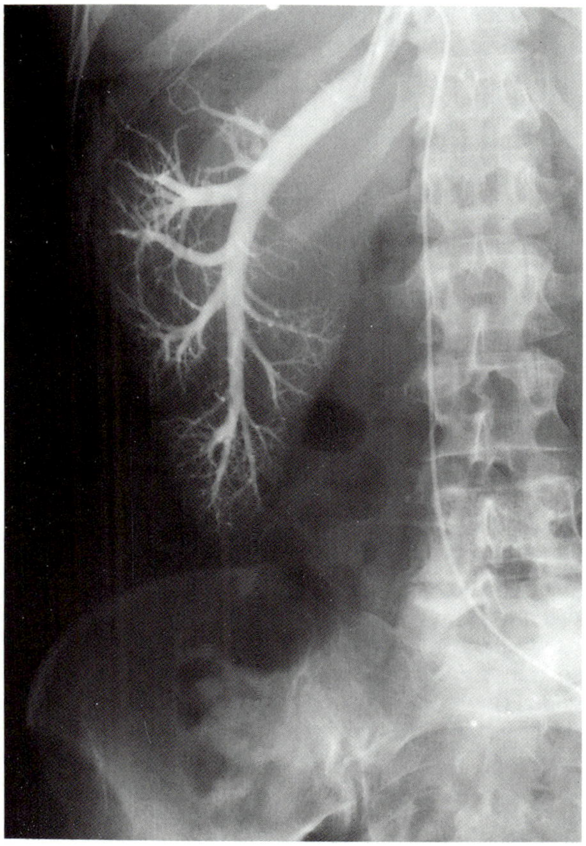

Fig. 11.**3** Selective angiography of the right hepatic vein. Retrograde contrast injection opacifies the venous tree out to small tributary branches

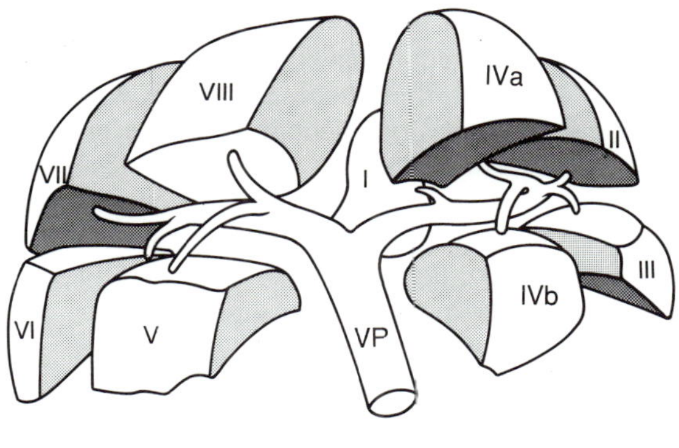

Fig. 11.**4** Hepatic segmentation. The liver is divided into eight segments according to the pattern of portal venous branching. Segments VI/VII and V/VIII are regarded as double segments separated by the right, middle, and left hepatic veins. VP = Portal vein

When examining the venous confluence, splenic vein, superior mesenteric vein, and superficial portal venous collaterals, a transducer with good near-field definition should be used. Minimal pressure should be exerted, because the splenic vein and mesenteric vein are easily obliterated in thin patients.

The portal vein can be imaged from the front by tracing it from the porta hepatis, but a right lateral intercostal approach is often more favorable because the smaller beam–vessel angle allows for better assessment of portal venous flow. The splenic vein is examined in transverse planes from an anterior approach. These views are then supplemented by transsplenic imaging from the left side.

The superior mesenteric vein is best demonstrated by following the vessel distally from its junction with the portal vein in transverse plane. It lies to the right of the homonymous artery and is easily recognized by its continuous flow pattern in the color-encoded image.

The flow in the abdominal veins is slower than in the arteries, so a medium velocity scale should be used. The color gain and threshold should be adjusted so that color artifacts are eliminated and color-encoded flow signals do not transgress the vessel lumen. If intraluminal flow is not detected, the velocity scale and Doppler angle should be checked. If the vessel axis is perpendicular to the transducer, as in the case of the vena cava, good intraluminal color can be achieved only by insonating at various angles or by using a sector-type probe. Although a standoff wedge is useful for scanning the peripheral vessels, a transducer with beam steering is advantageous for intra-abdominal examinations.

In instruments with adjustable wall filters, a threshold of 100 Hz should not be exceeded in portal vein examinations to ensure the detection of slow flow. Other problems can result from a faulty position of the focus (should be below to the examined vessel!) and from vigorous intestinal peristalsis, which creates a troublesome color mosaic. Often the only recourse in this situation is to administer an antispasmodic agent (e. g., scopolamine).

11.2.2.2 Documentation

Documentation requirements depend on the clinical question. In the search for thromboses and occlusions of the inferior vena cava, documentation should include the diameter of the vessel, respiratory and cardiac flow changes, and any intraluminal flow voids. Examination in two planes is mandatory. If renal vein thrombosis is suspected, the examiner should record exact kidney size, parenchymal pattern, and the prominence of the renal pyramids as compared with the contralateral side. The renal veins are documented in color-encoded flow from the anterior side using standard planes of section. If a tumor nephrectomy is planned, it is sufficient to document the terminal 3 cm of each vein along with the inferior vena cava. If a tumor enucleation is planned, the entire length of the renal vein should be examined. If the purpose of the examination is to identify the cause of splenomegaly or portal hypertension, the portal vein and splenic vein should be documented as completely as possible. Occlusive and nonocclusive thrombi in the portal venous or mesenteric system should be documented in two planes. In patients with known liver disease, flow direction and velocity, should be determined after appropriate angle correction. It is important to make an accurate record of the accessibility of the individual vascular segments and any limiting factors. The use of a standard report sheet is recommended.

11.3 Normal Findings

11.3.1 Inferior Vena Cava, Lumbar Veins, and Renal Veins

The upper portion of the inferior vena cava can be visualized in almost all patients by using the liver as an acoustic window. Its diameter ranges from 2 to 3 cm and fluctuates with respiration and cardiac acitvity. The vessel may collapse during inspiration with its diameter increasing again during apnea and expiration. As in all vessels, the lumen of the inferior vena cava should appear echo-free in the gray-scale image. When color flow encoding is switched on, color should completely and uniformly fill the vena cava during apnea (Fig. 11.**5**), signifying flow toward the heart. Rapid inspiration creates a suction effect in the chest causing increased flow and turbulence; the flow again becomes laminar during apnea. Turbulent zones, with their mosaic-like color signature, occur physiologically at the sites where the hepatic and renal veins open into the vena cava. Doppler spectra from the center of the vessel show two brief flow peaks directed toward the heart at the start of ventricular systole and during opening of the a–v valves (1, 49). The flow ceases or temporarily reverses during atrial contraction. Appearing as a brief color reversal on the flow image, this is a physiological phenomenon also seen in the right renal vein and hepatic veins.

The left renal vein, by contrast, usually exhibits continuous flow, which in thin patients may briefly be synchronous with aortic pulsations. This is probably due to constriction of the vein between the aorta and superior mesenteric artery. Venous expansion is apparent distal to the aorticomesenteric angle (Fig. 11.**6a**, **b**).

The distal portion of the inferior vena cava and the lumina of the common and external iliac veins are often obscured in the gray-scale image by scattering artifacts. Scanning through the distended bladder, however, can demonstrate the pelvic veins as color-filled vascular bands, even under poor examining conditions. The lumbar and gonadal veins can occasionally be imaged in thin patients as continuously perfused vessels with a band-like spectrum.

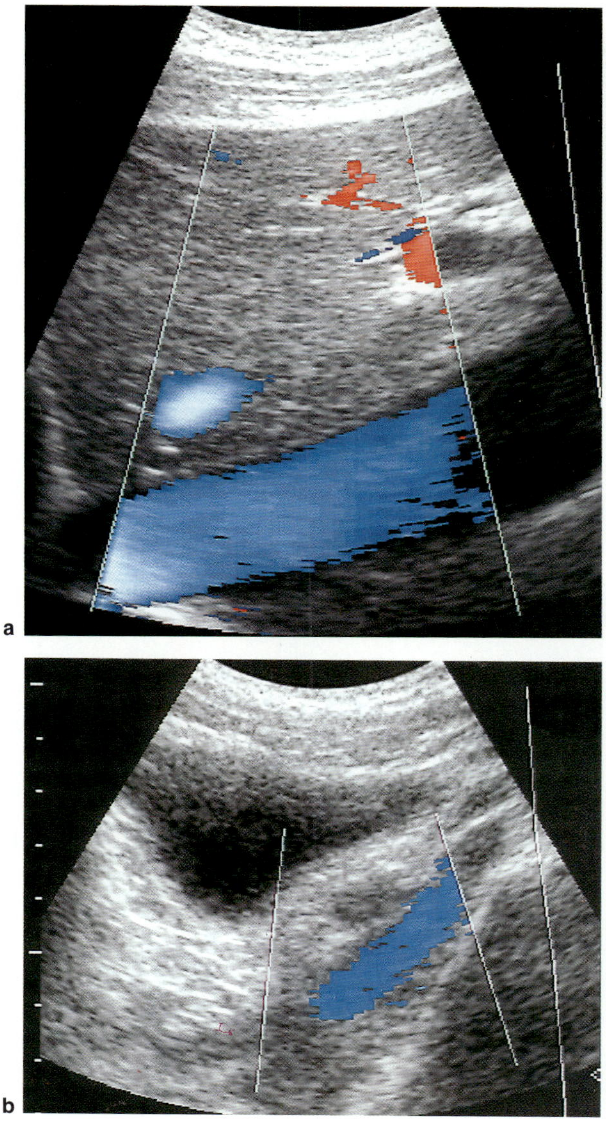

Fig. 11.**5a, b** Longitudinal views of the inferior vena cava and external iliac vein
a Proximal portion of a normal inferior vena cava. The image plane traverses the liver and portal vein (red)
b Normal left external iliac vein. Despite patient obesity, a normal color-encoded image of the vessel is obtained by applying careful compression and using the partially filled bladder as an acoustic window

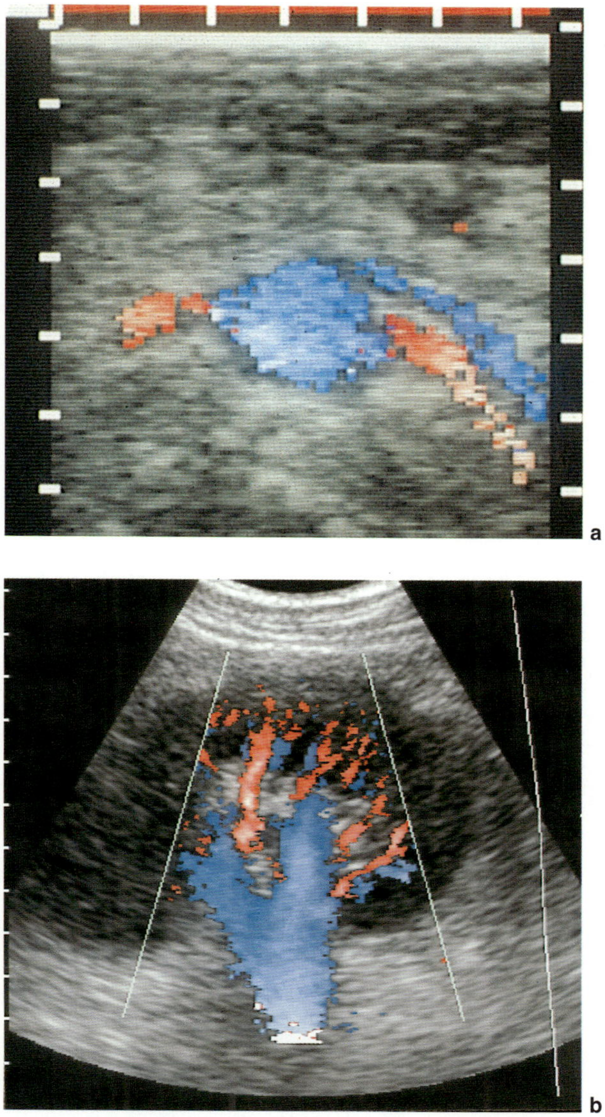

Fig. 11.**6a, b** Normal left renal vein
a Transverse image demonstrates the aorta (encoded blue), the left and right renal artery (encoded red), and the left renal vein (encoded blue)
b Longitudinal scan through the left kidney from the lateral side demonstrates individual interlobar veins converging via segmental veins to the main trunk of the renal vein (encoded blue). The segmental and interlobar arteries coursing toward the transducer appear red

11.3.2 Hepatic Veins and Portal Venous System

The hepatic veins are best visualized in an oblique subcostal scan and in longitudinal scans through the left and right lobes of the liver (Fig. 11.**7**). In a healthy liver the hepatic veins run in a smooth arc from the periphery of the liver to the inferior vena cava, their tributaries converging at angles of less than 45°. The normal veins present smooth, sharp borders with an echo-free lumen. The main hepatic veins can be tracked to the level of their second- and third-order tributaries in the color duplex image. Their flow normally shows cardiac modulation with a brief cessation or reversal of flow during atrial systole (Fig. 11.**8a**, **b**). Flattened tracings without triphasic flow patterns are seen in less than 9% of normal patients (50).

The normal portal vein presents in the gray-scale image as a smoothly marginated echo-free band, which may appear hypoechoic in more obese patients

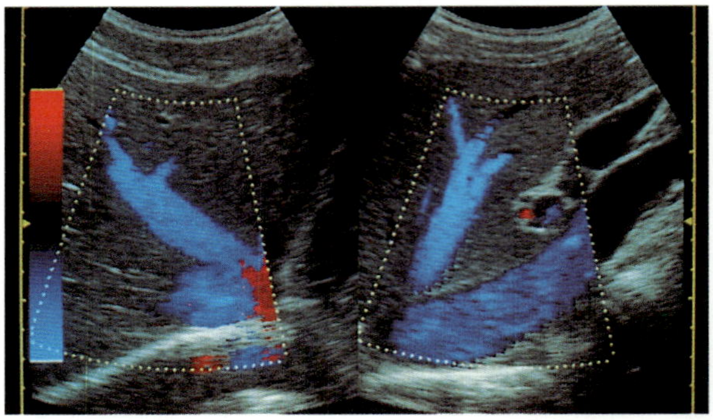

Fig. 11.**7** Normal inferior vena cava and hepatic veins. Oblique subcostal scan (left image) shows the middle hepatic vein, and the longitudinal scan (right image) shows the inferior vena cava and right hepatic vein

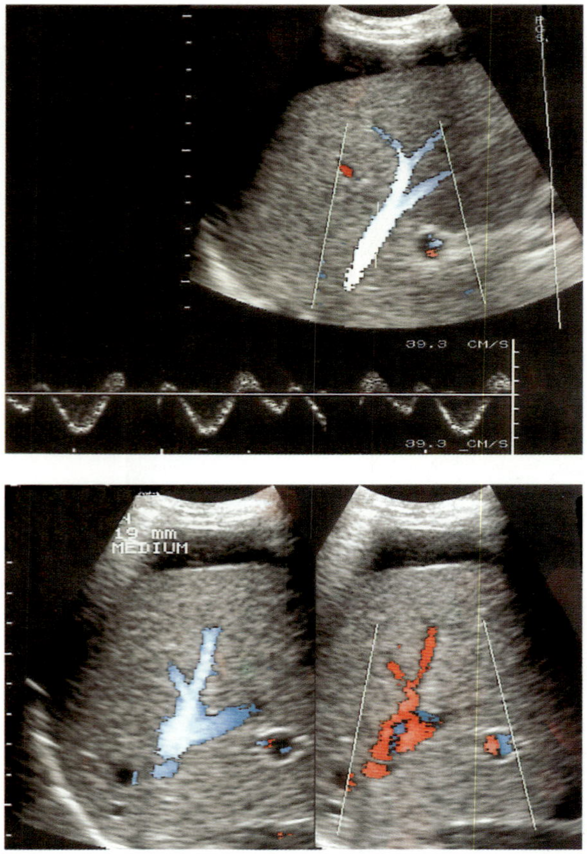

a

b

Fig. 11.**8a, b** Normal right hepatic vein with phasic flow in a patient with ascites

a Flow in the hepatic vein is encoded blue (above). Cardiac modulation (small reverse flow component during atrial contraction) produces double peaks in the Doppler spectrum (below)

b Color-encoded flow representation of the flow phases as shown in the Doppler spectrum (see **a**, below). The left image shows flow directed toward the heart (encoded blue), while the right image shows the brief retrograde flow that occurs during atrial contraction (encoded red)

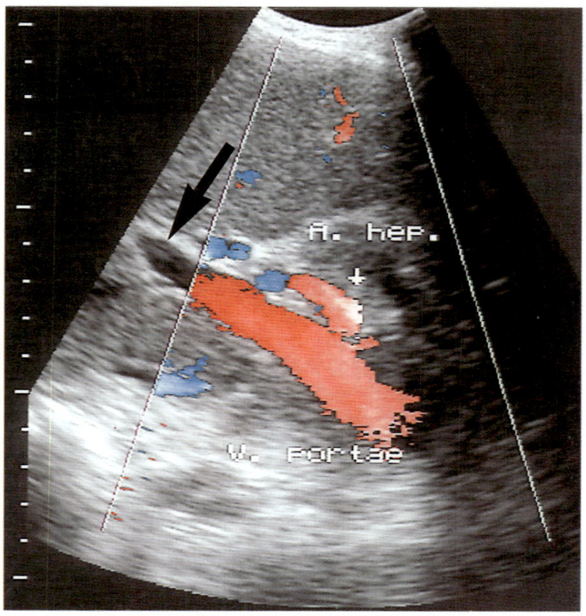

Fig. 11.**9** Normal-appearing porta hepatis with portal vein and hepatic artery. Anterior to the portal vein (= V. portae) is the proper hepatic artery (= A. hep.), both vessels are encoded in red = same flow direction. The "window technique" (straight white lines) accounts for the apparent flow void in the left part of the portal vein image (black arrow)

due to scattering effects. Unlike the inferior vena cava, whose patency can often be confirmed in the gray-scale image from its typical respiratory lumen changes and cardiac modulation (double-beat pattern), the portal vein shows only slight respiratory variations in caliber.

Color-encoded flow signals fill the portal vein completely and uniformly in the CDS image (Fig. 11.**9**). Portal venous flow is directed toward the liver, showing respiratory and cardiac modulations that can usually be appreciated only in a Doppler spectral recording. Velocity measurements normally show a range of 10 to 25 cm/s (49), but the maximum velocity may exceed 40 cm/s postprandially. A full-length examination of the portal vein can be accomplished in about 80% of cases from an anterior approach. Scanning from a right lateral intercostal approach can almost always demonstrate the entire vessel.

The major sonographically definable tributaries of the portal vein are the splenic vein and the superior mesenteric vein. Both can be evaluated in most patients. The inferior mesenteric vein is often completely or partially obscured by overlying gas. Usually the gastric coronary vein is the only nondistended, preformed collateral that can be visualized; its flow direction can be evaluated with color duplex. All the vessels demonstrate a continuous, hepatopetal, usually laminar flow like that observed in the portal vein (Fig. 11.**10a–d**).

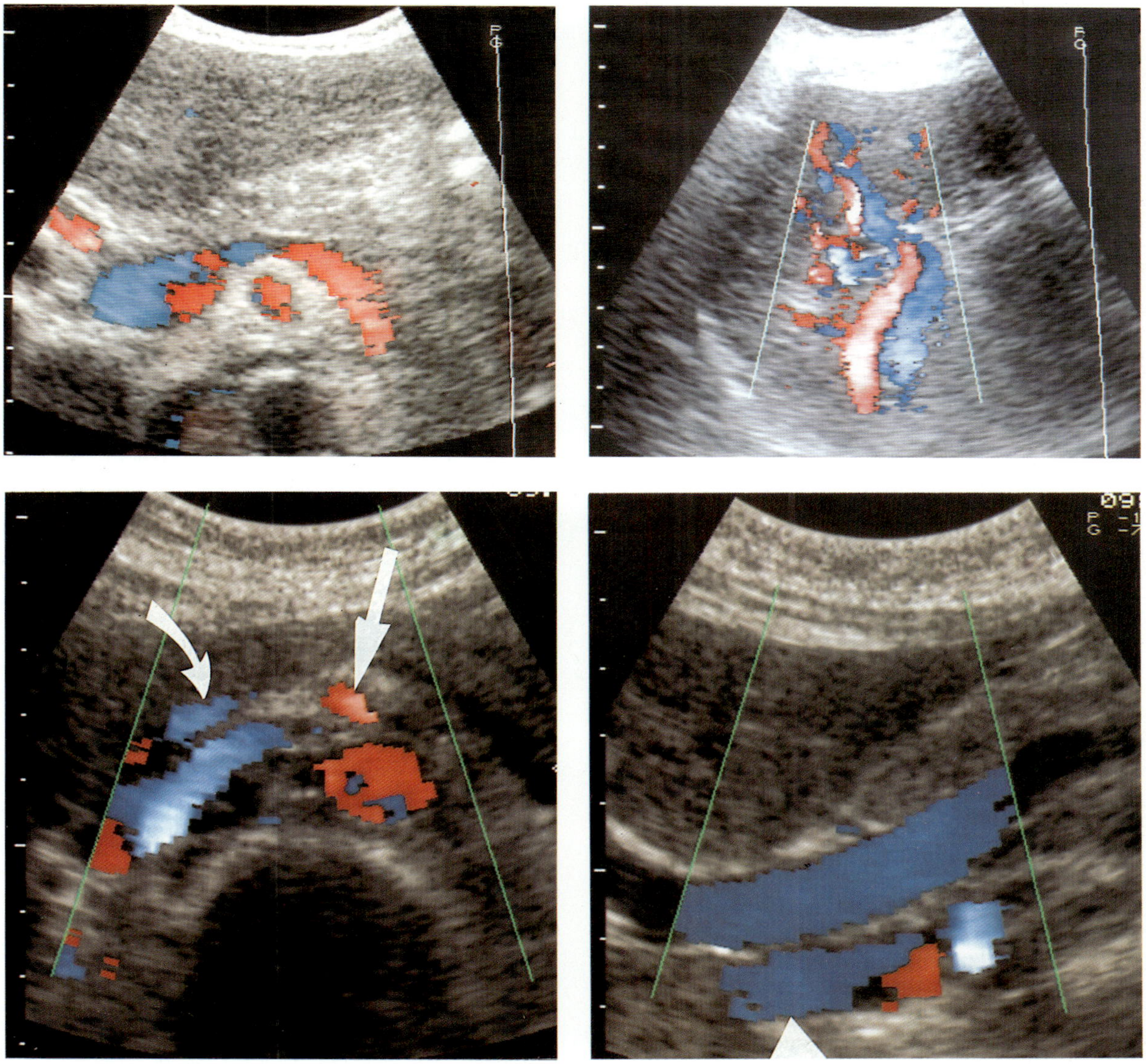

Fig. 11.**10a–d** Normal splenic vein and superior mesenteric vein

a Transverse midabdominal scan shows typical splenic-vein color changes from red (flow toward the transducer) to a relative color void at the vessel apex (Doppler angle = 90°) to blue (flow away from the transducer). Mixed red and blue signals appear at the junction with the superior mesenteric vein, while red appears in the superior mesenteric artery, which is cut transversely by the image plane (absence of color encoding in the aorta is a phase-dependent phenomenon)

b Scan from a lateral approach demonstrates the perihilar portions of the splenic artery and vein along with intrasplenic vessels

c Transverse midabdominal scan shows the aorta (red) and inferior vena cava (blue) with the terminal portion of the left renal vein. Anterior to the vena cava and aorta are the superior mesenteric vein (curved arrow) and superior mesenteric artery (straight artery). The blue-encoded areas in the aorta indicate the start of late systolic flow reversal

d Longitudinal oblique scan demonstrates the superior mesenteric vein with its junction with the portal vein. A segment of the inferior vena cava (arrowhead at bottom) is imaged posterior to the mesenteric vein

Color reversal is noted in the splenic vein due to the curvature of the vessel relative to the transducer face. Flow is not detected in segments in a parallel orientation to the transducer (see Chapters 1 and 4). Vorticity occurs normally at the confluence of the splenic and superior mesenteric veins and does not signify pathology. The distal third of the splenic vein, often obscured by meteorism when examined from the front, can generally be visualized from a lateral approach together with the larger intrasplenic vessels (Fig. 11.**10a–d**). The superior mesenteric vein likewise exhibits continuous flow but shows a moderate flow increase during expiration. Even slight pressure from the transducer is sufficient to compress the vein. A careful search with CDS demonstrates individual jejunal and ileal veins that can enlarge to form important collaterals in response to mesenteric vein thrombosis.

11.4 Pathologic Findings

11.4.1 Pathophysiologic Aspects

The venous system, like the arterial system, is subject to numerous disorders that involve the vasculature primarily or secondarily. The most important is thrombosis, whose significance is frequently underestimated in the abdomen. Primary thrombosis can originate at any site in the venous or portal venous system, or thrombosis may ascend to that level secondarily from a deep venous thrombosis in the lower extremity.

Thrombosis is an etiologically diverse disease. If the endothelial layer of the vessel is disrupted due to degenerative, hypoxic, toxic, or allergic–hypergic processes, blood comes in contact with collagen of the subendothelial matrix. Adherent and activated platelets then release mediators that potentiate fibrin coagulation, which is simultaneously induced. Shock, cardiac failure, and hypoxic injury can lead to slowing of blood flow with platelet and monocyte adhesion. Other risk factors for thrombosis are neoplasms and paraneoplastic syndromes, hematologic disorders such as polycythemia vera, antithrombin-III deficiency and, increasingly, contraceptive use in women who smoke.

The clinical symptoms of thrombosis depend on the location and caliber of the vessel and the rapidity of the process. Slowly progressive occlusions with good collateralization or concomitant recanalization may remain asymptomatic. This section describes the most important disorders of the inferior vena cava, renal veins, and portal venous system that can be detected sonographically and by CDS imaging.

11.4.2 Inferior Vena Cava, Lumbar Veins, and Renal Veins

11.4.2.1 Variants and Malformations

Given the complexity of its embryologic development, the venous system is subject to numerous anatomical variations and malformations (Fig. 11.**11 a–f**). The spectrum of findings ranges from partial aplasia to duplication of the vena cava (section 11.2.1). Most of these anomalies are asymptomatic, but their detection can be of vital importance in candidates for major abdominal surgery or the insertion of vena caval filters. Patients with complete aplasia of the vena cava or an azygos or hemiazygos continuation syndrome should be evaluated for associated cardiac disease.

The diagnosis can often be made from the grayscale image. But CDS is helpful for differentiating atypical, slowly perfused vessels from lymph nodes,

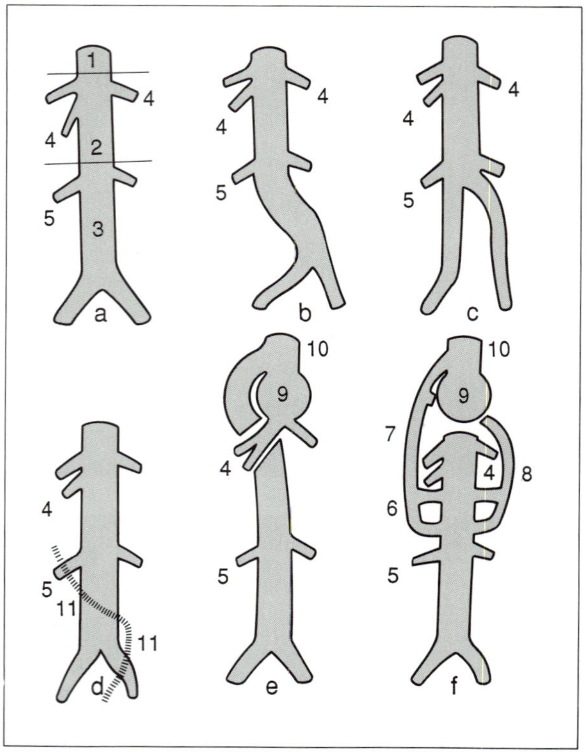

Fig. 11.**11 a–f** Variants of the inferior vena cava (after [39]): **a** normal development, **b** left-sided vena cava, **c** duplication, **d** retrocaval ureter, **e** partial agenesis, **f** congenital obstruction. (1) Hepatic part, (2) subcardinal part, (3) supracardinal part, (4) hepatic veins, (5) renal veins, (6) lumbar veins, (7) azygos vein, (8) hemiazygos vein, (9) right atrium, (10) superior vena cava, (11) ureter

and visualization of flow velocity and direction is helpful for the analysis of more complex anomalies and malformations.

A rare anomaly of the thoracic venous system that can be diagnosed by abdominal sonography is scimitar syndrome, first described in 1836. Anomalous pulmonary veins pass downward through the diaphragm and open into the inferior vena cava. Patients may be asymptomatic, but, progressive cardiac failure may develop if the shunt volume is large. Often there are many associated abnormalities of the cardiopulmonary system. The chest roentgenogram typically shows a crescent-shaped right paracardiac density. The atypical veins can be imaged by angling the transducer cephalad. Once considered rare, this anomaly is being demonstrated with increasing frequency through the use of color flow imaging (14, 28, 47).

Other anomalies are obstructive valves of the vena cave, leading to a Budd–Chiari-like syndrome, and aortocaval fistulas (see Chapter 9). CDS confirms the diagnosis by demonstrating venous dilatation, increased flow with arterialization, and massive localized vibrational artifacts (see Chapter 4) (7).

11.4.2.2 Stenoses, Occlusions, and Tumor Compression

Stenoses and occlusions of the vena cava are most commonly caused by malignant disease. Extrinsic compression of the vena cava can occur at any level due to retroperitoneal lymph nodes, renal and adrenal neoplasms (especially in children), hepatomegaly, pancreatic tumors, aneurysms, retroperitoneal fibrosis, and massive ascites.

Lymph nodes and lobulated tumors are marked by visible pressure defects, while a smoothly marginated, tubular stenosis suggests a fibrotic process. Uncomplicated tumor compression cannot always be distinguished sonographically from invasion of the vessel wall. The detection of a hyperechoic fat layer surrounding or adjacent to the vena cava or renal vein suggests that a safety margin is still present between the tumor and the inferior vena cava. With subtotal stenosis, CDS is helpful for identifying the residual lumen and evaluating the extent and pattern of collateralization.

Intrinsic obstruction may be caused by thrombosis or by intraluminal tumors or tumor extensions. An inferior vena cava thrombosis may ascend from the pelvis or lower extremity (apposition thrombus) or may result from local thrombus formation (e. g., following abdominal surgery). Thrombus formation may be followed within hours by a hemolysis that starts centrally and spreads toward the periphery. With hyalinization and organization of the clot by cellular invasion from the vessel wall and retraction of the fibrin filaments, the thrombus acquires a nonhomogeneously hyperechoic structure. Old thrombi may partially calcify. Renal vein thrombosis has a distinctive pathogenesis and tends to develop in the setting of nephrotic syndrome, glomerulonephritis (31), collagen diseases, amyloidoses, and dehydration or sepsis in children (Table 11.**2**). A CDS evaluation should be performed whenever the early warning signs of flank pain and renal enlargement are noted. Early diagnosis is imperative for survival of the kidney.

Table 11.**2** Renal vein thrombosis: causes and predisposing factors

I Primary thrombosis due to hypercoagulability

- Nephrotic syndrome, antithrombin III deficiency
- Dehydration, sepsis
- Pregnancy, contraceptive use
- Paraneoplastc syndrome
- Steroid use

II Secondary thrombosis due to impaired renal blood flow

- Extension of renal tumor
- Ascending thrombosis of the vena cava
- Outflow obstruction by aortic aneurysm or paraaortic lymph node metastasis
- Trauma

Primary intraluminal tumors of the vena cava are a rare cause of intrinsic obstruction. The main causative lesions are leiomyoma and leiomyosarcoma, malignant mesenchymal tumors that originate from the smooth muscle of the vessel wall. The tumors and their extensions present a sonodense pattern that is well appreciated even in gray-scale images of the inferior vena cava.

Invasion of the vena cava may be seen in association with hepatocellular carcinoma, retroperitoneal sarcoma, and renal and adrenal carcinoma, which tend to invade the renal veins. The detection of these tumor thrombi is of major importance in the planning of operative treatment. A four-stage classification of intracaval tumor extension is commonly used:

- Stage I involves a button-like projection of tumor from the renal vein into the inferior vena cava
- In stage II the upper tumor margin is still below the cranial border of the renal vein orifice
- Stage III involves tumor extension to the level of the hepatic vein
- Stage IV involves tumor extension to the atrium

In contrast to intraluminal tumors, tumor thrombosis, and older thrombi, which are frequently echogenic (Fig. 11.**12a**, **b**) and can be diagnosed in the gray-scale image, acute thrombosis usually appears hypoechoic to echo-free in the B-mode image and is likely to be missed initially, especially in muscular or obese patients. It can be reliably detected only by CDS (Fig. 11.**13**). A complete occlusion is confirmed by the absence of flow, while the finding of patency excludes a presumed thrombosis. An indirect sign of acute renal vein thrombosis in the arterial spectrum is loss or transient reversal of the diastolic flow component. This is attributed to a reflex vasoconstriction and resembles the findings associated with vascular rejection (see Chapter 12).

Often diagnosed too late, ovarian vein thrombosis most commonly occurs during or shortly after pregnancy (3). The complaints are nonspecific and are usually localized to the lower abdomen. Differentiation from appendicitis can be quite difficult. Sonography demonstrates thickening of the adnexa and a distended, nonperfused ovarian vein (2, 3). There is often an associated inflammatory response with thickened perivascular tissues. The thrombosis may propagate cephalad into the vena cava, and its extent is clearly defined on the B-mode image. The role of CDS remains unclear.

CDS is helpful in the planning and follow-up of vena caval filter insertions. Stainless steel basket filter devices have various designs and are introduced percutaneously for the prevention of pulmonary embolism or deep pelvic or lower extremity venous thrombosis. They are placed below the termination of the renal veins. The metal struts of the filter appear on the gray-scale image as hyperechoic band-like structures that may cast an acoustic shadow, depending on the filter design. The filter causes turbulent blood flow that is plainly demonstrated in the CDS image.

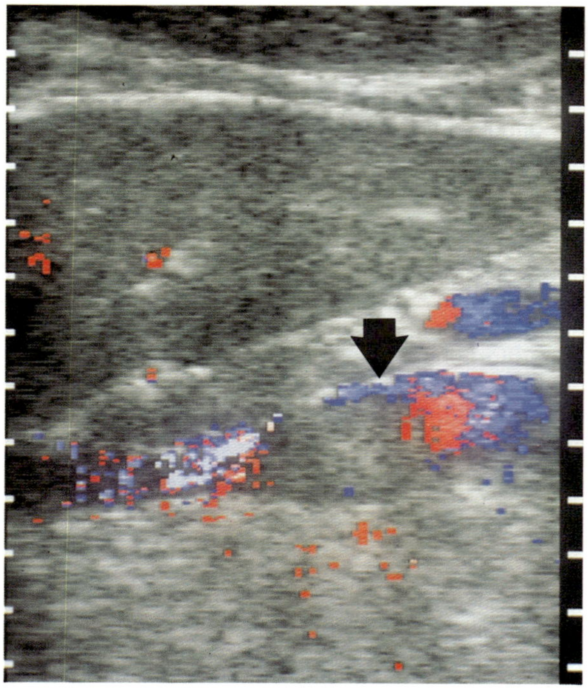

a

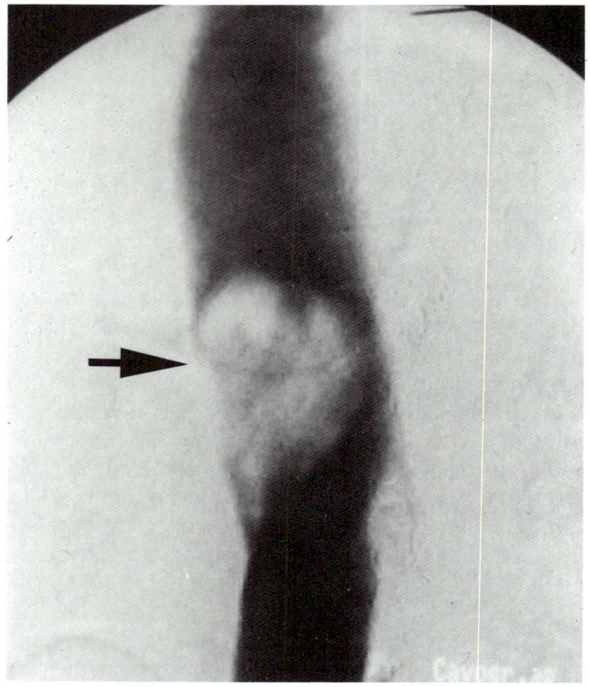

b

Fig. 11.**12a, b** Carcinoma of the right kidney with renal venous extension into the inferior vena cava (stage II)
a Longitudinal CDS scan through the inferior vena cava shows a moderately echogenic mass almost completely filling the vein lumen. Residual flow appears at the anterior vessel wall (arrow), and there is turbulence cranial to the mass (mixed red and blue signals)
b Cavography (DSA) demonstrates a filling defect caused by the tumor extension (arrow)

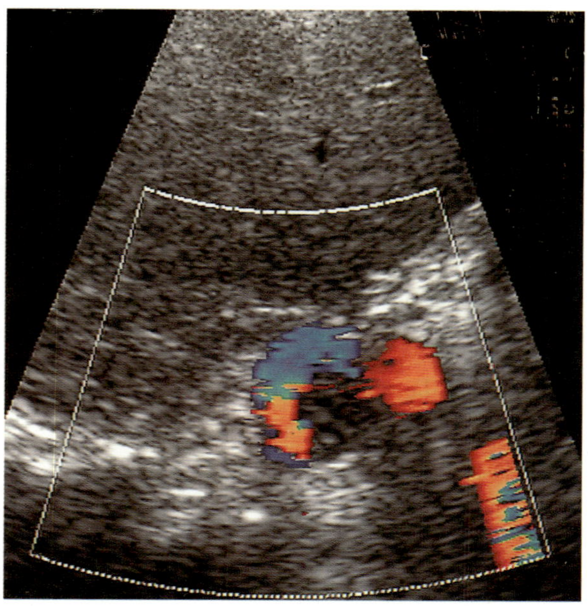

Fig. 11.**13** Partial thrombosis of the inferior vena cava. Transverse scan through the middle portion of the liver. The vena cava presents an incompressible lumen whose right lateral and ventral portion contains residual flow signals (encoded red and blue). Normal red encoding of the aorta

11.4.2.3 Collateral Circulations and Varices

A slowly progressive occlusion of the inferior vena cava evokes the development of collateral pathways that may become very extensive and fully compensate for the occlusion. The most important collateral circulations are the vertebral and paravertebral pathways, which carry blood to the superior vena cava through anastomoses with the lumbar, right azygos, and left hemiazygos veins. This central collateral circulation has the greatest functional importance.

Clinical complaints and the pattern of collateralization depend on the level of the occlusion. A distal occlusion frequently results from compression or systemic vascular disease. As in bilateral pelvic venous syndrome, the patient complains of leg edema, secondary varicose veins and, in severe cases, chronic venous insufficiency. Usually the occlusion does not extent cephalad past the orifice of the renal veins, because the high inflow at that level inhibits the further progression of thrombus growth.

A vena cava occlusion at the level of the renal veins is most commonly due to neoplastic disease or prior radiotherapy. The most important collateral routes besides renolumbar anastomoses are the central collateral pathways and the portal collateral circulation. Concomitant renal vein involvement is manifested by constant pain in the renal area.

A high occlusion may be congenital (agenesis, webs) or neoplastic. Most of the venous outflow is handled by the paravertebral plexus and ascending lumbar vein–azygos system (central collateral circulation) and by the superficial veins of the abdominal wall.

A common feature of all types of occlusion is pronounced venous congestion in the trunk and lower extremities. A chronic occlusion is asymptomatic and is often detected incidentally. The partially thrombosed collaterals present as masses of low echogenicity and are difficult to detect even by contrast-enhanced CT. Color duplex can localize the site of the flow obstruction. The distended collaterals show characteristic low-velocity color flow encoding, and the further course of their outflow can be tracked on the color flow image (Fig. 11.**14a**, **b**). The flow may be so slow that it is detectable only by using the lowest velocity scale and wall filter (< 100 Hz). Artifacts from peristaltic activity at these settings can be eliminated by administering an antispasmodic drug (e.g. scopolamine).

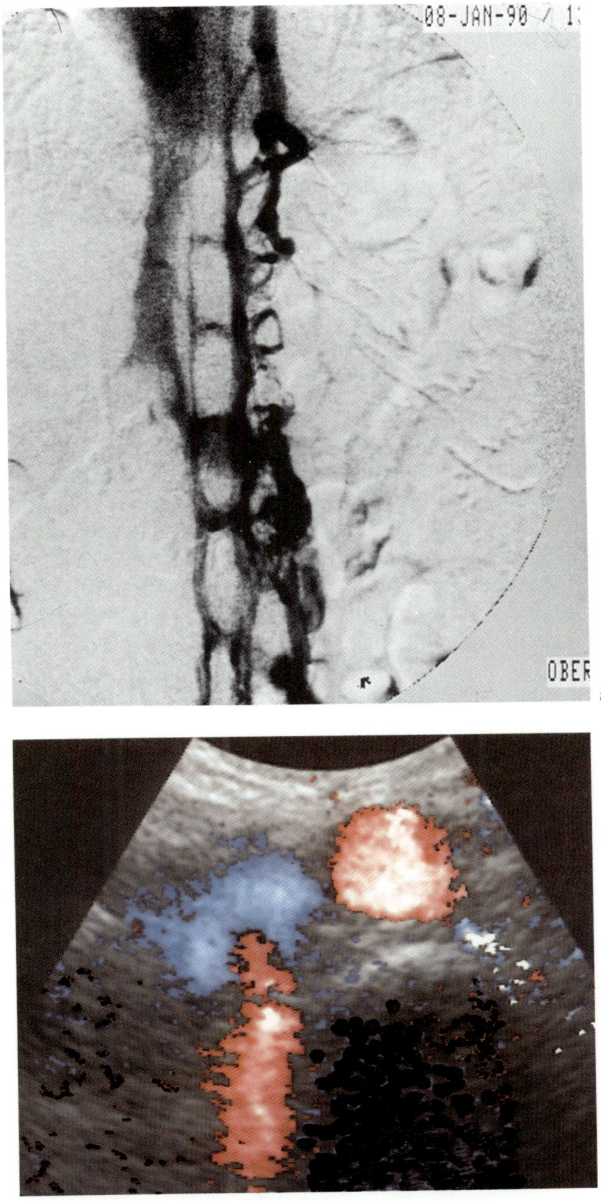

a

b

Fig. 11.**14a, b** Distal occlusion of the inferior vena cava with central collateralization

a Venogram demonstrates a complete occlusion of the inferior vena cava circumvented by vertebral and paravertebral venous collateralization. The collaterals reestablish communication with the patent portion of the vena cava below the diaphragm *(top)*

b Transverse CDS scan at the level of the patent vena cava (blue) shows the entry of a large-caliber segmental vein (red) that normally is not visible

11.4.3 Hepatic Veins and Portal Venous System

The main indication for selective ultrasonography of the portal venous system, besides the detection of mesenteric vein thrombosis and the diagnosis of neoplastic and parenchymal liver disease, is portal hypertension. This may result either from an increase in hepatopetal flow (hypercirculation, arterioportal fistula) or from increased resistance in the portal venous circulation (51).

11.4.3.1 Variants, Malformations, Aneurysms, and Fistulas

Positional variants and malformations of the portal vein and its tributaries have rarely been described. They may represent disturbances of embryologic venous development or may result from, and thus signify, an anomaly of bowel rotation.

Malrotation is invariably present if the superior mesenteric vein is to the left of the superior mesenteric artery, and it is present in 28% of cases where the vein is anterior to the artery (20). The converse is not always true, since a normal course of the superior mesenteric vein is observed in 4% of patients with malrotation. Nevertheless this positional anomaly, easily detectable by CDS imaging, is a very useful indicator of malrotation of the bowel.

Other anomalies involve atypical connections with the pulmonary veins. The range of possible findings include anomalous termination of the pulmonary veins in the extrahepatic or intrahepatic portal vein branches (14), in the inferior vena cava (see section 11.4.2.1), or directly in the hepatic veins (47). Duplication, strictures, obstructive valves, atresia, and hypoplasia of the portal vein are rare. There are increasing reports, however, of congenital shunts connecting the hepatic veins with one another or with portal venous branches. These shunts may spontaneously regress in infancy or may persist (27, 35). There are only isolated reports describing congenital extrahepatic portocaval shunts (32, 52). Portal venous inflow is absent, and blood from the spleen and mesentery is channeled into the renal vein or directly into the inferior vena cava instead of to the liver. In patients with complete shunting of the portal venous inflow, examination of the liver frequently reveals multiple adenomas and sites of focal nodular hyperplasia (32, 35).

The sonographic hallmark is the presence of a connection between the splenic vein, superior mesenteric vein, and inferior vena cava. The caliber of the vena cava increases toward the shunt orifice, and CDS provides direct visualization of the inflow. The intrahepatic branches of the portal vein are absent, and the portal venous trunk is either not visualized or opens directly into the inferior vena cava. The hepatic artery is hypertrophied, and its branches can be tracked far into the periphery. Doppler spectra indicating cardiac modulation of superior mesenteric and splenic venous flow, similar to that in the inferior vena cava, provide indirect evidence of the shunt.

Aneurysms of the portal venous system, once considered rare, have been diagnosed more frequently since the advent of color duplex imaging. They can develop at any age and occur either just above the confluence or farther distally in the portal venous branches. Their etiology is controversial. Congenital and iatrogenic causes are recognized (4), but there is also evidence that portal venous aneurysms can result from portal hypertension. The compressive effect of the aneurysm can cause biliary stasis.

Sonography demonstrates a cystic lesion that may be mistaken for a pancreatic pseudocyst, hepatic cyst, or choledochal cyst, depending on its location. The aneurysm, filled with turbulent flow, can be detected at once in the color-encoded flow image (Fig. 11.**15**) (54). The examination is completed by evaluating the flow in the splenic vein, confluence, and portal venous trunk and determining the relation of the aneurysm to the biliary tract (stasis, etc.).

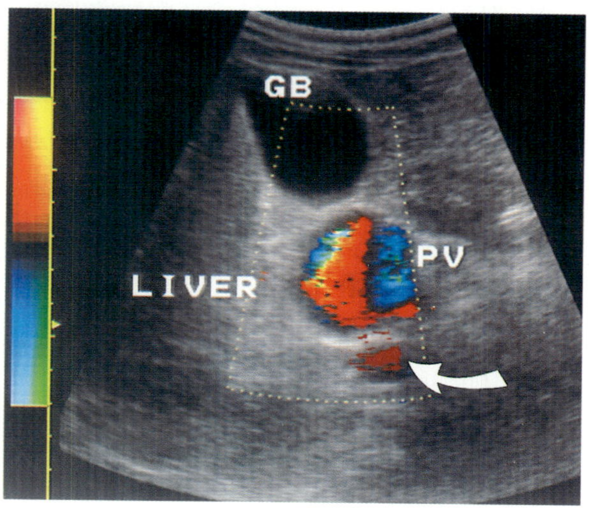

Fig. 11.**15** Portal vein aneurysm. CDS demonstrates a 3.5-cm saccular portal vein aneurysm with turbulent flow in the porta hepatis. GB = Gallbladder, PV = portal vein. The image plane cuts the inferior vena cava (arrow) posterior to the portal vein

Extrahepatic arterioportal fistulas most commonly result from trauma or surgery. They lead to an elevation of pressure in the portal venous system. A high-flow fistula can incite aneurysmal dilatation of the portal vein with obstruction of venous outflow from the mesenteric system.

CDS demonstrates a fusiform dilatation of the portal vein with conspicuous turbulence (Fig. 11.**16a**, **b**). There may be no evidence of the mosaic-like color artifact that typically occurs with peripheral a–v fistulae. If the pressure elevation is substantial, decreased or retrograde flow will be found in the portal vein trunk and the superior mesenteric vein.

11.4.3.2 Portal Hypertension—Stenoses and Occlusions

The hemodynamic changes in portal hypertension are complex. The pressure in the portal vein is normally 2–3 mmHg higher than in the inferior vena cava. It depends on the inflow from the splanchnic vessels, the intrahepatic resistance, the tonus of the portal vein, and the outflow through the hepatic veins and inferior vena cava. The sphincters at the level of the hepatic sinusoids additionally influence the relative blood flow occurring between the arterial and portal venous branches. Any significant imbalance in these factors leads to portal hypertension.

Portal hypertension is defined as a sustained pressure elevation of more than 11 mmHg. The cause may be excessive inflow due to hypercirculation or arteriovenous fistulas or an increased resistance in the portal circulation caused by post-, intra-, or presinusoidal stenoses and occlusions (Table 11.**3**). "Segmental" portal hypertension, like that associated with isolated splenic vein occlusion, is present when the pressure elevation affects only certain regions of the portal venous system. If portal hypertension is presumed to exist, a systematic survey should be made of ther intrahepatic vessels, splenoportal axis, mesenteric veins, and the region of potential collaterals. Portal vein dilatation in itself has little importance as a diagnostic sign. Criteria helpful for early diagnosis include loss of elliptical vessel cross section, dilated hepatic arteries, an engorged superior mesenteric vein with disappearance of normal respiratory variations in caliber, and a coronary vein diameter >4 mm. In patients with portal hypertension and hepatofugal flow in the coronary vein there is a higher incidence of variceal hemorrhage than in patients with hepatofugal flow (59).

Postsinusoidal portal hypertension is based on an obstruction of the hepatic veins. The truncal form (Budd–Chiari) chiefly involves the large hepatic veins and the proximal portions of the inferior vena cava. The most common causes of obstruction are

Table 11.**3** Causes and classification of portal hypertension

I Presinusoidal

- *Extrahepatic*
  - Portal vein thrombosis, compression, congenital stenosis
  - Increased inflow from the spleen, hypercirculation
  - Arterioportal fistula
- *Intrahepatic*
  - Infiltration of the portal tracts, myeloproliferative and lymphoreticular diseases, granulomas, schistosomiasis
  - Portal sclerosis, congenital hepatic fibrosis, early stage of primary biliary cirrhosis (PBC)
  - Toxic and pharmacologic insults

II Sinusoidal

- Acute and chronic hepatitis
- Hepatic cirrhosis

III Postsinusoidal

- *Intrahepatic*
  - Hepatic cirrhosis
  - Veno-occlusive disease (VOD)
- *Posthepatic*
  - Budd-Chiari syndrome, membranous stenosis of the vena cava
  - Tumor compression and vena cava thrombosis

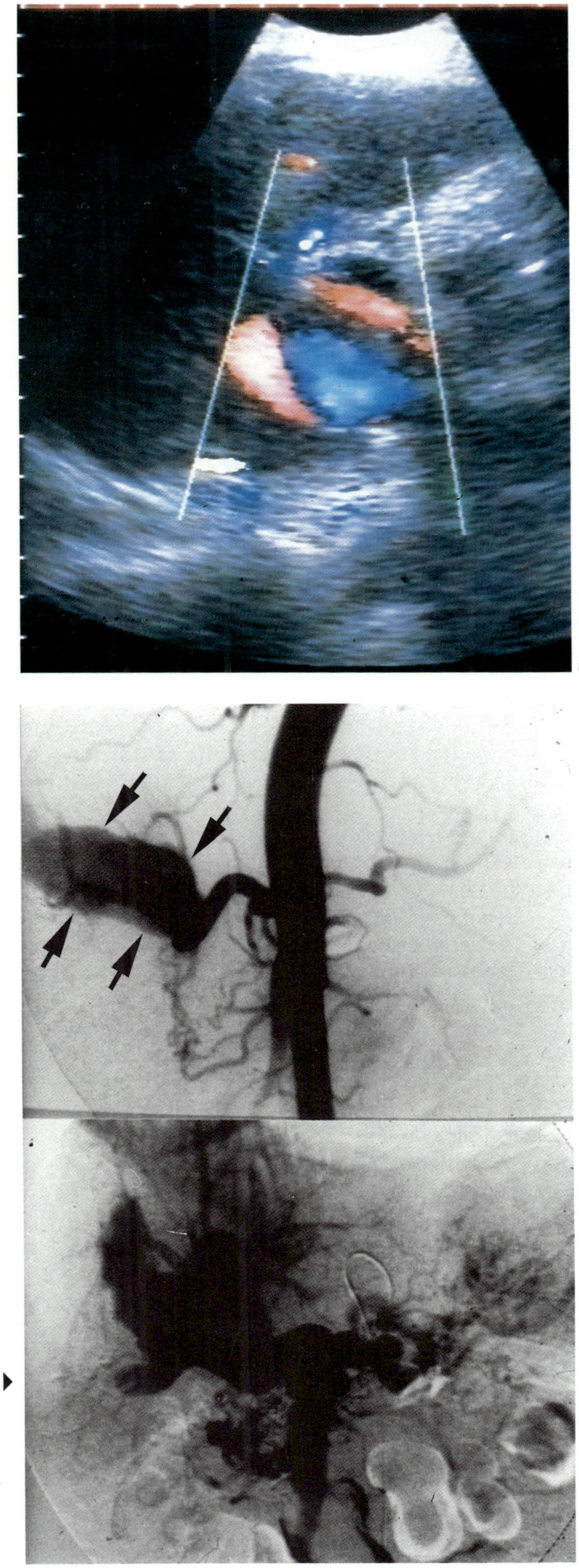

a

b

Fig. 11.**16a, b** Arterioportal fistula with portal vein ectasia ▶

a CDS shows a fusiform dilatation of the portal vein with pronounced turbulence

b Angiogram in the early arterial phase (upper frame) already shows opacification of the markedly distended portal vein (arrows) with reflux into the mesenteric venous system (lower frame) thrombosis, tumor compression, and in rare cases congenital anomalies such as obstructive valves or paroxysmal nocturnal hemoglobinuria (48). The radicular forms include intrahepatic phlebitis, usually caused by bacterial infection or sepsis (endophlebitis hepatica obliterans), and hepatic veno-occlusive disease (VOD). The latter process begins in the epithelium of the central and sublobular veins and culminates in complete fibrous obliteration of the venous branches. Precipitating factors are alkaloid use, contraceptive use, and irradiation. VOD is a common feature of polycythemia vera and is a very frequent complication of chemotherapy and radiation used in bone marrow transplantation patients. The truncal and radicular forms take different courses, but patients tent to present with the same clinical picture of hepatic congestion and portal hypertension, depending on the acuteness of the occlusion.

Acutely thrombosed hepatic veins appear enlarged and hypoechoic at sonography. Often the diagnosis cannot be established from the gray-scale image, and color duplex is required (25). With a complete occlusion, flow is no longer detectable. With partial thrombosis or early recanalization, the partially occlusive thrombus appears as a color void. The chronic form of the disease can be problematic. Despite nonvisualization of the major hepatic veins, differentiation from hepatic cirrhosis or structural alteration with rarefaction of the vascular tree can be difficult, especially in the absence of serial follow-up. Doubts are resolved by contrast venography, which can clearly demonstrate the occlusion and spidery collaterals.

In patients selected for bone marrow transplantation, the early detection of VOD is aided by performing a baseline examination prior to the operation, followed by postoperative examinations under standardized conditions (9, 20). The results are controversial, however. While Brown (9) noted a continuous decline of Doppler-measured flow velocities in the portal vein in one case of VOD and reversed or alternating portal venous flow in three cases, Herbetko (26) could not confirm these findings in a larger series of 65 cases. However, 19 of 20 episodes of VOD were associated with a rise in hepatic arterial resistance. The RI of 0.8 in these VOD patients was higher than the 0.7 value measured in controls. This might reflect a counterregulatory process at the central or sinusoidal level, but further research is needed in larger series before definite conclusions can be drawn.

If the portal venous branches and hepatic veins are patent, a specific search should be made for intrahepatic causes of the portal hypertension (Table 11.**3**). These causes may involve arterioportal fistulas, toxic or pharmacologic insults, granulomas, myeloproliferative disease, congenital hepatic fibrosis, chronic active hepatitis, hepatic cirrhosis, noncirrhotic nodules in the Felty syndrome, nodular regenerative hyperplasia, and rarer entities such as partial nodular transformation (51).

Structural alteration of the liver initially affects the vessels only indirectly. The earliest sonographic manifestation is hepatic venous changes, which can be appreciated in the gray-scale image. The hepatic veins show decreased filling and indistinct margins. Deviations from a straight linear course correlate with the extent of fibrosis. With further alteration, the tissue texture becomes heterogeneous, and the hepatic surface becomes irregular and nodulated with a sometimes dense, discontinuous capsular echo.

With progression of portal hypertension, the portal vein appears engorged, and the average flow velocity declines (49). Respiratory variations in caliber are no longer detected. Doppler spectra from the portal vein may show persistence of antegrade flow, alternating flow, or retrograde flow past a pressure of 30 mmHg. Analysis of hepatic venous flow in cirrhosis of the liver shows a loss of the physiologic triphasic pattern (Fig. 11.**7 a**, **b**). First the reverse flow component disappears, then the spectrum becomes band-like (8). These changes are also detectable by color duplex and should correlate with the Child–Pugh classification of liver disease severity (51). While structural alteration of the liver can usually be diagnosed from the B-mode image, color duplex is a useful adjunct for monitoring the progression of portal hypertension and for the early detection of complications such as portal vein thrombosis.

The most common prehepatic cause of portal hypertension is primary or secondary thrombotic occlusion of the portal vein or the superior mesenteric and splenic veins. Precipitating factors are toxic endothelial damage, slowing of blood flow due to hepatic cirrhosis or tumor invasion, abscess, cholangitis, purulent lymphadenitis, inflammatory bowel disease, pancreatitis, umbilical cord infection, and the risk factors stated in section 11.4.1. Clinical complaints are diverse, ranging from nonspecific abdominal pain with fever and an elevated WBC to an acute abdomen. A complete occlusion can be life threatening when acute, whereas gradual obstruction evokes the rapid development of an adequate collateral circulation. The therapeutic approach is controversial. It depends upon clinical features and includes anticoagulant therapy or a combination of thrombectomy and regional thrombolysis (19).

Typical sonographic features of portal vein, splenic and superior mesenteric vein thrombosis are initially hypoechoic or heterogeneous thrombic masses with dilatation of the affected vascular segment (Fig. 11.**17 a**, **b**), reduced compressibility, and disappearance of respiratory variations in caliber. CDS confirms complete thrombosis by demonstrating the absence of flow, or partial thrombosis by the visualization of residual flow channels. With passage of time the thrombotic material decreases in volume, becomes more echogenic, and shows less contrast with the hepatic tissue (Fig. 11.**17 a**, **b**). The thrombosed vein may be partially or completely recanalized. Mural residuae may remain detectable for some time and can cause local turbulence if there is sufficient residual narrowing (Figs. 11.**18**, 11.**19 a**–**c**).

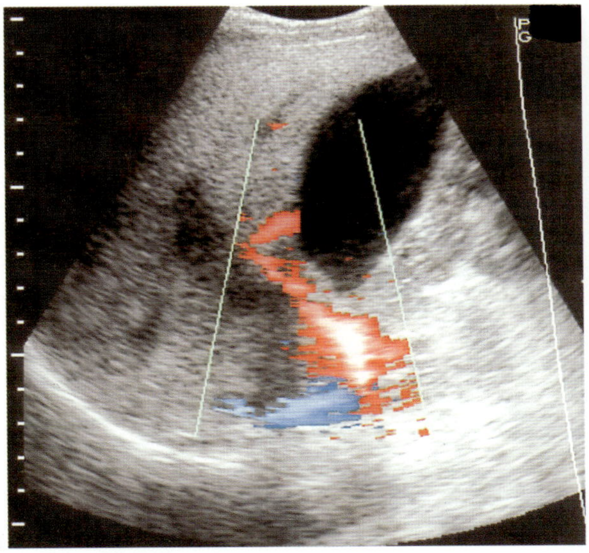

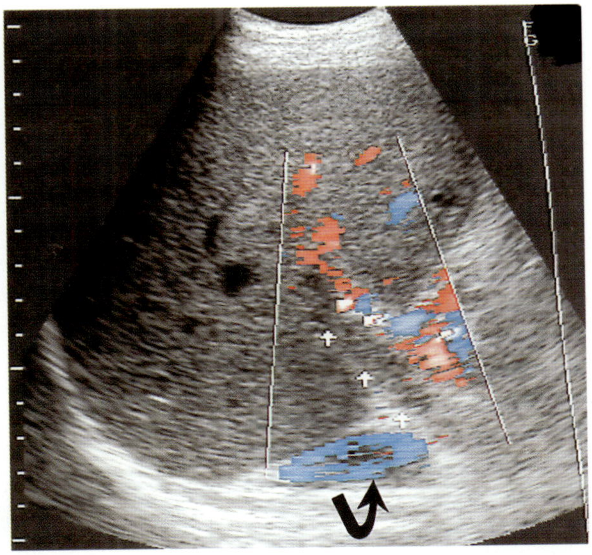

Fig. 11.**17 a, b** Portal vein thromboses
a Fresh occlusion with a hypoechoic vessel lumen showing no evidence of flow. Flow in the collateral veins is encoded red
b An older occlusion is moderately echogenic with indistinct boundaries and a small vascular diameter (arrows). Many small collaterals are demonstrated. Flow in the vena cava is encoded blue (curved arrow)

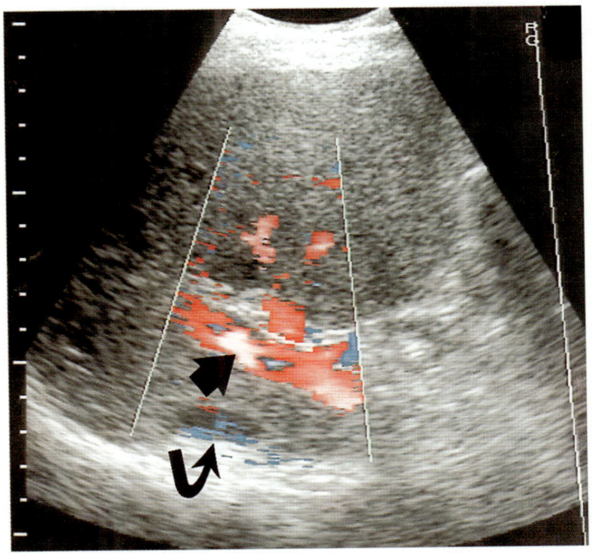

Fig. 11.**18** Recanalized portal vein with a patent lumen. There are small residual mural thrombi causing turbulence and localized flow acceleration (arrow). The posterior portion of the vena cava cut by the scan plane (curved arrow) shows minimal color flow (blue) due to the position of the transducer

Besides the sonographic criteria with dilatation and incompressibility of the superior mesenteric vein, dilated side branches are observed upstream from an isolated thrombosis, while the portal vein exhibits a reduced caliber downstream, and edematous bowel loops may produce bull's-eye figures depending on the stages of the disease (58). The thrombosis can be confirmed with CDS and its progress monitored noninvasively. The hallmark of acute thrombosis is a distended, nonperfused vessel. Compared with angiography, CDS permits the detection of partially occlusive thrombi and an accurate analysis of the collateral circulation (Fig. 11.**20 a–c**).

Cavernous transformation of the portal vein results from the structural alteration of a thrombosed portal vein, characterized by partial recanalization and the development of periportal collaterals. An aggregation of worm-like channels develops for the purpose of circumventing the occlusion (Fig. 11.**19**). The portal vein itself is no longer visualized.

The most reliable proof of portal hypertension is the detection of collaterals. The pattern or distribution of the collaterals depends on the site of the occlusion. Variable in their size and extent, the collaterals may be sufficiently developed to drain all of the portal venous blood. Their course should be systematically ana-

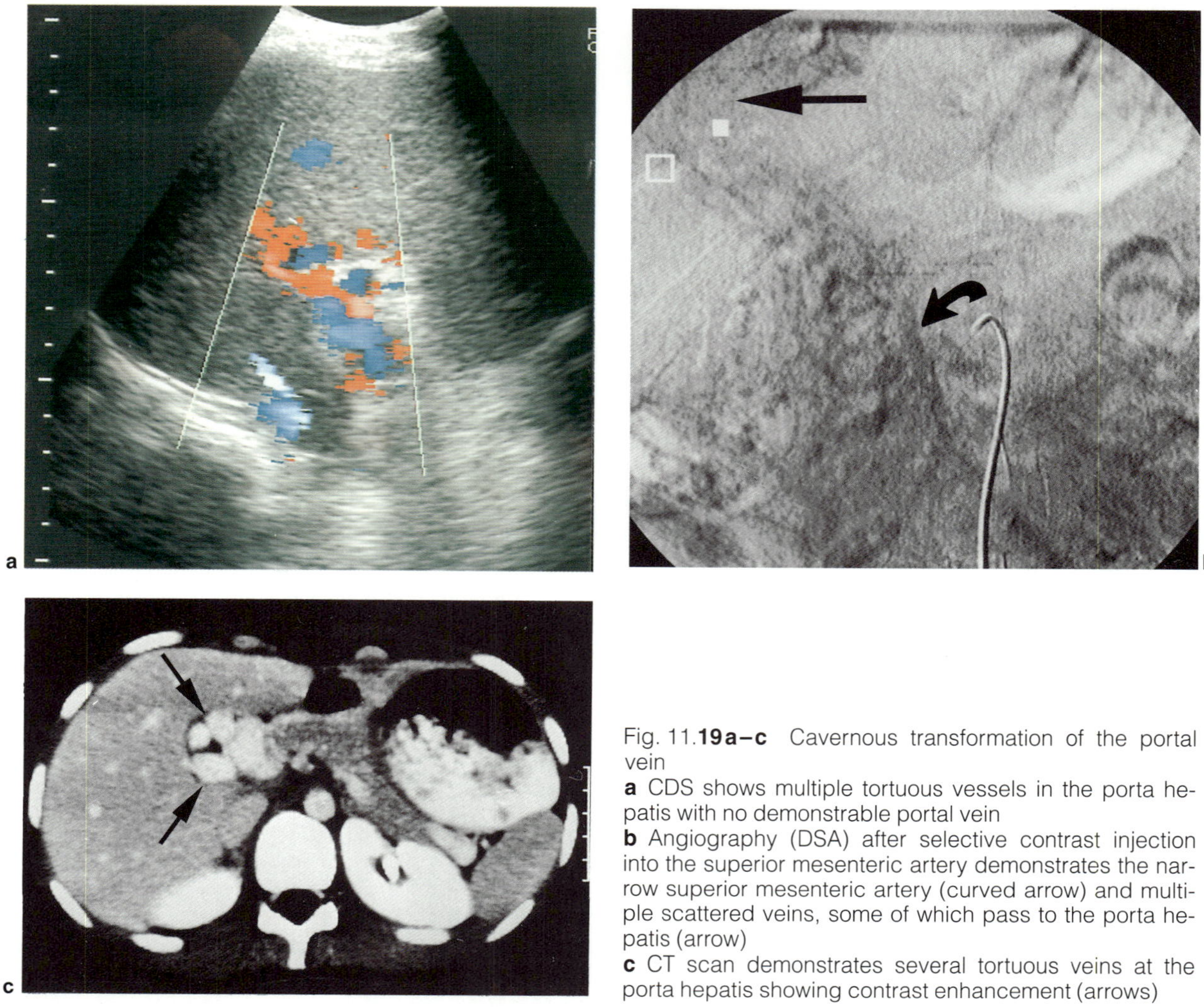

Fig. 11.**19a–c** Cavernous transformation of the portal vein
a CDS shows multiple tortuous vessels in the porta hepatis with no demonstrable portal vein
b Angiography (DSA) after selective contrast injection into the superior mesenteric artery demonstrates the narrow superior mesenteric artery (curved arrow) and multiple scattered veins, some of which pass to the porta hepatis (arrow)
c CT scan demonstrates several tortuous veins at the porta hepatis showing contrast enhancement (arrows)

lyzed to assess the direction and extent of the shunt flow (Fig. 11.**21a–c**). Sonographic visualization of the dilated paraumbilical veins in the falciform ligament provides the most sensitive indicator of portal hypertension. These vessels drain blood from the left portal vein branch caudad through the falciform ligament and anastomose with the external iliac vein via the epigastric veins.

The coronary vein and short gastric veins transport blood cephalad to the esophagus. They connect the stomach, esophageal venous plexus, and paraesophageal vessels with the portal vein. The detection of these veins is pathognomonic for portal hypertension. A coronary vein lumen larger than 6 mm is a reliable predictor of esophageal and gastric fundus varices. Gastric varices are easily recognized in the color duplex image (Fig. 11.**21a–c**). CDS cannot differentiate nonbleeding paraesophageal veins from esophageal varices, however.

Other very effective collaterals are gastrorenal and splenorenal anastomoses, which appear as convoluted vessels at the splenic hilum, at the inferior pole of the spleen, and toward the left kidney (Fig. 11.**21**). The pancreaticoduodenal veins drain the colon, duodenum, and pancreas and communicate with the inferior vena cava. Together with the peripancreatic veins that interconnect the splenic vein, portal vein, and superior mesenteric vein, these vessels can circumvent a partial thrombosis of the superior mesenteric vein.

With an isolated occlusion of the splenic vein, collateralization is established through three channels. The first route leads through the gastroepiploic veins along the greater curvature of the stomach to the superior mesenteric vein; this route is often not detectable by CDS. Far more effective is the connection through the short gastric veins and gastric venous plexus to the coronary vein, which shunts the blood to the portal vein. If this venous orifice is involved by the occlusion, esophageal varices will develop.

Besides the large preformed collaterals, the general pressure rise associated with portal vein occlu-

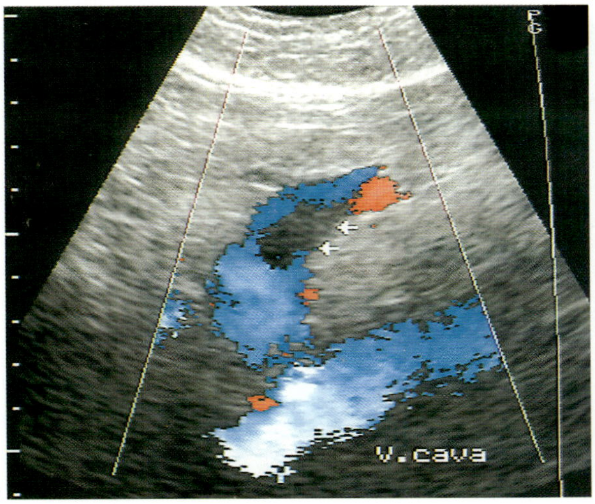

a

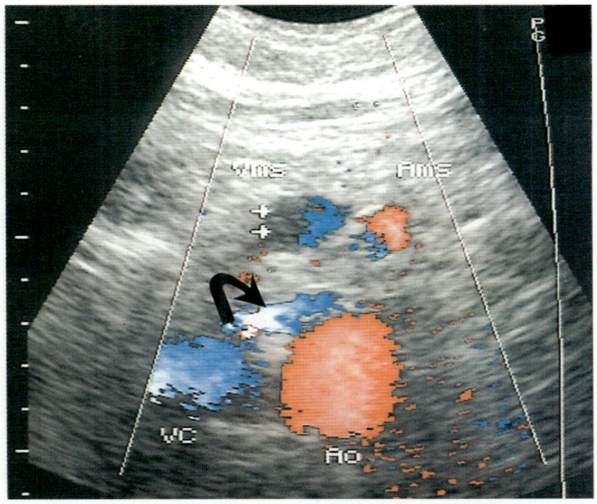

b

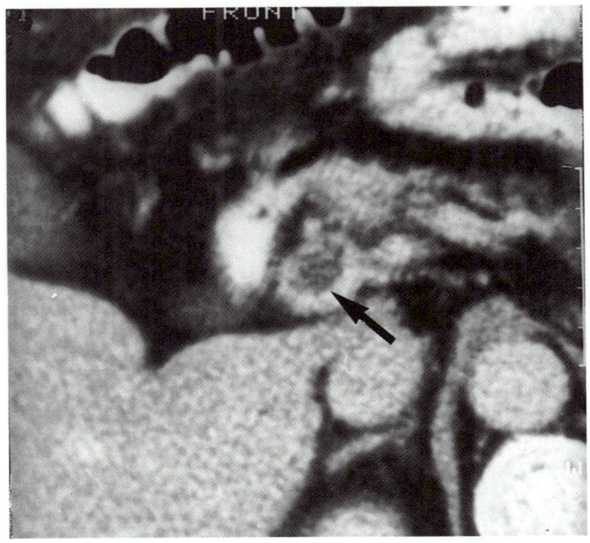
c

Fig. 11.**20 a–c** Isolated, partially occlusive thrombosis of the superior mesenteric vein
a Longitudinal scan through the superior mesenteric vein shows the vena cava and confluence and the partially occlusive thrombus (arrows) adherent to the posterior vein wall
b Transverse scan demonstrates the inferior vena cava (VC), aorta (Ao), left renal vein (curved arrow), and superior mesenteric artery (Ams). A left lateral residual flow lumen appears alongside the thrombus (arrows) in the superior mesenteric vein (Vms)
c CT after intravenous contrast injection shows a filling defect in the superior mesenteric vein caused by the thrombus (arrow)

sion evokes hypertrophy in smaller existing veins that surround the lymphatic and biliary system. These veins are visible as a fine network (Fig. 11.**19 a**, **b**). Part of their hepatopetal flow is routed through varicose vessels in the gallbladder wall (Fig. 11.**21 a–c**) and through the gallbladder bed into the intrahepatic branches of the portal vein. These collaterals are detectable by CDS imaging in 30% of patient with portal hypertension (12) and can be distinguished from other changes that are associated with thickening of the gallbladder wall (12, 30, 43, 61).

11.4.4 Diagnosis of Focal Hepatic Lesions

Ultrasound has been used since the late 1970s for the detection and preoperative staging of focal hepatic lesions. Its sensitivity depends on the sonomorphology of the lesion: Echogenic or cystic masses that contrast well with the surrounding liver tissue can be detected when no larger than 3–5 mm, whereas nonuniformly hypoechoic or isoechoic masses such as focal nodular hyperplasia (FNH) may be undetectable. The mass may be evidenced only by a curvilinear displacement of adjacent blood vessels. In most cases, based on its sonographic appearance, it cannot be determined whether a lesion is benign or malignant, and frequently the question of vascular involvement cannot be resolved.

CDS is useful for assessing the perfusion of focal hepatic lesions. Because the tumor-feeding vessels are generally too small to be defined in the gray-scale image, color-encoded flow permits only a qualitative assessment in relation to the normal surrounding hepatic tissue. CDS can also demonstrate the compression or infiltration of larger intrahepatic vessels (Figs. 11.**22**, 11.**23 a**, **b**). There is controversy regarding the use of tumor vascularity as a criterion for the benign/malignant differentiation of hepatic masses. Some authors have described typical perfusion patterns associated with hepatocellular carcinoma. Hypervascularity is seen in hepatocellular carcinoma, cholangio-

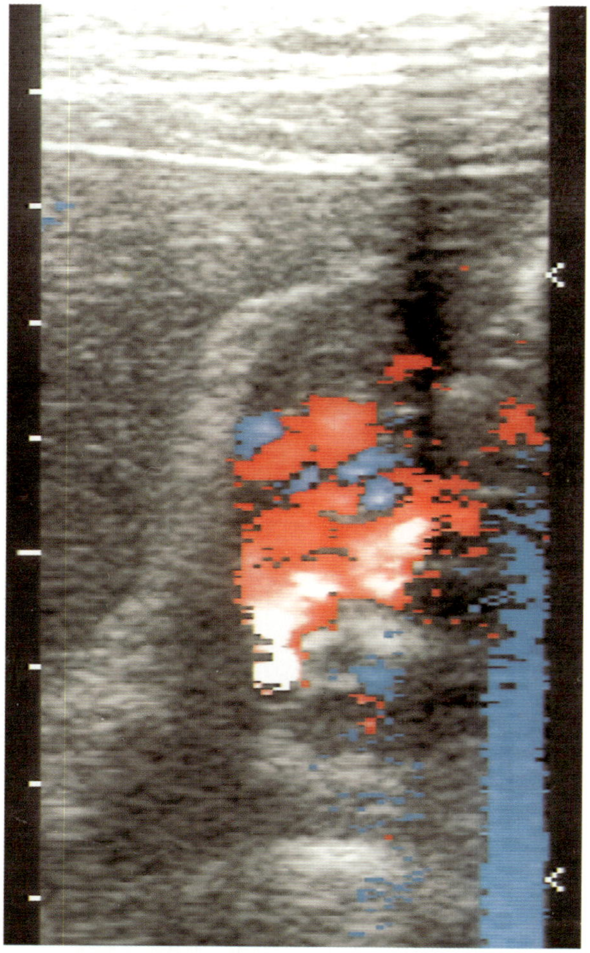
a

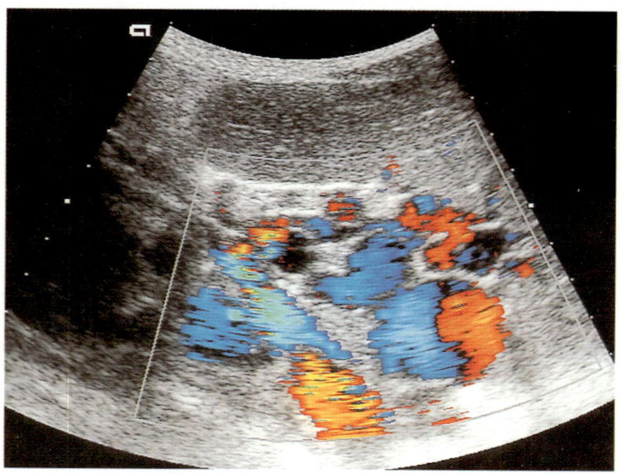
b

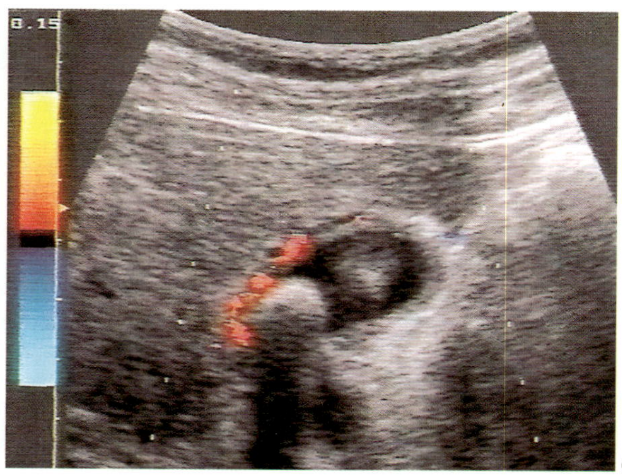
c

Fig. 11.**21** CDS appearance of venous collaterals in portal hypertension

a Gastric wall varices in cavernous transformation of the portal vein (see also Fig. 11.**18**)

b Multiple tortuous, grossly dilated collaterals in the hilum of the spleen

c Dilated veins in the superior gallbladder wall. A gallstone with a posterior acoustic shadow is present as an associated finding

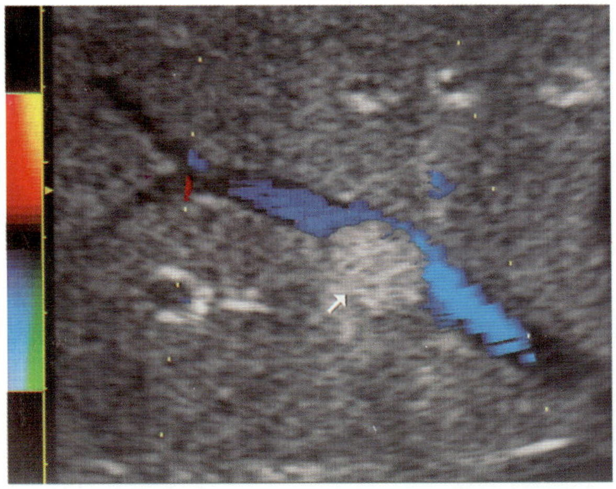

Fig. 11.**22** Hepatic tumor causing compression of the right hepatic vein. The mass (arrow) is slightly hyperechoic to the surrounding liver parenchyma, has indistinct margins, and causes stenosis of the hepatic vein

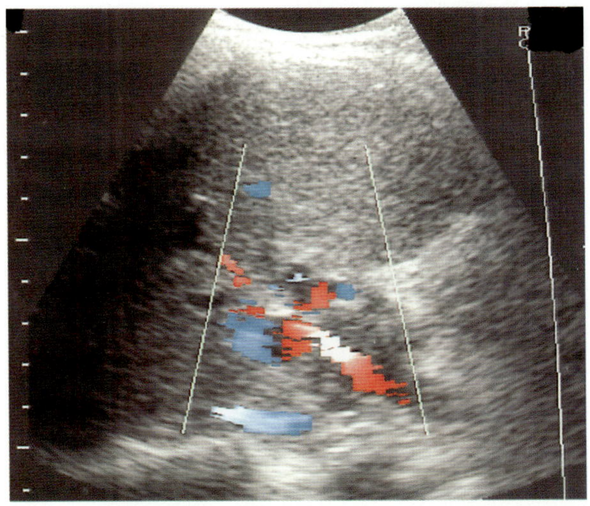

a

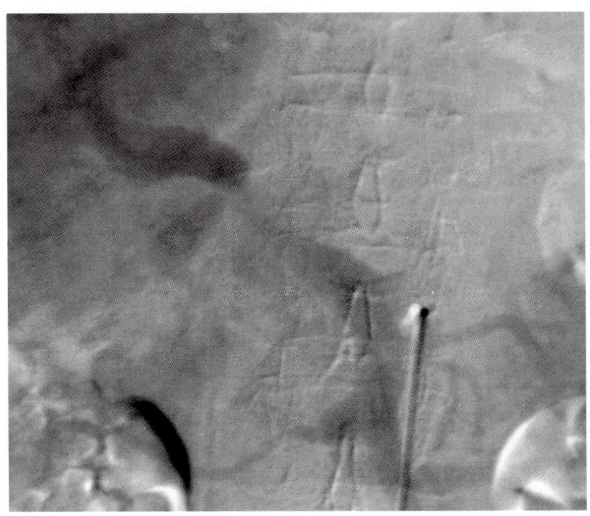

b

Fig. 11.**23 a, b** Tumor stenosis of the portal vein
a Scan through the porta hepatis shows severe narrowing of about a 1-cm segment of the portal vein by a heterogeneous mass (arrows) that is almost isoechoic to the liver. Flow acceleration (encoded almost white) is produced by the stenosis
b Corresponding angiogram (DSA) shows displacement and high-grade stenosis of the portal vein

cell carcinoma, FNH, adenomas, neuroendocrine tumors, and in some metastases (60). Flow pattern can be central or peripheral (36, 55). The blood supply of hemangiomas is also controversial. Reports of a consistently identifiable increase in vascularity conflict with other studies that found detectable blood flow only in hemangiomas that attain a certain size (23). This finding is consistent with the CT documentation of very slow blood flow in hepatic hemangiomas. Larger studies and our own experience indicate that the range of overlap between benign and malignant lesions is so large that a reliable differential diagnosis cannot be made (Fig. 11. **24a–c**) (6, 23, 24, 37, 42). It does not appear that frequency analysis contributes to benign/malignant differentation. CDS imaging is helpful for the identification of heavily vascularized tumors. Increased blood flow permits the visualization of lesions that have previously escaped sonographic detection.

Other observations that may have clinical relevance suggest that the vascularity of lymphomas decreases in response to successful therapy, and that residual tumor perfusion following therapeutic embolization can be effectively monitored noninvasively. There is also evidence that hypervascularized metastases respond better to regional chemotherapy.

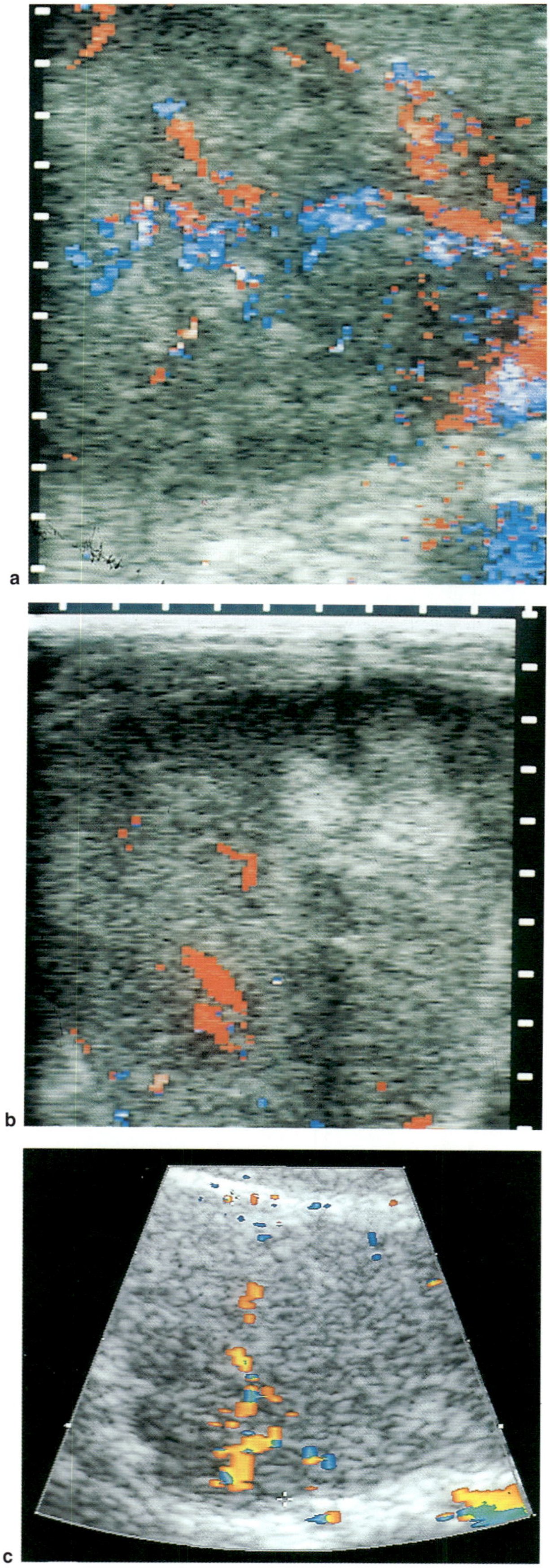

Fig. 11.**24a–c** Focal hepatic lesions
a Cholangiocarcinoma presents as a heterogeneous mass with indistinct margins and diffusely increased vascularity compared with normal liver tissue
b Hyperechoic metastases of gastric carcinoma in the ventral part of the liver show no change in perfusion relative to the surrounding tissue
c Focal nodular hyperplasia (FNH) of the liver is evidenced mainly by its increased vascularity in the grayscale image

11.4.5 Special Preoperative, Postoperative, and Postinterventional Studies

CDS is of established value in orthotopic liver transplantations (17, 40, 45). It allows for accurate preoperative and postoperative evaluation of the portal venous system and permits the simple, rapid detection of portal venous or hepatic venous occlusion.

Surgical shunts have become less common in the last 15 years owing to wide practice of endoscopic sclerotherapy for esophageal varices. Two main types of shunt are used (Fig. 11.**25a–f**):

- Nonselective shunts decompress the entire portal venous system. They are simpler in terms of operative technique, but they can compromise the residual blood flow of the liver. The most common types are the end-to-side or side-to-side portocaval shunt, the proximal splenorenal shunt, and the mesocaval shunt with an interposition graft.
- The most common selective shunt is the distal splenorenal shunt (Warren). The splenic vein is mobilized and divided. The central part is occluded, and the distal part is anastomosed to the left renal vein. Despite the pressure reduction on the gastroesophageal and gastrosplenic axis, hepatic blood flow is largely preserved (44).

CDS can be used for preoperative evaluation and postoperative follow-up (16, 33). Before performing the operation, the surgeon requires accurate information on the patency of the portal, mesenteric, and splenic veins. CDS can generally furnish this information without difficulty for the portal vein, confluence, and mesenteric vein. The weakness of CDS is that it may be unable to define the entire length of the splenic vein.

The nonselective shunts are well demonstrated sonographically. The direct criterion for patency is the detection of flow in the shunt (Fig. 11.**26a**, **b**). A "jet-like" flow acceleration may be associated with a narrow shunt orifice. Significant vorticity is observed at the site where the shunt enters the inferior vena cava. Indirect signs are an abrupt increase in the diameter of the vena cava above the shunt and cardiac modulation in the perianastomotic portal venous limb, producing a double-beat pattern in the B-mode image and Doppler spectrum (see section 11.3.1).

Examination of a distal splenorenal shunt demonstrates hepatofugal flow in the splenic vein and a large renal vein carrying flow toward the vena cava. The shunt site itself may not be seen in the color duplex image because of overlying bowel gas. Normal perfusion in the perihilar portions of the splenic vein, however (which can always be visualized), serves to confirm shunt patency.

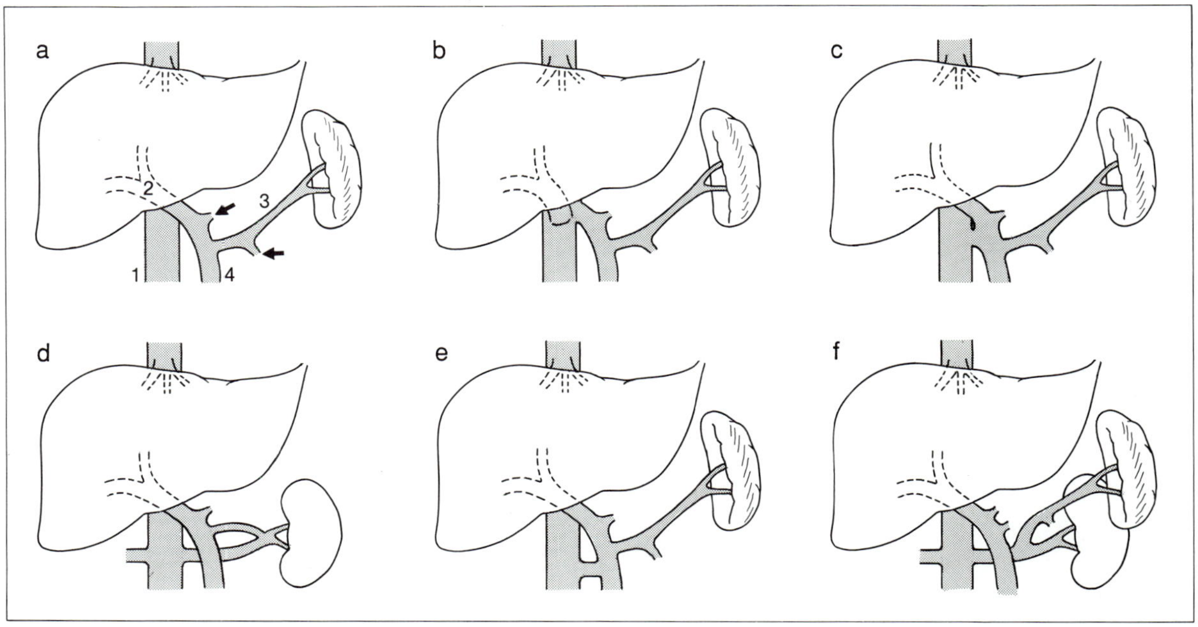

Fig. 11.**25a–f** Most common types of portosystemic shunt used in patients with portal hypertension (after Rikkers)

a Normal inferior vena cava (1), portal vein (2), splenic vein (3), and superior mesenteric vein (4). The terminations of the coronary vein and inferior mesenteric vein are shown (arrows)

b Classic end-to-side portocaval shunt

c Side-to-side portocaval shunt

d Distal splenorenal Linton shunt. The spleen is removed, followed by end-to-side anastomosis of the splenic vein to the left renal vein

e Mesocaval shunt with interposition of a synthetic graft (after Drapanas)

f Distal (central) splenorenal Warren shunt

Another option for the treatment of portal hypertension, only recently accepted as routine, is the transjugular placement of an intrahepatic portosystemic shunt with a stent (TIPSS): Following transjugular catheterization of the right hepatic vein, the portal vein is punctured through the hepatic parenchyma close to the porta hepatis under sonographic guidance, and the access tract is dilated and kept open with a metallic stent (Fig. 11.**27**). The efficacy of the hepatic–portal venous shunt in producing portal decompression depends on the caliber and long-term patency of the shunt. Experience has shown that even curved portosystemic shunts more than 9 cm in length can be constructed and kept open with the stents currently available (21, 38, 63).

The use of CDS during the intervention can simplify the technique (38). The ability to visualize the hepatic veins, portal vein branches, and needle tip enables the surgeon to select the shortest possible puncture route while avoiding the inadvertent puncture of biliary ducts. CDS can be used after the procedure to confirm shunt patency.

a
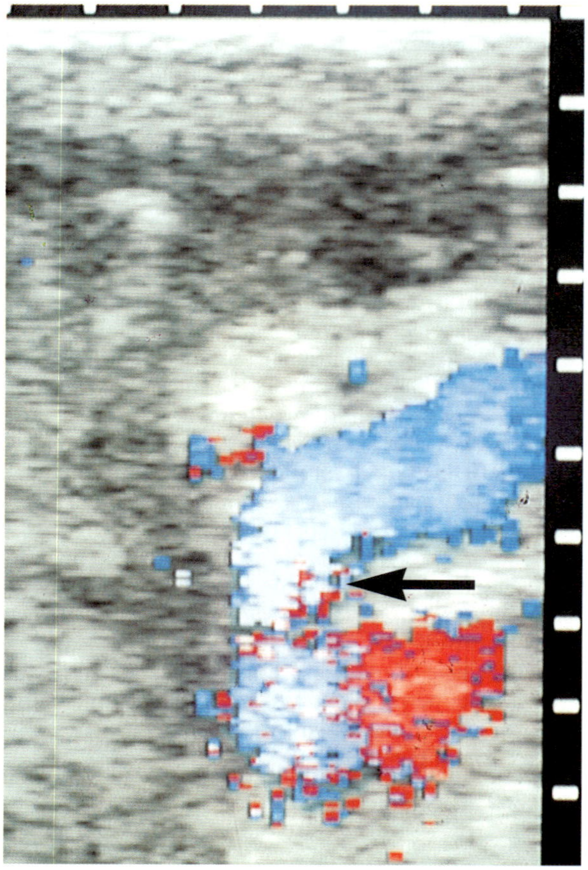

b
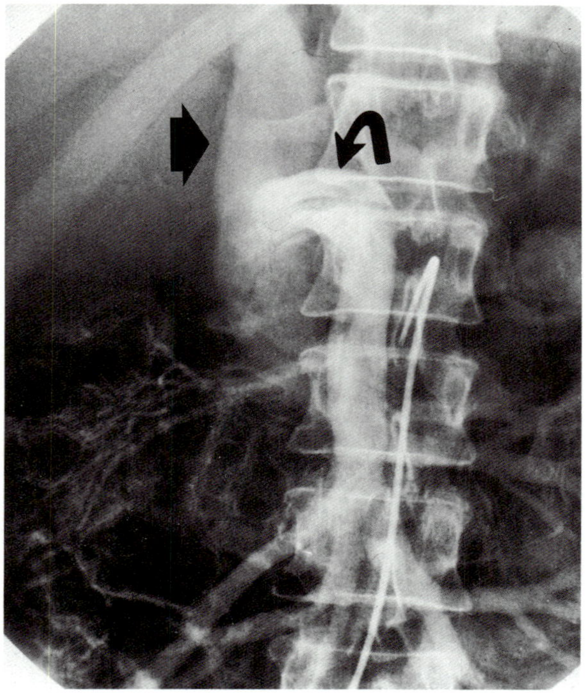

Fig. 11.**26 a, b** Portocaval shunt
a Transverse CDS scan at the level of the anastomosis (arrow) shows blue-encoded flow in the portal vein and vorticity (mixed red and blue) at the site where the portal flow enters the vena cava
b Angiography in the venous phase after selective catheterization of the superior mesenteric artery: blood from the superior mesenteric vein flows through the short trunk of the portal vein (curved arrow) into the inferior vena cava (short arrow)

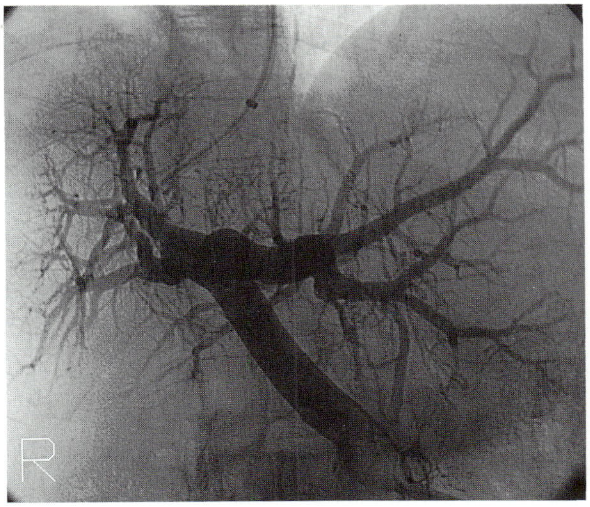

a

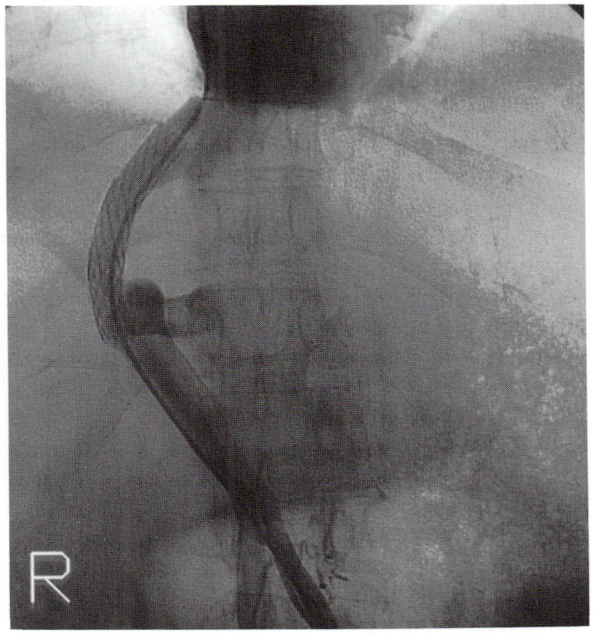

b

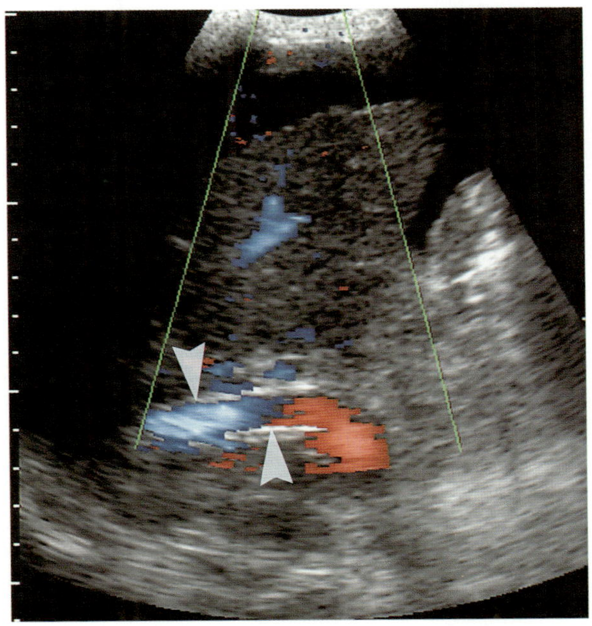

c

Fig. 11.**27a–c** Transjugular intrahepatic portosystemic shunt with stent (TIPSS).
a Direct portogram after puncture of the portal vein via a right hepatic vein: antegrade filling of the extrahepatic and the intrahepatic portal veins
b After stent placement blood flows directly from the portal vein via the intrahepatic shunt to the right hepatic vein. No contrast filling of the intrahepatic portal veins
c Transverse CDS scan through the liver shows streaky hyperechoic lines produced by the metallic stent (arrows) and color-encoded flow from the portal vein (red) through the shunt (blue). Massive ascites.

11.5 Diagnostic Value of Color Duplex Sonography in Relation to Other Diagnostic Procedures

11.5.1 Inferior Vena Cava, Renal Veins, and Lumbar Veins

The traditional procedures of choice for evaluating the inferior vena cava and its tributaries have been lower-extremity venography and cavography. Both methods require the injection of radiographic contrast medium into the dorsal pedal veins or femoral veins on one or both sides. The hepatic and renal veins can partially be identified on survey cavograms by inducing reflux into the terminal portions of the veins with a Valsalva maneuver or by noting the intraluminal voids produced by the entry of venous blood. Venography is not useful for detailed evaluations, especially the detection of partial thrombosis or intrarenal venous tumor extension.

The role of CDS in relation to venography and cavography can be understood in terms of the three main indications for its use in venous diagnosis:

1. In patients with pelvic and lower-extremity venous thrombosis, CDS defines the upper limit of an ascending thrombosis better and at less cost than contrast radiography. Evaluation of the inferior vena cava is feasible in more than 95% of cases.
2. As in extremity veins, CDS is useful for the primary evaluation of intra-abdominal thrombosis. Its usefulness depends, however, on the examination conditions and the therapeutic implications: thromboses and tumor thrombi are easily demonstrated in the inferior vena cava and the central portions of the renal veins. In our experience, difficulties are encountered only in the detection of small, hemodynamically insignificant mural thrombi. CDS is an adequate study in patients selected for tumor nephrectomy. If a tumor enucleation is planned, however, it is important to detect partial occlusions and the invasion of smaller intrarenal vessels. This is best accomplished by cavography with selective opacification of the renal veins. CDS is already an established modality for diagnosing thrombosis in neonatology and pediatrics (53) (see Chapter 9).
3. In patients with an occlusion of the inferior vena cava or anomalies, dilution effects can hamper the venographic detection of collaterals and atypical vessels. CDS has proven valuable in cases of this kind. The incidence of variants, once considered rare, has increased markedly since the advent of routine CDS imaging (11, 14, 28).

Alternative imaging procedures include contrast-enhanced CT. If sonographic evaluation of the pelvic or abdominal vessels is not possible in a muscular or obese patient, this modality is the method of choice used as a complement to CDS. Thrombi or venous occlusions appear as filling defects on contrast CT scans. Another modality is MRI, which can demonstrate thrombi without the use of contrast medium. The role of MRI is still controversial, and availability and high cost are limiting factors.

11.5.2 Hepatic Veins and Portal Venous System

As recently as the early 1960s, radionuclide scanning was the only noninvasive study available to image liver pathology, but since then ultrasound, CT, and MRI (22) have become established as imaging procedures. Initially, ultrasound was used mainly to screen for tumors and gallstones. But since the advent of duplex scanning and CDS, a complete evaluation of the hepatic venous system has become possible. The role of the various modalities is a function of indication:

1. Conventional B-mode ultrasound is the most important modality for the detection of hepatic diseases and portal hypertension, but CDS can greatly simplify the detection of tumor-related thromboses and stenoses as well as acute thrombosis in the portal venous system. Thrombosis can be excluded in less than 5 min, largely eliminating the need for direct or indirect splenoportography (49, 56). The same applies to cavernous transformation of the portal vein and the detection and analysis of collaterals.
2. The detection of a acute occlusion of the hepatic veins requires the use of duplex sonography or, preferably, CDS. These occlusions can be seen in the gray-scale image only after organization of the thrombotic material. Budd–Chiari syndrome is easily diagnosed in the initially healthy liver (e. g., thrombosis related to oral contraceptive use in young women). In a liver with preexisting disease, especially cirrhosis, compression or rarefaction of the hepatic veins due to structural alterations in the liver can lead to false-positive findings, so that differentiation from chronic Budd–Chiari syndrome requires hepatic venography.
3. Despite the methodologic problems involved in quantitative studies, flow measurements in the portal vein can be useful for recognizing pathophysiologic changes in hepatic blood flow: patients with cirrhosis show a significant reduction of blood flow in the portal vein which, to a degree, correlates with the severity of disease. Portal venous inflow decreases with propanolol, isosorbide-5-mononitrate, vasopressin and somatostatin, and it increases in response to eating and glucagon (38, 40, 50, 57). The latter response is diagnostically useful, because a significant difference is noted between individuals with a healthy liver and patients with portal hypertension.

Currently, the main indications for the routine clinical use of CDS are exclusion of thrombosis, monitoring of blood flow and collateralization in portal hypertension, monitoring of shunt flow, detection of variants and anomalies, and preprocedural and postprocedural studies in operations and interventional procedures.

11.6 References

1 Abu-Youssef, M.M.: Normal and respiratory variations of the hepatic and portal venous duplex Doppler waveforms with simultaneous electocardiographic correlation. J. Ultrasound Med. 11 (1992) 263–268

2 Baka, J.J., A.S. Lev-Toaff, A.C. Friedman, P.D. Radecki, D.F. Caroline: Ovarian vein thrombosis with atypical presentation: role of sonography and duplex Doppler. Obstet. Gynecol. 73 (1989) 887–889

3 Baran, G.W., K.M. Frisch: Duplex Doppler evaluation of puerperal ovarian vein thrombosis. Amer. J. Roentgenol. 149 (1987) 321–322

4 Bezzi, M., D.G. Mitchell, L. Needleman, B.B. Goldberg: Iatrogenic aneurysmal portal-hepatic venous fistula. Diagnosis by color Doppler imaging. J. Ultrasound Med. 7 (1988) 457–461

5 Bismuth, H.: Surgical anatomy and anatomical surgery of the liver. In Blumgart, L.H. (Ed.): Surgery of the Liver and Biliary tract. Churchill Livingstone, Edinburgh (1988)

6 Boerner, N., T. Clement, P. Herzog, K.F. Kreitner, H. Miltenberger, H. Schild, J. Meyer: Farbcodierte Dopplersonographie (FD-Sonographie) primaerer und sekundärer Lebertumoren. Ultraschall in Med. 11 (1990) 274–280

7 Bolognesi, R., D. Tsialtas, C. Manca: Diagnosis of an aorto-caval fistula by echo 2D color Doppler flow imaging and echocardiographic probe. Cardiology 79 (1991) 151–155

8 Bolondi, L., S.L. Bassi, S. Gaiani, G. Zironi, G. Benzi, V. Santi, L. Barbara: Liver cirrhosis: Changes in Doppler waveform of hepatic veins. Radiology 178 (1991) 513–516

9 Brown, B.P., M. Abu-Youssef, R. Farner, D. LaBrecque, R. Gingrich: Doppler Sonography: A noninvasive method for evaluation of hepatic venoocclusive disease. Amer. J. Roentgenol. 154 (1990) 721–724

10 Calliada, F., M. Bergonzi, C. Passamonti, R. Campani, O. Bottinelli, A. Bozzini, G. Beluffi, G. Corsi, G.B. Raimondi, F. Pollini, et al.: L'ipertensione portale di origine epatica. Valutazione qualitativa mediante color ed eco Doppler. Radiol. med. 79 (1990) 339–345

11 Cessot, F., D. Sautereau, P. Lacroix, P. Berry, A. Le Sidaner, B. Devalois, J.C. Bourras, B. Descottes, B. Pillegand: Diaphragme de la veine cave inferieure associe a un syndrome de Budd–Chiari. Apport de l'echographie et du Doppler couleur. Gastroenterol. clin. biol. 15 (1991) 548–550

12 Chawla, Y., J.B. Dilawari, S. Katariya: Gallbladder varices in portal vein thrombosis. Amer. J. Roentgenol. 162 (1994) 643–645

13 Chermet, J., J.M. Bigot: Venography of the Inferior Vena Cava and its Branches. Springer, Heidelberg (1980)

14 Chevalier, J.M., M. Jimenez, F. Sorain, A. Choussat, E. Baudet: Retour veineux pulmonaire anormal total infracardiaque. Interet de l'echocardiographie Doppler couleur. Arch. franc. Pediat. 47 (1990) 515–518

15 Chuang, V.P., C.E. Mena, P.A. Hoskins: Congenital anomalies of the inferior vena cava. Review of embryogenesis and presentation of a simplified classification. Brit. J. Radiol. 47 (1974) 206–213

16 Colletti, J., M. Halls: Color Doppler sonography of portocaval shunts. J. clin. Ultrasound 18 (1990) 379–381

17 Corbally, M.T., N. Heaton, M. Rela, G. Mieli-Vergani, B. Portmann, A. Mowat, R. Williams, K.C. Tan: Emergency liver transplantation after Kasai portoenterostomy. Arch. Dis. Childh. 70 (1994) 147–148

18 Couinaud, C.: Le foie: Etudes Anatomiques et Chirurgicale. Masson, Paris (1957)

19 Demertzis, S., B. Ringe, D. Gulba, H. Rosenthal, R. Pichlmayr: Treatment of portal vein thrombosis by thrombectomy and regional thrombolysis. Surgery 115 (1994) 389–393

20 Dufour, D., M.H. Delaet, M. Dassonville, S. Cadranel, N. Perlmutter: Midgut malrotation, the reliability of sonographic diagnosis. Pediat. Radiol. 22 (1992) 21–23

21 Ferral, H., M.C. Foshager, H. Bjarnason, D.E. Finlay, D.W. Hunter, W.R. Castaneda-Zuniga, J.G. Letourneau: Early sonographic evaluation of the transjugular intrahepatic portosystemic shunt (TIPS). Cardiovasc. intervent. Radiol. (1993) 275–279

22 Finn, J.P., R.A. Kane, R.R. Edelman, R.L. Jenkins, W.D. Lewis, M. Muller, H.E. Longmaid: Imaging of the portal venous system in patients with cirrhosis: MR angiography vs duplex Doppler sonography. Amer. J. Roentgenol. 161 (1993) 989–994

23 Fobbe, F., M. El-Bedewi, H. Kleinau, D. Wallrabe, K.-J. Wolf: Farbkodierte Duplexsonographie von Lebertumoren – erlaubt die Blutversorgung eine Aussage zur Dignität? Radiologe 32 (1992) 207–210

24 Golli, M., J.T. Van Nhieu, D. Mathieu, E.S. Zafrani, D. Cherqui, D. Dhumeaux, N. Vasile, A. Rahmouni: Hepatocellular adenoma: color Doppler US and pathologic correlations. Radiology 190 (1994) 741–744

25 Grant, E.G., R. Perrella, F.N. Tessler, J. Lois, R. Busuttil: Budd–Chiari syndrome: the results of duplex and color Doppler imaging. Amer. J. Roentgenol. 152 (1989) 377–381

26 Herbetko, J., A.P. Grigg, A.R. Buckley, G.L. Phillips: Venoocclusive liver disease after bone marrow transplantation: findings at duplex sonography. Amer. J. Roentgenol. 158 (1992) 1001–1005

27 Jabra, A.A., G.A. Taylor: Ultrasound diagnosis of congenital intrahepatic portosystemic venous shunt. Pediat. Radiol. 21 (1991) 529–530

28 Jimenez, M., E. Hery, N.H. van Doesburg, R. Guerin, S. Spier: Inferior vena cava stenosis in scimitar syndrome: a case report. J. Amer. Soc. Echocardiogr. 1 (1988) 152–154

29 Kadir, S.: Atlas of Normal and Variant Angiographic Anatomy. Saunders, Philadelphia (1991)

30 Kainberger, F.M., K.A. Vergesslich, M. Eilenberger, S. Poeltner, W. Ponhold: Color-coded Doppler evaluation of cholecystic varices in portal hypertension. Pediat. Radiol. 21 (1990) 71–72

31 Keusch, G.: Thrombotische Komplikationen beim nephrotischen Syndrom. Schweiz. med. Wschr. 119 (1989) 1080–1085

32 Kubale, R., F.-J. Vonnahme, Ch. Broelsch, W. Burdelski: Der kongenitale portokavale Shunt – eine seltene Variante. Ultraschall Klin. Prax. (Suppl.) 1 (1987) 8

33 Lafortune, M., H. Patriquin, G. Pomier, P.M. Huet, A. Weber, P. Lavoie, P. Blanchard, G. Breton: Hemodynamic changes after portosystemic shunts: Use of duplex sonography in 43 patients. Amer. J. Roentgenol. 149 (1987) 701–706

34 Lafortune, M., F. Madore, H. Patriquin, G. Breton: Segmental anatomy of the liver: A sonographic approach to the Couinaud nomenclature. Radiology 181 (1991) 443–448

35 Lalonde, L., B. Van Beers, J.P. Trigaux, M. Delos, M. Melange, J. Pringot: Focal nodular hyperplasia in association with spontaneous intrahepatic portosystemic venous shunt. Gastrointest. Radiol. 17 (1992) 154–156

36 Learch, T.J., P.W. Ralls, M.B. Johnson, R.B. Jeffrey, M. Nino-Murcia, K.P. Lee, D.R. Radin: Hepatic focal nodular hyperplasia: findings with color Doppler sonography. J. Ultrasound Med. 12 (1993) 541–544

37 Leen, E., J.A. Goldberg, J. Robertson, G.R. Sutherland, D.M. Hemingway, T.G. Cooke, C.S. McArdle: Detection of hepatic metastases using duplex/color Doppler sonography. Ann. Surg. 214 (1991) 599–604

38 Longo, J.M., J.I. Bilbao, H.P. Rousseau, F.G. Joffre, J.P. Vinel, L. Garcia-Villareal, B. Sangro: Color Doppler guidance in transjugular placement of intrahepatic portosystemic shunt. Radiology 184 (1992) 281–283

39 Lusza, G.: Röntgenanatomie des Gefäßsystems. Budapest (1972)

40 Mondragon, R.S., J.B. Karani, N.D. Heaton, S. Thomas, P.Y. Wong, J.G. O'Grady, K.C. Tan, R. Williams: The use of percutaneous transluminal angioplasty in hepatic artery stenosis after transplantation. Transplantation 57 (1994) 228–231

41 Ohta, M., M. Hashizume, M. Tomikawa, K. Ueno, K. Tanoue, K. Sugimachi: Analysis of hepatic vein waveform by Doppler ultrasonography in 100 patients with portal hypertension. Amer. J. Gastroenterol. 89 (1994) 170–175

42 Ralls, P.W., M.B. Johnson, K.P. Lee, D.R. Radin, J. Halls: Color Doppler sonography in hepatocellular carcinoma. Amer. J. physiol. Imag. 6 (1991) 57–61

43 Ralls, P.W., D.S. Mayekawa, K.P. Lee, P.M. Colletti, M.B. Johnson, J.M. Halls: Gallbladder wall varices: diagnosis with color flow Doppler sonography. J. clin. Ultrasound 16 (1988) 595–598

44 Rikkers, L.: Surgical complications of cirrhosis and portal hypertension. In Sabiston, D.C. (Ed.): Textbook of Surgery. Saunders (1991) 1015–1029

45 Rosh, J.R., S.B. Ritter, K.J. Benkov, C.M. Miller, A.H. Schwersenz, M. Schwartz, E. Katz, Y. McFarlane-Ferreira, N.S. LeLeiko: Endoscopic color Doppler assessment of portal and hepatic vasculature after orthotopic liver transplantation. Gastrointest. Endosc. 37 (1991) 190–191

46 Sabba, C., G. Ferraioli, P. Genecin, L. Colombato, P. Buanamico, E. Lerner, K.J.W. Taylor, R.J. Groszmann: Evaluation of postprandial hyperaemia in superior mesenteric artery and portal vein in healthy and cirrhotic humans: An operator-blind echo-Doppler study. Hepatology 13 (1991) 114–118
47 Satomi, G., A. Takao, K. Momma, M. Ando, K. Toyama et al.: Detection of drainage site in anomalous pulmonary venous connections by two-dimensional Doppler color flow mapping echocardiography. Heart and Vess. 2 (1986) 41–44
48 Schmets, L., H. Hagege, C. Merlet, H. Zylberberg, M. Chousterman: Double thrombose porte et hepatique revelatrice d'une hemoglobinurie paroxystique nocturne et regressive sous heparinotherapie (Porto-hepatic thrombosis, revealing paroxysmal nocturnal hemoglobinuria, followed by regression induced by heparin therapy). Gastroenterol. clin. biol. 17 (1993) 955–958
49 Seitz, K.H., R. Kubale: Duplexsonographie der abdominellen und retroperitonealen Gefäße. VCH, Weinheim (1988)
50 Shapiro, R.S., F. Winsberg, C. Maldjian, A. Stancato-Pasik: Variability of hepatic vein Doppler tracings in normal subjects. J. Ultrasound Med. 12 (1993) 701–703
51 Sherlock, S.: Diseases of the Liver and Biliary System, 7th ed. Blackwell, Oxford (1985)
52 Sie, A., M.B. Johnson, K.P. Lee, P.W. Ralls: Color Doppler sonography in spontaneous splenorenal portosystemic shunts. J. Ultrasound Med. 10 (1991) 167–169
53 Stringer, D.A., J. Krysl, D. Manson, C. Babiak, A. Daneman, P. Liu: The value of Doppler sonography in the detection of major vessel thrombosis in the neonatal abdomen. Pediat. Radiol. 21 (1990) 30–33
54 Tanaka, S., T. Kitamura, M. Fujita, H. Iishi, H. Kasugai, K. Nakanishi, S. Okuda: Intrahepatic venous and portal venous aneurysms examined by color Doppler flow imaging. J. clin. Ultrasound 20 (1992) 89–98
55 Tanaka, S., T. Kitamura, M. Fujita, K. Nakanishi, S. Okuda: Color Doppler flow imaging of liver tumors. Amer. J. Roentgenol. 154 (1990) 509–514
56 Tessler, F.N., B.J. Gehring, A.S. Gomes, R.R. Perrella, N. Ragavendra, R.W. Busuttil, E.G. Grant: Diagnosis of portal vein thrombosis: value of color Doppler imaging. Amer. J. Roentgenol. 157 (1991) 293–296
57 Tincani, E., G. Cioni, A. Cristani, P. D'Alimonte, A. Vignoli, G. Abbati, P. Ventura, R. Romagnoli, E. Ventura: Duplex Doppler ultrasonographic comparison of the effects of propranolol and isosorbide-5-mononitrate on portal hemodynamics. J. Ultrasound Med. 12 (1993) 525–529
58 Tranquet, T., J.M. Bescos, B. Reparaz: Noninvasive methods in the diagnosis of isolated superior mesenteric vein thrombosis: US and CT. Gastrointest. Radiol. 14 (1989) 321–325
59 Wachsberg, R.H., M.Z. Simmons: Coronary vein diameter and flow direction in patients with portal hypertension: evaluation with duplex sonography and correlation with variceal bleeding. Amer. J. Roentgenol. 162 (1994) 637–641
60 Weimann, A., H. Repp, J. Klempnauer, M. Gebel, H. Lang, B. Ringe, R. Pichlmayr: Diagnostic value of color Doppler sonography in primary liver tumors – a trend study. Imaging 60 (1993) 140–143
61 West, M.S., B.S. Garra, S.C. Horii, W.S. Hayes, C. Cooper, P.M. Silverman, R.K. Zeman: Gallbladder varices: imaging findings in patients with portal hypertension. Radiology 179 (1991) 179–182
62 Williams, P.L., R. Warwick, M. Dyson, L.H. Bannister (Eds.): Gray's Anatomy, 37th ed. Churchill Livingstone, Edinburgh (1989)
63 Zemel, G., G.J. Becker, J.W. Bancroft, J.F. Benenati, B.T. Katzen: Technical advances in transjugular intrahepatic portosystemic shunts. Radiographics 12 (1992) 615–622, 623–624

12 Renal Transplants

F. Fobbe

12.1 General Remarks

Renal transplants are threatened by a number of complications, especially in the immediate postoperative period, that can jeopardize graft and patient survival. These include thrombotic occlusion of the transplant vein or artery, acute tubular necrosis, transplant rejection, cyclosporin nephrotoxicity, and urinary tract obstruction. Anuria is often the predominant or only sign of potential complications. A method is needed for evaluating the renal transplant that is simple, noninvasive, and well tolerated by the vulnerable allograft and by the patient. Color duplex sonography satisfies almost all these requirements in comparison with other modalities.

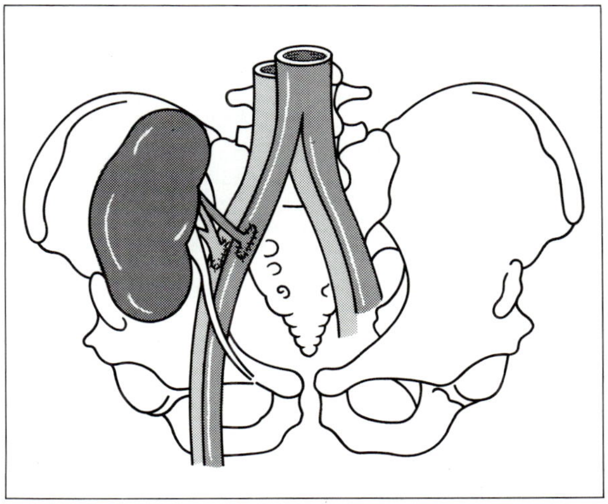

Fig. 12.**1** Schematic drawing of a renal transplant, showing allograft location and sites of vascular anastomosis

12.2 Normal Anatomy, Common Variants, Examination Technique, and Documentation

12.2.1 Normal Anatomy

The renal allograft is implanted retroperitoneally into the iliac fossa. It relates to the iliacus muscle behind and the peritoneum in front. The donor renal vessels are anastomosed end-to-side with the ipsilateral external iliac vessels, and the donor ureter is implanted into the bladder wall (Fig. 12.**1**). If the transplant is supplied by multiple arteries, the smaller renal arteries may be anastomosed to the largest arteries before the implantation, or they may be separately anastomosed to the external iliac artery. If multiple allograft renal veins are present, generally only the largest vein is joined to the external iliac vein, and the rest are occluded. An end-to-end anastomosis of the transplant artery to the internal iliac artery is rarely practiced today.

12.2.2 Examination Technique

The patient is examined in the supine position. In obese patients it is helpful to turn the patient about 20° to the opposite side to displace the soft tissues away from the transplant. This position is also useful in the immediate postoperative period, as the kidney can be imaged through an acoustic window lateral to the operative wound; the wound itself need not be exposed. Drainage tubes brought out laterally through the skin can hamper the examination, so it is better to route the drains medially if at all possible. As a precaution against infection from the transducer, the skin should be moistened with an antiseptic (or sterile gel) rather than standard ultrasound gel. Covering the wound with a sterile film has proven unsatisfactory, because air trapped between the film and skin can significantly degrade the image. To date there have been no reported instances of wound infection due to the ultrasound examination of renal allografts.

Most patients can be examined with a 5-MHz transducer (without standoff). A lower-frequency transducer is necessary only in very obese patients. Following the usual adjustments of the gray-scale and color-encoded flow images (color flow is set to encode frequencies $>$ 100 Hz when a 5-MHz probe is used), the transplant morphology (size, prominence, echogenicity of parenchyma and pyramids, width of the pyelocaliceal system), and peritransplant soft tissues are evaluated. Color-encoded flow is then used to assess allograft perfusion. Flow signals are followed from the large hilar vessels to the renal periphery (Fig. 12.**2**). If the allograft perfusion is uniform, a Doppler spectrum is sampled from a segmental artery (Fig. 12.**3**). The sample volume size, if adjustable, should be as small as possible to avoid interference from adja-

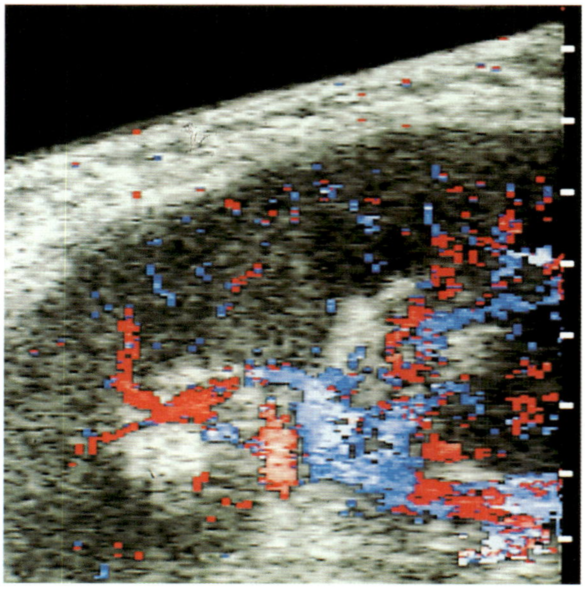

Fig. 12.**2** Longitudinal image of a normal renal transplant. Typical perfusion is observed throughout the kidney. Flow signals are detectable even in the distal renal parenchyma

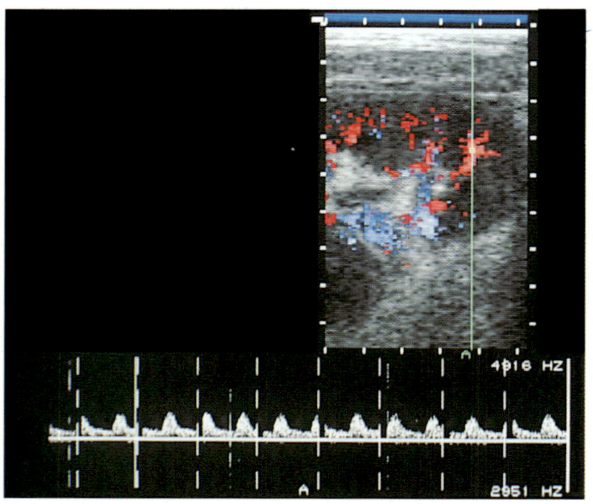

Fig. 12.**3** CDS image and Doppler spectrum of a normal renal transplant. The spectrum shows a normal waveform with antegrade diastolic flow (Pourcelot index = 0.7)

cent vessels. This spectrum is used to calculate the Pourcelot index (resistance index) and perhaps the pulsatility index (see Chapter 3). To avoid errors, an artifact-free spectrum should be used for the index calculations. This is especially important when calculating the pulsatility index (the mean frequency shift over a cardiac cycle is used in the calculation, so artifacts lead to a greater error than in the single-point measurement for the Pourcelot index). If transplant perfusion is nonuniform, spectra should be sampled at various sites. If perfusion is reduced, arterial spectral analysis is supplemented by examining the flow in a large central vein and in the distal iliac vein (to exclude renal vein thrombosis) (see Chapter 8).

For examination of the extrarenal portions of the transplant vessels, the artery and vein may be identified at the renal hilum and followed centrally in the real-time image, or the distal external iliac artery can be located and followed cephalad to the anastomosis of the allograft vessels. Uniform color encoding along the entire course of the vessels is sufficient to exclude stenosis. But the transplant vessels often show significant tortuosity, especially near the anastomotic sites. The direction changes in the vessels can mimic a stenosis. If turbulent blood flow (mixed red and blue signals) or a significant increase in frequency shift (color saturation toward white) is demonstrated, a frequency analysis with angle correction should be performed (see Chapter 6). In most cases, however, the vascular anastomoses cannot be visualized in the early post-transplantation period because of the surgical wound, soft-tissue edema, bowel gas and the air trapped in the tissue surrounding the transplant.

12.2.3 Documentation

Documentation should cover the morphology and the perfusion of the renal allograft. This includes a general view of the kidney showing its greatest longitudinal diameter (composite images may be formed) and a spectrum sampled from an artery. The spectral documentation should specify the location of the sample volume to facilitate follow-up. Extrarenal changes (e. g., hematoma, urinoma) should be documented separately in two planes. A local perfusion deficit should be documented on videotape (a static image does not permit an accurate assessment of perfusion).

12.3 Normal Findings

The renal transplant is located within the iliac fossa. It is oriented somewhat obliquely compared with the orthotopic kidney, but its margins can be clearly defined. A small perinephric fluid collection may be seen postoperatively. The parenchyma shows a uniformly moderate echogenicity, and the pyramids often appear enlarged and hypoechoic (much as in children and adolescents). The renal pelvis and calyces also may appear broader than in the native kidney. The color-encoded flow image shows uniform perfusion throughout the organ. Flow signals generally are easier to detect in the veins than in the arteries, especially in the proximal venous segments, owing to their larger calibers. If a decrease or absence of perfusion is noted in certain areas, those areas should be reexamined from a different position or after angling the transducer to obtain a more favorable Doppler angle (see Chapter 4). Arterial signals are clearly distinguishable from venous signals by Doppler frequency analysis. The arterial spectrum shows a narrow systolic peak and antegrade diastolic flow with a Pourcelot index less than 0.9. The pulsatility index should be less than 1.6 (4, 9, 10, 26, 27, 31). The flow in the renal veins is monophasic but may occasionally show slight modulation by pulsations transmitted from an adjacent artery. Due to the absorption and scattering of sound waves by very obese patients or by early postoperative edema or air in the soft tissues, it may be possible to evaluate blood flow only in vascular segments close to the hilum. Frequency analysis is especially important for differential diagnosis in these cases.

12.4 Pathologic Findings

Renal transplantation may be followed by a number of severe complications that threaten the integrity of the graft. These complications are discussed below in the order of their importance for the transplant, the timing of their occurrence, and their differentiation from other complications.

12.4.1 Acute Renal Failure vs. Occlusion of the Transplant Artery or Vein

Failure of a transplanted renal allograft to function may reflect renal failure due to perioperative ischemia or may result from a postoperative loss of sufficient transplant perfusion. Absence of perfusion in the initial hours following the operation is most frequently caused by occlusion of the transplant renal artery. An acute renal vein occlusion is more likely to occur during the first few days (2). In the case of acute renal failure (usually caused by acute tubular necrosis in the renal allograft), CDS demonstrates normal transplant perfusion and a normal Doppler spectrum. Acute renal failure is attributed to ischemia prior to transplantation and/or faulty handling to the allograft during transport.

No significant morphologic changes are apparent in the early stage of an acute transplant renal arterial occlusion. CDS, however, shows an absence of perfusion in all renal segments. Whereas the capsular arteries can maintain perfusion in a native kidney following acute renal artery occlusion, this is not possible in a fresh renal allograft. Given the importance of the diagnosis for the patient, the examiner should check the blood flow in a normally perfused structure (e. g., the femoral vessels) to rule out faulty instrument settings or a malfunction. The most common cause of allograft arterial occlusion is believed to be kinking of the vessel due to a change in the position of the transplant. Thrombotic occlusion of the transplant vein may result from kinking or extrinsic compression (e. g., by a hematoma, urinoma, or lymphocele). If the vein is totally occluded, either of two findings may be observed:

1. Due to the lack of outflow, the renal artery also becomes thrombosed, and CDS shows an absence of transplant perfusion (just as in a primary arterial occlusion).
2. The renal artery remains patent despite the absence of outflow. In this case flow signals can be detected in the renal artery and perhaps in the proximal segmental arteries. The Doppler spectrum shows a relatively typical pattern marked by a very narrow and sharp systolic peak followed at once by a sharp decline to a negative peak that may approach the amplitude of the positive peak (Fig. 12.**4d**). This "alternating flow" in the large renal arteries is due to a reflex vasoconstriction evoked by the absence of venous drainage. Much as in an elastic tube occluded at one end, the blood column is forced into the tube during systole and is then expelled by the rebounding vessel walls (25). CDS imaging of this alternating flow shows a rapid alternation between red and blue. Frequency analysis is necessary for an accurate evaluation. If the hilar region can be clearly visualized, the thrombosed vein itself appears as a hypoechoic, band-like structure that is unaffected by compression. The transplant may exhibit nonspecific morphologic changes with an edematous, heterogeneous parenchymal echo pattern and very prominent pyramids.

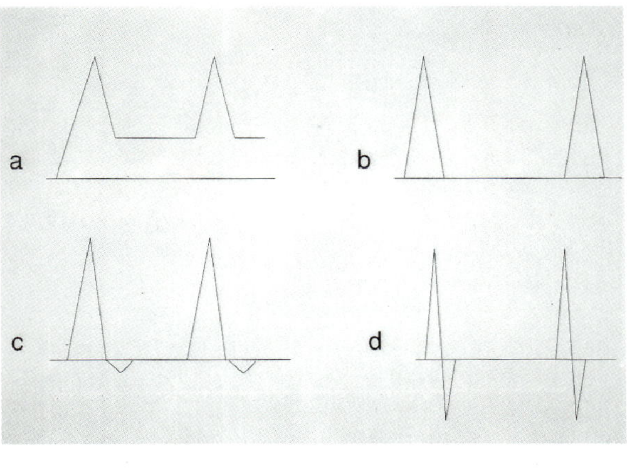

Fig. 12.**4a–d** Schematic diagram of various spectral waveforms occurring in renal transplants
a Normal spectrum with antegrade diastolic flow
b Transplant rejection with narrow systolic peak and absence of diastolic flow
c Severe rejection with slight, transient early diastolic flow reversal (negative diastolic flow)
d Alternating flow as in renal vein thrombosis. Spectrum shows a very narrow systolic peak followed at once by an almost equal downstroke

12.4.2 Acute Rejection vs. Acute Renal Failure

Rejection is another potential cause of renal allograft dysfunction. The rejection may be classified as hyperacute, acute, or chronic. Hyperacute rejection occurs in the immediate posttransplantation period and is believed to be mediated by circulating antibodies against the graft (2). This type of rejection has become rare in recent years as a result of improved patient selection. Acute rejection may develop during the first few days after renal transplantation. The rejection may be classified as predominantly interstitial or predominantly vascular, according to its histologic features. Renal function impairment is invariably present and may be associated with fever, weakness, and a painful swelling of the graft. Besides enlargement, the morphologic features of acute rejection include nonhomogeneous echogenicity of the parenchyma, very prominent and hypoechoic pyramids with ill-defined margins, and broadening of the wall of the renal pelvis. All these changes are nonspecific, however, and may occur in other complications (5, 14, 17). Transplant perfusion is severely reduced in hyperacute rejection and shows varying degrees of impairment in acute rejection depending on the type of rejection that occurs.

Generally, a reduction in perfusion can be diagnosed with CDS only by comparison with previous examinations (due to individual differences in acoustic absorption and scattering; see also section 12.3). The perfusion is reduced by an increase in peripheral resistance. This elevated resistance in turn is caused by edema and cellular infiltration of the renal tissue in the interstitial form of acute rejection. The vascular form is characterized by a primary thickening of the vessel wall. Doppler frequency analysis is an essential aid to differentiation. The spectrum in acute rejection typically shows decreased or absent flow in diastole, and brief diastolic flow reversal may occur in rare cases (Fig. 12.**4a**, **b**, Fig. 12.**5**). The Pourcelot resistance index is then greater than or equal to 0.9, and the pulsatility index is 1.6 or higher. If the kidney is uniformly perfused, a segmental artery offers the best site for spectral sampling. If a weak signal is obtained, several sites should be sampled, and the waveform with the highest frequency shift and best graphic representation should be used for the evaluation. Doppler spectra from different areas of the transplant show only slight discrepancies that are not diagnostically significant (8, 9). The reported sensitivity and specificity of Doppler spectral changes for differentiating rejection from acute renal failure are 60–80% and 80–100%, respectively (see section 12.5).

12.4.3 Renal Vein Thrombosis vs. Acute Rejection

In cases of a severe rejection (based on clinical signs), the differential diagnosis includes acute renal vein thrombosis. Each condition is associated with similar clinical signs and morphologic changes, and in each case transplant perfusion is significantly reduced. But the nature of the perfusion can provide a useful differentiating feature: in severe rejection, weak flow signals can still be detected in the renal parenchyma, the spectrum showing an absence of antegrade diastolic flow or even a slight negative diastolic component. In renal vein thrombosis, on the other hand, flow signals, if present at all, are detectable only in the major hilar vessels. Also, the spectrum shows the typical signs of "alternating flow" in which sharp, narrow systolic peaks alternate with sharp, prominent diastolic downstrokes (Fig. 12.**4c**, **d**).

12.4.4 Chronic Rejection

Occurring weeks after renal transplantation, chronic rejection may represent the continuation of an acute rejection, or it may arise in a transplant that initially exhibits normal function. Also, acute rejection may supervene on chronic rejection.

Transplant perfusion in chronic rejection may appear normal or moderately reduced on CDS. The spectrum manifests no specific changes. We have found that renal perfusion may appear completely normal even in cases where the transplant has failed to function for months and the patient has been placed on dialysis. Often the only apparent morphologic changes are a slight decrease in renal size and increased transplant echogenicity. This may result from fibrotic degeneration of the parenchyma and the development of intraparenchymal arteriovenous connections.

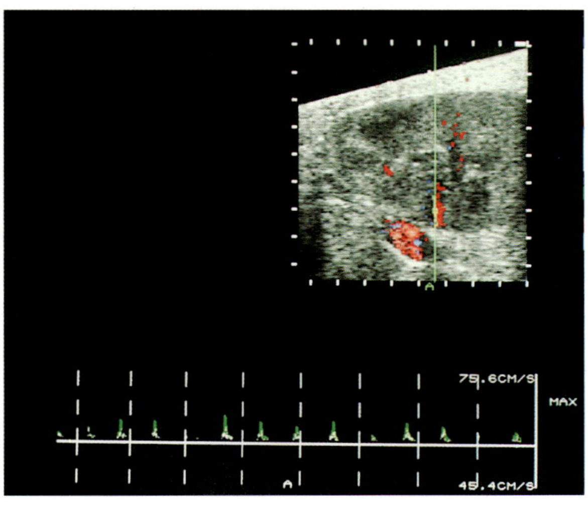

Fig. 12.**5** Renal transplant rejection is manifested by parenchymal edema, decreased perfusion, and the spectral features of a narrow systolic peak and absence of diastolic flow (Pourcelot index = 1)

12.4.5 Cyclosporin Nephrotoxicity

Cyclosporin is routinely administered postoperatively to renal transplant patients as a means of inhibiting rejection. But the drug itself is nephrotoxic and can cause impairment of renal function. Cyclosporin toxicity is clinically indistinguishable from acute transplant rejection, and even blood levels and histologic findings often cannot provide a definitive diagnosis (4, 23). There are no known sonographic features that are specific for cyclosporin toxicity. Given the difficulty of diagnosis, only a few studies have been done in relatively small numbers of patients with confirmed cyclosporin nephrotoxicity. In the majority of cases, cyclosporin did not lead to a rise in peripheral resistance (4, 9). Thus, normal resistance indices found in patients with initially good transplant function that deteriorates within days after the operation are suggestive of cyclosporin nephrotoxicity.

12.4.6 Extracapsular and Subcapsular Hemorrhage

The posttransplant complications of extracapsular and subcapsular hemorrhage are promoted by coagulopathy in the setting of uremia and by anticoagulation during hemodialysis. Extracapsular hemorrhage can originate from small capsular arteries in the donor kidney, from the anastomotic sites, or from inadequately secured vessels in the transplant bed. Ultrasound demonstrates a hypoechoic structure completely or partially surrounding the kidney. Generally the bleeding site is occluded by pressure from the hematoma, so flow signals are not detected. Subcapsular hemorrhage can occur after biopsy or during severe rejection. Rapid swelling of the transplant in severe acute rejection can disrupt the renal tissue and capsule, causing a diffuse hemorrhage into surrounding tissues (2, 3, 18).

Sonography demonstrates a heterogeneous, ill-defined disruption of echogenicity in the allograft itself and, with a capsule rupture, in the area surrounding the graft. In severe cases the renal substance is indistinguishable from its surroundings due to diffuse hemorrhage. An initially profuse hemorrhage may be arrested by tamponade, or some oozing may persist. Hence, CDS is not helpful for identifying the source of the bleeding. Ultrasound image quality is degraded due to heavy absorption and scattering of the sound waves. CT with contrast injection can furnish a definitive diagnosis in suspicious cases.

12.4.7 Arteriovenous Fistulas and Aneurysms

Arteriovenous fistula and pseudoaneurysm are potential complications of renal allograft biopsy. Arteriovenous fistulas are usually clinically occult, are not visible in the gray-scale image, and are detected with increasing frequency by CDS imaging. Severe cases, however, can lead to hematuria (connection with calyces), hypertension, impairment of allograft function (steal effect due to high volume flow through the fistula), and cardiac failure (6, 22). Typical changes are apparent with CDS, most notably a patchy, cloud-like mixture of red and blue pixels at the site of the fistula (Fig. 12.**6a**, **b**). This "color cloud" is caused by vibrations of the vessel wall induced by the high blood flow velocity. An elevated flow velocity with a low resistance pattern is detectable in the supplying artery (compared with vessels in normal areas), and the signal in the draining vein is arterialized (see also Chapter 6). A severe fistula is associated with a marked reduction of perfusion in the other renal segments.

Pseudoaneurysms produce symptoms only in the rare cases where they rupture into the perinephric space or renal collecting system. The gray-scale image reveals a cyst-like mass, and CDS demonstrates either turbulent flow or a constant, swirling flow pattern within the pseudoaneurysm cavity (Fig. 12.**7**). The afferent artery spectrum shows an elevated flow velocity and low-resistance pattern that is less pronounced than with an a–v fistula. The CDS features of a–v fistula and pseudoaneurysm are unmistakable. Angiography is necessary only if therapeutic intervention (embolization of the supplying artery) is required (6, 13, 22, 32).

12.4.8 Urinary Stasis, Lymphocele, Urinoma

Urinary stasis, lymphocele, and urinoma are other potential causes of renal allograft dysfunction. Urinary stasis can result from kinking of the ureter, obstruction of the ureter by a blood clot, or edema at the ureterovesical junction. Lymphocele and urinoma can exert an extrinsic pressure sufficient to cause urinary stasis and/or outflow obstruction in the pelvic veins, leading to swelling of the lower extremities. Urinary stasis is readily detected in the gray-scale image by the dilatation of the pyelocalyceal system. Lymphocele and urinoma both appear as extrarenal, homogeneously anechoic, unperfused structures with smooth margins. In pronounced cases, however, urinary stasis may be indistinguishable from lymphocele or urinoma, and needle aspiration is required for differentiation. With urinary stasis of acute onset, reflex vasoconstriction leads to a potentially severe rise in peripheral resistance (with loss of diastolic flow or even a negative diastolic flow component in the spectrum). This increase of the peripheral resistance may be mistaken for that associated with acute rejection.

12.4.9 Transplant Renal Artery Stenosis

Approximately 50–60% of patients who undergo renal transplantation subsequently develop hypertension. The percentage of patients whose hypertension is caused by transplant renal artery stenosis is not pre-

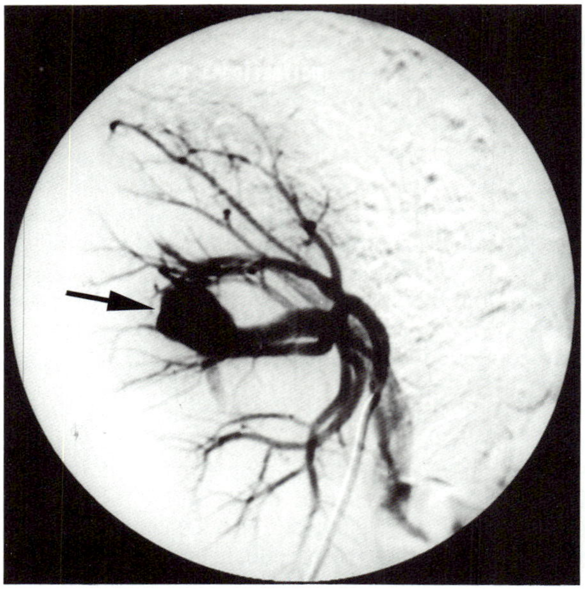

a

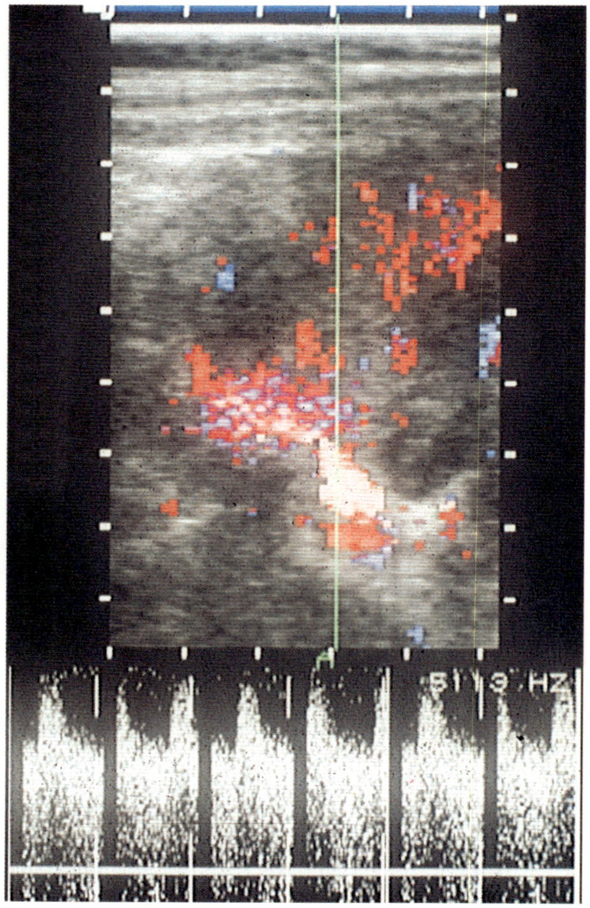

b

Fig. 12.**6a, b** Arteriovenous fistula in a renal transplant secondary to needle biopsy
a Selective arterial angiography shows immediate opacification of the renal vein through the large a–v fistula. The fistula also communicates with a renal calyx (arrow)
b CDS shows a marked, circumscribed frequency shift increase in the afferent arterial vessel (encoded almost white) and mottled red and blue signals ("color cloud") at the fistula. The Doppler spectrum (sampled in the afferent artery) shows a high-frequency shift with only slight cyclic variation

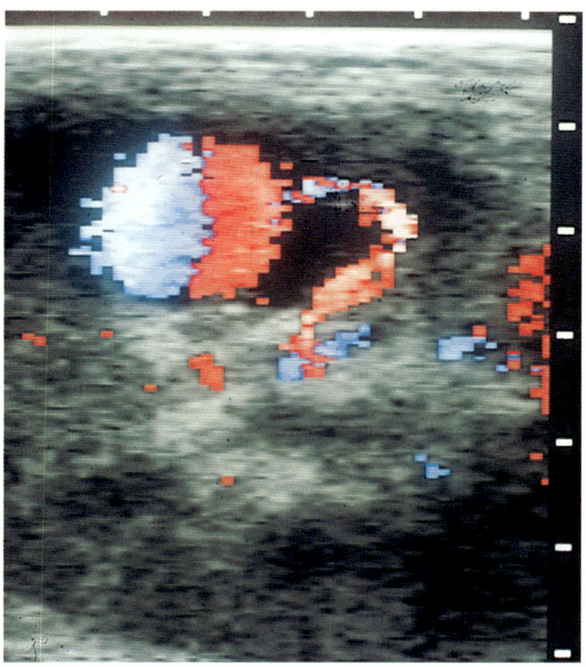

Fig. 12.**7** Postbiopsy pseudoaneurysm appears as a round structure with "swirling" blood flow (sharp line of separation between red and blue) and an increased frequency shift (color encoding nearly white) in the supplying artery

cisely known. But renal artery stenosis has been reported to occur in 30% of patients whose posttransplant hypertension is difficult to control (3, 18, 28). In most patients, renal artery stenosis develops within 3 years after transplantation. The stenosis most commonly affects the perianastomotic portion of the vessel (28). After wound healing is complete, the transplant artery can be clearly visualized with CDS from its anastomosis with the external iliac artery to the renal hilum. It is evaluated using the same criteria applied in native kidneys (laminar versus turbulent flow, ratio of prestenotic and intrastenotic maximum frequency shifts, disappearance of cyclic variations in the spectrum, see Chapter 9). Because most stenoses occur at the anastomotic site, and the renal artery passes to the anastomosis in an arc of at least 90°, in most cases it is possible only to establish that the stenosis is hemodynamically significant; a further grading of the severity in quantitative terms is not possible (6, 13, 21).

12.5 Diagnostic Value of Color Duplex Sonography in Relation to Other Diagnostic Procedures

Renal transplantation involves substantial logistical and technical costs and represents a radical change of life for the recipient. Corresponding diligence is called for in providing appropriate postoperative care. This includes selecting a diagnostic method that is easy to perform and can detect potential complications without causing harm to the patient or the transplant. Gray-scale sonography is unquestionably the method of choice for the detection of urinary stasis, lymphocele, and urinoma.

An occlusion of the transplant renal artery or vein can be excluded by radionuclide scanning, contrast angiography, or color duplex sonography.

Radionuclide scanning and angiography are very costly and time-consuming studies. Angiography requires arterial access and poses a risk of contrast-induced nephropathy. Radionuclide imaging cannot reliably distinguish severe rejection from vascular occlusion. CDS, on the other hand, can be performed at bedside in minutes. The experience of recent years has shown that CDS can definitely answer the question of transplant perfusion. If the study demonstrates nonperfusion and corresponding clinical symptoms are present, immediate surgery is indicated (6, 10). Only in ambiguous findings (e. g., an inexperienced examiner, massive obesity) is it reasonable to proceed with angiography. In the majority of cases however, CDS is sufficient to diagnose or exclude a major disruption of the transplant perfusion.

If urinary outflow obstruction and nonperfusion have been excluded as possible causes of allograft failure, the remaining possibilities include acute renal failure, rejection, and cyclosporin toxicity. The diagnostic options include CDS, radionuclide imaging, MR imaging, and NMR spectroscopy. Radionuclide imaging can differentiate acute renal failure from rejection with a sensitivity of 70–80% (16, 29). It cannot differentiate these conditions from cyclosporin toxicity, however. In MRI, the degree of corticomedullary differentiation has been cited as an indicator of transplant rejection. Accuracy rates up to 98% were reported in older publications (16). With improvements in image quality, however, it has been found that the definition of the corticomedullary junction in the transplant can vary as a function of the imaging technique. As a result, rejection cannot be reliably diagnosed on the basis of corticomedullary differentiation (20). NMR spectroscopy permits a noninvasive evaluation of metabolic parameters. Initial studies have shown that rejection is associated with a specific shift in the distribution of certain metabolic parameters (15). But a number of technical problems remain to be solved before this method can be used routinely. On the whole, magnetic resonance technology, whether used for imaging or spectroscopic analysis, is not suitable at present for the surveillance of renal transplants.

Besides radionuclide imaging, duplex sonography has been the longest-used method for the surveillance of renal allografts. The difference between duplex sonography and CDS lies in the detection and representation of blood movement. Duplex sonography represents blood flow as a waveform sampled from a selected site in the gray-scale image, while CDS displays color-encoded flow data from vessels throughout the image field. Both techniques employ the same criteria for differentiating between rejection and renal failure. But real-time color-encoded flow imaging permits more rapid and precise positioning of the sample volume for frequency analysis. Color encoding is also necessary for the diagnosis of segmental perfusion deficits.

The appraisal of the Doppler frequency analysis in its ability to discriminate between acute renal failure and rejection has changed in recent years. Initially the increase in peripheral resistance, which can be reproducibly determined using ratios calculated from the Doppler spectrum, was considered a reliable indicator of renal allograft rejection. Investigators (working with relatively small case numbers) reported sensitivity rates as high as 95% (30). These claims have been moderated, however, as more experience has been gained (10, 11, 12, 31). The contributions of Grant and Perrella (12) and Taylor and Marks (31) are of interest in this regard. While Grant and Perrella considered the Doppler spectrum to be of little value in the diagnosis of rejection, Taylor and Marks reached the opposite conclusion. They affirm the value of Doppler sonography in differential diagnosis when combined with the clinical examination.

Rejection is not the only condition associated with a rise in peripheral resistance. Similar spectral changes are seen with acute urinary stasis (7). Moreover, it is difficult to define the cutoff point be-

Tabel 12.**1** Comparison of the results of several studies using the Pourcelot index (resistive index = RI) to differentiate between acute renal failure and rejection. Cutoff = definition of the point between normal and rejection. Number = number of patients examined

Author	Number	Cutoff	Sensitivity	Specificity
Allen (1)	56	0,75	76%	83%
Genkins (11)	77	0,9	9%	–
Rifkin (26)	81	0,9	13%	100%
Rigsby (27)	24	?	60%	90%
Fobbe (9)	50	0,9	56%	86%

tween normal and abnormal values: when Rifkin et al. (26) used a Pourcelot resistive index (RI) of 0.5 as a cutoff, they determined acute rejection with a sensitivity of 100% and a specificity of 0%. An RI of 0.9 or greater was 100% specific but only 13% sensitive for acute rejection. Our own prospective studies in nonselected patients using an RI cutoff of 0.9 indicated a sensitivity of 56% and specificity of 86% (9, 10) (Table 12.**1**). However, sensitivity is improved when clinical parameters are evaluated in conjunction with the CDS findings (24).

A cutoff of 0.9 is an arbitrary choice. It may be justified by assuming that a Pourcelot index of 0.9 is associated with minimal antegrade diastolic flow (1 = no diastolic flow, > 1 = reverse diastolic flow). The ratio in a Doppler spectrum from a healthy native kidney is between 0.5 and 0.8. Thus, a value of 0.9 represents a marked elevation of intrarenal peripheral resistance. A survey of the literature shows that this is the value most commonly used (26). Besides the RI, the pulsatility index (PI) is also used for renal allograft evaluations. The PI is derived not just from measurements at two points (see Chapter 3) but from the entire spectral waveform (27). In theory, this provides greater sensitivity in the detection of spectral changes. However, calculation of the PI is considerably more complex (involving integration below the waveform) and more susceptible to interference (e. g., from an adjacent venous waveform). As a result, the calculated values are more dependent on the quality of the examination and less reproducible than the RI, which is the parameter recommended for routine use.

These ratios are not useful for distinguishing cyclosporin toxicity from acute allograft failure. Neither complication is probably associated with a rise in peripheral resistance (4, 9, 10, 23). It should be added that even histologic examination cannot always establish a definitive cause for renal allograft dysfunction (19, 23). Acute renal failure, acute rejection, and cyclosporin nephrotoxicity may occur separately or concomitantly in the same transplant. Thus analysis of the peripheral vascular resistance is useful only when combined with an analysis of clinical and laboratory findings. If clinical data raise suspicion of rejection and Doppler frequency analysis indicates a rise in peripheral resistance (relative to the previous examination), rejection is very probable, and appropriate treatment should be instituted without delay (24). Given the complexity of differential diagnosis, however, biopsy is generally unavoidable for an accurate evaluation.

In summary, color duplex sonography provides a convenient, low-cost method for answering many questions that arise after renal transplantation. The morphology and perfusion of the renal allograft can be evaluated, and rejection can be diagnosed by interpreting the CDS findings within the context of the clinical presentation, laboratory findings, and previous baseline examination. Computed tomography is indicated if allograft rupture is suspected, and contrast angiography is necessary only for the treatment of transplant renal artery stenosis or an a–v fistula.

12.6 References

1 Allen, K.S., D.K. Jorkarsky, P.H. Arger, M.G. Velchik, K. Grumbach, B.G. Coleman, M.C. Mintz, S.E. Betsch, L.J. Perloff: Renal allografts: prospective analysis of Doppler sonography. Radiology 169 (1988) 371–376

2 Barker, C.F., A. Naji, D.C. Dafoe, L.J. Perloff: Renal transplantation. In Sabiston, D.C. (Ed.): Textbook of Surgery. Saunders, Philadelphia (1991) 374

3 Belzer, F.O., N. Glass, H. Sollinger: Technical complications after renal transplantation. In Morris, P.J. (Ed.): Kidney Transplantation. Saunders, Philadelphia (1988) 511

4 Buckley, A.R., P.L. Cooperberg, C.E. Reeve, A.B. Magil: The distinction between acute renal transplant rejection and cyclosporin nephrotoxicity: value of Duplex sonography. Amer. J. Roentgenol. 149 (1987) 521–525

5 Cochlin, D.L.L., A. Wake, J.R. Salaman, P.J.A. Griffin: Ultrasound changes in the transplant kidney. Clin. Radiol. 39 (1988) 373–376

6 Dodd, G.D., M.E. Tublin, A.B. Zajko: Imaging of vascular complications associated with renal transplants. Amer. J. Roentgenol. 157 (1991) 449–459

7 Don, S., K.K. Kopecky, R.S. Filo, S.B. Leapman, J.V. Thomalla, J.A. Jones, E.C. Klatte: Duplex Doppler US of renal allografts: causes of elevated resitive index. Radiology 171 (1989) 709–712

8 Flückiger, F., M. Ratschek, H. Steiner: Farbkodierte Duplexsonographie von Nierentransplantaten mit Dysfunktion. Radiologe 31 (1991) 51–55

9 Fobbe, F., L. Schudrowitsch, M. Dietzel, K.-J. Wolf: Verlaufskontrolle von Nierentransplantaten mit der farbkodierten Duplexsonographie. Fortschr. Röntgenstr. 150 (1989) 76–79

10 Fobbe, F.: Farbkodierte Duplexsonographie (FKDS) bei Transplantatnieren. Z. Transplant Med. 2 (1990) 23–30

11 Genkins, S.M., F.P. Sanfilippo, B.A. Caroll: Duplex Doppler sonography of renal transplants: lack of sensitivity and specificity in establishing pathologic diagnosis. Amer. J. Roentgenol. 152 (1988) 535–539

12 Grant, E.G., R.R. Perrella: Wishing won't make it so: Duplex Doppler sonography in the evaluation of renal transplant dysfunction. Amer. J. Roentgenol. 155 (1990) 538–539

13 Grenier, N., C. Douws, D. Morel, J.-M. Ferriere, M.L. Guillou, L. Potaux, J. Broussin: Detection of vascular complications in renal allografts with color Doppler flow imaging. Radiology 178 (1991) 217–223

14 Griffin, J.F., C.D. Short, W. Lawler, N.P. Mallick, R.W.G. Johnson: Diagnosis of disease in renal allografts: correlation between ultrasound and histology. Clin. Radiol. 37 (1986) 59–62

15 Grist, T.M., H.C. Charles, H.D. Sostman: Renal transplant rejection: diagnosis with ^{31}P MR spectroscopy. Amer. J. Roentgenol. 156 (1991) 105–112

16 Hricak, H., F. Terrier, M. Marotti, B.L. Engelstad, R.A. Filly, F. Vincenti, R.M. Duca, P.N. Bretan, C.B. Higgins, N. Feduska: Posttransplant renal rejection: comparison of quantitative scintigraphy, US, and MR imaging. Radiology 162 (1987) 685–688

17 Kelcz, F., M.A. Pozniak, J.D. Pirsch, T.D. Oberly: Pyramidal appearance and resistive index: insensitive and nonspecific sonographic indicators of renal transplant rejection. Amer. J. Roentgenol. 155 (1990) 531–535
18 Kirkman, R.L., N.L. Tilney: Surgical complications in the transplant recipient. In Milford, E.L., B.M. Brenner, J.U. Stein (Ed.): Renal Transplantation. Churchill Livingstone, New York (1989) 231
19 Krause, P.H.: Die Histologie des Nierentransplantates. Z. Transplant Med. 2 (1990) 3–10
20 Liou, J.T., J.K.T. Lee, J.P. Heiken, W.G. Totty, P.L. Molina, W.M. Flye: Renal transplants: can acute rejection and acute tubular necrosis be differentiated with MR imaging? Radiology 179 (1991) 61–65
21 McGee, G.S., L. Peterson-Kennedy, P. Astleford, J.S.T. Yao: Duplex assessment of the renal transplant. Clin. N. Amer. 70 (1990) 133–141
22 Middleton, W.D., G.M. Kellman, G.L. Melson, B.L. Madrazo: Postbiobsy renal transplant arteriovenous fistulas: color Doppler US characterisation. Radiology 171 (1989) 253–257
23 Mihatsch, M.J., G. Thiel, B. Ruffel: Morphology of cyclosporin nephropathy. Progr. Allergy 38 (1986) 447–465
24 Mizrahi, S., J.L. Hussey, D.H. Hayes, J.P. Boudreaux, C.R.B. Merrit, E.I. Bluth: Protocol Doppler color flow imaging immediatly after kidney transplantation. Sth. med. J. 86 (1993) 1126–1128
25 Reuther, G., D. Wanjura, H. Bauer: Acute renal vein thrombosis in renal allografts: detection with duplex doppler US. Radiology 170 (1989) 557–558
26 Rifkin, M.D., L. Needlemann, M.E. Pasto, A.B. Kurtz, P.M. Foy, E. McGlynn, C. Canino, O.H. Baltarowich, R.G. Pennell, B.B. Goldberg: Evaluation of renal transplant rejection by duplex doppler examination. Amer. J. Roentgenol. 148 (1987) 759–762
27 Rigsby, C.M., P.N. Burns, G.G. Weltin, B. Chen, M. Bis, K.J.W. Taylor: Doppler signal quantitation in renal allografts: comparison in normal and rejecting transplants, with pathologic correlation. Radiology 162 (1987) 39–42
28 Roberts, J.P., N.L. Ascher, D.S. Fryd, D.W. Hunter, D.L. Dunn, W.D. Payne, D.E.R. Sutherland, W. Castaneda-Zunica, J.S. Najarian: Transplant renal artey stenosis. Transplantation 48 (1989) 580–583
29 Staab, E.V., F. Whittier, D.D. Patton, E.H. Ginn, J.R. Ackermann: Early evaluation of cadaver renal allotransplant by means of radionuclide imaging. Radiology 106 (1973) 147–151
30 Steinberg, H.V., R.C. Nelson, F.B. Murphy, J.L. Chezmar, B.R. Baumgartner, V.B. Delany, J.D. Whelchel, M.E. Bernadino: Renal allograft rejection: evaluation by Doppler US and MR imaging. Radiology 162 (1987) 337–342
31 Taylor, K.J.W., W.H. Marks: Use of Doppler imaging for evaluation of dysfunction in renal allografts. Amer. J. Roentgenol. 155 (1990) 536–537
32 Tobben, P.J., A.B. Zajko, J.H. Sumkin, A.D. Bowen, C.R. Fuhrman, M.L. Skolnick, K.M. Bron, C.O. Esquivel, T.E. Starzl: Pseudoaneurysmas complicating organ transplantation: roles of CT, duplex sonography, and angiography. Radiology 169 (1988) 65–70

13 Scrotum

F. Fobbe

13.1 General Remarks

When combined with the history and clinical examination, real-time ultrasound scanning is a proven method for the evaluation of scrotal disorders. But ultrasound morphology and clinical data cannot always discriminate among the various causes of an "acute scrotum." Especially in younger patients, scrotal pain of acute onset requires differentiation of testicular torsion and epididymo-orchitis. Both disorders can present similar morphologic features on ultrasound examination. Often the testis cannot be examined by palpation following severe scrotal trauma, where it is necessary to assess the extent of the testicular injury and the status of testicular perfusion.

Varicocele also presents diagnostic difficulties. While larger varicoceles can be diagnosed by palpation and B-mode imaging, less pronounced "subclinical" (= "functional") varicoceles cannot be reliably detected. But varicocele is one of the few treatable causes of male infertility. This underscores the need for a simple, noninvasive, reliable diagnostic procedure.

13.2 Normal Anatomy and Examination Technique

13.2.1 Normal Anatomy

The scrotum represents an evagination of the anterior abdominal wall. It contains the testes, the epididymides, the spermatic cords, nerves, and blood vessels. The tunica vaginalis lines the inside of the scrotal wall. It forms a closed sac (cavum serosum testis) in which the testis and epididymis are suspended cranially by the spermatic cord but are otherwise freely mobile. The testis is an ovoid gland that in adults measures approximately 4–5 cm in length and 2.5–3 cm in diameter; it weighs 10–14 g. The left testis usually hangs somewhat lower than the right. The testis is enveloped by a fibrous capsule, the tunica albuginea, from which fibrous septa radiate into the parenchyma, dividing it into 200–300 lobules. Each lobule contains up to four seminiferous tubules. Each seminiferous tubule can be described as a convoluted loop opening at both ends into the rete testis via the tubuli recti. The rete testis is part of the mediastinum testis, which appears sonographically as a highly echogenic band inside the testis. The rete testis terminates superiorly in 10–15 efferent ductules, which open into the epididymis (11, 18).

The epididymis forms a cap-like structure on the posterolateral aspect of the testis. It consists of a superior portion (head), central portion (body), and inferior portion (tail). The tail of the epididymis is continuous with the ductus deferens (Fig. 13.**1**).

Attached to the upper third of the testis and epididymis are "appendices," sometimes referred to as "hydatids." These structures are of clinical interest only because a sudden disturbance in the blood supply to one of these appendages can produce symptoms similar to those of testicular torsion.

The intrascrotal organs are supplied predominantly by the testicular artery. Generally both testicular arteries arise from the aorta slightly below the renal arteries. The artery enters the spermatic cord at the deep inguinal ring. After giving off branches to the epididymis and ductus deferens, the vessel enters the testis at the hilum. Skirting the tunica albuginea, the artery first runs inferiorly on the testicular surface, winds around the lower pole of the testis, turns upward again and terminates at the upper pole of the testis. The individual branches pass into the interior of the testis with the lobular septa (Figs. 13.**1**, 13.**2**). The venous drainage likewise shows an outside-to-inside arrangement. The veins converge in the mediastinum testis and unite with the tributaries from the epididymis to form the pampiniform plexus. This venous network constitutes the major portion of the spermatic cord. The plexus reduces to three or four veins at the level of the external inguinal ring, and at the internal ring there is usually only one major vessel, the testicular vein (internal spermatic vein). Additional small accompanying veins, which either follow the main vessel upward or pass to other retroperitoneal organs, communicate with one another at the level of the internal inguinal ring. The number, course, and termination of the veins accompanying the testicular vein are highly variable. The left testicular vein opens into the left renal vein, while the right testicular vein opens into the vena cava just below the termination of the right renal vein (5, 11, 18).

The spermatic cord consists basically of the ductus deferens, the testicular artery, the pampiniform plexus, the cremaster muscle, nerves, lymphatics, and fatty tissue. The spermatic cord is formed by the descent of the testis through the abdominal wall. The

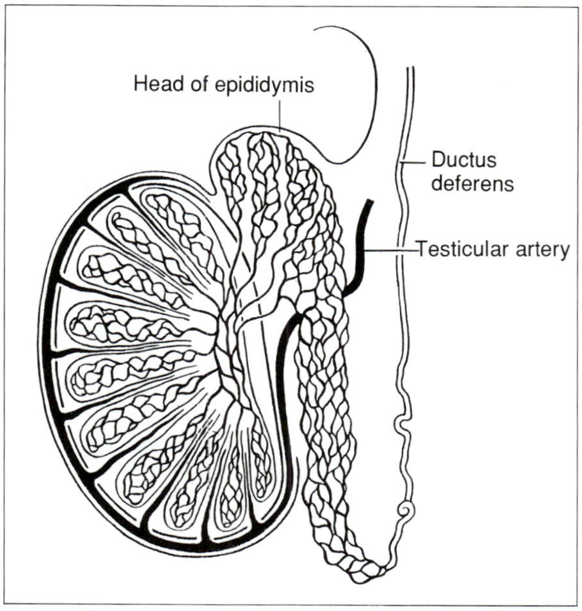

Fig. 13.**1** Schematic drawing of the scrotal contents (modified from Williams [18])

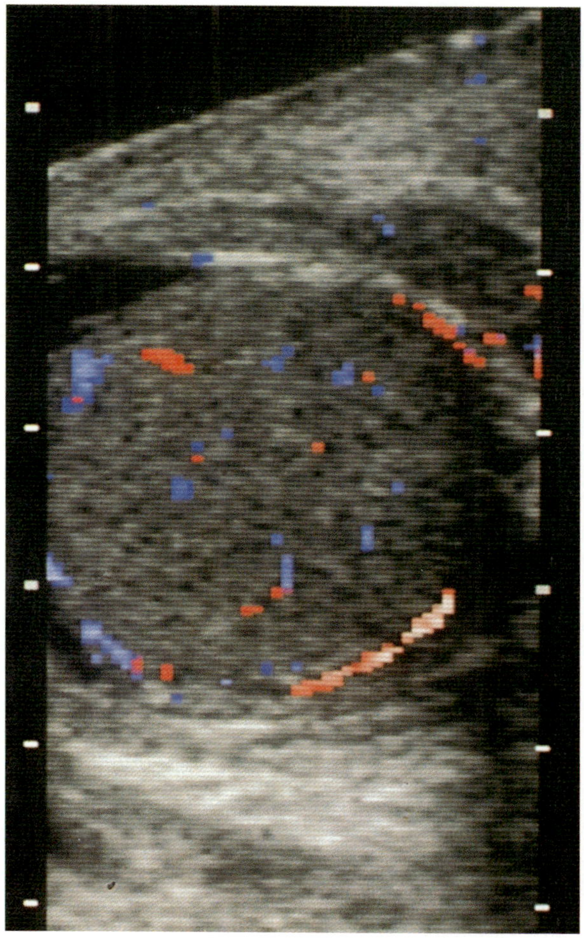

Fig. 13.**2** Transverse CDS scan of a normal testis shows moderate, uniform echogenicity. The vessels encircle the testis like a ring and give off centripetal branches that pass into the parenchyma of the testis (see Fig. 13.**1**)

various structures of the spermatic cord pass together through the inguinal canal and diverge just above the hilum testis (11, 18).

13.2.2 Examination Technique

A synthesis of the history, palpable findings, sonomorphology, and perfusion is essential for the accurate diagnosis of scrotal abnormalities. Diagnosis begins, therefore, with a thorough history and manual examination. For the ultrasound examination, the patient is placed in a relaxed supine position with the legs adducted. In this position the scrotum is easily accessible from the front, the adducted thighs providing a convenient support surface. The patient holds the penis upward against the abdominal wall. Occasionally, as in the search for a varicocele, an upright examination may be performed to supplement the supine examination. The transducer is manipulated with a light, gentle touch, and the patient lies quietly to avoid color artifacts. Sedation may occasionally be required in infants, but generally this can be dispensed with as follows: The child is fasted before it is brought in for examination. The accompanying adult then takes the child into his or her lap and feeds it. The ultrasound contact gel should be warmed so that the child is not frightened or startled. When these precautions are followed, most children can be examined without undue difficulty. The examiner should be comfortably seated and should rest his elbow on the patient's thigh to facilitate precise, gentle handling of the transducer.

In adults, the rugae and pilosity of the scrotal skin cause air trapping that can seriously interfere with the examination. A copious volume of contact gel should be applied, therefore. The transducer operating frequency should be at least 5 MHz, but 7.5 MHz is preferred. For visualization of the scrotal skin, the use of a standoff pad is recommended to improve the definition of superficial structures. The grayscale image is adjusted so that the normal testis displays a homogeneous, moderate echogenicity throughout. Color-encoded flow parameters are adjusted to ensure the detection of slow-moving blood. Especially in examinations of infants, the threshold for color-encoded frequency shifts should be set as low as possible. If a 7.5-MHz transducer is used, the threshold for color encoding should be set so that a frequency shift of 40 Hz is detected (this will display a velocity of 1.4 cm/s at an insonation angle of 72°). One result of this sensitive setting is that even slow movements of the transducer on the skin will produce color-encoded artifacts. The examiner may first try a higher threshold and proceed to the lower threshold if the initial setting fails to demonstrate testicular perfusion.

After the instrument settings have been optimized (see Chapter 4), both testes and epididymides are completely surveyed in longitudinal and transverse planes, and the previous palpable findings are correlated with the ultrasound findings. Both the morphology and the perfusion of the testis and epididymis are evaluated in a side-to-side comparison, maintaining the same instrument settings for both sides. The pampiniform plexus is best evaluated in a longitudinal or transverse scan performed cranial and slightly lateral to the head of the epididymis. After the spermatic cord has been located, the patient is instructed to perform a Valsalva maneuver while the examiner observes the change in the blood flow signals. Again it is advisable to compare the findings with the opposite side. If findings are equivocal, it may also be necessary to image the pampiniform plexus with the patient standing and braced against the examination table. The rest of the examination proceeds as in the supine position. In patients with an indeterminate scrotal mass, the para-aortic region should be examined in the same sitting to exclude lymphoma. The total length of the examination, including the history and palpation, is approximately 15 minutes.

13.2.3 Documentation

Each testis should be separately documented in its greatest longitudinal and transverse dimension. A view of the head of the epididymis should demonstrate the size and position of the epididymis in relation to the testis; this is best accomplished with a longitudinal scan. For side-to-side comparison, both testes should be documented in one transverse view. The pampiniform plexus should be documented during the Valsalva maneuver. A reproducible projection is obtained by defining the upper pole of the testis on the right side of the image and rotating the transducer slightly laterally from the sagittal plane. Pathologic findings are additionally documented in two planes.

13.3 Normal Findings

The testis of the postpubertal male is oval, smoothly demarcated from its surroundings, and displays uniform, medium-level echogenicity throughout its substance. The homogeneous texture of the normal testis is interrupted only by the mediastinum testis, which appears as a narrow, hyperechoic band traversing the long axis of the testis in a slightly off-center position. Additionally, a large vein may occasionally be seen at the border of the testis. The testis has a hypoechoic texture in children and becomes moderately echogenic with sexual maturity (8).

CDS demonstrates flow signals scattered throughout the testis. Aside from larger veins, the vessels producing these signals are too small to be definable in the gray-scale image. The detectable extent of perfusion in the color-encoded flow image depends on the quality of the instrument, the instrument settings, the transducer frequency, and the absorption and scattering of the sound waves in the tissue. As a result, perfusion can be evaluated in qualitative but not quantitative terms. Perfusion abnormalities are recognized by comparison with the opposite side.

The epididymis borders directly on the testis. The testis and epididymis are easily distinguished sonographically by the intervening fibrous sheath. The head of the epididymis covers the upper pole of the testis like a cap. Its greatest diameter ranges from 5 to 12 mm. The body and tail of the healthy epididymis are so slender, however, that they cannot be differentiated from surrounding structures (11). The echogenicity of the epididymis is equal to or slightly greater than that of the testicular tissue (Fig. 13.**2**). Due to its small size, little or no color-encoded flow is visible within the epididymis. The appendices of the testis and epididymis are small and normally are not visualized. The small amount of fluid present in the cavum serosum appears as a narrow, echo-free rim surrounding the testis and epididymis.

The spermatic cord is heterogeneously echogenic and so is difficult to distinguish from surrounding fat in the gray-scale image. The Valsalva maneuver produces a slight longitudinal shift of the structures in the inguinal canal. Normally the vessels of the spermatic cord are too small to be seen in the grayscale image, but perfusion can be appreciated in the color-encoded flow image. The arterial flow signals are synchronous with the pulse, while venous flow signals from the pampiniform plexus are weak, irregular, and show no significant Valsalva response.

13.4 Pathologic Findings

13.4.1 Inflammation

13.4.1.1 Epididymis

Acute epididymitis is the most common disease of the scrotal organs. The patient complains of rapidly increasing pain with swelling of the corresponding hemiscrotum. The severe pain makes scrotal palpation difficult. The degree of the sonographic changes can vary from one site to another. For example, there may be isolated, nonhomogeneous enlargement of the tail of the epididymis while the rest of the epididymis appears normal. Besides enlargement and a mixture of hyperechoicity and hypoechoicity, acute inflammation is associated with a marked increase in perfusion (Fig. 13.**3a**, **b**). If liquefaction occurs in the course of the epididymitis (Fig. 13.**4**), it can be detected early (i. e., before the development of an abscess) by the local absence of perfusion. The inflammation may be

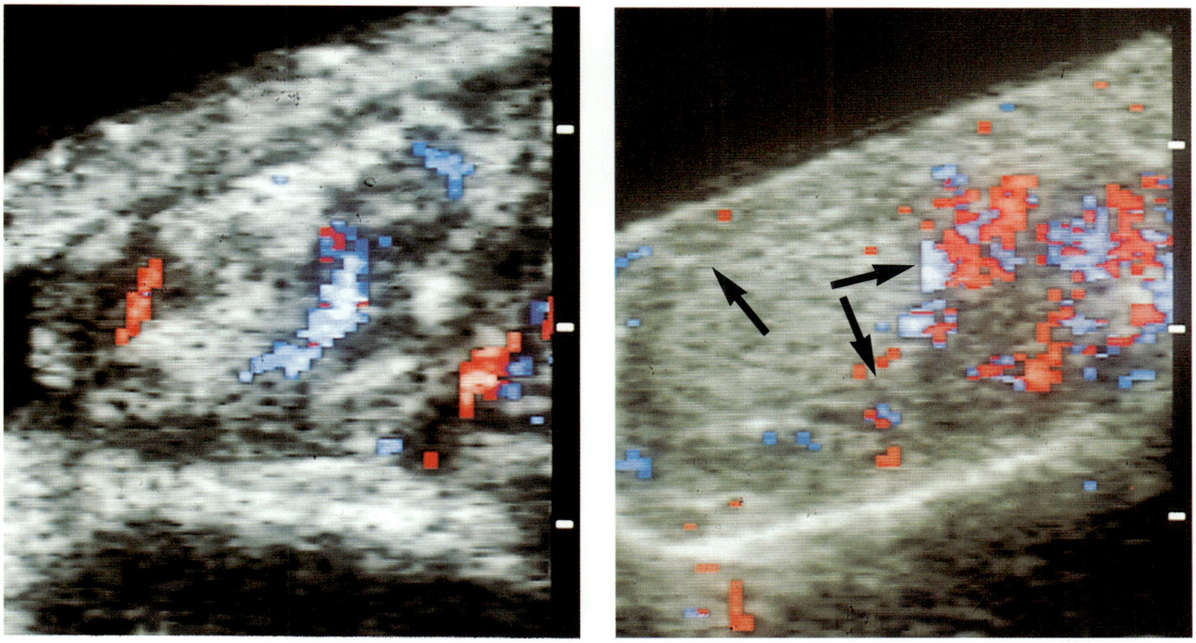

a b

Fig. 13.**3 a, b** Epididymitis

a Longitudinal scan shows significant enlargement of the head of the epididymis with heterogeneous echogenicity and increased perfusion

b Longitudinal scan, the epididymis is generally enlarged with a prominent tail and clear demarcation from the testis (arrows). The tail of the epididymis shows a marked, diffuse increase of perfusion. The testis shows normal echogenicity and normal perfusion

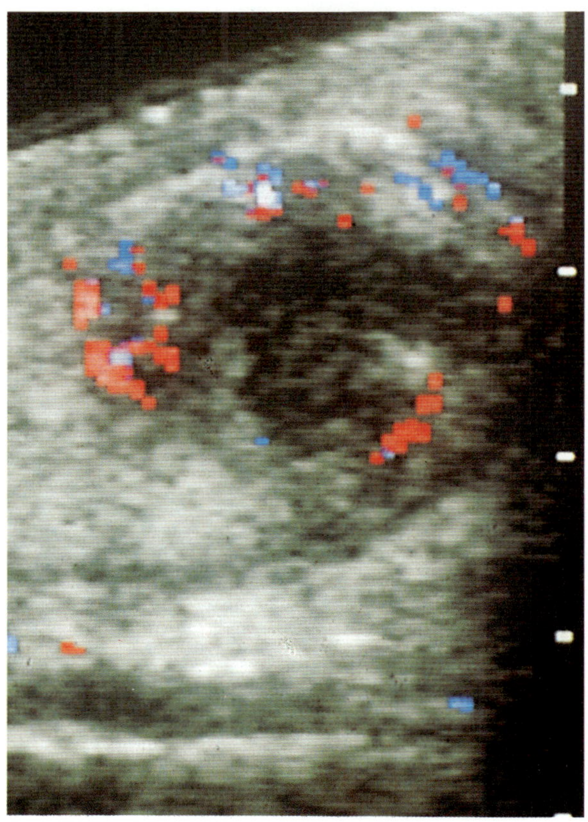

Fig. 13.**4** Abscess following severe epididymitis predominantly affecting the tail of the epididymis. CDS shows significant enlargement of the tail of the epididymis with mixed echogenicity and a central, rounded, almost echo-free structure that shows markedly increased perfusion only at its border

accompanied by a hydrocele (increased fluid in the cavum serosum) and thickening of a scrotal skin. With severe inflammation, increased blood flow can be demonstrated in the thickened scrotal skin. These changes are not specific, however. In most cases the inflammation affects only the epididymis and perhaps portions of the spermatic cord, but concomitant testicular involvement can occur (epididymo-orchitis).

Chronic epididymitis is characterized by persistent bouts of recurring pain. The epididymis is accessible to palpation. Sonography shows slight enlargement of part of the epididymis with a homogeneous or heterogeneous echo pattern and no more than a moderate increase in perfusion (compared with the opposite side).

13.4.1.2 Testis

Isolated orchitis is relatively rare (e. g., as a complication of mumps). Most cases occur as an accompanying feature of epididymitis. The presence of an accompanying orchitis is difficult to establish clinically. Sonography shows an enlarged gland with heterogeneously decreased echogenicity. Comparison with the healthy opposite side makes the extent of the changes clear. As in the epididymis, part or all of the testis may be involved. In these cases differentiation from an underlying testicular tumor is occasionally difficult (serial examinations!). Perfusion in the inflamed areas is diffusely distributed and markedly increased (Fig. 13.**5a**, **b**). The whole testis may exhibit a relatively uniform perfusion increase, or the increases may be localized. As in the epididymis, liquefaction can be detected early by the absence of flow signals.

The sonographic features of the testis may return to normal following a bout of acute orchitis. In other cases the testis remains hypoechoic but returns to a normal size. Severe orchitis may lead to testicular atrophy with replacement of the parenchyma by scar tissue. At ultrasound, the atrophic testis appears markedly smaller than its counterpart and presents a heterogeneous, hypoechoic structure. The perfusion of the affected testis is reduced (always relative to the opposite side). The testis may feel normal or indurated on palpation. Differentiation from a "burned-out" testicular tumor is difficult and must rely on the history and comparison with previous examinations.

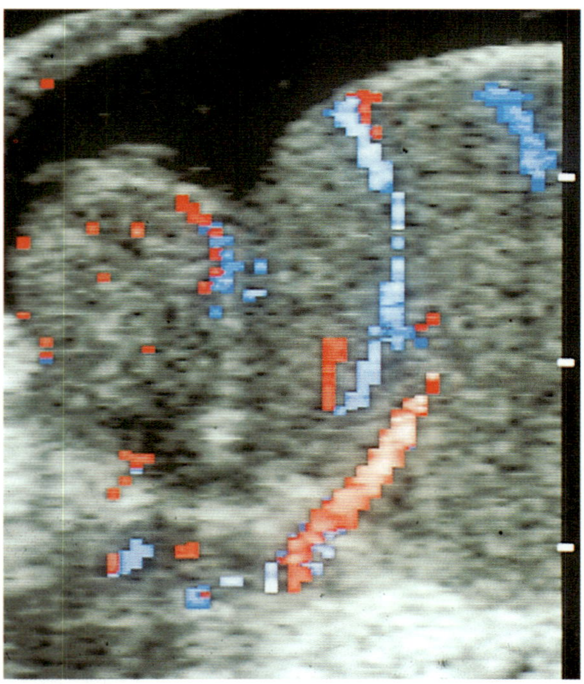
a

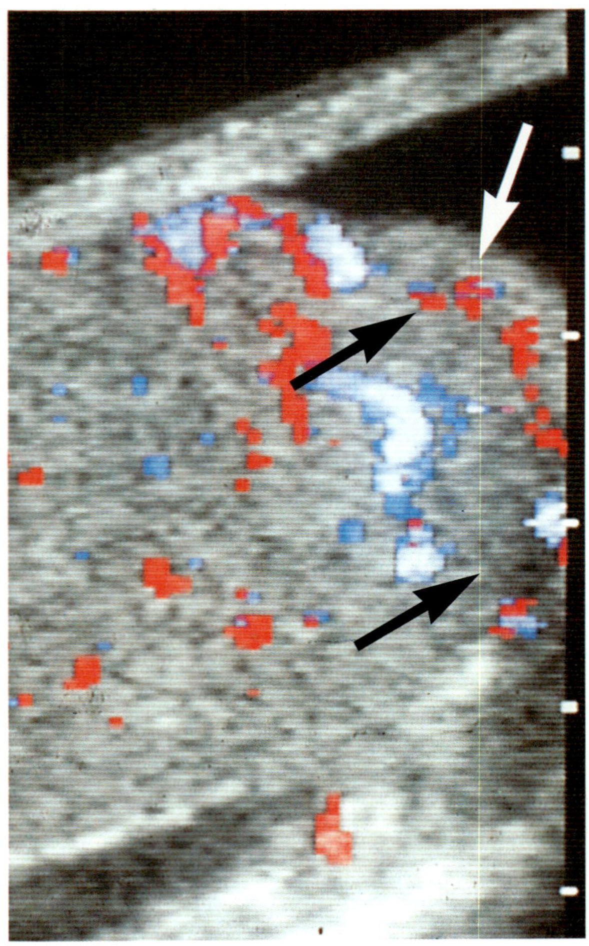
b

Fig. 13.**5a, b** Epididymo-orchitis (two different patients)
a Longitudinal scan of the superior pole of the testis and the head of the epididymis. The enlarged testis and epididymis show mixed echogenicity and increased perfusion. A moderate hydrocele is also present
b Longitudinal scan of the inferior pole of the testis shows mixed echogenicity and an enlarged tail of the epididymis (arrows), which is poorly demarcated from the testis. Increased perfusion is apparent in the testis and epididymis

13.4.2 Tumors

13.4.2.1 Testis

Approximately 95% of intrascrotal tumors are malignant. Almost all of these malignancies are intratesticular (11). With few exceptions, then, every testicular tumor requires histologic evaluation. Testicular tumors may present any conceivable shape on sonographic examination. No correlation can be drawn between sonographic appearance and histologic type. The most common presentation is a solid, uniformly hypoechoic mass that is sharply demarcated from the surrounding testicular tissue. But the tumor may involve the entire gland and may exhibit a combination of solid and cystic elements and calcifications. Tumors in advanced stages may transgress the gland boundaries and infiltrate the epididymis and spermatic cord. The perfusion of testicular tumors is variable. The vascularity may be uniformly or nonuniformly increased, or it may be reduced. Malignant and benign tumors exhibit no specific pattern of vascularity. Neither the sonographic features nor the perfusion pattern are useful for the benign/malignant differentiation of testicular tumors (4). The major value of ultrasound lies in its ability to discriminate between intratesticular and extratesticular lesions.

Other intrascrotal masses are intratesticular cysts and tunica albuginea fibrosis. Nonpalpable, smoothly marginated, homogeneously echo-free masses that abut on the tunica albuginea or mediastinum testis and do not disturb the surrounding tissue are regarded as benign testicular cysts. Biopsy is unnecessary in such cases, and surveillance is adequate (7). Fibrosis of the tunica albuginea may be secondary to trauma or inflammation. The lesions are palpable as circumscribed, approximately lentil-sized, firm, nontender nodules on the surface of the testis. Often these lesions can be seen sonographically only when imaging is assisted by palpation. The definite absence of a structural abnormality in the testis must be confirmed before tunica albuginea fibrosis is diagnosed.

13.4.2.2 Epididymis

Tumors of the epididymis are very rare (11). The benign adenomatoid tumor is the most common epididymal neoplasm. Its usual site of occurrence is the tail of the epididymis. Palpation reveals a firm, essentially nontender mass. CDS shows a rounded, well-demarcated lesion that usually shows a nonuniformly decreased echogenicity and a diffusely distributed, moderately increased perfusion (compared with the normal epididymis). This increased perfusion serves to differentiate the lesion from a sperm granuloma or chronic granulomatous inflammation, which have similar sonographic features but do not exhibit increased blood flow.

13.4.3 Acute Scrotum

"Acute scrotum" is a collective term applied to any scrotal pain of acute onset, possibly accompanied by swelling and erythema. This is not a specific disease entity but a symptom complex. The main importance of acute scrotum is that it calls for prompt action to exclude a disorder that would necessitate surgery. The possible causes of acute scrotum include testicular torsion, hydatid torsion, epididymitis or epididymo-orchitis, acute hydrocele, a strangulated hernia, an abscess, or traumatic testicular rupture (11, 16). In many cases these disorders cannot be differentiated on the basis of the history, clinical presentation, and laboratory studies.

13.4.4 Testicular Torsion

Testicular torsion refers to the twisting of the testis and epididymis about their longitudinal axis, causing occlusion of the efferent and/or afferent blood vessels with consequent ischemia. Testicular torsion may be intravaginal or extravaginal. The more common intravaginal type is most prevalent between 12 and 16 years of age. Supravaginal torsion, in which the vessels are occluded at the level of the external inguinal ring, is most commonly reported in newborns (11, 16). Regardless of type, ultrasound demonstrates a homogeneous or nonhomogeneous hypoechoic enlargement of the testis and epididymis, similar to the changes seen in epididymo-orchitis. There may be associated hydrocele formation and thickening of the scrotal skin. Thus, in the acute stage, the gray-scale image alone cannot differentiate testicular torsion from inflammation. If the torsion is several days old, evidence of necrosis or secondary hemorrhage may be apparent in the B-mode image. Necrosis presents as a mildly tender, nonhomogeneously hypoechoic to echo-free mass in the testis, while hemorrhage typically appears hyperechoic. Testicular torsion can be excluded in the gray-scale image only if pathologic changes are confined to the epididymis (signifying epididymitis), and the testis is completely normal (compared with the opposite side!). But if changes are noted in both the testis and epididymis, torsion cannot be ruled out on the basis of sonomorphologic features.

With a fresh testicular torsion (less than 1 hour old), CDS demonstrates an absence of blood flow in both the testis and epididymis. This is the essential criterion for differentiating testicular torsion from epididymitis, in which blood flow is increased. If perfusion is not detected with the standard settings, the instrument should be set to the lowest possible threshold for color-encoded flow detection. If blood flow still is not detected and morphologic changes are noted in the testis and epididymis, the diagnosis of torsion is considered to be established (Table 13.**1**). Reexamination several hours later will show increased perfusion in the peritesticular tissue and especially in the scrotal skin (Fig. 13.**6a–c**). This increased blood

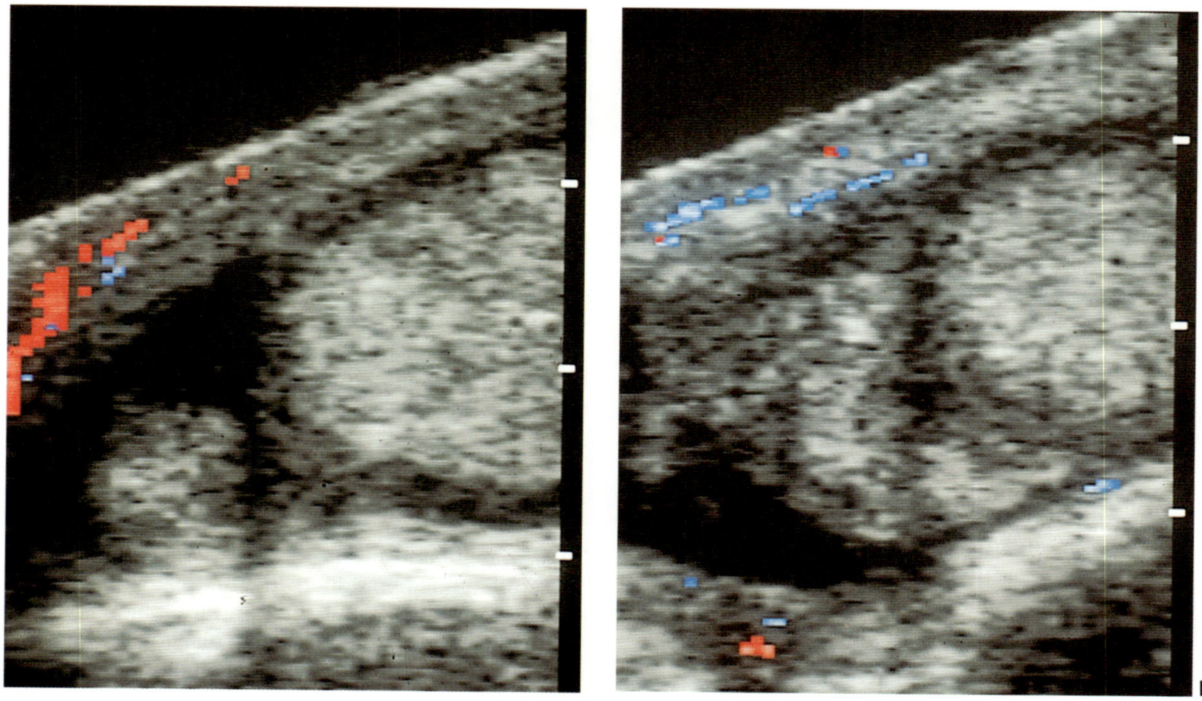

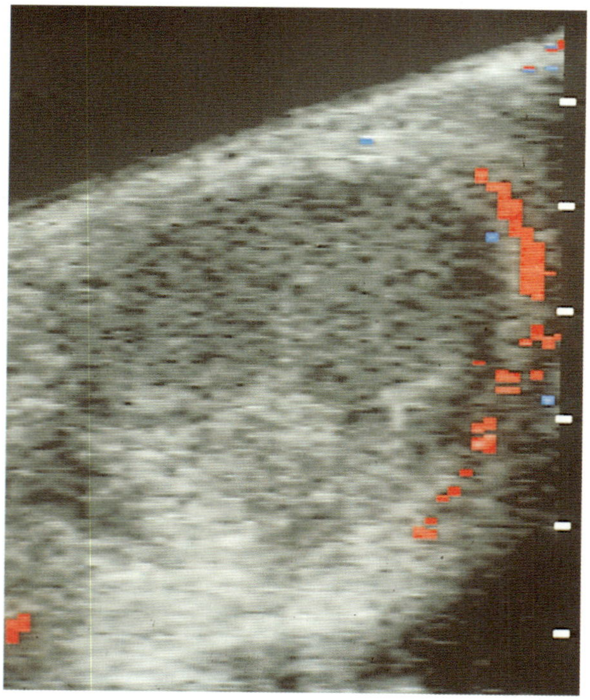

Fig. 13.**6a–c** Testicular torsion (three different patients)
a Longitudinal scan through the head of the epididymis and the superior pole of the testis. The epididymis is moderately enlarged and shows, together with the testis, an inhomogeneous echogenicity. Perfusion is not detected in the epididymis or testis, but flow signals (red) are detected in the moderately thickened scrotal skin
b The head of the epididymis is markedly enlarged, and the epididymis and superior pole of the testis (right side of image) show mixed echogenicity. Perfusion is detected only in the scrotal skin (blue)
c The testis in transverse section displays a nonhomogeneous, partially increased echogenicity with no evidence of intratesticular perfusion. Blood flow is detected only in the paratesticular tissue (red)

flow in the scrotal skin is fairly characteristic of torsion, through it may also occur in severe epididymitis (in which case the associated increase in epididymal perfusion is an aid to differentiation). Peritesticular flow increases with the duration of ischemia. After several days have passed, these vessels may be found supplying a small amount of flow to the outer portions of the testis. This "neovascularization" is always confined to isolated, peripheral portions of the testis and should not be confused with the increased blood flow evoked by inflammation. Thus, testicular torsion can be diagnosed with high confidence based on the combined evaluation of morphology and perfusion.

Besides complete testicular torsion, which generally is easy to recognize and is associated with an absence of perfusion, intermediate stages can occur that require a differentiated assessment. "Partial torsion" is associated with incomplete vascular occlusion and

Table 13.**1** Comparison of the ultrasound morphology and perfusion of the testis and their importance in the diagnosis of acute testicular torsion: − = testicular torsion unlikely, + = testicular torsion possible or certain, (+) = possible torsion with spontaneous lysis, 0 = faulty instrument setting

Morphology	Perfusion: Normal	Increased	Diminished	Absent
– Normal	−	(+)	0	0
– Enlarged	−	−	+	+
– Homogeneous	−	−	+	+
– Nonhomogeneous	−	−	+	+

may compromise the artery and vein in different degrees. The clinical symptoms are similar to those of complete torsion. Sonography may show only subtle changes in the testis and epididymis. Diagnosis relies mainly on a side-to-side comparison of blood flow, CDS demonstrating a decreased testicular and epididymal flow on the affected side. Isolated occlusion of the vein is associated with marked testicular enlargement and weak arterial signals at the immediate subcapsular level. These findings necessitate surgical exploration.

Torsion with spontaneous detorsion is even more difficult to diagnose. There is the usual sudden onset of severe scrotal pain, but the complaints improve or resolve completely by the time of examination. Sonography demonstrates minimal or no morphologic abnormalities, but increased perfusion is noted on the affected side (relative to the opposite side!). This increased blood flow represents a reactive hyperemia evoked by the previous perfusion deficit.

13.4.5 Appendiceal Torsion

Appendiceal torsion is most prevalent during puberty. The pain is variable in degree but may be quite severe. Often there are no palpable abnormalities, especially when symptoms first appear. Occasionally a small blue nodule may be visible through the scrotal skin (representing the twisted adnexa). Palpation becomes difficult within a few hours due to secondary changes such as hydrocele formation. CDS imaging demonstrates normal morphology and perfusion of the testis and epididymis. The twisted appendices may occasionally be demonstrable in the symptomatic hydrocele. Scans show a pedunculated, hyperechoic structure adjacent to the testis or epididymis. The mass usually measures up to 1 cm in its greatest longitudinal dimension and shows no evidence of perfusion. The primary task of CDS in these cases is the exclusion of testicular torsion.

13.4.6 Testicular Trauma

Palpation following testicular trauma (intrascrotal hemorrhage, swelling, severe pain) is not helpful for evaluating the condition of the testis. Some types of trauma (e. g., crushing of the testis against the pubic bone) cause tearing of the tunica albuginea that may extend to involve the parenchyma. The hemorrhage and edema lead to a pressure increase causing extrusion of the testicular parenchyma through the tunica rupture. Early diagnosis is necessary in order to salvage the testis. Knowledge of the extent and location of the rupture and hematoma and the perfusion of the fragments is necessary for optimum treatment planning. Sonographic examination of testicular rupture shows an interruption of the parenchyma by a structure of high or low echogenicity (due to hemorrhage). The interruption may be partial or complete, and fragmentation of the testis may be present in very severe cases. Even moderate intrascrotal hemorrhage following a rupture can compromise the perfusion of the remaining testicular tissue. In these cases as in testicular torsion, CDS can differentiate the perfused and nonperfused areas (Fig. 13.**7**). This is particularly helpful in the follow-up of conservatively managed cases.

13.4.7 Varicocele

Varicocele is the most common treatable cause of male infertility. The lesions represent a dilatation of the veins of the pampiniform plexus and most commonly occur on the left side. The cause of idiopathic varicocele is unknown, and several causes have been postulated: absent or incompetent valves in the testicular vein, entry of the left testicular vein into the renal vein at a hemodynamically unfavorable 90° angle, and compression of the left renal vein between the aorta and superior mesenteric artery with damming back of blood into the testicular vein.

Besides grading severity, contrast venography can assign varicoceles to one of five types (14) based on the course of the testicular vein in the retroperitoneum (cranial to the internal inguinal ring). This classification has been used in the past as a means of selecting patients for sclerotherapy. The various groups cannot be distinguished sonographically, but this is unnecessary for two reasons: First, the purpose of CDS is simply to diagnose the varicocele. Regardless of the varicocele type, this finding has therapeutic implications in terms of selecting sclerotherapy or surgery. Second, the five-part classification of varicoceles was introduced at a time when sclerotherapy was applied to the superior portion of the testicular vein (14). But with modern coaxial catheter systems, the testicular vein can be catheterized to its point of entry into the internal inguinal ring. Injecting the agent at that site will sclerose all the accompanying veins, regardless of the course of the retroperitoneal portions of the vein (3, 5). Thus the traditional classification of varicoceles is obsolete, and the ability to

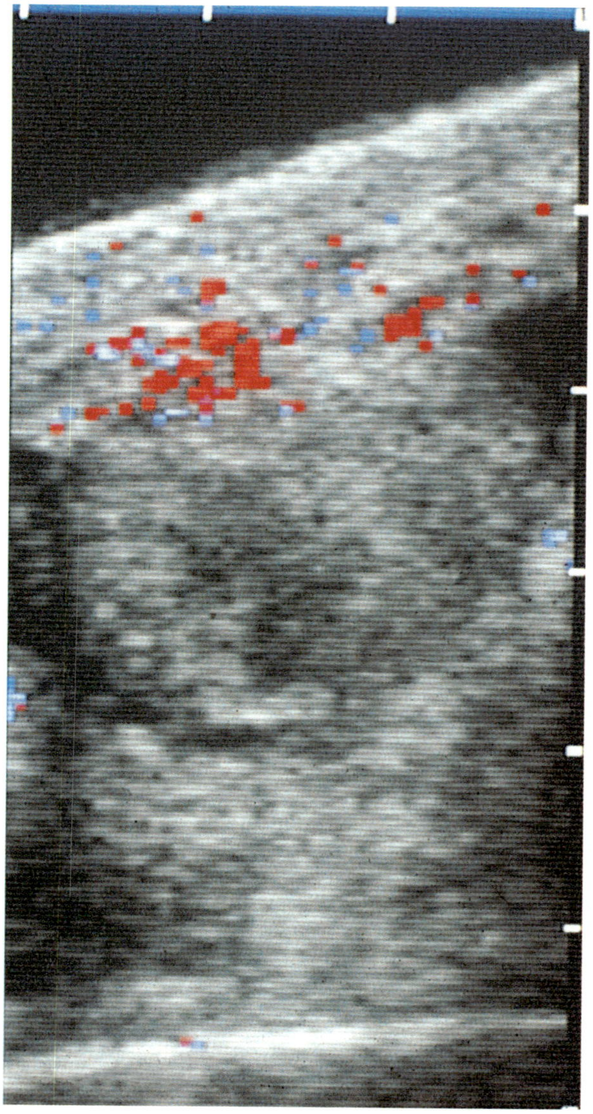

Fig. 13.**7** Transverse scan of an avascular testis following trauma and rupture of the tunica albuginea and the testicular parenchyma shows a nonhomogenous hypoechoic structure in the testis (rupture with hemorrhage) with no evidence of perfusion. Increased perfusion is apparent in the scrotal skin (red and blue)

catheterize the testicular vein is the only question that needs to concern the therapist.

It has been reported that even mild "subclinical" varicoceles can produce an abnormal semen analysis. Subclinical varicoceles are also referred to as "functional varicoceles" (11), i. e., varicoceles that are not palpable and can be detected only by methods such as sonography and venography.

Varicoceles rarely cause complaints aside from occasional pain on standing and after exertion. Their clinical significance lies in their potential for causing infertility. Larger varicoceles reportedly can cause developmental abnormalities of the testis, and prophylactic therapy (with corresponding follow-up) has been advocated in children. A simple, reliable, and noninvasive diagnostic method is desirable, therefore.

Symptomatic varicoceles result from obstruction of the testicular vein or renal vein. The most common obstructive lesion is a renal tumor. Especially in patients with varicoceles of sudden onset and spontaneous reflux in a relaxed resting position, the sonographic workup should include an examination of the kidneys.

With idiopathic varicocele, the veins of the pampiniform plexus are distended. Sonographic criteria support a diagnosis of varicocele when the caliber of the veins is greater than 2 mm at rest and increases when the patient stands upright or performs a Valsalva maneuver (6). This definition covers only pronounced varicoceles, however, and troublesome "subclinical varicoceles" are not diagnosed. CDS can detect varicoceles using the same criterion applied in contrast venography: retrograde blood flow in response to a Valsalva maneuver. In the supine position and during quiet respiration, CDS shows only isolated flow signals in the veins of the pampiniform plexus. When any degree of varicocele is present, retrograde blood flow can be demonstrated at the very start of the Valsalva maneuver (Fig. 13.**8a**, **b**). The veins return to their initial state at the completion of the maneuver. In some patients a slight longitudinal displacement of the spermatic cord occurs at the start of the Valsalva maneuver. If this movement exceeds a certain velocity, it will produce color encoding that may be mistaken for varicocele. Generally this movement is very brief, however. In doubtful cases it is helpful to compare the findings with the opposite side (no retrograde blood flow during the Valsalva maneuver) or repeat the examination in the standing position. Standing usually accentuates the varicocele, making it easier to detect.

CDS is also useful for follow-up after caudal sclerotherapy (sclerosant applied at the level of the internal inguinal ring). This treatment may be followed by thrombosis of the veins of the pampiniform plexus. All the veins appear distended and hypoechoic in the gray-scale image. If varicocele persists due to incomplete sclerosis, the color-encoded flow image makes it easy to distinguish thrombosed from nonthrombosed veins. However, it has to be remembered that CDS displays only the perfusion in the pampiniform plexus and does not give information about the quality of the semen. There is only a limited correlation between the posttherapeutic semen analysis and the diagnosis of a persistent successfully treated varicocele (2).

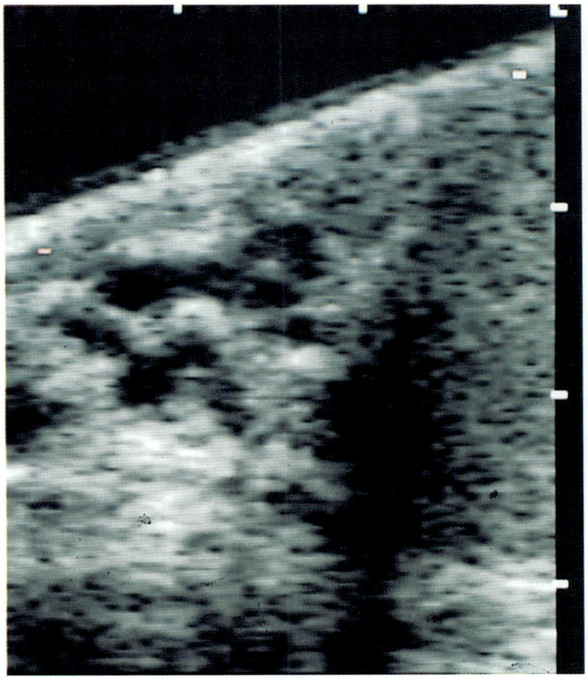

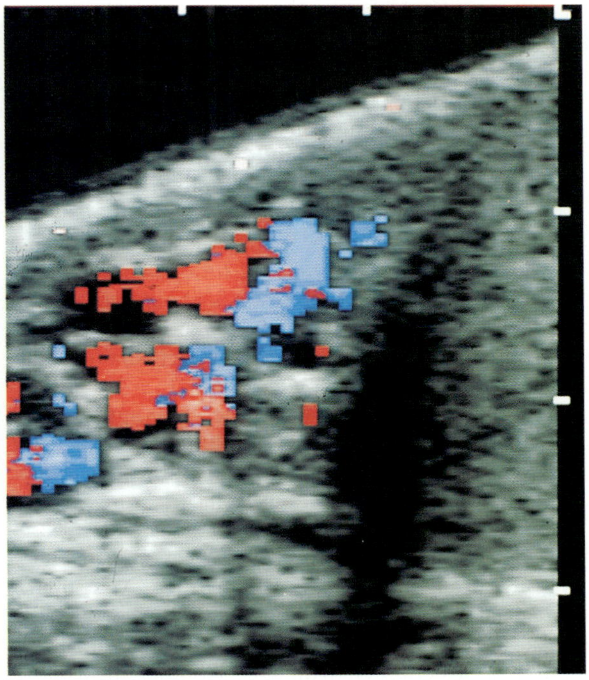

Fig. 13.**8a, b** Longitudinal scan through the upper pole of the testis (right side of image) in a patient with varicocele **a** During normal respiration the veins of the pampiniform plexus are dilated and tortuous and show almost no evidence of flow

b The Valsalva maneuver evokes marked retrograde flow in the veins (red and blue). This typical phenomen of retrograde flow during the Valsalva maneuver is displayed even in small "subclinical" varicoceles

13.5 Diagnostic value of Color Duplex Sonography in Relation to other Diagnostic Procedures

Ultrasound is the method of choice for scrotal examinations when correlated with the history and palpable findings. The following are the indications for the use of scrotal ultrasound (after [11]):

- Indeterminate scrotal mass (identifying the mass as testicular or epididymal, solid or cystic)
- Scrotum that cannot be examined by palpation (e. g., due to hydrocele or severe pain)
- Suspicion of testicular tumor (e. g., in gynecomastia or retroperitoneal lymphomas of undetermined nature, carcinophobia)
- Localization of undescended testis
- Follow-up of severe inflammation (check for abscess formation)
- Testicular trauma
- Suspected testicular torsion
- Diagnosed of varicoceles

It is important to consider the particular indications in which information on perfusion (i. e., the use of CDS imaging) is necessary in reaching a diagnosis. A morphologic (gray-scale) examination is sufficient for evaluating or localizing a scrotal mass. A knowledge of perfusion does not contribute to the differentiation of testicular tumors (4, 10). Nor is vascularity a significant concern in the localization of undescended testes. Thus, CDS does not have a significant role in the first four indications listed above.

Blood flow imaging is essential, however, in patients with severe testicular trauma or suspicion of testicular torsion. The perfusion status in these cases must be known in order to make an accurate diagnosis, and CDS imaging offers an alternative to surgical exploration (1, 4, 12). It is the only method that permits an accurate, noninvasive assessment of testicular and peritesticular perfusion. To avoid misinterpretation, it is again emphasized that CDS can provide a qualitative but not a quantitative assessment of blood flow. Consequently, perfusion is always evaluated in comparison with the unaffected side. This is important especially in cases of partial torsion and torsion with spontaneous detorsion. Here the diagnosis is only possible by combining and comparing the morphologic findings and the perfusion status of both testicles. The relatively low sensitivity in diagnosing a testicular torsion reported in some publications (e. g. 13, 15, 17) could be due to examining only the affected testicle without comparing the result with the scrotal contents of the contralateral side. In addition, it is essential to remember that an adequate examination of the scrotal contents in a case of suspected testicular torsion requires the use of a transducer frequency of at least 7.5 MHz. This is especially true for the examination of infants and children. To display the very slow blood movement in the small testicles of these patients, the CDS machine has to be adjusted to its highest flow encoding sensitivity, and the examination must be performed with the utmost skill .

An alternative diagnostic modality in patients with suspected testicular torsion is radionuclide imaging. But this procedure has several disadvantages compared with CDS: It is relatively time-consuming (the warm ischemia time of the testis is about two hours!), provides only indirect visualization of flow (testicular and peritesticular flow are indistinguishable), and does not display morphologic details (e. g., an abscess and chronic torsion have much the same appearance). Radionuclide scanning also involves a small degree of radiation exposure. CW Doppler ultrasound can be used in the acute scrotum, but it likewise provides no morphologic information. An absence of detectable flow on examination of the spermatic cord is suggestive of torsion, but our experience with CDS scanning indicates that torsion is followed rather early by an increase in peritesticular flow. The source of this flow cannot be ascertained with CW Doppler ultrasound. Nor can this method detect partial testicular torsion (11). Conventional duplex scanning provides a combination of morphologic and flow information, but frequency shifts can be sampled from only one site in the gray-scale image. Given the small size of the blood vessels, the sample volume would have to be slowly advanced through the region of interested until a flow signal is detected. In practice, orchitis can be detected by this method under favorable conditions, but an absence of perfusion cannot be diagnosed with the necessary confidence.

An abscess that forms in the setting of severe epididymitis or epididymo-orchitis is detectable by gray-scale imaging. But the color-encoded flow image can establish the diagnosis earlier by demonstrating an absence of perfusion during initial liquefaction (Table 13.**2**; [4, 9]).

Table 13.**2** List of the most common disorders of the scrotal contents: + = additional information on perfusion is important for diagnosis, (+) = additional information on perfusion is of slight importance for diagnosis, – = additional information on perfusion is unimportant for diagnosis

Inflammation epididymis/testis	(+)
Tumor Testis/epididymis	–
Torsion Testicular/appendiceal	+
Trauma	+
Varicocele	+

Varicoceles can be detected by the combined use of telethermography and gray-scale ultrasound (6). Telethermography is very sensitive in detecting the hyperthermia associated with varicocele, but its specificity is low. To exclude inflammation, therefore, it must be supplemented by ultrasound. The advantage of CDS is that it can define the morphology of the scrotal contents while simultaneously displaying typical varicocele-associated changes with a high degree of sensitivity and specificity (4). The same factors that limit the usefulness of CW Doppler and conventional duplex in the acute scrotum also limit their value in the diagnosis of varicoceles.

Sonography is a valuable and now established method for examination of the scrotal contents. For certain inquiries, however, a knowledge of morphologic details must be supplemented by a knowledge of perfusion status. Only CDS can furnish both types of information noninvasively and with acceptable accuracy. CDS is the diagnostic procedure of choice in patients with suspected testicular torsion, severe trauma, or suspicion of varicocele.

13.6 References

1 Burks, D.D., B.J. Markey, T.K. Burkhard, Z.N. Balsara, M.M. Haluszka, D.A. Canning: Suspected testicular torsion and ischemia: evaluation with color Doppler sonography. Radiology 175 (1990) 815–821

2 Cvatanic, O.A., J.J. Cronan, M. Sigman, S.T. Landau: Varicoceles: postoperative prevalence – a prospective study with color Doppler US. Radiology 187 (1993) 711–714

3 Fobbe, F., B. Hamm, R. Sörensen, D. Felsenberg: Percutaneous transluminal treatment of varicoceles: where to occlude the internal spermatic vein. Amer. J. Roentgenol. 149 (1987) 983–987

4 Fobbe, F., P. Heidt, B. Hamm, H.-C. Koennecke, G. Hauck, K.-P. Dieckmann, K.-J. Wolf: Verbesserung der Diagnostik skrotaler Erkrankungen mit der farbkodierten Duplexsonographie. Fortschr. Röntgenstr. 150 (1989) 629–634

5 Gösfay, S.: Untersuchungen der Vena spermatica interna durch retrograde Phlebographie bei Kranken mit Varikozele. Z. Urol. 2 (1959) 105–115

6 Hamm, B., F. Fobbe, R. Sörensen, D. Felsenberg: Varicoceles: combined sonography and thermography in diagnosis and posttherapeutic evaluation. Radiology 160 (1986) 419–424

7 Hamm, B., F. Fobbe, V. Loy: Testicular cysts: differentiation with US and clinical findings. Radiology 168 (1988) 19–23

8 Hamm, B., F. Fobbe: Maturation of the testis: ultrasound evaluation. Ultrasound Med. Biol. (in press)

9 Hostman, W.G., W.D. Middleton, G.L. Melson: Scrotal inflammatory disease: color Doppler US findings. Radiology 179 (1991) 55–59

10 Hostman, W.G., G.L. Melson, W.D. Middleton, G.L. Andriole: Testicular tumors: findings with color Doppler US. Radiology 185 (1992) 733–737

11 Hricak, H., B. Hamm, B. Kimm (Eds.): Imaging of the scrotum. Raven Press (1995) (in press)

12 Middleton, W.D., B.A. Siegel, G.L. Melson, C.K. Yates, G.L. Andriole: Acute scrotal disorders: prospective comparison of color Doppler US and testicular scintigraphy. Radiology 177 (1990) 177–181

13 Pariquin, H.B., S. Yazbeck, B. Trinh, S. Jequier, P.N. Burns, A. Grignom, D. Filitault, L. Garel, J. Dubois: Testicular torsion in infants and children: diagnosis with Doppler sonography. Radiology 188 (1993) 781–785

14 Sigmund, G., H. Gall, W. Bähren: Stop-type and shunt-type varicocels: venographic findings. Radiology 163 (1987) 105–110

15 Steinhardt, G.F., S. Boyarsky, R. Mackey: Testicular torsion: pitfalls of color Doppler sonography. J. Urol. 150 (1993) 461–462
16 Stewart, R., B.A. Caroll: The scrotum. In Rumack, C.M., S.R. Wilson, J.W. Charboneau (Eds.): Diagnostic Ultrasound. Mosby, St. Louis (1991) 565–589
17 Wilbert, D.M., C.W. Schärfe, W.D. Stern, W.L. Strohmaier, K.H. Bichler: Evaluation of the acute scrotum by color coded Doppler ultrasonography. J. Urol. 149 (1993) 1475–1477
18 Williams, P.L., R. Warwick, M. Dyson, L.H. Bannister: Gray's Anatomy, 37th ed. Churchill Livingstone, Edinburgh (1989) 1424

14 Penile Vessels—Erectile Dysfunction

P. Landwehr

14.1 General Remarks

Erectile dysfunction is a common disorder in males. According to a Mayo Clinic estimate, approximately 10 million men in the United States suffer from erectile dysfunction (9, 21). Due to lack of awareness of the physiology and pathophysiology of erection, psychologic factors were long regarded as the main underlying cause of erectile dysfunction. For example, it was assumed for many years that 80–95% of cases of erectile dysfunction had a psychopathologic basis (29, 46). It is only in the last 20 years that intensive research has been done on the physiologic processes involved in penile erection. As more was learned about erectile function and its disorders, it became possible to develop the first effective therapeutic approaches to male impotence. It is believed now that only about 5–15% of cases of erectile dysfunction have a purely psychogenic cause. Even today, however, it is difficult to establish the causes of erectile dysfunction because many cases have a multifactorial etiology, and primary organic erectile disturbances may be compounded by secondary psychologic changes (18).

Most organic cases of erectile impotence are referable to vascular disease. The classic radiographic procedures for the evaluation of vasculogenic impotence are penile angiography (4, 36) and cavernosometry combined with cavernosography (15, 49) assisted by pharmacologically induced penile tumescence. In recent years, Doppler ultrasound techniques combined with pharmacologic tests have gained an established place in the routine evaluation of erectile dysfunction (8, 15, 20, 30, 41, 43). The present chapter deals with the capabilities of CDS in the diagnosis of erectile dysfunction.

14.2 Normal Anatomy, Common Anatomic Variants, Physiology of Erection, and Examination Technique

14.2.1 The Erectile Unit

The "erectile unit" consists of the paired, communicating corpora cavernosa and the corpus spongiosum, which is traversed by the urethra and is expanded at its distal end to form the glans penis. The entire penis is covered by the superficial penile fascia and the deep fascia (Buck fascia, continuous with the inferior fascia of the urogenital diaphragm). The corpora cavernosa are separated from the rest of the penile tissue by the rigid tunica albuginea (Fig. 14.**1**). The base of the penis is fixed to the pubic bone, ischium, and urogenital diaphragm by the ischiocavernosus and bulbospongiosus muscles.

The erectile bodies themselves consist of a network of smooth muscle cells and collagenous connec-

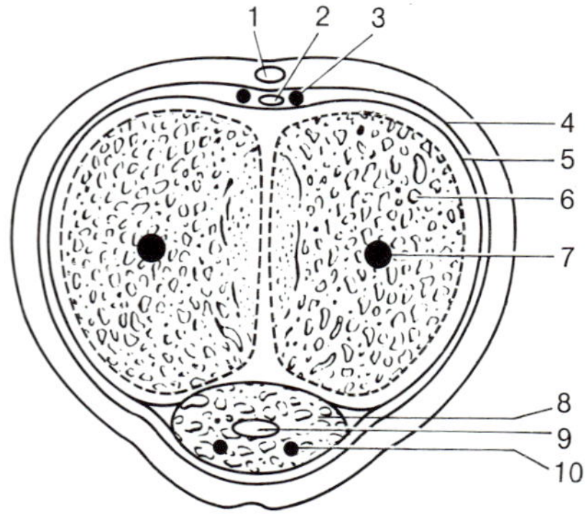

Fig. 14.**1** Normal cross sectional anatomy of the penis. 1 = Dorsal penile vein, 2 = deep dorsal penile vein, 3 = dorsal penile artery, 4 = deep penile fascia, 5 = tunica albuginea of the corpus cavernosum, 6 = corpus cavernosum, 7 = deep penile artery, 8 = corpus spongiosum, 9 = urethra, 10 = urethral artery

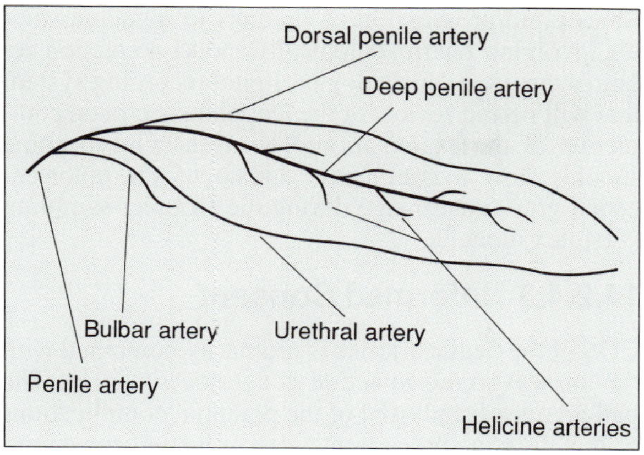

Fig. 14.2 Schematic diagram of the penile arterial supply (on one side)

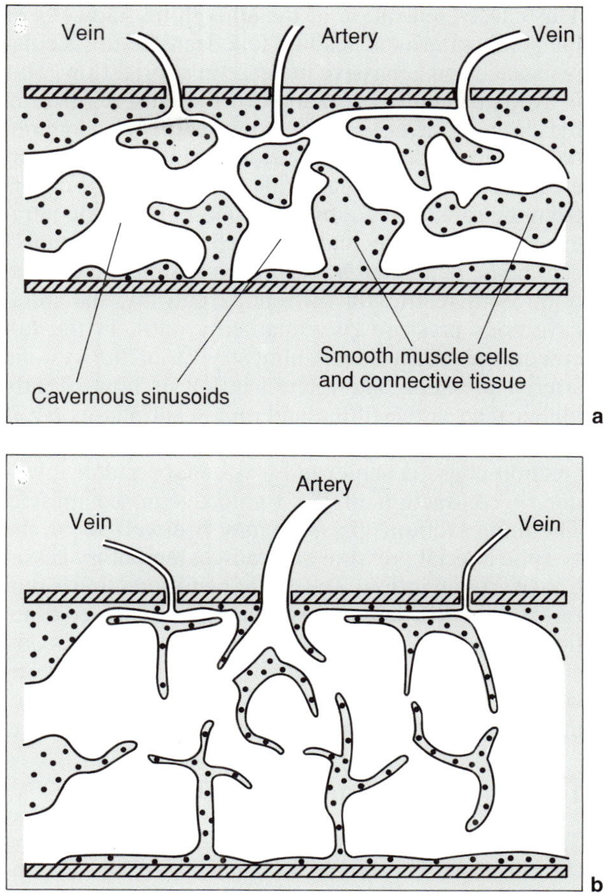

Fig. 14.3a, b Mechanism of erection at the level of the corpus cavernosum (schematic drawing)
a In the flaccid state there is maximum contraction of the sinusoidal muscle cells and free venous drainage from the sinusoids
b Erection is marked by dilatation of the supplying artery and relaxation of the muscle cells. Venous outflow is decreased by expansion of the sinusoids, and the intracavernosal pressure rises

tive tissue permeated by cavernous spaces (Fig. 14.**3a, b**) with an endothelial lining. These "sinusoids" represent active contractile units and are sensitive to neurologic stimuli (1, 28).

14.2.2 Penile Vascular System

The penis is supplied by paired arteries derived from the internal iliac system (Figs. 14.**1**, 14.**2**). The penile artery arises in continuity with the internal pudendal artery. It quickly gives off branches to the bulb of the penis and the corpus spongiosum before dividing into the cavernosal (deep) and dorsal penile arteries. The cavernosal artery supplies the principal erectile body, the corpus cavernosum, through numerous corkscrew-like side branches called the helicine arteries. Interconnecting channels between the corpora cavernosa ensure a uniform arterial inflow. The penile skin and glans are supplied mainly by the dorsal penile artery, which also may send small branches to the corpus cavernosum.

The arterial supply of the penis is subject to numerous variations that do not necessarily compromise perfusion of the erectile tissues. Angiographic studies indicate that the "classic" arterial anatomy is present in only about 40% of cases (4). Possible variants include duplication of the cavernosal artery, anastomoses between the dorsal and cavernosal arteries or between the cavernosal and urethral arteries, intercommunication of both cavernosal arteries, and hypoplasia of the dorsal or cavernosal artery (4, 13). Severe hypoplasia and aplasia are no longer considered normal variants, but pathologic anomalies that underlie primary arteriogenic erectile dysfunction (44).

Venous drainage is accomplished by the deep penile veins and the superficial and deep dorsal veins, which drain into the periprostatic venous plexus and the internal and external pudendal venous system.

The nerve supply of the penis, beyond our present scope, is reviewed in (2).

14.2.3 Physiology of Erection

The process of penile erection can be divided into six phases (2). The flaccid phase (resting phase) is characterized by slight arterial and venous blood flow corresponding to a minimum maintenance flow. In response to cognitive-emotional stimuli, the cavernosal nerves are stimulated in a process mediated by the limbic system and thoracic and sacral erection centers, triggering the release of neurotransmitters (3, 6, 19).

This causes relaxation of the smooth muscle cells of the penile arterioles, leading to a decrease in vascular resistance and a massive increase in arterial flow. This is accompanied by relaxation of the muscle fibers in the corpora cavernosa, creating space to accommodate the increased arterial inflow. This initial phase of erection is called the latent or filling phase. It differs from the subsequent tumescent phase in that the intracavernous pressure remains unchanged. The tumescent phase is marked by penile expansion and elongation. With restriction of venous outflow, the intracavernous pressure rises markedly until, in the full erection phase, it equals almost 90% of the systolic arterial pressure. The arterial inflow is now slightly higher than in the filling and tumescent phases but is markedly higher than in the flaccid state. The rigid erection phase is achieved by voluntary and/or involuntary contraction of the ischiocavernosus muscle. The intracavernous pressure may rise well above the systolic arterial pressure and cause a temporary cessation of arterial inflow. The end of penile erection is represented by the detumescent phase, in which contraction of the smooth muscles around the sinusoids and arterioles restricts the arterial inflow while greatly increasing the venous outflow. This leads to a rapid reduction in penile volume and intracavernous pressure.

14.2.4 Examination Technique

The reader is referred to Chapter 4 for information on the basic techniques and instrument settings for optimum vascular imaging with CDS. The special circumstances of penile arterial examinations are discussed below.

14.2.4.1 Preliminary Studies

Given the frequent multifactorial etiology of erectile dysfunction (ED), the diagnostic evaluation of ED is a multidisciplinary undertaking that can involve the specialties of urology, radiology, internal medicine, neurology, psychiatry, and dermatology (43). The preliminary workup includes a detailed general history with emphasis on risk factors (e.g., drugs, previous surgery and trauma, metabolic disorders, nicotine abuse, neurologic disorders, vascular disorders) and a sexual history. A comprehensive workup includes the clinical examination (e.g., to detect malformations, penile deviations, or absent inguinal pulses) and laboratory tests (e.g., to check for diabetes mellitus or a hormonal disorder). The workup may include measurements of nocturnal penile tumescence and recording of the bulbocavernosus reflex.

14.2.4.2 Instrument Requirements

The penile vessels are best examined with a high-frequency linear-array transducer with a frequency of at least 7 MHz. The low blood flow velocities in patients with arterial insufficiency require the use of an instrument that is sensitive to low flow. The sometimes rapid progression of findings in dynamic studies involving pharmacologically induced erection requires the use of an analog or digital recording system that will permit review of the Doppler spectra on completion of the examination. The ultrasound machine should allow a continuous update of the color-encoded grey scale image during the Doppler-sampling ("Triplex mode").

14.2.4.3 Informed Consent

CDS of the penile arteries is ordinarily combined with the intracavernous injection of a vasoactive drug. The patient must be advised of the potential complications of this invasive procedure and give his informed consent. Pain and a feeling of tension are possible intraprocedural effects that may cause subjective discomfort. But particular emphasis is placed on the potential risks of priapism, hematoma, fibrosis, cardiac complications (e.g., angina pectoris), urethral injury, and infection. The patient should understand that, if priapism occurs, it may conceivably lead to irreversible impotence. He should also be advised of the extremely remote possibility of a lethal outcome of pharmacologically induced tumescence (survey in [33]). Prolonged priapism can be avoided by early therapeutic intervention. The patient must be aware that treatment is necessary if the erection does not subside within 3 hours or if significant pain occurs. Irreversible damage to the erectile bodies has been observed only in cases where priapism persisted longer than 24 hours after the examination (35).

14.2.4.4 Position of the Patient and Examiner

The examination should be performed in a quiet atmosphere that respects the emotionally stressful nature of the situation. The patient is placed in a comfortable supine position. The penis may be examined in a normal resting position, or the dorsum may be held against the abdomen with the ventrum exposed. The examiner sits next to the patient. It may be advantageous to have an assistant present during the examination to help with the injection and record findings. This makes it easier to start the examination immediately after the injection and makes for a more efficient postprocedural evaluation.

14.2.4.5 Examination Protocol

The penile vessels can be scanned from a dorsal (Figs. 14.**4**, 14.**5**) or ventral approach. The ventral approach is advantageous at maximum erection, as it allows the penis to remain in a physiologic position. A lateral approach is useful for demonstrating both cavernosal arteries in the same image (Fig. 14.**6a**).

The examination begins with longitudinal and transverse scans in the flaccid state. The dorsal and cavernosal arteries are first identified at the base of the penis in the color flow image and are tracked distally. A maximum sensitivity setting is used to detect

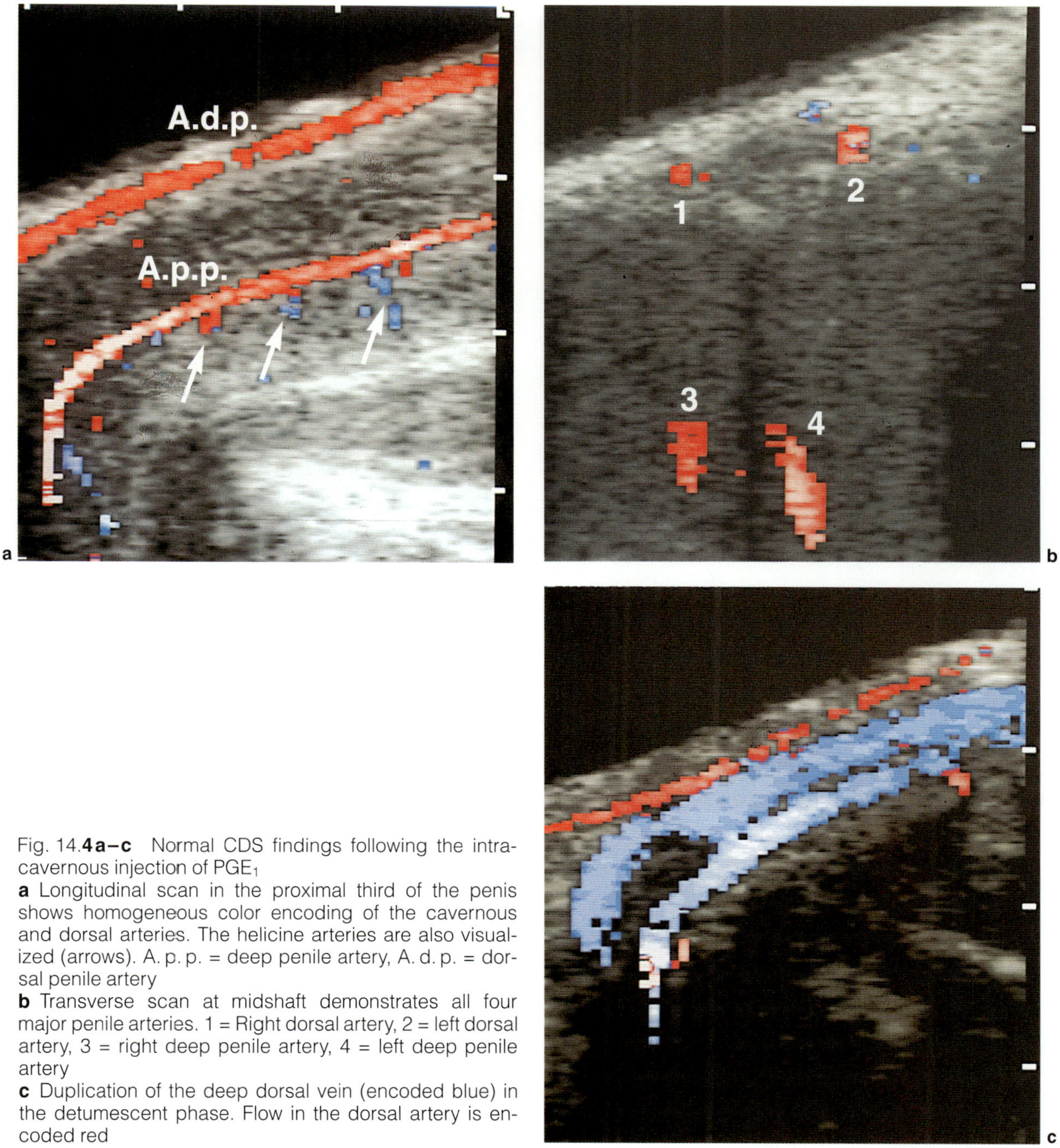

Fig. 14.**4a–c** Normal CDS findings following the intracavernous injection of PGE_1
a Longitudinal scan in the proximal third of the penis shows homogeneous color encoding of the cavernous and dorsal arteries. The helicine arteries are also visualized (arrows). A. p. p. = deep penile artery, A. d. p. = dorsal penile artery
b Transverse scan at midshaft demonstrates all four major penile arteries. 1 = Right dorsal artery, 2 = left dorsal artery, 3 = right deep penile artery, 4 = left deep penile artery
c Duplication of the deep dorsal vein (encoded blue) in the detumescent phase. Flow in the dorsal artery is encoded red

the very low flow in the flaccid penis. Doppler spectra should be recorded from all four penile arteries in a longitudinal scan at the base of the penis. The corpora cavernosa are examined for structural nonhomogeneities and especially for hyperechoic areas (calcification, fibrosis).

After initial scanning, a vasoactive drug is injected into the corpus cavernosum. Erection may be induced with prostaglandin E_1 (PGE_1), papaverine, or a combination of papaverine and phentolamine. Lately PGE_1 has been the agent of choice, especially in Europe, because the intracavernous injection of papaverine or the papaverine–phentolamine mixture is associated with a higher complication rate than PGE_1 (11, 25, 33, 34, 42). This particularly applies to the development of priapism, which is significantly more common after papaverine and its combinations than after PGE_1. The injection of 20 μg PGE_1 in 1 ml of saline solution is recommended as an initial test dose, and 10 μg is considered adequate by some. The US literature as of 1993 still reflects a preference for papaverine injection in the diagnosis and treatment of erectile dysfunction. Most authors recommend an initial test dose of 60 mg (8, 12, 23, 37, 38).

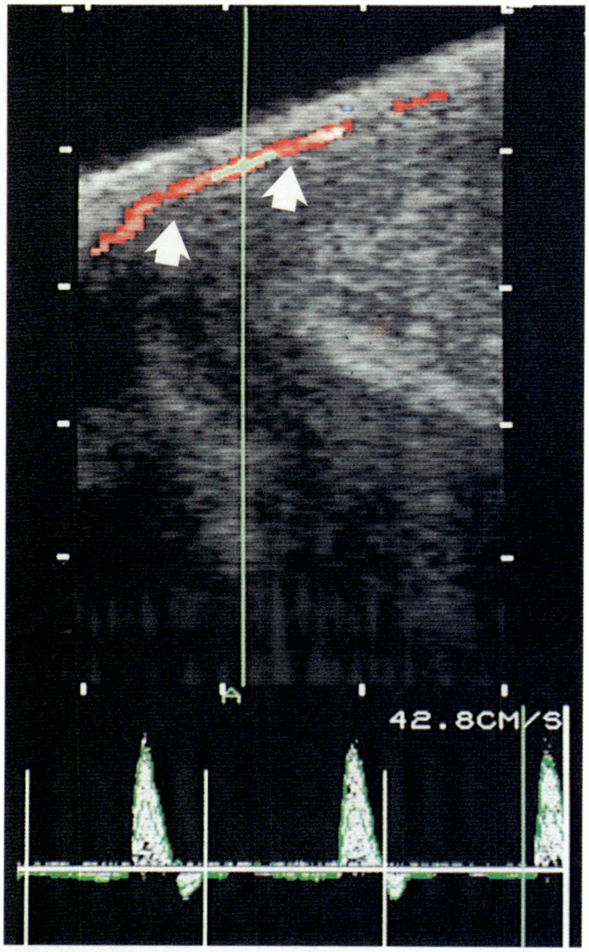

Fig. 14.**5** Longitudinal CDS image of the dorsal penile artery (arrows) and Doppler spectrum show normal features in the full erection phase after the intracavernous injection of PGE_1. Flow direction is from left to right. The spectrum indicates a high peripheral vascular resistance

The drug is injected into the side of the corpus cavernosum using a 26- or 28-gauge needle. A unilateral injection is sufficient owing to the anatomic connections between the corpora. After the injection, the injection site should be briefly compressed, and the patient is instructed to massage the penis briefly at the base using light manual pressure to improve the distribution of the drug.

After the time of the injection is documented, the cavernosal arteries are imaged in longitudinal section, and Doppler spectra are acquired. Spectral recording begins as soon after the injection as possible to trace the dynamics of penile blood flow during the erectile process (Figs. 14.**7b**, 14.**8b**), and additional spectra are recorded at 1-min intervals for 10 min. At that point scanning is repeated at 2-min intervals for a total of 30 min postinjection or until full erection is achieved (12). If a uniform response pattern is noted in both cavernosal arteries during the early phase, the subsequent examination may be limited to one of the arteries. If different patterns are noted, the larger of the two arteries should be examined further, but spectra should still be acquired from the other artery at 5, 10, 20, and 30 min. Because the dorsal arteries are of little primary importance in erection, it is sufficient to sample their spectra at 5, 10, 20, and 30 min. If both cavernosal arteries are occluded, the dorsal arteries should be scanned at more frequent intervals (Fig. 14.**5**).

If the spectral waveform characteristics become constant for a certain period during the tumescent or erection phase, there is time to make a systematic arterial and venous survey in longitudinal and transverse planes, giving particular attention to variants in the course of the vessels, vascular cutoffs, and caliber variations. The presence or absence of flow in the four major arteries should be recorded in the proximal, middle, and distal thirds of the penis. While imaging the arteries, the examiner should check to see whether the large venous vessels (dorsal veins) are visualized (Fig. 14.**4c**). It is unnecessary to record spectra from the penile veins.

If marked tumescence is achieved 10–15 min after the injection but a rigid erection does not occur, the examiner should briefly interrupt the examination and leave the patient alone for several minutes. It has been our experience that this brief recess can often relieve the psychogenic inhibition of full erection that commonly affects younger males under the intimidating conditions of the examination. Additionally, there

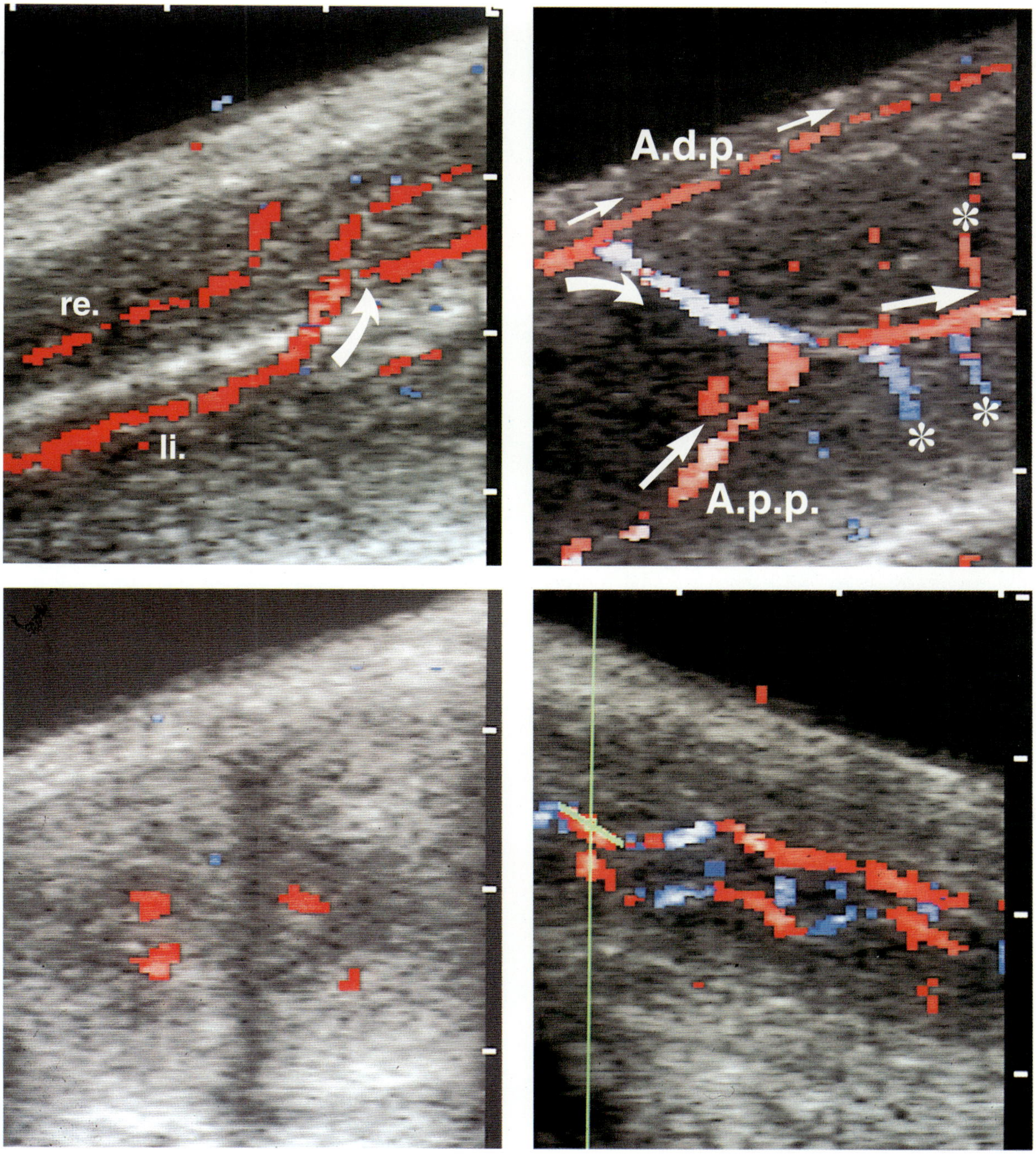

Fig. 14.**6 a–d** Variants of the penile arteries

a Longitudinal scan from the right side demonstrates hypoplasia of the right cavernosal artery (re.) with termination of the color-encoded lumen in the middle third of the penis. A very large-caliber left cavernosal artery (li.) is seen crossing the intercavernous septum (arrow)

b Communication (curved arrow) between the dorsal penile artery (A. d. p.) and deep penile artery (A. p. p.). Large-caliber helicine arteries (asterisks) are also seen. Straight arrows = flow direction in the dorsal penile artery and deep penile artery

c Transverse scan at midpenis shows duplication of the cavernosal artery. Signals are displayed from four arterial vessels in the corpora cavernosa, but there is no evidence of perfusion in a dorsal penile artery on either side (aplasia of both vessels?)

d Longitudinal scan in the same patient (see Fig. 14.**6 c**) shows duplication of the cavernosal arteries, which are tortuous and of large caliber

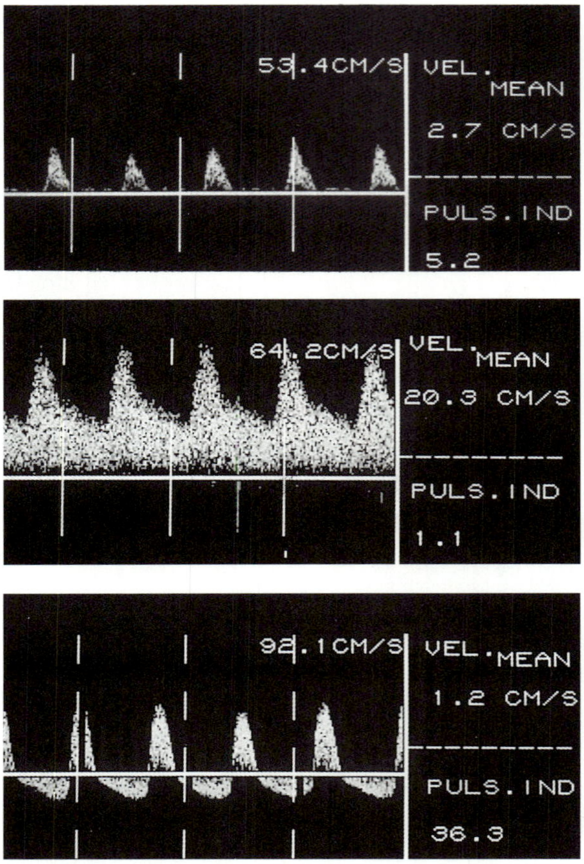

Fig. 14.**7a–c** Doppler spectra in different phases of normal penile erection. Spectra were sampled from the cavernosal artery before and after the intracavernous injection of 10 µg PGE_1

a Spectrum in the flaccid state shows a steep systolic upstroke with a peak velocity of 18 cm/s. There is minimal antegrade flow in diastole (high peripheral vascular resistance, PI = 5.2). The time-integrated mean flow velocity is 2.7 cm/s

b Spectrum in the filling phase at 30 s postinjection shows a rise in the peak systolic velocity to 61 cm/s and pronounced diastolic forward flow reflecting the low peripheral resistance (PI = 1.1). The mean flow velocity is increased to 20.3 cm/s (approximately 7 times the initial value)

c Spectrum in the rigid erection phase at 15 min postinjection shows a decrease in peak systolic velocity to 45 cm/s and significant diastolic reverse flow (peripheral resistance higher than in the flaccid state, PI = 36.3). The integral flow velocity (1.2 cm/s) is less than the resting value, signifying low maintenance flow at maximum erection

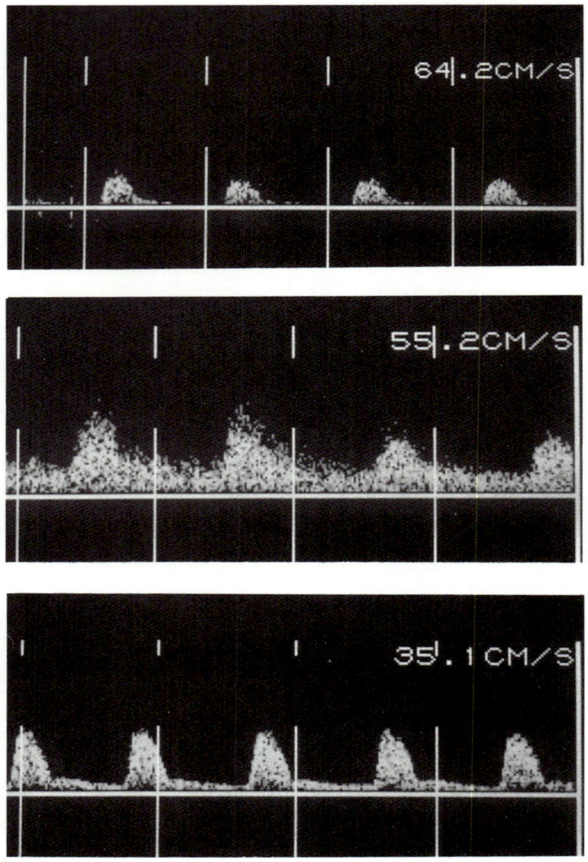

Fig. 14.**8a–c** Doppler spectra recorded in a patient with arteriogenic erectile dysfunction

a Poststenotic spectrum from the left cavernosal artery in the flaccid state before injection of PGE_1 shows a broadened systolic peak with a maximum velocity of 12 cm/s

b Spectrum at 30 s postinjection shows only a moderate rise of peak systolic velocity to 22 cm/s with a decreased peripheral resistance

c At 17.5 min postinjection the peak systolic velocity is still below the 25 cm/s threshold are reports in the literature of using manual, visual, or fantasized erotic stimuli for the augmentation of pharmacologic tumescence (40, 41).

If arterial insufficiency is present, the pelvic arteries should also be examined by CDS (see Chapter 6). Although the internal iliac territory cannot be directly evaluated with CDS, it is possible to detect stenoses or occlusions of the common iliac artery or aorta that may have causal significance in penile arterial insufficiency.

At the end of the examination the patient is again instructed to see a urologist if the erection is painful or persists for more than 3 hours.

Interpretation of the Doppler spectra involves determining the angle-corrected maximum systolic velocity (V_{max}) and minimum diastolic velocity (V_{min}) in the cavernosal arteries. Because the maximum peak systolic velocity and minimum diastolic velocity can occur at different time intervals despite an identical dose of vasoactive drug (12), it is frequently necessary to review the entire videotape record of the examination. This review is facilitated by noting during the examination the time intervals at which the apparent maximum peak systolic velocity and minimum diastolic velocity occurred.

14.2.4.6 Documentation

The diagnostic evaluation of erectile dysfunction relies critically on a complete and detailed record of the changes in penile hemodynamics following injection of the vasoactive drug. Documentation of the spectral traces, especially those acquired from the cavernosal arteries, should begin as soon after the injection as possible and should be repeated at frequent intervals. During later evaluation it should be possible to correlate a particular spectrum with time after injection, so reproducible labeling of specific video segments (vessel, side, time) is essential.

Besides the frequently recorded Doppler spectra described above, the following video documentation should be obtained in the tumescent and erection phases:

- Longitudinal view of the four main arteries
- Transverse views in the proximal, middle, and distal thirds of the penis
- Views of any vascular anomalies or occlusions that are observed

After the spectral evaluation, the following documentation should be obtained for review:

- Longitudinal scan of the four main arteries in the tumescent phase
- Transverse scans in the proximal, middle, and distal thirds
- Scans of any vascular anomalies or occlusions that are observed
- Doppler spectrum from one of the cavernosal arteries at the time of maximum systolic velocity, with documentation of the velocity measurement and time
- Doppler spectrum from one of the cavernosal arteries at the time of minimum diastolic velocity, with documentation of the velocity measurement and time

Written documentation may be freely formulated or entered in a standard report form that includes notation of the measured velocities and drawings of the observed vascular anatomy. The time of occurrence and extent of maximum erection should also be documented.

14.3 Normal Findings

Different spectral waveform characteristics are seen in the different phases of erection. The normal flaccid state is characterized by an "extremity" type of spectral pattern with high pulsatility and low diastolic flow or even brief diastolic flow reversal (Fig. 14.**7a**). The systolic peak is steep and of short duration. There are no normal values of absolute velocity in the resting state, nor is it likely that such values would be determinable or diagnostically useful. Due to the low arterial flow velocities in the flaccid state, CDS imaging often can demonstrate the vessels only at the base of the penis. An apparent absence of blood flow at rest should never be mistaken for a vascular occlusion. The large penile arteries usually take a tortuous course in the flaccid or minimally tumescent penis, and they become straighter as the penis expands and elongates during erection. The helicine arteries generally cannot be visualized in the flaccid state.

The intracavernous injection of a vasoactive drug is followed very rapidly by a dramatic qualitative and quantitative change in penile blood flow. With the progression of peripheral vasodilation, the peripheral resistance falls, arterial inflow greatly increases, and the Doppler spectrum shows a parenchymal type of flow pattern with marked antegrade flow in diastole. Meanwhile the peak systolic velocity increases (Fig. 14.**7b**). This flow pattern is present to varying degrees in the filling and tumescent phases and reflects rapid filling of the cavernosal sinusoids. The penile vessels are demonstrated most clearly by CDS in this phase, because the flow rate is highest (Fig. 14.**4**). Even the helicine arteries can be visualized.

As the intracavernous pressure rises in the late tumescent phase and especially in the full erection phase, the peak systolic velocity remains elevated while the diastolic flow declines and finally assumes negative values in the rigid erection phase, producing maximum pulsatility of the spectral waveform (Fig. 14.**7c**). The intracavernous pressure is maximal at this stage, and there is very little net inflow of blood. CDS imaging of the main arteries demonstrates forward flow in systole and reverse flow in diastole. The helicine arteries are much less prominent than in the tumescent phase.

The detumescent phase is characterized by a marked reduction of arterial inflow and a slight elevation of diastolic flow due to reopening of the venous channels. Normally the larger veins can be identified in the color-encoded flow image (Fig. 14.**4c**).

In most duplex studies performed to date (all using papaverine), a peak systolic velocity of less than 25 cm/s is used as the threshold for diagnosing arterial insufficiency (12, 14, 26, 27, 28, 32). Higher velocities are usually observed in normal populations (e.g., 47 ± 9 cm/s) (7, 8). A minimum diastolic velocity of 5 cm/s has been used in recent studies as the threshold for predicting venous incompetence (12, 37).

The diameter of the penile arteries increases significantly after injection of the vasoactive drug. A caliber increase of approximately 0.6 mm is obtained in healthy subjects (20). The amount of this increase does not appear to hold diagnostic significance, however, and an accurate distance measurement cannot be performed at this scale using conventional 7.5-MHz transducers.

Transient dorsal vein flow can be observed during the initial minutes after the intracorporeal injection. If dorsal vein flow persists for more than 10 min after the initial 5-min postinjection interval, venous leakage is probably present (12).

14.4 Pathologic Findings

14.4.1 Preliminary Remarks

The etiology of erectile dysfunction (ED) is potentially diverse and often multifactorial. Vascular (arterial, venous, or mixed), neurogenic, hormonal, pharmacologic, psychogenic, and anatomic causes have been identified. Vascular disorders represent the most common cause of ED, which is due predominantly to arterial insufficiency in about two-thirds of cases and venous incompetence in the remaining third (48).

Erectile dysfunction may be primary or secondary. Primary ED refers to erectile impotence that has been present since childhood or puberty. A prevalence of 0.4% has been reported in an unselected population of males under 25 years of age (22). Arterial and venous malformations are a frequent cause of primary ED (44).

Secondary ED arises in a patient who has previously had normal erectile function. Any of the factors listed above can have causal significance.

In the sections that follow, we shall focus our attention on arterial and venous causes of ED. In patients with nonvasculogenic ED, all Doppler techniques can do no more than exclude a vascular cause. A specific diagnosis must be established within the framework of a multidisciplinary diagnostic approach.

14.4.2 Erectile Dysfunction Due to Arterial Insufficiency

Deficient arterial perfusion of the penis can have various causes ranging from congenital vascular hypoplasia or aplasia and traumatic vascular lesions to atherosclerosis and its associated risk factors (4, 5).

The arterial obstruction leading to ED may be located anywhere in the vessels supplying the penis or within the penis itself. Stenoses and occlusions at any level from the aorta and iliac arteries to the pudendal artery and individual penile arteries can produce basically the same symptoms. But as elsewhere in the circulation, stenoses and occlusions can evoke the development of collateral systems that can functionally compensate for the obstructive lesion. For example, a unilateral stenosis of the common iliac artery would not be expected to produce ED with an otherwise intact arterial system. However, bilateral pudendal artery stenosis would be very likely to produce arteriogenic ED due to an inherent lack of collateral capacity at that level. All Doppler-based techniques, including CDS, can only evaluate arterial perfusion in the target organ, which represents the net result of the original circulation plus the collateral channels. Even if occlusive lesions are demonstrated at the penile level, there may be a coexisting proximal arterial obstruction.

Occlusions and positional anomalies of the penile arteries are easily detected with CDS after pharmacologic stimulation (Fig. 14.**6a–d**). Perfusion deficits exhibit an abnormal pattern that is particularly well documented by Doppler frequency analysis. The maximum systolic velocity shows a significantly smaller increase after the injection than in normal subjects (Figs. 14.**8a–c**, 14.**9b**). A value of 25 cm/s is consistently reported for the peak systolic velocity threshold (7, 12, 14, 26–28, 32). Experience has shown that it is not sufficient to acquire velocity data during the first 5 min after the injection (8, 26, 37) or at a time based on the clinical progression of tumescence and rigidity (31, 41). Only about 75% of patients achieve their peak systolic velocity during the first 5 min after injection of the vasoactive drug. While normal subjects show only slight velocity differences between both cavernosal arteries, a discrepancy of more than 10 cm/s between the cavernosal arteries is believed to indicate incipient arterial insufficiency (8).

All the studies cited above used papaverine or a papaverine–phentolamine mixture for induction of tumescence. Threshold values for intracavernous PGE_1 have not yet been published.

14.4.3 Erectile Dysfunction Due to Venous Incompetence (Venous Leakage)

Rigid erection is made possible by the effective restriction of venous outflow from the penis. It also requires maximum, unimpaired arterial inflow and maximum

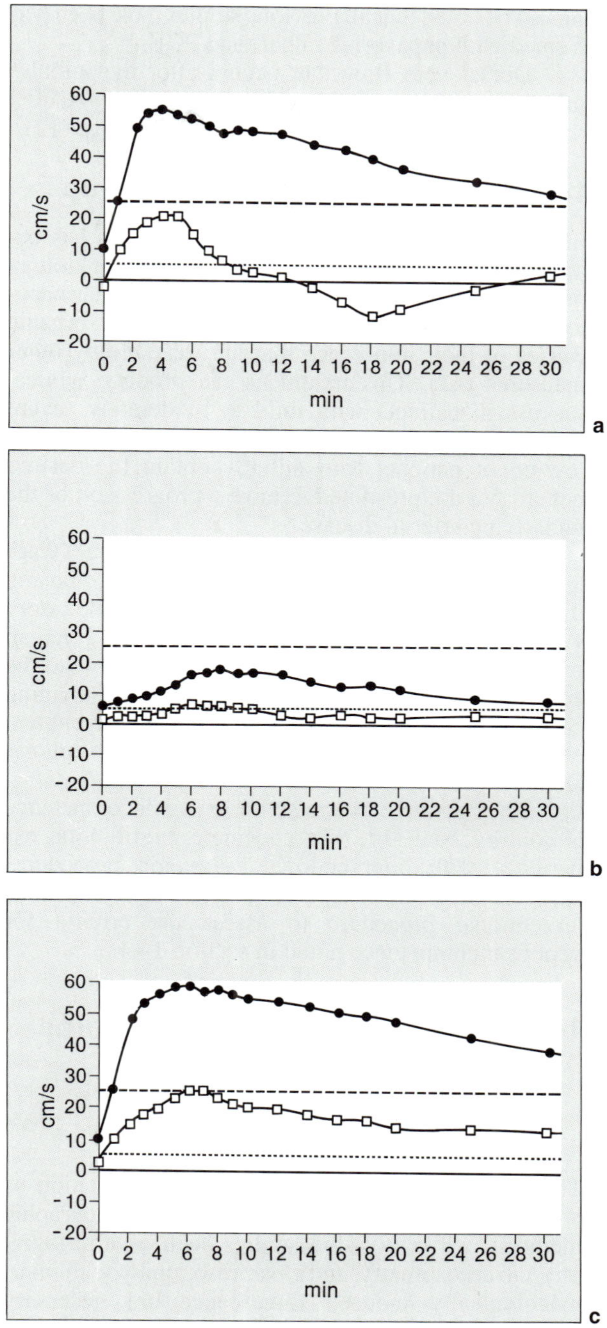

Fig. 14.**9a–c** Progression of maximum systolic flow velocity (upper curve) and minimum diastolic flow velocity (lower curve) during pharmacologically induced erection. Lines indicate the systolic threshold of 25 cm/s for arteriogenic ED and the diastolic threshold of 5 cm/s for venous leak (see text). Intracavernous injection performed at time 0

a Normal finding: The maximum systolic velocity of 56 cm/s is reached at 4 min. After an initial rise in the filling and tumescent phases, the diastolic velocity falls to negative values. Maximum erection is attained at about 15 min

b Severe arteriogenic ED: The maximum systolic velocity rises to no more than 18 cm/s. Due to the deficient arterial inflow, the flow rate shows very little change in diastole (see also Fig. 14.**8**)

c Erectile dysfunction due to venous leak: The minimum diastolic velocity is well above the threshold value of 5 cm/s throughout the examination. Because of the increased venous outflow, systolic perfusion remains elevated for a longer period than when full erection is achieved. Even the injection of 40 µm PGE_1 induces only moderate tumescence (findings confirmed by cavernosography and cavernosometry)

relaxation of the smooth muscle cells in the sinusoids of the erectile tissues. Incompetence of the venous occlusive mechanism ("venous leakage") may occur at the level of the sinusoids, the subcutaneous venous plexuses, or the deep cavernosal veins. Despite adequate arterial inflow, full erection is not achieved because the intracavernous pressure cannot rise sufficiently. Patients with venous incompetence do not develop an adequate erection in response to pharmacologic testing ("nonresponders") (49).

Excessive venous drainage with adequate systolic inflow is associated with a fall in peripheral resistance that produces a characteristic arterial Doppler spectrum on pharmacologic testing. There is a persistence of diastolic forward flow, and the pulsatility remains relatively low (Fig. 14.**9 c**). A diastolic velocity greater than 5 cm/s is suspicious for venous leakage (37). As with arterial insufficiency, the diagnosis of venous incompetence requires extended flow sampling well beyond the initial 5-min interval (up to 30 min postinjection) in patients who do not achieve a full erection. When these conditions are met, the 5 cm/s threshold is 95% sensitive and 83% specific for the diagnosis of venous incompetence (12), though it should be noted that all previous studies have been performed with papaverine rather than PGE_1.

Dorsal vein flow that occurs after the initial 5 min or persists longer than 10 min appears to be 80% sensitive and 100% specific for venous leakage (12).

14.4.4 Posttherapeutic Follow-up

Intracavernous autoinjection therapy (ICAT) has become an increasingly important treatment option in patients who show positive response to pharmacologic testing and have no psychogenic or organic causes of their impotence that are treatable by other measures (45). This treatment can produce clinical success in patients with mild to moderately severe arteriogenic impotence. CDS is important in the follow-up of patients who initially obtain the desired benefit but are presumed to have a progression of the underlying arterial disease.

Surgical revascularization can improve symptoms in selected patients. For example, anastomosing the inferior epigastric artery to a dorsal penile artery while connecting the latter to the deep dorsal vein can provide significant improvement of blood flow to the erectile tissue (17). During follow-up, CDS imaging can be used to confirm the patency of the afferent and efferent vessels and the integrity of the anastomosis (16).

The operative treatment of venous incompetence is controversial (17, 47), and there is still little experience with interventional radiologic procedures (10, 39). CDS can be used after open surgery or an interventional procedure to assess the criteria for venous incompetence noted in section 14.4.3.

14.5 Diagnostic value of Color Duplex Sonography in Relation to Other Procedures

The diagnostic imaging and functional evaluation of erectile dysfunction rely increasingly on sonographic methods, while invasive studies such as arteriography, cavernosometry, and cavernosography with pharmacologically induced tumescence are necessary only after an extensive preliminary workup in cases where invasive treatment is proposed. Nevertheless, these radiologic procedures continue to be the diagnostic gold standard in vasculogenic impotence, for they alone can provide direct information on the integrity of the blood vessels supplying the penis, especially in the pelvic region.

CDS is the most recent addition to the armamentarium of imaging procedures in erectile dysfunction (12, 16, 24, 37, 40, 51). Conventional duplex scanning and CW Doppler ultrasound have a considerably longer history of clinical use (8, 15, 20, 23, 26, 30, 31, 36, 38, 41). Virtually all Doppler studies of erectile dysfunction are aided by the pharmacologic induction of erection.

The advantage of CW Doppler sonography lies in its universal availability and low equipment costs. However, CW Doppler is not useful in itself for quantitative determination (velocity measurement), as this requires morphologic information on the course of the vessel.

Duplex techniques allow for correction of the Doppler angle based on the longitudinal orientation of the vessel. This permits the measurement of absolute flow velocities. The key advantage of CDS over conventional (noncolor) duplex is that it permits a significantly easier and more rapid identification of blood vessels in the real-time image. Course anomalies and occlusions are easily visualized, and Doppler frequency analysis can be performed at more frequent intervals after intracavernous injections, providing greater accuracy in the monitoring of blood flow dynamics during tumescence and erection. Previous studies leave no doubt that CDS is advantageous over conventional duplex in the evaluation of erectile dysfunction. But available studies fail to answer the essential question: Is the absolute measurement of blood flow velocities by duplex scanning necessary for the effective diagnosis of erectile dysfunction? There have been no prospective studies comparing CDS imaging and CW Doppler ultrasound. Given the significantly higher costs of the procedure and its still-limited availability compared with CW Doppler, CDS with pharmacologically induced tumescence cannot be used as a primary screening study at the present time. The procedure is indicated for the exclusion of penile vascular anomalies in patients with primary erectile dysfunction, in all cases of etiologically obscure organic impotence that would require higher doses for ICAT testing that are recommended for primary testing (especially patients with severe arterial insufficiency), and in all ICAT nonresponders with a suspected venous leak. Additionally, CDS scanning should be routinely performed whenever an invasive diagnostic procedure (arteriography, cavernosometry, or cavernosography with pharmacologically induced tumescence) or invasive therapeutic procedure (arterial revascularization, venous surgery, radiologic venous occlusion) is planned.

The problem of velocity measurements in the penile arteries has not yet satisfactorily resolved. Local velocity increases relating to penile vascular stenoses can lead to false-negative results when only one site is examined. Velocity measurements in one vessel cannot adequately take into account the complex collateralization at the penile level. The momentary cardiac output also influences penile blood flow. Combinations of arterial and venous changes are superimposed and cannot always be adequately resolved by Doppler frequency analysis in terms of their relative significance. Systolic and diastolic velocity thresholds published in previous studies have been based on papaverine stimulation. Prostaglandin E_1 is preferable, however, as it causes fewer side effects. We have found that the rate of false-positive results in the diagnosis of venous incompetence is higher with PGE_1

(even at higher doses) than with papaverine, possibly because the stress induced by the examination technique tends to inhibit the response to (the more physiologic) PGE_1 more than to papaverine.

Compared with many other applications (carotid system, extremity arteries, etc.) in which duplex technology can furnish a definitive diagnosis and is often the final diagnostic study before treatment, CDS represents a less critical, though not unimportant, component in the workup of erectile dysfunction. Its capabilities in the detection of organic causes of impotence can narrow the scope of the differential diagnosis. CDS in itself cannot provide a complete workup of erectile dysfunction, however, and must be supplemented by other investigations. Larger prospective studies are needed before we can definitively assess the role of CDS in the evaluation of erectile dysfunction.

14.6 References

1 Aboseif, S. R., T. F. Lue: Hemodynamics of penile erection. Urol. Clin. Amer. 15 (1988) 1–7

2 Aboseif, S. R., T. F. Lue: Fundamentals and hemodynamics of penile erection. Cardiovasc. intervent. Radiol. 11 (1988) 185–190

3 Andersson, K. E., H. Helund, A. Mattiasson: Relaxation of isolated human corpus spongiosum induced by vasoactive intestinal polypeptide, substance P, carbachol and electrical field stimulation. Wld. J. Urol. (1983) 203–208

4 Bähren, W., H. Gall, W. Scherb, C. Stief, W. Thon: Arterial anatomy and arteriographic diagnosis of arteriogenic impotence. Cardiovasc. intervent. Radiol. 11 (1988) 195–210

5 Bähren, W., W. Scherb, H. Gall, A. Gallwitz, J. E. Altwein: Selektive Arteriographie der A. pudenda interna bei posttraumatischer erektiler Dysfunktion. Fortschr. Röntgenstr. 143 (1985) 334–341

6 Benson, G. S., J. A. McConnell, W. A. Schmidt: Penile polsters: functional structures or atherosclerotic changes? J. Urol. 125 (1981) 800–803

7 Benson, C. B., J. E. Aruny, M. A. Vickers: Correlation of duplex sonography with arteriography in patients with erectile dysfunction. Amer. J. Roentgenol. 160 (1993) 71 –73

8 Benson, C. B., M. A. Vickers: Sexual impotence caused by vascular disease: diagnosis with duplex sonography. Amer. J. Roentgenol. 153 (1989) 1149–1153

9 Collins, W. E., J. B. R. McKendry, M. Silverman, L. E. Krul, J. P. Collins, A. H. Irvine: Multidisciplinary survey of erectile impotence. Canad. med. Ass. J. 128 (1983) 1393–1399

10 Courtheoux, P., D. Maiza, J.-P. Henriet, C. D. Vaislic, C. Evrard, J. Theron: Erectile dysfunction caused by venous leakage: treatment with detachable balloons and coils. Radiology 161 (1986) 807–809

11 Earle, C. M., E. J. Keogh, Z. S. Wisniewski, A. G. S. Tulloch, D. J. Lord, G. R. Watters, C. Glatthaar: Prostaglandin E1 therapy for impotence, comparison with papaverine. J. Urol. 143 (1990) 57–59

12 Fitzgerald, S. W., S. J. Erickson, W. D. Foley, E. O. Lipchik, T. L. Lawson: Color Doppler sonography in the evaluation of erectile dysfunction. Amer. J. Roentgenol. 157 (1991) 331–336

13 Forster, A.: Beiträge zur Anatomie der äußeren männlichen Geschlechtsorgane des Menschen. Z. Morphol. Anthropol. 6 (1903) 435–501

14 Fried, J. J., B. C. Mellinger, E. D. Vaughan: Papaverine-induced penile blood flow acceleration in impotent men measured by duplex scanning. J. Urol. 141 (1989) 418

15 Gall, H., C. H. Sparwasser, C. G. Stief, W. Bähren, W. Scherb, G. Holzki: Diagnosis of venous incompetence in erectile dysfunction. Urology 35 (1990) 235–238

16 Gehl, H.-B., R. Sikora, K. Bohndorf, M. Sohn, D. Vorwerk: Darstellung von Penisgefäßanastomosen mittels farbkodierter Doppler-Sonographie: Vergleich mit CW-Dopplersonographie und Klinik. Ultraschall in Med. 11 (1990) 155–160

17 Hauri, D.: Operative Möglichkeiten in der Therapie der vaskulär bedingten erektilen Impotenz. Urologe, Ausg. A 28 (1989) 260–265

18 Iacono, F., S. Barra, T. Lotti: Evaluation of penile deep arteries in psychogenic impotence by means of duplex sonography. J. Urol. (1993) 1262–1264

19 Jünemann, K. P., J. A. Luo, N. L. Benowitz, E. A. Tanagho: The effect of cigarette smoking on penile erection. J. Urol. 137 (1987) 186

20 Jünemann, K.-P., M. Siegsmund, M. Löbelenz, P. Alken: Doppler-Sonographie der Penisarterien. Urologe, Ausg. A 29 (1990) 113–119

21 Kiely, J. M., H. D. Pohle: Impotenz in den USA – eine weitverbreitete und häufig erfolgreich behandelbare gesundheitliche Störung. Mayo Clin. Hlth Lett. 9 (1986) 1–9

22 Kinsey, A. C., W. B. Pomeroy, C. E. Martin: Sexual behavior in the human male. W. B. Saunders Co., Philadelphia (1948)

23 Krysiewicz, S., B. C. Mellinger: The role of imaging in the evaluation of impotence. Amer. J. Roentgenol. 153 (1989) 1133–1139

24 Landwehr, P., R. A. Zink: Farbkodierte Duplexsonographie des Penis bei erektiler Dysfunktion. Ultraschall. Klin. Prax. (Suppl.) 1 (1989) 134

25 Liu, L.-C., C.-C. Wu, L.-H. Liu, C.-P. Chiang, C. H. Huang, Y.-H. Chou, L.-B. Tan: Comparison of the effects of papaverine versus prostaglandin E1 on penile blood flow by color duplex sonography. Europ. Urol. 19 (1991) 49–53

26 Lue, T. F., H. Hricak, K. W. Marich, E. A. Tanagho: Vasculogenic impotence evaluated by high resolution ultrasonography and pulsed Doppler spectrum analysis. Radiology 155 (1989) 777–781

27 Lue, T. F., H. Hricak, K. W. Marich, E. A. Tanagho: Evaluation of arteriogenic impotence with intracorporeal injection of papaverine and the duplex ultrasound scanner. Semin. Urol. 3 (1985) 43–48

28 Lue, T. F., E. A. Tanagho: Physiology of erection and pharmacological management of impotence. J. Urol. 137 (1987) 829–836

29 Masters, W. H., V. E. Johnson: Human Sexual Inadequacy. Little Brown, Boston (1970)

30 Melman, A.: The evaluation of erectile dysfunction. Urol. Radiol. 10 (1988) 119–128

31 Müller, S. C., H. v. Wallenberg-Pachaly, G. E. Voges, H. H. Schild: Comparison of selective internal iliac pharmaco-angiography, penile brachial index and duplex sonography with pulsed Doppler analysis for the evaluation of vasculogenic (arteriogenic) impotence. J. Urol. 143 (1990) 928–932

32 Padma-Nathan, H., I. Goldstein, R. J. Krane: Evaluation of the impotent patient. Semin. Urol. 4 (1986) 225–232

33 Porst, H.: Prostaglandin E1 bei erektiler Dysfunktion. Urologe, Ausg. A 28 (1989) 94–98

34 Porst, H.: Stellenwert von Prostaglandin E1 (PGE1) in der Diagnostik der erektilen Dysfunktion (ED) im Vergleich zu Papaverin und Papaverin/Phentolamin bei 61 Patienten mit ED. Urologe, Ausg. A 27 (1988) 22–26

35 Porst, H., H. v. Ahlen: Pharmakon-induzierte Priapismen – ein Erfahrungsbericht über 101 Fälle. Urologe, Ausg. A 28 (1989) 84–87

36 Porst, H., H. v. Ahlen, O. Köster, K.-H. Schlolaut: Vergleich von Papaverin-induzierter Doppler-Sonographie und Angiographie in der Diagnostik der erektilen Dysfunktion. Urologe, Ausg. A 27 (1988) 8–13

37 Quam, J. P., B. F. King, E. M. James, R. W. Lewis, D. M. Brakke, D. M. Ilstrup, B. G. Parulkar, R. R. Hattery: Duplex and color Doppler sonographic evaluation of vasculogenic impotence. Amer. J. Roentgenol. 153 (1989) 1141–1147

38 Rajfer, J., V. Canan, F. J. Dorey, C. M. Mehringer: Correlation between penile angiography and duplex scanning of cavernous arteries in impotent men. J. Urol. 143 (1990) 1128–1130

39 Schild, H., S. C. Müller, R. A. Bürger, Th. Fritz: Transpenile Venenokklusion zur Therapie der erektilen Impotenz. Fortschr. Röntgenstr. 151 (1989) 470–472

40 Schwartz, A. N., K. Y. Wang, L. A. Mack, M. Lowe, R. E. Berger, D. R. Cyr, M. Feldman: Evaluation of normal erectile function with color flow Doppler sonography. Amer. J. Roentgenol. 153 (1989) 1155–1160

41 Shabsigh, R., I. J. Fishman, E. T. Quesada, C. K. Seale-Hawkins, J. K. Dunn: Evaluation of vasculogenic erectile impotence using penile duplex ultrasonography. J. Urol. 142 (1989) 1469–1474

42 Stackl, W., R. Hasun, M. Marberger: Intracavernous injection of prostaglandin E1 in impotent men. J. Urol. 140 (1988) 66–68

43 Stief, C. G., W. Bähren, H. Gall, W. Scherb: Functional evaluation of penile hemodynamics. J. Urol. 139 (1988) 734–737

44 Stief, C. G., W. Bähren, W. Scherb, H. Gall: Primary erectile dysfunction. J. Urol. 141 (1989) 315–319
45 Stief, C. G., H. Gall, W. Scherb, W. Bähren: Mid-term results of autoinjection therapy for erectile dysfunction. Urology 31 (1988) 483–485
46 Strauss, E. B.: Impotence from the psychiatric stand point. Brit. Med. J. 1 (1950) 697
47 Treiber, U., P. Gilbert: Venous surgery in erectile dysfunction: a critical report on 116 patients. Urology 34 (1989) 22–27
48 Virag, R., P. Bouilly, D. Frydman: Is impotence an arterial disorder? A study of arterial risk factors in 440 impotent men. Lancet I (1985) 181–184
49 Weiske, W.-H.: Pharmakokavernosometrie und Pharmakokavernosographie bei erektiler Dysfunktion. Urologe, Ausg. A 29 (1990) 126–134
50 Weiske, W.-H.: Drei Jahre Erfahrungen mit der Schwellkörperautoinjektionstherapie. Urologe, Ausg. A 28 (1989) 253–257
51 Zink, R. A., P. Landwehr: Color duplex sonography. A new tool in the evaluation of erectile dysfunction. J. Urol. 141 (1989) 187

15 Thyroid Gland

F. Fobbe

15.1 General Remarks

Thyroid disorders are endemic in many parts of the world. Diffuse thyroid enlargement, or goiter, is particularly widespread. Epidemiologic data indicate a prevalence of more than 10% in the general population (21). An autonomous adenoma can develop from a nodular goiter in the setting of alimentary iodine deficiency, especially in older patients. There is probably also a relationship between iodine deficiency and thyroid malignancies; at least there is a definite link between iodine deficiency and differentiation in carcinomas (10, 17). For these reasons, there is a need for simple, noninvasive, reproducible, and cost-effective methods of thyroid examination. Modern, high-resolution ultrasound imagers can define even small structural abnormalities in the thyroid gland. Unfortunately, the morphologic information supplied by gray-scale images does not permit the exclusion of autonomous adenoma or carcinoma in patients with thyroid enlargement. Thus the standard workup of thyroid disease has traditionally included radionuclide imaging and fine-needle aspiration biopsy in addition to the clinical examination and laboratory studies.

In 1976 Zachrisson (23) published the results of his angiographic studies in patients with thyroid disorders. He discovered that vascularity was a useful criterion for assessing thyroid function and predicting the benign or malignant nature of thyroid disease. CDS is another modality that can be used to assess the perfusion of parenchymatous organs. Our investigations have shown that this type of information is useful in the differential diagnosis of goiter.

15.2 Normal Anatomy, Common Variants, Examination Technique, and Documentation

15.2.1 Normal Anatomy and Common Variants

The thyroid gland consists of two elliptical lobes that appose to the anterolateral aspects of the trachea and lower larynx. A narrow region called the isthmus interconnects the right and left lobes in front of the trachea (second to third tracheal cartilage). Occasionally a narrow strip of tissue (the pyramidal lobe) ascends from the isthmus to the hyoid bone. Each lobe is about 5 cm long with a greatest transverse and anteroposterior dimension of about 2–3 cm. The lobes enlarge during menstruation and pregnancy.

The gland is ensheathed by a layer of the deep cervical fascia. It is covered anteriorly by the inferior hypoglossus muscles and anterolaterally by the sternocleidomastoid. At the posterolateral aspect of each lobe are, from medial to lateral, the common carotid artery, the vagus nerve, and the internal jugular vein. Four intracapsular parathyroid glands are usually related to the posterior border of the lobe. These bodies are about 6 mm long and 3–4 mm wide and deep. Besides these four, additional parathyroid glands may occur inside or outside the capsule.

The thyroid gland derives its blood supply from the paired inferior thyroid arteries, which arise from the thyrocervical trunk, and the superior thyroid arteries, which arise from the external carotid artery. Both arteries enter the gland through its inferior and superior poles. From there they course around the gland on the subcapsular plane and send branches toward the interior of the lobes. A fifth, unpaired artery, termed the thyroidea ima artery, is sometimes present. It may arise from either the aortic arch or the brachiocephalic (innominate) artery. The thyroid arteries are interlinked by numerous connecting channels. The veins form a plexus on the surface of the thyroid gland. This plexus gives origin to the paired superior, middle, and inferior thyroid veins. The superior and middle thyroid veins enter the internal jugular vein, while the inferior thyroid vein opens into the left brachiocephalic vein either separately or conjointly with the contralateral vessel. The thyroid vessels also supply the intracapsular parathyroid glands (7).

15.2.2 Examination Technique

The examination is best performed in the supine position. A pad is placed under the back to hyperextend the neck and facilitate access to the thyroid gland. The hyperextension tends to displace the gland upward so that its inferior portions can be examined more easily. Care is taken, however, to provide occipital head support. This is especially important in older patients with limited cervical spine mobility; otherwise muscle tension in the neck will make it difficult to adapt the transducer to the skin and will increase absorption and scattering of the sound waves. Each lobe of the thyroid gland is scanned completely in longitudinal and transverse planes. A 7.5-MHz transducer is best for obtaining the necessary spatial resolution. After the gray-scale image has been optimally adjusted, the color-encoded flow threshold is set to display frequency shifts of ≥ 80 Hz (when a 7.5-MHz transducer is used). At this setting the lumen of the carotid artery should be completely filled with color-encoded signals in systole. The examiner looks for any circumscribed or diffuse increase in flow signals, so the instrument parameters should not be changed during the examination. The transducer should be held perpendicular to the skin to obtain good gray-scale definition. Because the vessels in the thyroid parenchyma course in all directions, the transducer position does not interfere with the assessment of blood flow. A standoff pad facilitates adaptation of the transducer to the skin and improves the display of superficial structures.

15.2.3 Documentation

Each thyroid lobe and the isthmus should be documented in two planes (through their maximum dimension). Abnormalities also are documented in two planes. Tissue perfusion can be evaluated only in a real-time image, so flow is documented in videotape sequences. Also, instrument parameters (gray-scale image settings, color flow threshold and intensity) should be documented for purposes of follow-up.

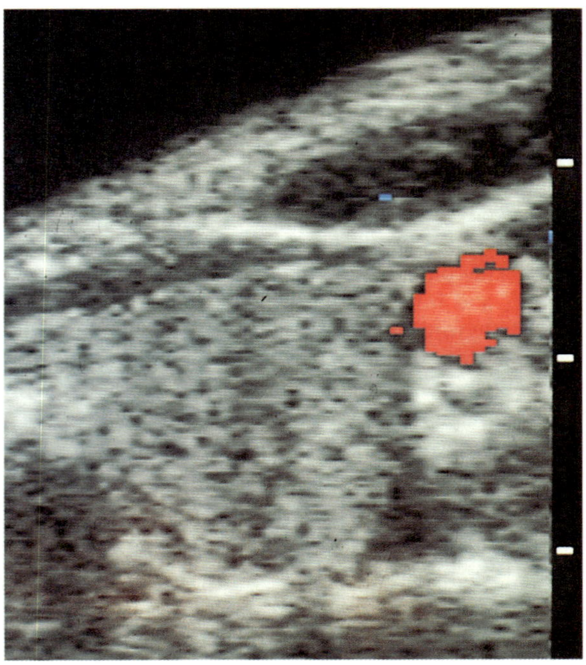

Fig. 15.**1** Transverse CDS scan of the normal left lobe of the thyroid gland shows normal configuration, size, and margins. The lobe is uniformly hyperechoic (relative to the sternocleidomastoid muscle) with uniformly scattered intrathyroidal color flow signals. Flow in the common carotid artery is encoded red

15.3 Normal Findings

The normal thyroid gland has smooth margins, is clearly demarcated from its surroundings, and shows a homogeneous echo pattern that is hyperechoic to the adjacent musculature. The volume of the thyroid gland is determined most easily (and with acceptable accuracy) with the simplified formula for calculating the volume of an ellipsoid (the greatest diameter in all three planes is multiplied by 0.5, making separate calculations for each thyroid lobe and for the isthmus) (3). The large inflow and outflow vessels at the poles of the thyroid lobes are clearly defined by their color-encoded flow signals. Only scattered flow signals are detected within the thyroid tissue (Fig. 15.**1**). These signals are distributed uniformly throughout the gland with no circumscribed increases in intrathyroidal flow.

15.4 Pathologic Findings

Diffuse or nodular goiter is endemic in many regions of the world. Seventy percent of patients have a simple goiter representing adaptive hyperplasia in response to an iodine deficiency. This condition does not involve a functional disturbance like that in hyperthyroidism or hypothyroidism. A hyperthyroid metabolic state is found in 5–10% of patients with adenomas (12).

Multinodular goiter can develop from a simple goiter just as autonomous foci or autonomous adenomas can develop in association with chronic goiters in iodine-deficient regions (13, 18). The histologic examination of goiter can differentiate true neoplasia (follicular adenoma) from follicular or nodular hyperplasia (4, 6). Nodular goiters are associated with a higher incidence of carcinoma. Depending on the region and study criteria, malignant transformation is reported to occur in 2–13% of patients with a nodular goiter, with women affected more frequently than men (10, 17, 20). The most common malignant thyroid tumor is papillary carcinoma (45–70% of cases) followed by follicular carcinoma (25%), anaplastic carcinoma (10–25%), and medullary carcinoma (5–10%). These intrinsic thyroid malignancies are distinguished from metastatic involvement or involvement by generalized lymphoma (6).

15.4.1 Diffuse and Nodular Goiter

Diffuse goiter is recognized mainly by its size. It is hyperechoic to the surrounding muscle and occasionally somewhat nonhomogeneous. Nodular goiter is characterized by one or more focal abnormalities in the thyroid tissue. In the early stage the nodule may be virtually isoechoic to the surrounding tissue and is defined only by a hypoechoic rim. In advanced cases both hyperechoic and hypoechoic nodules may be found. The lesions usually display a homogeneous echogenicity, but larger nodules are especially likely to contain nonhomogeneous elements and calcifications. These calcifications may occur singly or in clusters. In extreme cases the entire thyroid gland shows nodular transformation and normal thyroid tissue is no longer discernible. Solid nodules may undergo partial or complete degeneration and cystic transformation. These lesions are marked by an irregular cyst wall, and tissue rests can appear as hyperechoic areas within the lumen. Intracystic hemorrhage is relatively common and can have various sonographic presentations depending on the age of collection. A true epithelium-lined thyroid cyst is very rare (11).

The morphologic thyroid changes detectable with ultrasound—nodule composition (hyperechoic, hypoechoic, homogeneous, nonhomogeneous, calcifications), margination (sharp, indistinct), and size—are not useful for assessing functional status or excluding malignant transformation. Even the combination of ultrasound morphology and radionuclide imaging cannot establish or exclude malignant change (Table 15.**1**). Similarly, the familiar sonolucent "halo" around a nodule is not pathognomonic for a benign lesion (11, 16).

The perfusion of the thyroid gland in patients with a goiter or nodular goiter is indistinguishable from normal thyroid perfusion: Scattered blood flow signals are observed diffusely throughout the gland. Blood vessels coursing superficial to the gland, especially at the poles, are the only prominent features (Fig. 15.**2a, b**). During interpretation, it is important always to evaluate the overall perfusion of the gland while noting any circumscribed or diffuse areas in which blood flow is increased. This can occasionally

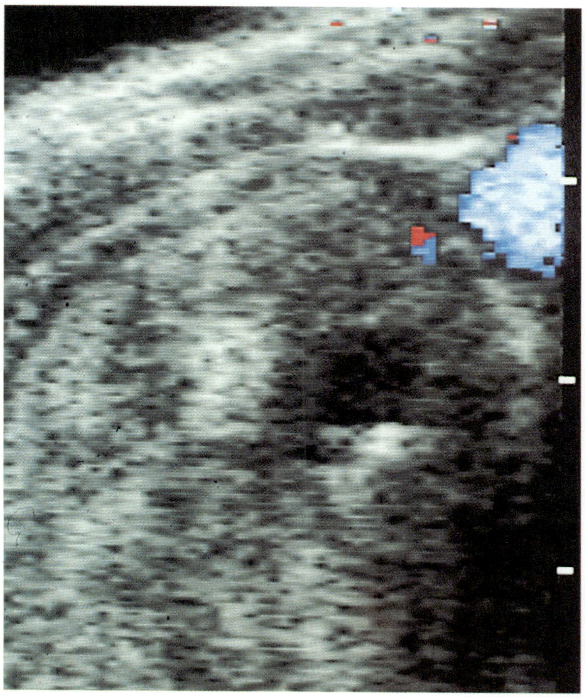

a

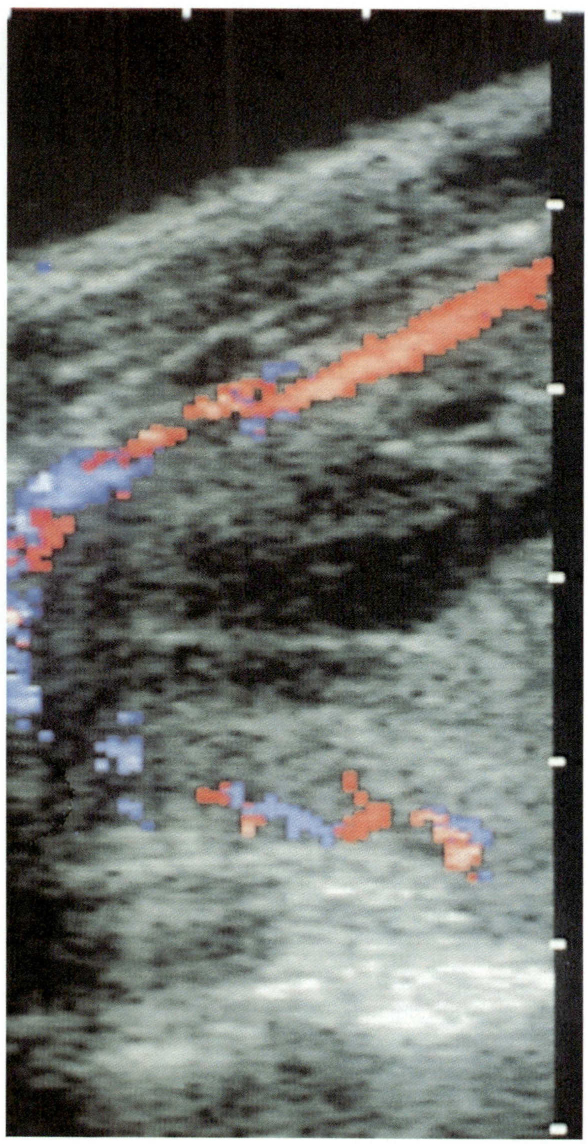

b

Fig. 15.**2a, b** Nodular goiter with normal perfusion
a Transverse scan through the left thyroid lobe demonstrates an enlarged, rounded gland showing nonhomogeneous echogenicity and a well-defined, uniformly echo-free mass in the lateral third with posterior acoustic enhancement (cyst). Scattered flow signals are evenly distributed throughout the gland. Flow in the common carotid artery is encoded blue
b Longitudinal scan through the superior pole of the thyroid gland shows very prominent vessels in the thyroid capsule with no evidence of increased intrathyroidal flow

Table 15.**1** Comparison of the sonographic morphologic criteria of thyroid nodules with radionuclide scanning ("cold" or "warm") and histology (after 16)

Ultrasound morphology	Cold		Warm
	Malignant n = 164 (%)	Benign n = 234 (%)	Benign n = 164 (%)
Solid	70	44	71
Liquid	26	47	28
Hypoechoic	75	29	77
Isoechoic/ hyperechoic	22	71	23
Halo	4	34	52
Sharp	20	20	41
Indistinct	40	30	7

be difficult in very large thyroid glands that have undergone complete nodular transformation, as there is no normal tissue for comparison, and the position and course of the large supplying vessels cannot be clearly defined.

15.4.2 Adenoma and Carcinoma

In contrast to follicular and nodular hyperplasia, the majority of adenomas and almost all autonomous adenomas show increased perfusion (Table 15.**2**). The increased blood flow is most apparent at the periphery of the nodule. This increased peripheral perfusion appears as a ring-like hypoechoic zone in the gray-scale image and probably corresponds to the "halo" described in the literature. When the nodule reaches a size of about 2 cm or more, increased blood flow is also noted in the interior of the lesion (Fig. 15.**3a–c**). Hypervascularization is also a feature of thyroid malignancies—intrinsic thyroid tumors as well as metastases (Table 15.**2**). The increased perfusion tends to be more diffuse in carcinomas and not confined to the surface as in small autonomous adenomas. Additionally, increased flow signals can be demonstrated in the morphologically normal tissue surrounding the carcinoma (Fig. 15.**4a–c**). In our experience, however, these differences in tumoral and peritumoral vascularization are not sufficient to distinguish an (autonomous) adenoma from a malignancy. The perfusion pattern is helpful only for distinguishing the normal blood flow of a benign nodular goiter from the increased flood flow of an autonomous adenoma or malignant tumor.

15.4.3 Graves Disease

Graves disease (diffuse toxic goiter) is the second most common thyroid disease after simple nodular goiter. It is characterized by the excessive production of thyroid hormones due to abnormal stimulation of the gland (21). The gland shows diffuse, general enlargement at ultrasound with a homogeneous, usually hypoechoic texture. In rare cases the gland may appear uniformly hyperechoic (similar to the structure of a normal thyroid gland). In patients with untreated Graves disease, intrathyroidal flow is diffusely and markedly increased throughout the gland (14). The increase in blood flow is so pronounced that it permits a confident diagnosis even without normal tissue for comparison (Fig. 15.**5**). However, the clinical manifestations, laboratory findings, and ultrasound morphology are generally clear-cut and are sufficient for the diagnosis. CDS scanning may be used for follow-up if required (response of perfusion to therapy).

Histology (and radionuclide scanning for autonomous adenoma)	n	Vascularization +	–
Follicular/nodular hyperplasia	61	29	32
Adenomas	35	29	6
Autonomous adenomas	37	33	4
Graves disease	13	12	1
Riedel struma	1	–	1
Papillary carcinomas	16	14	2
Follicular carcinomas	3	2	1
Anaplastic carcinomas	4	3	1
Medullary carcinomas	1	1	–
Malignant lymphomas	1	1	–
Metastases	2	2	–
	174	126	48

Table 15.**2** Comparison of blood flow at CDS imaging with histology and radionuclide scanning in strumectomized patients (n = 174): + = increased blood flow relative to surroundings, – = equal or diminished blood flow relative to surroundings

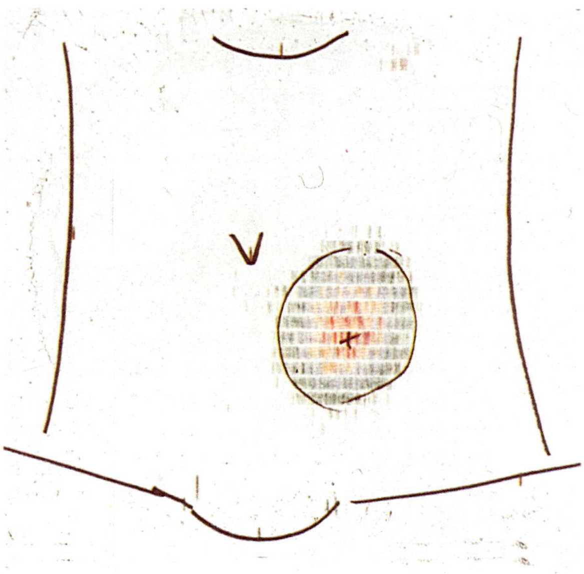

a

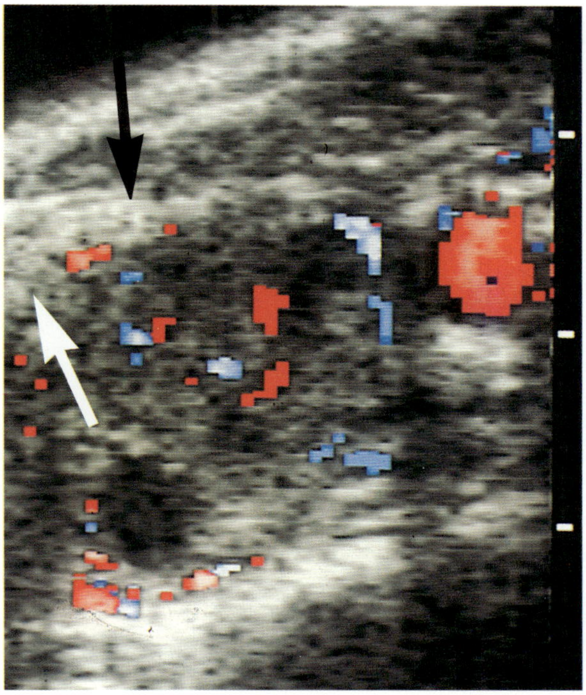

b

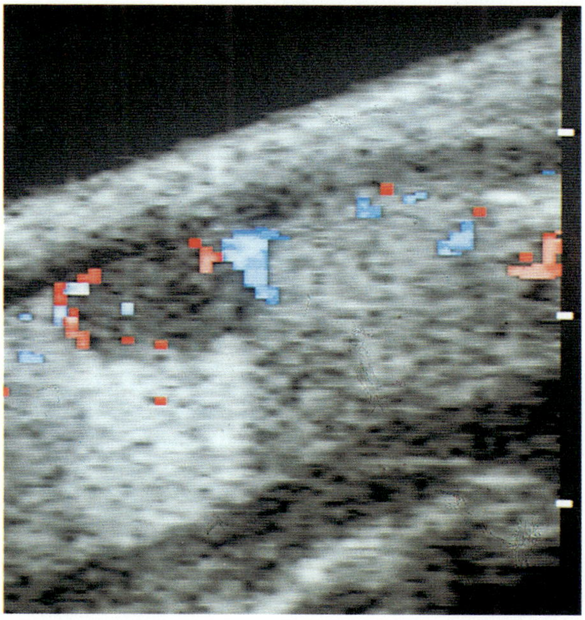

c

Fig. 15.**3a–c** Autonomous adenomas of the thyroid gland

a Radionuclide scan shows a circumscribed area of increased uptake in the left lobe of thyroid gland with suppression of uptake in the rest of the gland

b Transverse CDS scan shows a nonhomogeneous mass occupying almost the entire left lobe of the thyroid gland. Blood flow is most notably increased at the periphery of the mass. Normal thyroid tissue is only present anteromedially (arrows). Flow in the common carotid artery is encoded red

c Longitudinal CDS scan shows a superficial, elliptical, uniformly hypoechoic mass with a maximum diameter of about 1 cm and increased blood flow at its periphery

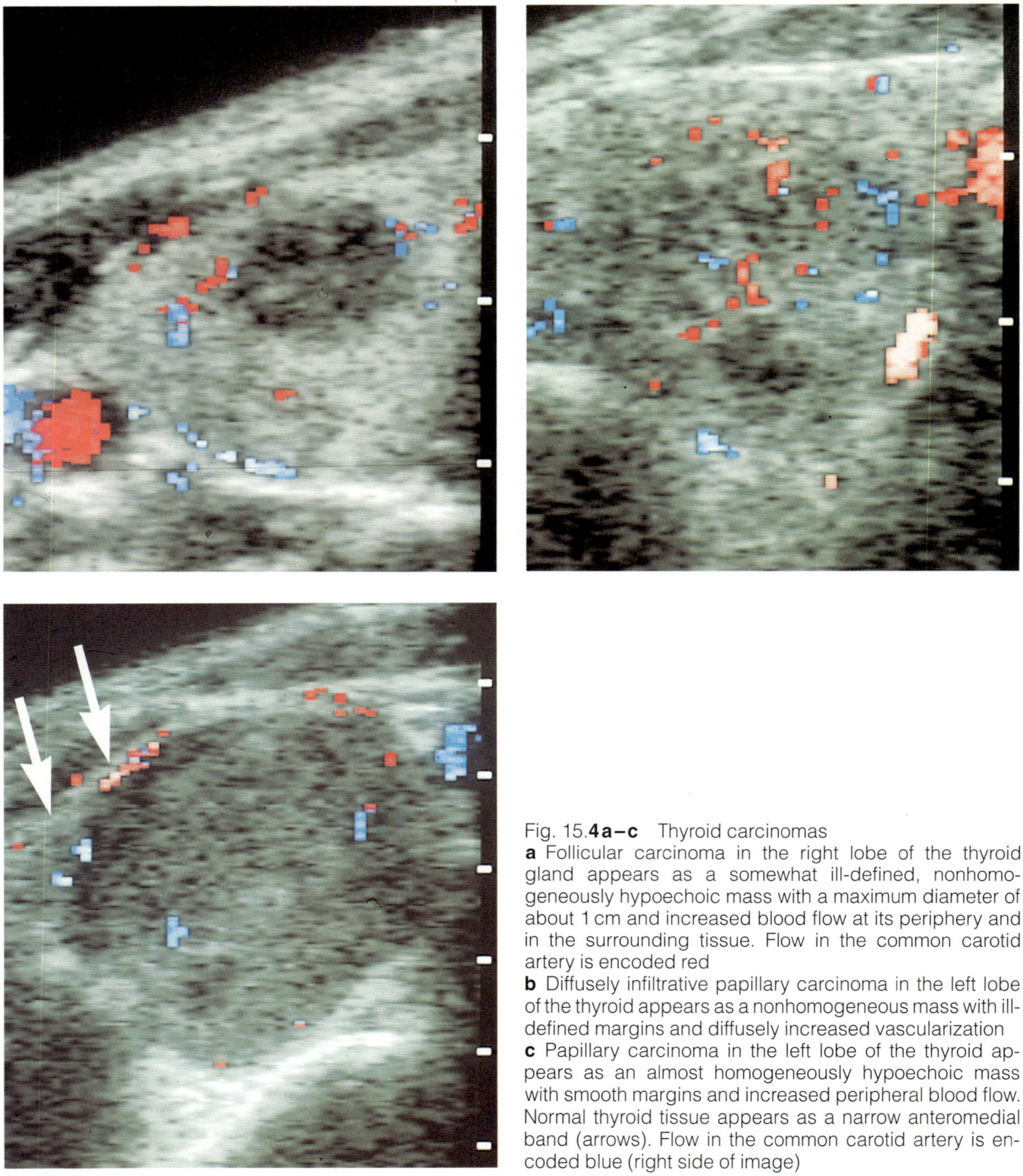

a b c

Fig. 15.**4 a–c** Thyroid carcinomas
a Follicular carcinoma in the right lobe of the thyroid gland appears as a somewhat ill-defined, nonhomogeneously hypoechoic mass with a maximum diameter of about 1 cm and increased blood flow at its periphery and in the surrounding tissue. Flow in the common carotid artery is encoded red
b Diffusely infiltrative papillary carcinoma in the left lobe of the thyroid appears as a nonhomogeneous mass with ill-defined margins and diffusely increased vascularization
c Papillary carcinoma in the left lobe of the thyroid appears as an almost homogeneously hypoechoic mass with smooth margins and increased peripheral blood flow. Normal thyroid tissue appears as a narrow anteromedial band (arrows). Flow in the common carotid artery is encoded blue (right side of image)

15.4.4 Thyroiditis

Inflammatory disorders of the thyroid gland include granulomatous thyroiditis (de Quervain subacute thyroiditis), lymphocytic thyroiditis (e.g., Hashimoto thyroiditis), invasive fibrous thyroiditis (Riedel thyroiditis), and acute suppurative thyroiditis. Inflammatory thyroid diseases are relatively rare, the granulomatous and lymphocytic forms being the most common. Acute suppurative thyroiditis is very rare, and invasive fibrous thyroiditis is extremely rare (20 cases in 42 000 thyroidectomized patients at the Mayo Clinic in Minnesota) (6).

The sonomorphologic features of thyroiditis are nonspecific. Scanning in newly diagnosed cases shows an enlarged, uniformly hypoechoic gland. In more chronic cases where thyroid parenchyma is replaced by scar tissue, ultrasound shows a small gland with a nonhomogeneous echo pattern. Similar changes in perfusion are observed, with acute cases

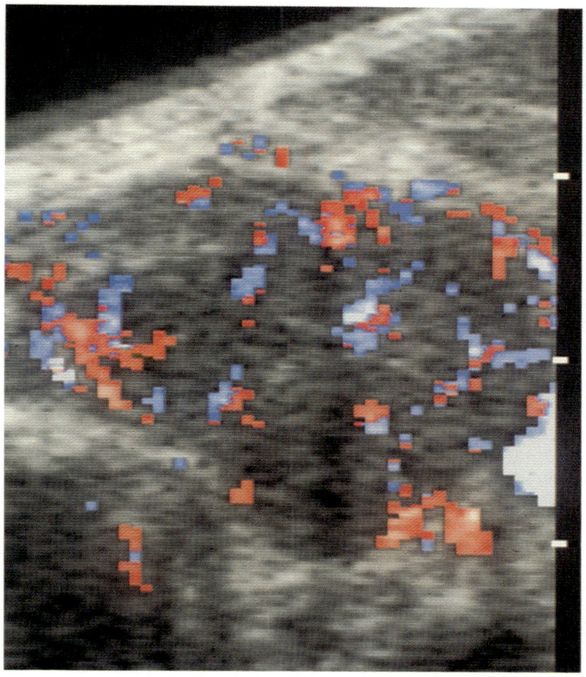

Fig. 15.**5** Transverse scan of the left thyroid lobe in a patient with Graves d sease. The thyroid tissue is of nonhomogeneous, low-level echogenicity with a marked, diffuse increase of blood flow throughout the gland

showing a diffuse perfusion increase (similar to Graves disease but less pronounced). Perfusion diminishes with scar-tissue replacement of the glandular tissue. Inflammatory thyroid diseases are rare, so there is only limited experience with their color duplex appearance, and a reliable evaluation is not possible at the present time (5, 14).

15.5 Diagnostic Value of Color Duplex Sonography in Relation to Other Procedures

The diagnosis of thyroid diseases is a major public health problem due to the frequency of these disorders. There is need for a diagnostic procedure that can detect lesions at an early stage, assess their functional status, and differentiate benign from malignant disease. Gray-scale sonography is highly sensitive in its ability to detect even very small morphologic changes (15), but it cannot discriminate between benign and malignant disease (11, 16). The same applies to function: an autonomous adenoma cannot be identified on the basis of gray-scale morphology (15).

Fine-needle aspiration biopsy provides a nonoperative means of investigating structural irregularities in the thyroid. Its accuracy depends, however, on the adequacy of the specimen, proper smear technique, the experience of the physician performing the biopsy, and proper cytologic interpretation. The reported incidence of false-negative results with fine-needle aspiration biopsy ranges from 1–8% (1, 2, 8). Besides the diagnostic uncertainty, one must also consider that fine-needle aspiration biopsy is an invasive procedure that can lead to complications such as infection and bleeding at the puncture site and can be psychologically distressful for the patient.

Radionuclide imaging with ^{99m}Tc pertechnetate or ^{123}I shows the distribution of isotope uptake as a means of assessing local thyroid function. It clearly differentiates between normal tissue, areas of no uptake ("cold nodules"), and areas of increased uptake ("hot nodules"). Thus this modality can provide information on metabolic state. One limitation, however, is the relatively low sensitivity of the method. The spatial resolution of radionuclide scanning can detect nodules $\geq$ 1 cm; cold spots smaller than 1 cm may be missed or obscured by normal overlying tissue. Another difficulty lies in the detection of compensated adenomas, which can be detected only in a suppression scintiscan. Also, as in conventional ultrasonography, the isotope scan is not useful for distinguishing benign from malignant nodules. Cold nodules may represent cystic or degenerative areas as well as carcinoma, lymphoma, or a metastatic tumor. A warm nodule may represent an autonomous adenoma or, in rare cases, a carcinoma (15). Thus, an abnormal radionuclide scan is an indication for further diagnostic studies.

The angiographic studies of Zachrisson in 1976 (23) demonstrated a high correlation between abnormal vascularity and autonomous adenomas and carcinomas. The clinical use of this method is contraindicated, however, by its invasiveness. Conventional Duplex scanning with Doppler spectral sampling (22) is not useful for differentiation due to theoretical considerations (the measured frequency shifts depends on the course and calibers of the intrathyroidal vessels, which mostly are indeterminate in the gray-scale image; see Chapter 4).

CDS can provide a qualitative assessment of intrathyroidal blood flow based on a comparison of different areas. It is unnecessary to make allowance for the size or course of a particular vessel. The results of the few studies performed to date indicate that qualitative perfusion correlates well with the functional status and benignancy of thyroid lesions (5, 19). Our examinations showed an increased blood flow in 88% of autonomous adenomas and in 85% of malignant tumors (histologic confirmation in surgical specimens) (Table 15.**2**). On the other hand, increased blood flow was also noted in 60% of non-hyperfunctioning adenomas. These results provide a basis for discussing the problems of the method:

1. A circumscribed or diffuse increase of perfusion in the thyroid tissue is useful only in detecting pathologic changes that go beyond a diffuse or nodular goiter. It is not useful for benign/malignant discrimination. For example, an autonomous adenoma cannot be distinguished from carcinoma on the basis

of perfusion. Every patient found to have increased intrathyroidal blood flow requires further diagnostic evaluation (5, 9, 19).

2. The size of the goiter: CDS evaluation is based on comparing the perfusion in different areas of the thyroid, so "normal" perfusion must be identified as a basis for comparison. The larger the goiter, however, the more difficult this becomes. The blood flow in very large goiters is nonhomogeneous and is generally increased due to the very size of the gland. This problem of defining normal blood flow accounts for the high false-positive rate in the diagnosis of adenomas. Four of 27 malignancies (our studies in strumectomized patients, Table 15.**2**) did not show an increase in perfusion. One of these cases involved a large, locally infiltrative carcinoma. The histologic workup of a second specimen revealed a small focal (about 2 mm) diffuse metastasis from a papillary carcinoma. Lesions on this scale are beyond the resolving capacity of ultrasound. Two other carcinomas with a diameter of 8 mm (oncocytoma) and 10 mm (follicular carcinoma) likewise showed no perfusion increase on CDS imaging. Patients with very large goiters are generally referred for strumectomy, so follow-up with color duplex is not an issue. The tendency of ultrasound to miss very small carcinomas remains a problem, however.

3. Instrument settings: The instrument settings must be optimally matched to the situation in order to demonstrate local perfusion differences. The frequency scale should be adjusted to permit adequate color encoding of slow-moving blood but should not be set so low that troublesome artifacts obscure perfusion disparities, especially in smaller areas. The instrument that we used for these investigations (QAD 1) was set to encode a frequency shift of ≥ 80 Hz (for a 7.5-MHz transducer). Because different machines detect perfusion with different degrees of sensitivity, the precise examination parameters and instrument sensitivity must be known so that the results in different groups can be compared.

4. Subjectivity: The difference between a homogeneously perfused thyroid gland and a gland with a circumscribed change in blood flow is not precisely defined. The local perfusion increase in most patients is so pronounced that it can be evaluated with a high degree of confidence. But the evaluation of subtle changes depends strongly on the experience of the examiner. As the size of the gland increases, the assessment becomes more difficult. This particularly applies to the superior and inferior poles of the thyroid, where the large thyroid vessels are bunched together and can mimic an increase in perfusion. Because increased perfusion is always declared to be present in doubtful cases, this leads to an increased rate of false-positive diagnoses.

In conclusion, an autonomous adenoma or malignant tumor can be excluded in goiter patients by the CDS evaluation of intrathyroid blood flow. Experience to date indicates that CDS imaging is useful in the surveillance of patients with a moderate goiter. As long as uniform thyroid perfusion is observed, it is unnecessary to proceed with further (invasive) diagnostic procedures. But all patients with a circumscribed change in perfusion and very large goiters should be referred for a complete diagnostic evaluation.

15.6 References

1 Al-Sayer, H. M., Z. H. Krukowski, V. M. M. Williams, N. A. Matheson: Fine needle aspiration cytology in isolated thyroid swellings: A prospective two year evaluation. Brit. Med. J. 20 (1985) 1490–1494

2 Boey, J., C. Hsu, R. J. Collins: False negative errors in fine-needle aspiration biopsy of dominant thyroid nodules: A prospective follow-up study. Wld J. Surg. 10 (1986) 623–630

3 Brunn, J., G. Block, G. Ruf, I. Bos, P. Kunze, C. Scriba: Volumetrie der Schilddrüsenlappen mittels Real-time-Sonographie. Dtsch. Med. Wschr. 106 (1981) 1338–1340

4 Desforges, J. F.: Management of a solitary thyroid nodule: N. Engl. J. Med. 328 (1993) 553–559

5 Fobbe, F., R. Finke, E. Reichenstein, H. Schleusener, K.-J. Wolf: Appearance of thyroid diseases using color-coded duplex sonography. Europ. J. Radiol. 9 (1989) 29–31

6 Franssila, K. O.: Thyroid gland. In Kissane, J. M. (Ed.): Anderson's Pathology, 9th ed. Mosby, St. Louis (1990) 1544–1569

7 Williams, P. L., R. Warwick, M. Dyson, L. H. Bannister (Eds.): Gray's Anatomy, 37th ed. Churchill Livingstone, Edinburgh (1989) 1459

8 Harsoulis, P., M. Leontsini, A. Economou, T. Gerasimidis, Smbarounis: Fine needle aspiration biopsy, cytology in the diagnosis of thyroid cancer: comparative study of 213 patients. Brit. J. Surg. 73 (1986) 461–464

9 Hübsch, P., B. Niederle, P. Barton, B. Pesau, M. Knittel, M. Schratter, M. Hermann, F. Längle: Farbkodierte Doppler-Sonographie der Schilddrüse: Ein Fortschritt in der Karzinomdiagnostik? Fortschr. Röntgenstr. 156 (1992) 125–129

10 Hurxthal, L. M., A. C. Heinemann: Nodular goiter and thyroid cancer. New Engl. J. Med. 258 (1958) 457–465

11 James, E. M., J. W. Charboneau, I. D. Hay: The thyroid. In Rumack, C. M., S. R. Wilson, J. W. Charboneau (Eds.): Diagnostic Ultrasound. Mosby, St. Louis (1991) 507

12 Leight, G. S.: Nodular goiter and benign and malignant neoplasms of the thyroid. In Sabiston, D. C. (Ed.): Textbook of Surgery, 14th ed. Saunders, Philadelphia (1991) 579–590

13 Peter, H. J., H. Studer, R. Forster, H. Gerber: The pathogenesis of "hot" and "cold" follicles in multinodular goiters. J. clin. Endocrinol. 55 (1982) 941–946

14 Ralls, P. W., D. S. Mayekawa, K. P. Lee, P. M. Colletti, D. R. Radin, W. D. Boswell, J. M. Halls: Color-flow Doppler sonography in Graves disease. Amer. J. Roentgenol. 150 (1988) 781–784

15 Rojeski, M. T., H. Gharib: Nodular thyroid disease. Evaluation and management. New Engl. J. Med. 313 (1985) 428–436

16 Sciuk, J., O. Schober: Die Sonographie der Schilddrüse. Radiologe 29 (1989) 95–102

17 Sokal, J. E.: The problem of malignancy in nodular goiter-recapitulation and a challenge. J. Amer. med. Ass. 170 (1959) 405–412

18 Studer, H., Ramelli, F.: Simple goiter and its variants: Euthyroid and hyperthyroid multinodular goiters. Endocr. Rev. 3 (1982) 40–61

19 Thomas, C., W. Bautz, W. Müller-Schauenburg, U. Feine: Angiodynographie bei umschriebenen Schilddrüsenveränderungen. Fortschr. Röntgenstr. 150 (1989) 72–75

20 Veith, F. J., J. R. Brooks, W. P. Grigsby, H. A. Selenkow: The nodular thyroid gland and cancer: a practical approach to the problem. New Engl. J. Med. 270 (1964) 431–436

21 Wartofsky, L., S. H. Ingbar: Diseases of the thyroid. In Wilson, J. D., E. Braunwals, K. J. Isselbacher, R. G. Petersdorf, J. B. Martin, A. S. Fauci, R. K. Root (Eds.): Harrison's Principles of Internal Medicine, 12th ed. McGraw-Hill, New York (1991) 1692

22 Woodcock, J. P., G. M. Owen, E. J. Shedden, K. J. Hodgson, A. MacGregor, A. Srivastava: Duplex scanning of the thyroid. Ultrasound Med. Biol. 11 (1985) 659–663

23 Zachrisson, B. F.: Thyroid angiography. Acta radiol. (Suppl.) 350, (1976) 1–112

16 Ultrasound Contrast Agents

F. Fobbe, J. Siegert

Ultrasound waves are attenuated as they pass through tissue. The degree of attenuation depends on the distance between the transducer and the object of interest, the transmission frequency, and the composition of the tissue. The more distant the transducer from the structure of interest, the weaker the signal intensity received by the transducer. Because the blood cells are significantly smaller than the wavelength of the transmitted ultrasound waves, they do not reflect the waves, but scatter them in all directions (see Chapters 1 and 17). As a result, the signal from the lumen of the blood vessel is considerably weaker than, say, the signal returned from the vessel wall (the vessel-wall structures are much larger than the ultrasound wavelength, so the waves are reflected far more than they are scattered). If the object of interest is distant from the transducer or if it is scanned through tissue that is a strong sound absorber, the soft-tissue structures may still be adequately defined in the gray-scale image, but the sound waves are so heavily reflected and scattered in the tissue that the signal from the vessel lumen is too weak for measurement of blood flow. One solution to this problem is to increase the acoustic power of the sound waves. But this would increase reflection at the vessel wall and only slightly increase the backscatter from the blood corpuscles. In any case, power output is subject to stringent controls due to the potential for biological effects (see Chapter 2). Another solution is to increase the intensity of the signals from the vessel lumen. This approach has prompted the development of ultrasound contrast agents. A substance is injected into the blood which will produce the highest possible impedance difference relative to surrounding structures. When a sound wave encounters this substance, a higher percentage of the energy is backscattered. The signal returned to the transducer has a higher amplitude and is more clearly distinguished from artifacts and ambient noise. Ultrasound contrast agents can also be used in cavities, such as the bladder and uterine tubes, that normally do not contain significant numbers of scatterers. The importance of ultrasound contrast agents, especially when combined with CDS imaging, will have an increasing role in the future. The present chapter deals with the basic physical principles and properties of ultrasound contrast agents as well as current clinical experience with contrast-enhanced color duplex imaging.

The term "ultrasound contrast agents" is somewhat misleading. In view of its mode of action, it seems more appropriate to call these products "echo enhancers." However, the term "ultrasound contrast agent" is widely accepted and will therefore be used in this book.

16.1 Principles and Preclinical Results

J. Siegert

16.1.1 Introduction

Since Gramiak and Shah (37) first described the use of an ultrasound contrast agent in the late 1960s (Fig. 16.**1**), there have been rapid advances in the contrast agents themselves and in ultrasound techniques. While only A-mode and M-mode ultrasound were available at that time, today there are high-resolution

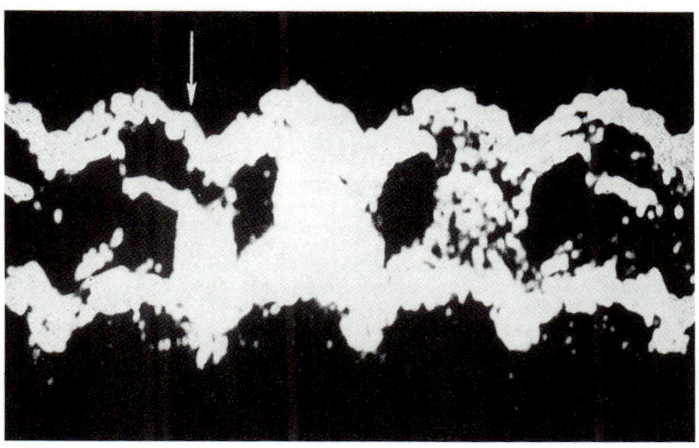

Fig. 16.**1** M-mode display during the intra-aortic injection of physiologic saline in a patient with a normal aortic valve (first publication on the use of ultrasound contrast agents from [37]). The arrow indicates the administration of the contrast agent

techniques that provide a simultaneous, two-dimensional display of soft tissue structures and color-encoded blood flow. The evolution of ultrasound contrast agents has progressed from the use of minute, often naturally occurring gas bubbles in solutions to experimental so-called "manual methods" (Tables 16.**1**, 16.**2**) to the development of standardized agents (Table 16.**3**). The first of these agents has already been approved for diagnostic use in humans. In "manual methods" that use gas as the mechanism for producing contrast echoes (Table 16.**1**), hand agitation (e.g., pumping the solution back and forth between two syringes through a three-way stopcock) or mechanical treatment (e.g. sonication) is used to produce free microbubbles in various solutions (saline, plasma expanders, X-ray contrast media, albumin solution). Microencapsulated gas bubbles also have been used, as well as agents that release microbubbles through a change in physical state (e.g., ether, which boils at body temperature and forms bubbles) or by chemical reactions (e.g., hydrogen peroxide, enzyme-mediated gas release).

Ultrasound contrast agents that use a mechanism other than gas to produce echo enhancement (Table 16.**2**) consist of microparticle systems (microspheres), solutions, and emulsions.

Perfluorochemicals (PFCs) are difficult to classify because their mechanism of action is not fully understood. These agents were developed as blood subtitutes with the ability to transport gases. It is unclear whether this property plays a role in producing the contrast effect, in which case the agent should be classified among the gas-containing systems. A notable feature of these agents is that a large dose is needed to produce the desired effect (2–3 g/kg body weight). This suggests that gas is not involved in the mechanism of action, since gases are highly efficient scatterers of sound (see section 16.1.2). The enhance-

Table 16.**1** Ultrasound contrast agents, "manual methods" using gas to produce echo enhancement

Agent	Organ (method)*	References
Physiologic saline (rapid injection)	Aortic root	37
Rapid injection of glucose solution	Heart (right ventricle)	78
Indocyanine-green 1–5%	Heart (right ventricle)	38
Vitamin solutions (with CO_2)	Heart (right ventricle)	12
Hydrogen peroxide	Heart (right and left ventricles), liver	90, 91
Ether, CO_2	Femoral artery (dog), heart (left ventricle)	55, 63, 93
Gelatin microcapsules filled with nitrogen	VX_2 tumor (rabbit), myocardium (catheter)	10
Microcapsules	Heart	44, 45
Water drunk through a straw	Stomach	92
Sonicated glucose solutions	Myocardium (catheter)	18
Sonicated albumin	Myocardium (injection into the aortic root)	19, 20, 47
Sonicated x-ray contrast media	Myocardium (catheter injection)	47, 58
Agitated plasma expander	Heart	94
Mixture of fat emulsion, plasma, expander, iron (III) salt solution agitated	Myocardium	5
Iodipamide ethyl ester with gas bubbles ("bubbicles")	Liver	62
Gas-filled liposomes ("aerosomes")	Heart (left ventricle, aorta)	84, 85
Lipid-coated microbubbles ("filmix")	Brain	77
Erythrocyte ghosts	Vessels	11

* Applications described in the literature (visualized structures, applied technique, experimental method)

Table 16.**2** Ultrasound contrast agents, "manual methods" using substances other than gas

Agent	Organ*	References
Gelatin microspheres	Liver (dog)	61
Collagen microspheres	Liver (dog)	60
Solutions (citrate, glucose, chelating, amino acid)	Mouse	83
Perfluorochemicals	Myocardium (dog), liver, spleen, kidney	56, 57
Barium sulfate	Intestinal tract	54
Iodipamide ethyl ester particles	Liver	82
Fat emulsion	Liver	23

* see Table 16.**1**

Table 16.**3** Ultrasound contrast agents in development

Agent	Organ (method)*	References
Standardized microbubbles (SHU 454 = Echovist)	Fallopian tube (sterility evaluation)	24, 71
	Vascular imaging (venous or catheter)	33, 89
	Myokardium (catheter)	64
	Liver (intraoperative)	16
	Stomach	22
Stabilized, standardized microbubbles (SHU 508, proposed trade name: Levovist)	Heart (right and left ventricles)	69, 79,
	(Organ)perfusion	25, 74
	Color Doppler	7
	CDS imaging	35, 75
Albumin-stabilized microbubbles (Albunex)	Heart (right and left ventricles)	21, 46
	Myocardium	48
	Liver	34
	Doppler	8, 42
Gas microparticles	Liver, spleen, perfusion	81
Polyaminodicarboxylic acid coimide with gas	Heart (left ventricle)	17
Microfoam (By 20)	Heart	50, 68, 72

* see Table 16.**1**

ment of the ultrasound waves probably depends on the high density and the low acoustic velocity of the substance (33, 36, 39, 65).

Besides the "manual methods" noted above, efforts are underway to develop standardized ultrasound contrast agents for diagnostic use. Considerable progress has been made in the development of agents that contain free bubbles (standardized microbubbles) or stabilized bubbles (stabilized and standardized microbubbles, albumin-stabilized microbubbles). Microparticle systems containing gas are still in an early experimental stage (Table 16.**3**).

16.1.2 Physical Basis

To assess the suitability of substances as ultrasound contrast agents, it is necessary to consider the principles governing the reflection and scattering of sound. The echogenicity of scattering objects depends on the size of the scatterer in relation to the wavelength of the incident sound wave, which is determined by the frequency of the sound wave and its propagation speed in the medium (about 1540 m/s for tissues other than lung and bone). A scatterer in the acoustic field may be significantly smaller than, approximately equal to, or significantly larger than the wavelength of the sound. The frequencies of

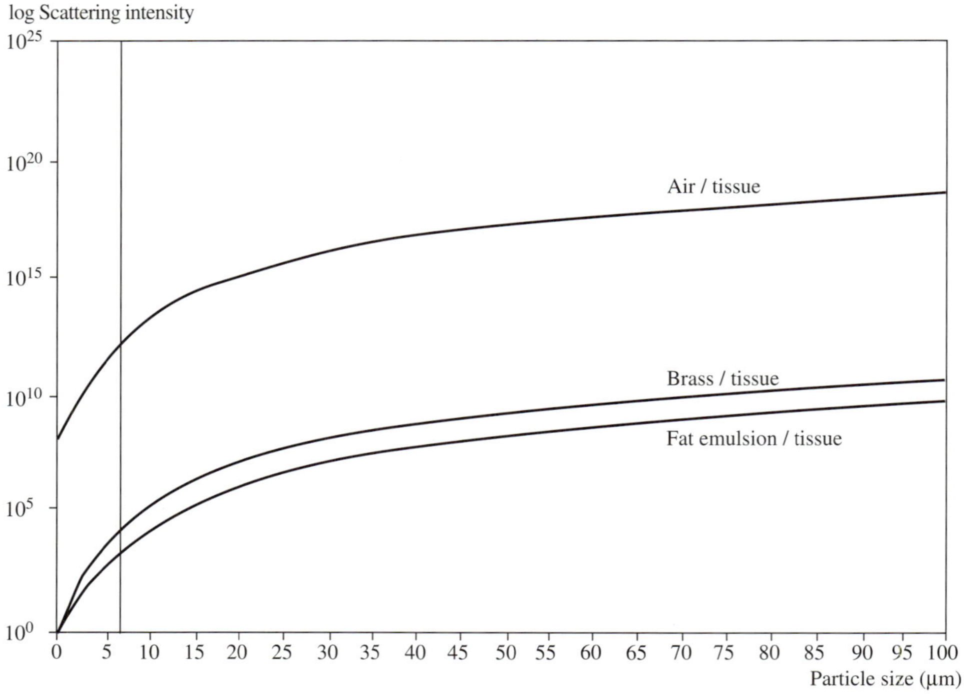

Fig. 16.**2** Relationship between particle size and scattering intensity, calculated for air–tissue, brass–tissue, and fat emulsion–tissue interfaces (for a transducer frequency of 5 MHz in a parenchymatous organ). Scattering intensity at the air–tissue interface is several orders of magnitude higher than at the other interfaces

1–10 MHz used in diagnostic ultrasound are associated with wavelengths in the range of 1540–154 μm. Scatterers for intravascular use have to be smaller than the circulating erythrocytes so that they will not produce hemodynamic effects. Thus an acceptable intraluminal contrast agent has to contain scatterers that are significantly smaller than the wavelength of the ultrasound. Only agents for use in the gastrointestinal tract may contain scatterers with a size comparable to or greater than the ultrasound wavelength.

Therefore we may limit our attention to scatterers that are significantly smaller than the wavelength of ultrasound. The scattering intensity of particles is a function of the particle diameter, the ultrasound frequency, and the properties of the interface between a particle and the surrounding medium (impedance difference). Figure 16.**2** shows the relationship between particle size and scattering intensity (dimensionless) for various substances interfacing with biologic tissue. The air–tissue interface was selected to illustrate a low-density medium with a low sound velocity. The brass–tissue interface illustrates the conditions for a high-density material with a relatively high sound velocity, while the fat emulsion–tissue interface illustrates a relatively close match in density and sound velocity between the interfacing media. The data were calculated for a frequency of 5 MHz and plotted in log scale.

It is apparent from Figure 16.**2** that gas bubbles are much more effective scatterers under the defined conditions than substances with a high density and relatively high sound velocity. When the contiguous media have similar densities and sound velocities, they also have similar scattering intensities, resulting in low echogenicity. To compensate, significantly larger particle diameters (30–50 μm) are necessary at interfaces other than gas–tissue. Due to physiological reasons such a particle size is unsuitable for intravascular use. Other possible solutions, such as increasing the concentration or using a higher transducer frequency (to increase the scattering intensity) are also unacceptable due to technical or medical problems.

Therefore we have to conclude that only gas-containing systems are capable of producing a medically safe and diagnostically useful increase in the echogenicity of intravascular structures. All ultrasound contrast agents approved for diagnostic use and currently under development are based on this principle.

16.1.2.1 Significance of Echogenicity Enhancement by Contrast Agents in Color-Encoded Flow Imaging Techniques

Doppler techniques involve measurement of the frequency shift between the emitted ultrasound and the backscatted signal from the moving object (e.g., red blood cells). The frequency shift is proportional to the velocity of the insonated object (see Chapter 17).

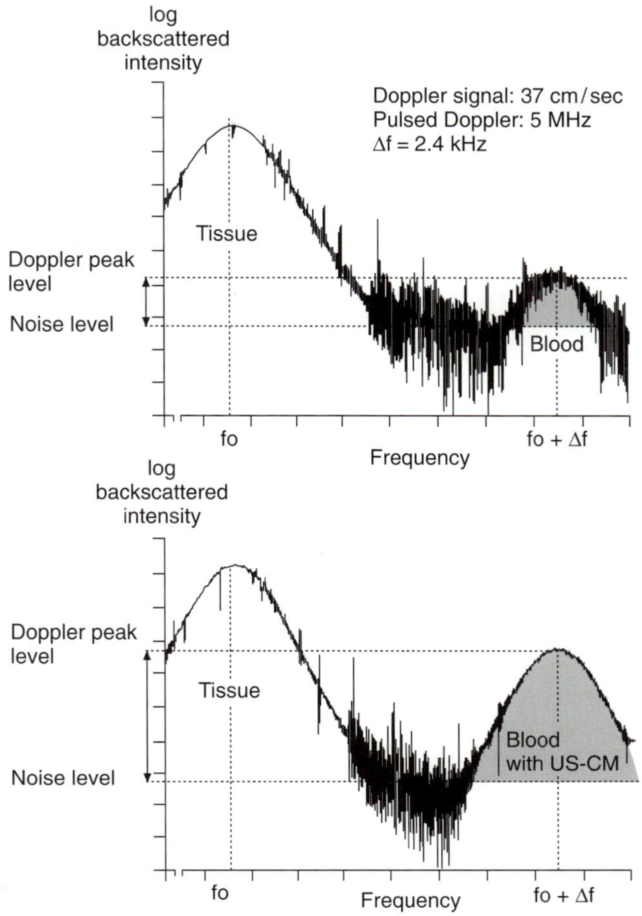

Fig. 16.**3** Graphic representation of a Doppler signal for low-volume flow in a small vessel. In the native situation (= without contrast medium) *(top)* the Doppler signal is poorly differentiated or indistinguishable from noise. After the administration of contrast medium *(bottom),* signal definition is significantly improved.
f_0 = Transmission frequency, Δf = frequency shift ("Doppler shift"), ↕ = technically useful component of signal intensity

In the imaging of low-volume flow and/or slow flow and in the detection of blood flow at greater depths, the low signal-to-noise ratio creates problems in the detection of frequency shifts and thus in the Doppler display. Ultrasound contrast agents improve the signal-to-noise ratio by increasing the intensity of the backscattered signal, thereby improving the ability of the ultrasound instrument to detect and display the signal. These effects are graphically illustrated in Figures 16.**3** and 16.**4**.

Time domain processing (TDP) differs from conventional Doppler techniques in that it does not utilize information on frequency or phase shifts. In this method data sets of characteristic signal components in designated volume elements are cross-correlated at successive, closely spaced points in time. Flow velocities can be calculated from the movement of these characteristic signal components in designated time intervals (see Chapter 1 and 17). Because this method uses the same signals as Doppler but simply interprets them in a different way, a poor signal-to-noise ratio (e.g., due to a large distance between transducer and vessel, low-volume flow, or difficult anatomic conditions) again leads to an unsatisfactory flow image. As in Doppler technology, the use of ultrasound contrast agents can improve the signal-to-noise ratio and thus improve the detection of certain signals or even enable the detection of signals that would be missed otherwise.

Without contrast enhancement, color-encoded ultrasound techniques are unable to demonstrate motion in cavities (e.g., fallopian tubes, ureters, urethra) that are not perfused by acoustic scatterers such as red cells. The instillation of an ultrasound contrast agent into these cavities produces a flow of scatterers that can be visualized in the color-encoded image.

The effect of ultrasound contrast agents in CDS imaging techniques (Doppler, TDP) is based on the enhanced echogenicity. A larger percentage of the ultrasound energy is scattered back, and the signal-to-noise ratio is improved (Fig. 16.**5a, b**).

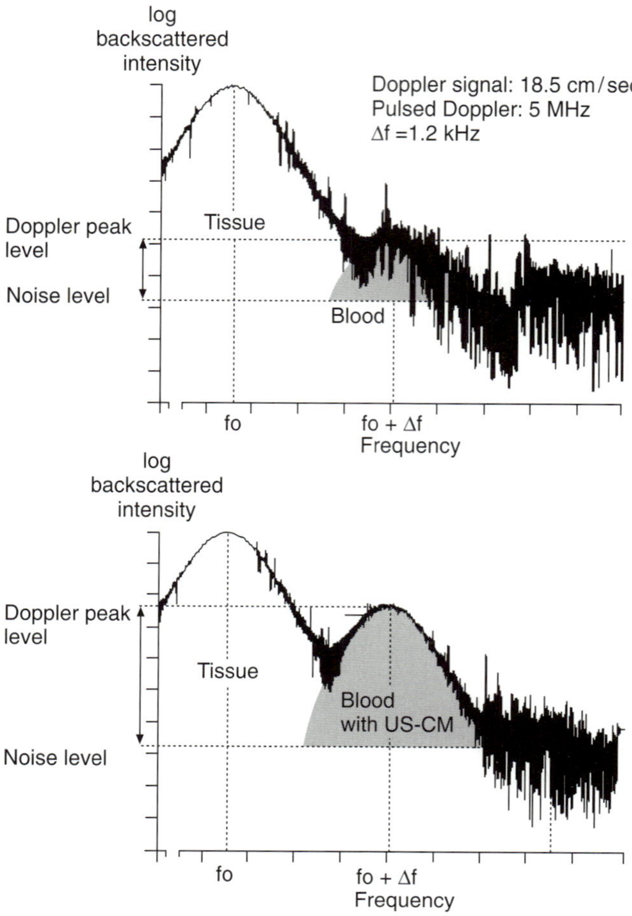

Fig. 16.**4** Graphic representation of a Doppler signal for low-velocity flow (low-frequency shift). In the native situation, the Doppler signal is poorly distinguishable from the stationary-tissue signal. After administration on the contrast agent, the intensity of the Doppler signal is increased, and the frequency-shifted component is easier to detect
f_0 = Transmission frequency, Δf = frequency shift ("Doppler shift"), ↕ = technically useful component of signal intensity

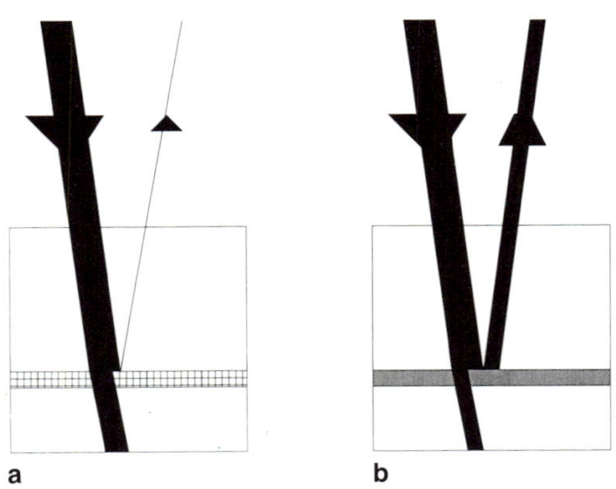

Fig. 16.**5 a, b** Schematic diagram illustrating the effect of an ultrasound contrast agent on signal intensity
a In a native scan, only a small portion of the incident energy is backscattered as the sound wave passes through the vessel lumen
b After administration of the ultrasound contrast agent, the amplitude of the wave backscattered to the transducer is increased

16.1.3 Properties of Ultrasound Contrast Agents (Approved or in Development)

The development of ultrasound contrast agents of the type listed in Tables 16.**1** and 16.**2** ("manual methods") is limited due to lack of reproducibility and homogeneity of the ultrasound contrast effects, resulting in inherent resistance of these methods to standardization (52). Moreover, the safety of these agents is unproven, and side effects related to inadequate standardization have been reported (53). Finally, the poor scattering properties of the agents listed in Table 16.**2** lead to poor efficacy under physiologic conditions.

To solve these problems, several contrast agents have been developed in recent years which utilize gas to produce echo enhancement. These agents are listed in Table 16.**3**. The first three agents are either in clinical development or have already been approved (at least in Germany) for specific indications. These agents can be divided into two classes: (1) "right-heart contrast agents," which are destroyed or filtered during their first passage through the lung after peripheral intravenous application, and (2) "left-heart" or "transpulmonary" contrast agents, which survive pulmonary transit when administered by the same route and produce Doppler signal enhancement in the arterial system. Gas microparticles and polyaminodicarboxylic acid coimidenes with gas are relatively new experimental approaches that are not yet available for clinical use. There are virtually no recent data (since 1988) on microfoam (By 20). These approaches are omitted from the following discussions, therefore.

16.1.3.1 Right-Heart Contrast Agents

One agent in this group, Echovist, has already been approved for echocardiographic use in Germany. This ultrasound contrast agent consists of a two-vial system. One vial contains microparticles (median diameter 3.5 μm, 99% smaller than 12 μm [29]), which in the dry state are aggregated to form small spherical granules (Fig. 16.**6**). These granules disintegrate into separate microparticles when suspended with the suspension medium. A second vial contains the suspension medium (galactose solution). Prior to use, the necessary amount of suspension medium is transferred into the vial with the microparticles, and the vial is shaken to produce a milky suspension that is ready for use. The suspension is stable for at least 5 min at room temperature (51). The contrast effect is produced by gas microbubbles adherent to the galactose microparticles and depends on the particle concentration (mg/mL) (26). The gas content per ml of suspension is less than 40 μL (1 g of the agent contains less than 100 μL gas).

Comprehensive studies have shown no evidence of toxicity problems with this agent (27). Animal studies have proven the efficacy of the agent for imaging of the right ventricle (52, 79), myocardium (40, 66, 67), and liver and in gynecologic and urologic applications (27). Tests in large clinical series have been conducted for various indications in cardiology, urology, and gynecology (29). Echovist is available as an approved contrast agent for opacification of the right heart, and further applications are currently under investigation and will be forthcoming.

16.1.3.2 Transpulmonary Contrast Agents

At present there are two agents of this group in clinical trials. One (SHU 508, hereafter referred to by its proposed trade name of Levovist) is a preparation based on Echovist (see above). The second, Albunex, consists of albumin-stabilized microspheres.

Levovist is composed of galactose microparticles (galactose content >99%, median <2 μm, 99% <7 μm) with stable, standardized gas microbubbles adherent to their surface. These microbubbles are stabilized to the galactose microparticles by the addition of a physiologically occurring fatty acid (content <0.5%). One milliliter of suspension with a concentration of 400 mg/mL contains approximately $2 \cdot 10^{10}$ microbubbles above 1 μm in diameter. The microparticles are suspended in water for injection, and the

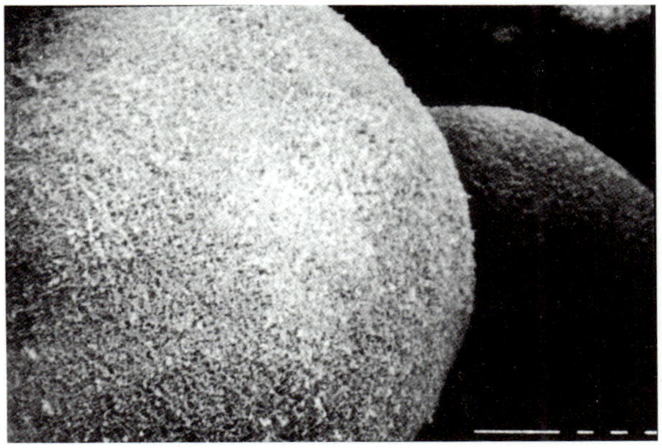

Fig. 16.**6** Electron micrograph of Echovist granules. Galactose microparticles are visible on the surface of the two magnified granules. The interspaces contain gas

volume of water used to suspend the microparticles determines the concentration of the suspension. The freshly prepared suspension remains stable for more than 15 min. The gas volume of the suspension is approximately equal to that in Echovist. The usual microparticle concentration ranges from 50 to 400 mg/mL.

Comprehensive tolerance studies in experimental animals (acute and subacute toxicity with extensive histologic evaluation, local tolerance, embryotoxicity, genotoxicity, measurement of hemodynamic parameters after intravenous and intra-arterial injection, direct observation of the microcirculation) have demonstrated no medically significant adverse effects related to the system (33). The diagnostic efficacy of Levovist has been confirmed in both B-mode and Doppler studies in animals (24, 25, 28, 30, 31, 34, 35).

Albumin-stabilized microspheres (Albunex). Albunex is produced by the sonication of 5% human albumin solution, forming stable, gas-filled proteinaceous shells that do not dissolve in albumin solution (2–4). Parts of the proteinaceous shells show properties that differ from native albumin (isoelectric point, anion binding) (4). The estimated particle concentration is 437 million/mL (48), with a wall thickness of 40–50 nm (3) and diameter of 1.4–18.3 μm (median 4.0 μm, 90% < 10 μm) (14, 21). Reports on the shelf life of Albunex range from 6 to 12 months (when stored at 4–22 °C (3, 48). Following intravenous administration of this agent, gray-scale signal enhancement is observed only in the left ventricle; there is no effect in the large arterial vessels downstream (46). Doppler signal enhancement is fully attenuated by the second capillary transit (13).

Numerous studies have been done on the safety of Albunex. Hemodynamic studies and clinical observation in dogs, apes, and human subjects showed no agent-related changes considered to be of clinical significance (19, 21, 88). Acute and subacute studies in rats, dogs, and monkeys showed no significant changes in hematologic or serologic parameters or urinary composition (2). The injection of Albunex in pigs led to marked increases in pulmonary arterial blood pressure, which could be prevented with high doses of indomethacin. It is known from immunologic studies (3) that the protein shell of Albunex acts as an antigen in certain species but not in humans or cynomolgus monkeys.

Studies also have been done on the contrast efficacy of Albunex for Doppler investigations of the liver and kidneys in woodchucks (9, 43) and for cardiac imaging in various animal species. Clinical studies have shown that an i.v. dose of approximately 0.05 mL/kg body weight produces right ventricular contrast effects in all patients, while a dose of 0.08 mL/kg produces left ventricular opacification in 90% of patients. Increasing the dose did not improve the results (21). In one clinical study contrast effects were observed in the myocardium after image processing (58).

The echocardiographic applications of Albunex are the most fully developed, and the documents for this application have been submitted to authorities in several countries (1) and are already approved for clinical use in Sweden and Japan. Additional applications are expected to be forthcoming (1).

16.1.3.3 Negative Contrast Agents for Imaging the Gut

Another type of contrast agents is currently being investigated that aims at avoiding artifacts due to gas in the gut. The agents contain hydrocolloids and/or polysiloxan (5, 41, 55, 86).

These agents are still under investigation and their clinical potential, especially in color-encoded techniques, has yet to be proven.

16.1.4 In Vitro Studies of Contrast Agents in Color Duplex Sonography

To test the validity of the theoretical considerations on the mode of action and potential applications of ultrasound contrast agents (see section 16.1.2.1), we performed flow imaging experiments with Echovist and Levovist in PTFE tubes embedded at various depths in an agar–agar/graphite phantom. Various pumps were used to generate both continuous and pulsatile blood flow (reconstituted erythrocyte concentrates) to simulate vascular perfusion. We found that when a portion of the perfusion volume was replaced with Echovist (200 mg/mL), we were able to detect flow signals that were undetectable without the agent (Fig. 16.7**a, b**). Use of the contrast agent lowered the velocity threshold of flow detection by a factor of from two to four.

To simulate the imaging of cavities that normally do not contain significant number of scatterers (e.g., ureters, urethra, fallopian tubes), we perfused the tubes in the phantom with physiologic saline solution and with pure contrast agent. The movement of the saline solution in the tubes produced little or no color flow activity (QAD I = Doppler system, Platinum = TDP system [Quantum, Philips]). But even low concentrations of contrast agent (50 mg/mL) generated prominent flow signals in the perfused tubing in both the Doppler and TDP studies.

These in vitro experiments confirmed the expectations raised by theoretical considerations. Additionally, it was shown that agents that did not have gas as their mechanism of action did not produce an acceptable contrast effect in the CDS systems (80).

16.1.5 Flow Imaging in Experimental Animals

Experiments were performed in beagle dogs to confirm the in vitro findings. The differences between native scans and postcontrast scans (after the i.v. injection of Levovist) were studied in perfusion images of the liver, kidney, and vessels using color duplex ultrasound techniques.

16.1.5.1 Transpulmonary Contrast Agents, Doppler Technique

Renal perfusion studies with CDS imaging (QAD I) showed that the i.v. injection of Levovist in a concentration of 300 mg/ml and a volume of 2 ml produced marked enhancement of perfusion in the kidney (Fig. 16.**8a, b**). In this situation the contrast agent led to almost complete color encoding of the perfused renal areas, while the unenhanced images demonstrated blood flow only in the large perihilar vessels. Further studies showed that even small intrarenal perfusion defects were reliably demonstrated by CDS following intravenous contrast injection (Levovist, 2 mL, 300 mg/mL). The perfusions defects detected with contrast-enhanced CDS showed good agreement with correlative angiograms (Fig. 16.**9a, b**). Following release of the experimental occlusion, a perfusion disturbance could be seen longer with contrast-enhanced CDS than with angiography. This may indicate that CDS with contrast enhancement is the more sensitive procedure in the detection of perfusion deficits.

Due to the vast absorption and scattering of sound in the canine skin, even superficial vessels are difficult to define in the B-mode image. Again, the i.v. injection of Levovist provided marked, dose-dependent enhancement of the color-encoded flow signals compared with the precontrast scans. In one dog the injection of 2 mL (300 mg/kg) Levovist produced excellent Doppler signal enhancement that persisted for approximately 3 min (Fig. 16.**10a, b**). The color-encoded signals completely filled the vessel lumen in systole, and no artifacts were observed at this dose level. Even after the second capillary transit, the contrast agent produced marked enhancement of the venous flow signals. Increasing the contrast dose tends to produce conspicuous artifacts, especially in the early postinjection period. The color-encoded signals transcend the vessel lumen, creating a perivascu-

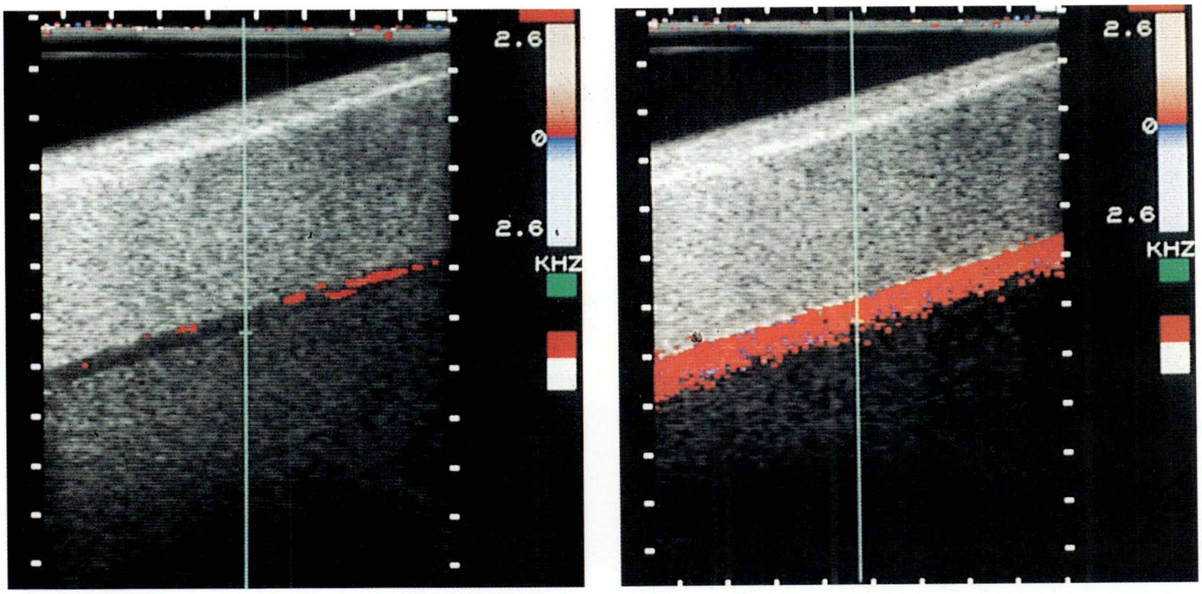

a b

Fig. 16.**7a, b** Color duplex study (QAD 1) of the perfusion of a plastic tube in an agar–agar/graphite phantom
a Perfusion with blood at a flow rate of 45 mL/min. The lumen of the tube appears as a hypoechoic structure. The green vertical line with the two horizontal bars represents the volume for quantitative measurement. Only isolated color-encoded flow signals are visible in the real-time image

b Same rate of flow, with 10% of the blood replaced by Echovist (200 mg/mL). Now the lumen is completely filled with color-encoded flow signals. The extraluminal signals at the bottom of the tube result from an excessive concentration of contrast agent

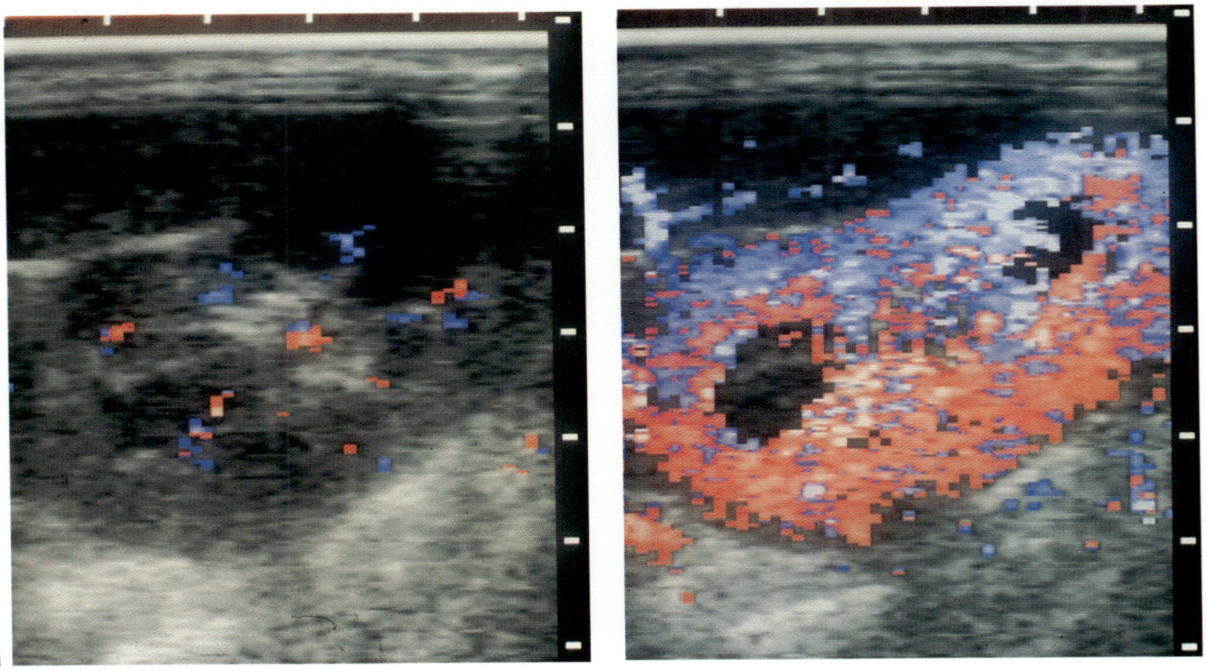

a b

Fig. 16.**8a, b** Normal left kidney of a dog (12 kg body weight) before and after the i. v. injection of ultrasound contrast agent (examination with QAD I)
a The plain image shows color-encoded flow signals only in the large vessels near the renal hilum

b After the injection of 2 mL Levovist (300 mg/mL), flow signals completely fill the renal parenchyma, sparing only the renal pelvis

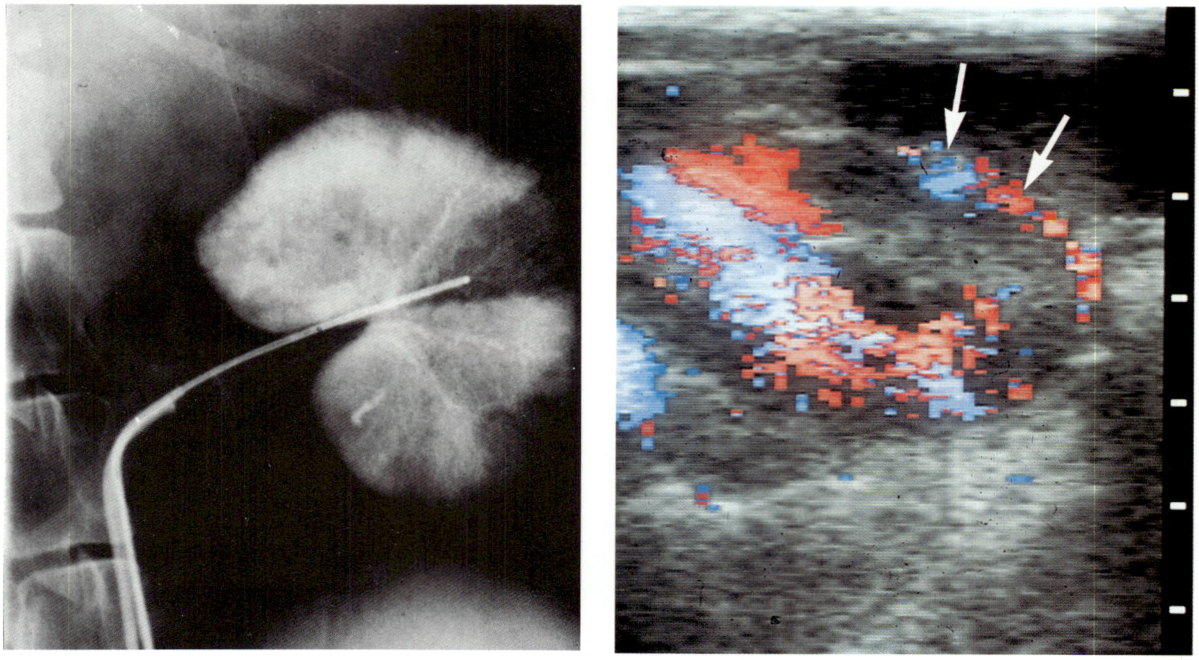

a b

Fig. 16.**9a, b** Experimentally induced temporary occlusion of renal segmental arteries in dog (12 kg body weight)
a Selective angiography in the parenchymal phase demonstrates wedge-shaped defects in the central and caudal portions of the kidney

b CDS (examination with QAD I) after i. v. contrast (2 mL [300 mg/mL] Levovist) shows wedge-shaped perfusion deficits (color voids) in the renal parenchyma similar to those in the angiogram. CDS also shows flow in renal capsular vessels (arrows) not visualized in the angiogram

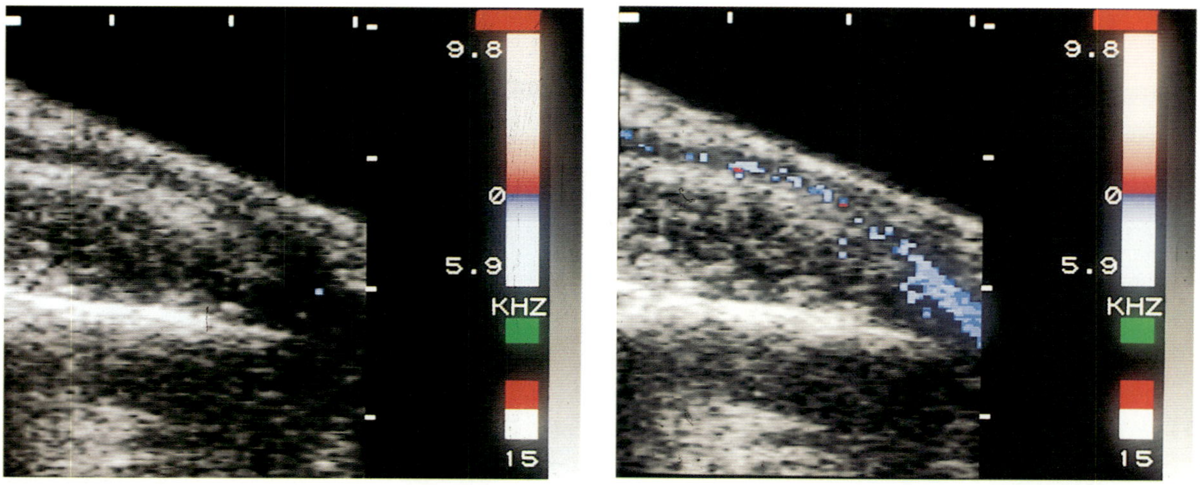

a b

Fig. 16.**10a, b** CDS scans (examinations with QAD I) of a superficial vein in the hind leg of a dog
a The vessel is defined on the precontrast scan, but flow signals are not visible at the selected setting

b Scan on the same plane after i. v. injection (brachial vein) of 2 mL (300 mg/mL) Levovist. Now the venous flow signals are prominently color-encoded without manipulation of the soft tissues. This degree of enhancement was obtained after the second capillary transit

lar "cloud" of mixed red and blue signals. These artifacts subside after an initial phase. In dogs with a proximal occlusion of the femoral artery (which was surgically ligated during previous studies), the i.v. injection of Levovist significantly improved visualization of the distal connecting vessels compared with the precontrast images. The vascular anatomy and lesion sites showed an obvious correlation with angiographic findings (i.v. DSA) (Fig. 16.**11 a, b**).

Intravenous Levovist also produced flow signal enhancement in the extracranial portions of the carotid artery. Because the blood flow in this region is

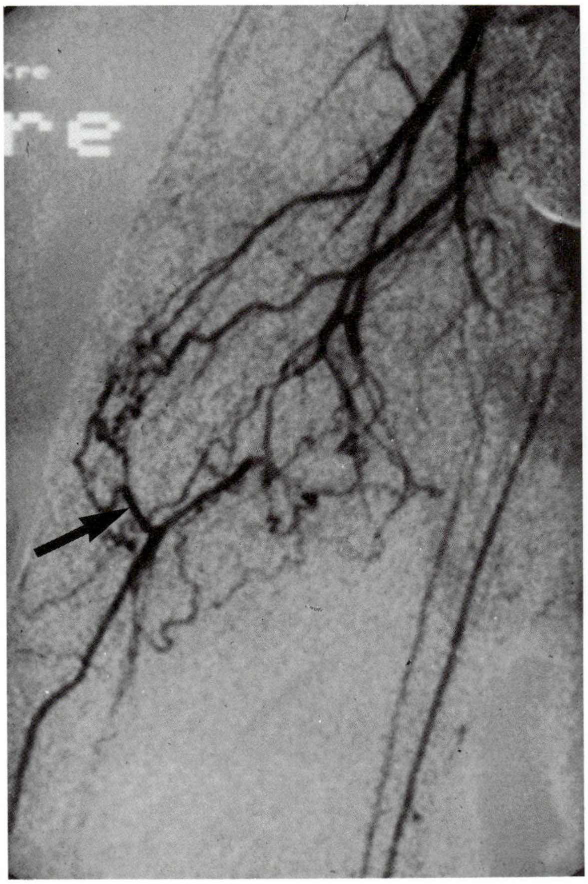

a

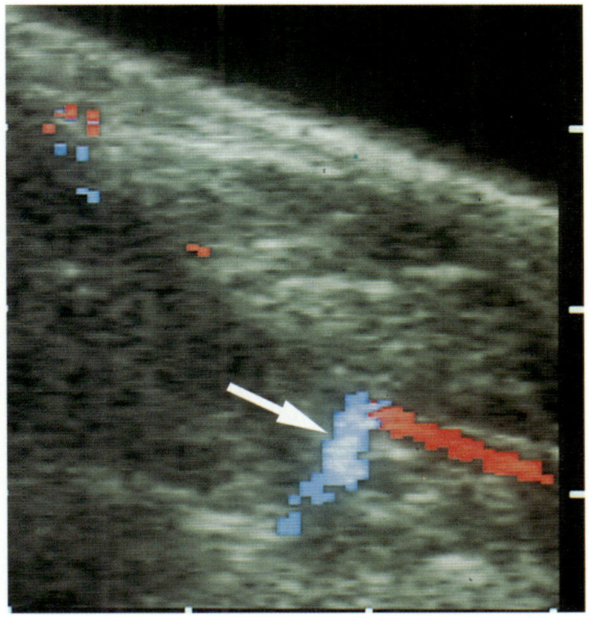

b

Fig. 16.**11 a, b** Proximal occlusion of the femoral artery in a dog (surgically ligated in a previous study)
a Intravenous DSA demonstrates a long occlusion of the femoral artery. A large collateral (arrow) reconstitutes flow to the popliteal artery in its proximal third
b CDS scan (examination with QAD I) after i. v. contrast injection (2 mL [300 mg/mL] Levovist). Enhanced color-encoded flow signals clearly demonstrate the collateral (arrow, not visible in the precontrast scan) and the connecting vessel

generally copious and rapid, there would seem to be little need for ultrasound contrast agents in extracranial carotid examinations. The intracranial vessels, however, present an unfavorable signal-to-noise ratio (transcranial Doppler sonography) that can be positively influenced by the use of a suitable ultrasound contrast agent. Initial animal studies in this area (transvitreous examination of retro-orbital perfusion in dogs) have shown that the use of contrast agents can expand the areas accessible to color flow imaging. This shows that a diagnostic gain can be achieved with the use of ultrasound contrast agents in transcranial Doppler techniques in humans.

Echovist has already been approved in Germany for use in cardiologic examinations. Ultrasound contrast agents can be beneficial in the evaluation of cardiac defects. These agents facilitates the detection of valvular defects or small atrial or ventricular septal defects (ASD, VSD). Figure 16.**12** shows a small regurgitant jet over a canine mitral valve that was virtually undetectable on the precontrast scan (left side of the M-mode image in the figure). In this case the i.v. injection of Levovist enabled the detection of mitral insufficiency (center of the M-mode image).

CDS imaging after intravenous Albunex provided enhanced visualization of hepatic tumors in rabbits (experimental VX_2 tumor) and of renal perfusion in woodchucks (43). Furthermore, signal enhancement was also described in Doppler recordings from the rabbit aorta following i.v. injections of Albunex (42).

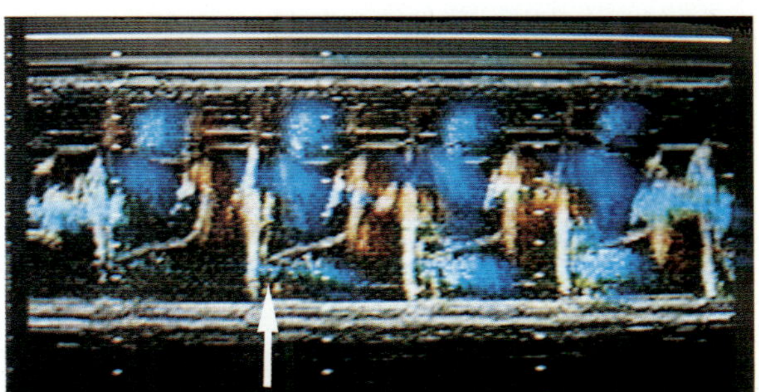

Fig. 16.**12** M-mode color Doppler echocardiogram in a dog with moderate mitral regurgitation. The blue-encoded reflux through the valve is detected (lower part of image) only after injection of the contrast agent (arrow)

16.1.5.2 Transpulmonary Contrast Agents, Time Domain Processed Imaging

Analogous to Doppler technique, the administration of Levovist produces significant, concentration-dependent enhancement of flow signals in the time domain processed image (TDP). This has been confirmed in in vitro experiments as well as animal models. The signal enhancement obtained in TDP is somewhat weaker than in the Doppler technique, however. Intravenous Levovist in dogs, for example, produced a two-peak pattern of enhancement in the color-encoded areas of the liver (Fig. 16.**13a, b**). The first, weaker peak resulted from the influx of the contrast agent through the artery and the second, stronger peak from additional inflow through the portal system. Further studies are needed, however, to make a valid assessment of the capabilities of contrast-enhanced CDS using the TDP technique.

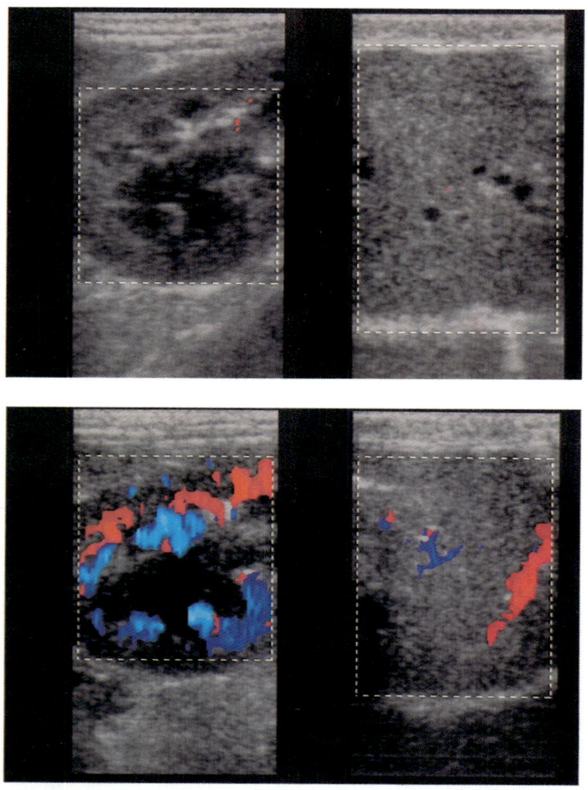

Fig. 16.**13a, b** Time domain processed images (Platinum) of a canine kidney and liver (see Chapter 17)
a Precontrast CV images show only isolated color-encoded flow signals in the kidney *(left)* and liver *(right)*
b The i.v. injection of 2 mL (300 mg/mL) Levovist enhances the flow images in both organs. Signal enhancement is significantly greater in the kidney than in the liver (due to the lower perfusion of that organ relative to total blood flow)

16.1.5.3 Assessment

In interpreting the results of the animal studies, it should be considered that the insonated vessels are generally smaller than the corresponding human vessels. In applying the results to humans, therefore, one can expect somewhat more favorable results in the larger human vessels.

Animal studies have demonstrated a positive effect of ultrasound contrast agents in the assessment of organ perfusion as well as peripheral vessels. Slow and/or relatively low-volume flows and signals in unfavorable anatomic conditions (high tissue attenuation, structures distant to the transducer) can be evaluated with much greater clarity following the intravenous injection of ultrasound contrast medium.

16.1.6 Cavity Imaging in Experimental Animals

Body cavities that normally contain no moving scatterers (erythrocytes) or very small quantities of scatterers (e.g., epithelial cells in the bladder) are poorly demonstrated by CDS techniques. The results of phantom experiments indicate, however, that cavitary structures such as the lower urinary tract or fallopian tubes can be visualized by instilling an ultrasound contrast agent into the structure (see section 16.1.4). In contrast to X-ray studies, in which the cavity is opacified by the contrast medium filling it, CDS demonstrates the flow of the contrast agent inside the cavity. Once again, studies were performed in experimental animals to check the results of the in vitro studies. Experiments with bladder imaging in dogs showed that CDS can detect and display the intravesical flow of contrast agent with a higher sensitivity than is achieved by gray-scale imaging of the contrast agent in a conventional B-mode scan. The instillation of Levovist into the bladder in low concentration (50 mg/mL, 10 mL) produced only marginal gray-scale enhancement when the bladder contents were stationary. When a circular flow pattern was introduced, prominent color-encoded flow signals filled the bladder lumen in the CDS display. Substantially higher concentrations of the contrast agent were needed to achieve stronger gray-scale enhancement in this model (200 mg/mL, 10 ml). In this case the circular flow pattern led to color encoding transcending the anatomical structures and artifacts that distorted the image (Fig. 16.**14a–d**).

In one dog with an experimentally induced unilateral vesicoureteral reflux (the ureter was detached and reimplanted outside the trigone), it was determined whether CDS could demonstrate the retrograde flow of contrast agent into the renal pelvis. The kidneys were alternately examined during instillation of the contrast suspension into the bladder. After the bladder was filled with a mixture of ultrasound contrast agent (Echovist or Levovist) and saline solution, color-encoded flow signals were detected only in the renal

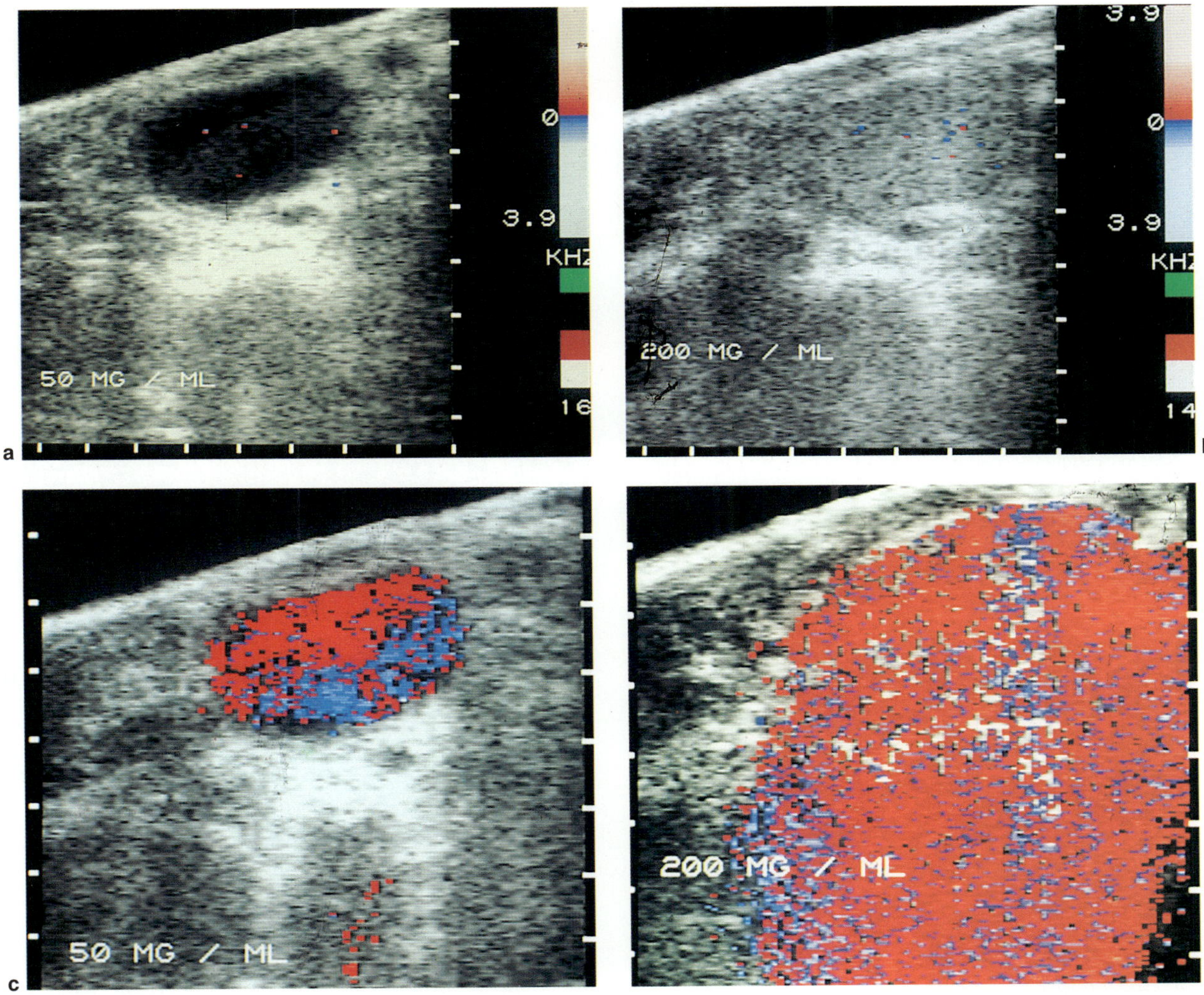

Fig. 16.**14a–d** Canine urinary bladder imaged with the QAD I
a, **b** The bladder was filled with 10 mL of Levovist suspension in a concentration of 50 mg/mL (**a**) and 200 mg/mL (**b**). 50 mg/mL of contrast agent produces minimal gray-scale enhancement in the bladder lumen, while 200 mg/mL produces a hyperechoic lumen
c, **d** The bladder is additionally filled with 0.9% saline solution, producing a circular movement of the bladder contents. The concentration of 50 mg/mL (**c**) yields color-encoded flow signals that are confined to the bladder lumen. The higher concentration (200 mg/mL) (**d**) produces massive artifacts that seriously hamper evaluation of the bladder

pelvis on the side of the radiographically confirmed reflux (Fig. 16.**15a–c**). No significant difference was noted between the contrast agents, although Levovist produced a better contrast effect at lower concentration than Echovist.

16.1.7 Summary

The combination of CDS and ultrasound contrast medium produces significant enhancement of blood flow signals in phantom experiments and animal models, thereby improving the visualization of slow and/or low-volume flow. This effect is particularly useful in situations where the signal-to-noise ratio is poor (examination of structures distant to the transducer, elevated absorption of sound waves by tissues). The instillation of contrast agent is necessary for the CDS imaging of cavities that do not contain moving scatterers.

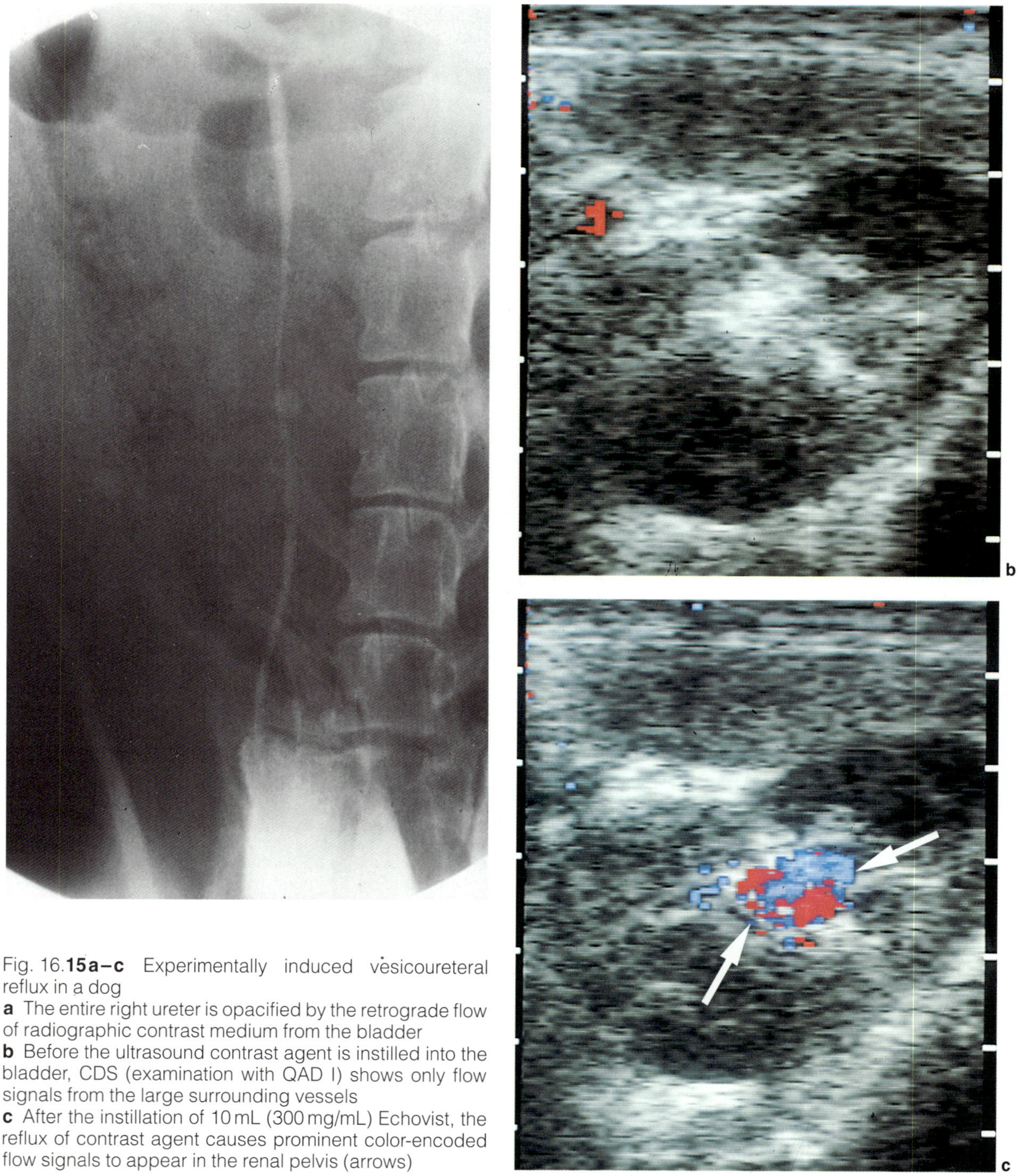

Fig. 16.**15a–c** Experimentally induced vesicoureteral reflux in a dog

a The entire right ureter is opacified by the retrograde flow of radiographic contrast medium from the bladder

b Before the ultrasound contrast agent is instilled into the bladder, CDS (examination with QAD I) shows only flow signals from the large surrounding vessels

c After the instillation of 10 mL (300 mg/mL) Echovist, the reflux of contrast agent causes prominent color-encoded flow signals to appear in the renal pelvis (arrows)

16.2 Clinical Application

F. Fobbe

16.2.1 Introduction

The results of phantom and animal experiments suggest that ultrasound contrast agents are a potentially valuable adjunct to CDS imaging. This particularly applies to agents that survive transpulmonary passage after peripheral intravenous injection and produce signal enhancement in the arterial system. The signal enhancement produced by the contrast agent is clearly apparent in the real-time CDS image and permits a full evaluation of the structure of interest. Despite numerous animal studies, clinical experience with contrast-enhanced CDS is still limited. This is due mainly to the limited availability of suitable contrast agents. To date, only one contrast agent has been approved in Germany for echocardiographic use (Echovist). This agent loses its contrast efficacy on its first passage through the lung, however. Presently there are two additional agents in the clinical testing stage (Levovist and Albunex) which retain their efficacy on crossing the lung and provide signal enhancement in the arterial system following peripheral venous injection. Most publications on the clinical application of these agents deal with their use in echocardiography (2, 3, 5, 10, 12). Nevertheless, previous clinical experience in the noncardiologic use of contrast-enhanced CDS imaging (Echovist and Levovist, still no known clinical studies with Albunex) is quite promising and will be discussed below. We shall review the principal results without attempting a complete description of the studies. The interested reader may consult the literature for further details.

16.2.2 Intravascular Use

16.2.2.1 Direct

The direct application of ultrasound contrast was investigated in patients with deep venous thrombosis of the lower extremity. The ultrasound contrast agent (Echovist) was injected into a dorsal pedal vein in the supine patient, just as in contrast venography, and the contrast runoff was followed by CDS imaging. The contrast agent was too concentrated for this procedure, however, and serious artifacts occurred. Also, most contrast runoff occurred through the nonthrombosed veins, and the volume of the contrast agent (10 mL) was too low. The only effect was a brief enhancement that was inadequate for evaluation of the lower leg veins, even in the absence of artifacts. This experience is consistent with the results of animal studies. Besides peripheral venous injections, the agent was also injected directly into arterial vessels. Again, this produced conspicuous artifacts that interfered with the evaluation.

16.2.2.2 Indirect

In an indirect contrast examination, the agent is injected into a peripheral vein, and the contrast effect in the systemic arteries is utilized after the agent has traversed the lung. This technique leads to a dose-dependent, and thus controllable, enhancement of the blood flow signals. The pulmonary transit distributes the agent in such a way that its contrast effect persists for 2–3 min even when the agent is administered by bolus injection. This technique was used clinically to examine the peripheral arteries of patients with significant chronic arterial occlusive disease. Injection of the contrast agent (Levovist) was always followed by enhancement of the Doppler signals from the blood. Even slow flow like that occurring distal to an occlusion could be clearly evaluated in the contrast enhanced images (Fig. 16.**16a–c**). Blood flow in small collateral vessels was also demonstrated. Signal enhancement in the lower extremity veins was still apparent after the second capillary transit (8). The indirect application of Levovist provided significant improvement of color-encoded flow visualization even under difficult examination conditions. Similar results as in peripheral arterieas of the leg were obtained in intracranial vessels (4, 6, 9).

16.2.3 Extravascular Use

Besides their intravascular use, ultrasound contrast agents can be used in cavities where normally occurring scatterers are too small or too sparse to produce detectable flow. This application has already been tested in the assessment of tubal patency in infertile women and in children with suspected vesicoureteral reflux.

In two studies a total of 27 infertile women were examined with Echovist-enhanced CDS, and the result was compared with X-ray hysterosalpingography (HSG). The ultrasound contrast agent was slowly instilled into the uterine cavity through a catheter. Seventeen women were examined transabdominally and 10 transvaginally. In women with freely patent tubes, prominent flow signals could be tracked through the fallopian tube in both techniques (Fig. 16.**17a, b**) with good agreement between the results of CDS and HSG (7, 11). Only about 5 mL of the contrast agent was required. This is considerably less than needed when gray-scale imaging alone is used (1). The transvaginal approach is advantageous in that it does not require bladder distention, and the uterus and ovaries are less obscured by overlying bowel. This simple, well-tolerated technique could replace X-ray HSG.

Vesicoureteral reflux (VUR) is the most common cause of recurrent urinary tract infections in children. In the past, radiographic techniques have been the only means available for diagnosing VUR with acceptable confidence. After positive results in animal experiments (see section 16.2), we initiated a study comparing Echovist-enhanced CDS images with voiding cystourethrography. However, we were

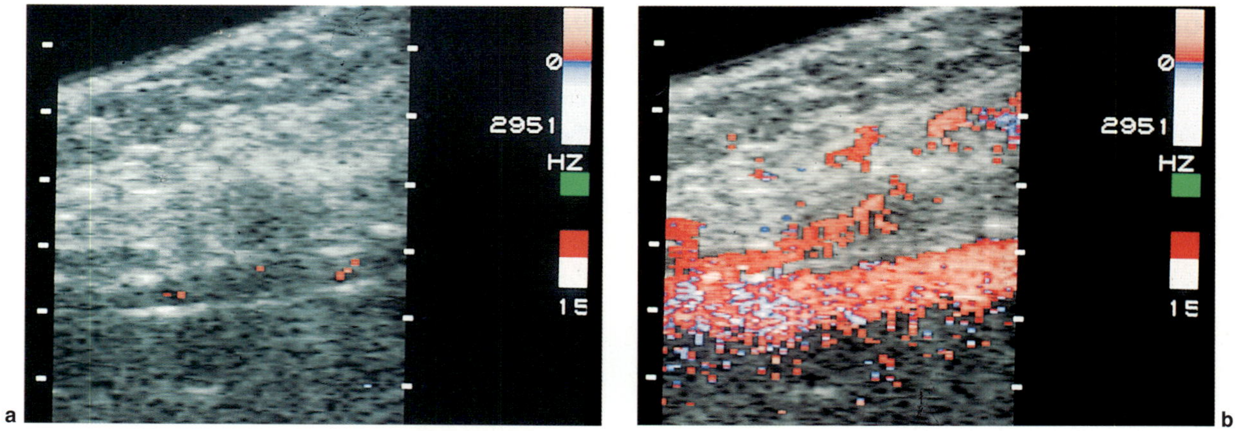

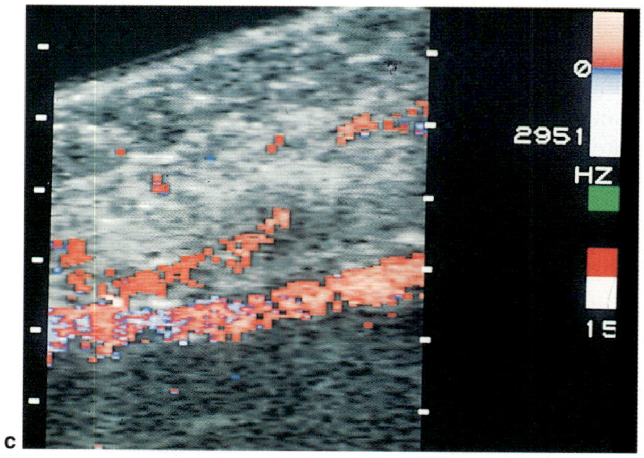

Fig. 16.**16a–c** CDS appearance (examination with QAD I) of the distal superficial femoral artery before and after the peripheral intravenous injection of an ultrasound contrast agent
a The vessel wall is defined on the precontrast image, but only isolated flow signals are detected
b In the initial phase after 10 mL of Levovist (300 mg/mL) there is excessive signal enhancement with artifacts and extraluminal color-encoded signals. Besides the femoral artery, signals from collateral vessels are also displayed
c Ideal enhancement is observed in the plateau phase. Color-encoded signals precisely fill the vessel lumen, demonstrating luminal narrowing with flow disturbance (mixed red and blue signals) distal to the origin of a side branch in the cranial part (left side) of the vessel

unable to duplicate the good results of the animal experiments due to the inadequate half-life (5 min) and rapid sedimentation of the contrast agent in the bladder. Levovist, a newer contrast agent with a longer stability and slower sedimentation, is probably better suited for the detection of vesicouretral reflux. So far, however, no clinical studies have been done on this application of Levovist.

16.2.4 Future Outlook

When combined with CDS, ultrasound contrast agents can expand the diagnostic capabilities of ultrasound. Contrast-enhanced CDS imaging has already been used for infertility evaluation in women and in patients with significant peripheral arterial occlusive disease, and many other applications are conceivable. The diagnostic improvement anticipated with ultrasound contrast agents generally pertains to organs or organ systems that are consistently or occasionally difficult to evaluate by "plain" CDS imaging. This would include the detection of perfusion deficits in the orthotopic kidney and liver of obese patients, complete survey of the renal artery to exclude stenosis, and flow imaging of the portal system in the presence of ascites. Contrast-enhanced CDS imaging could increase the sensitivity of ultrasound in the detection of focal liver lesions (by displaying the different vascularisation of normal liver tissue and focal lesions). Available results indicate that when the proper application technique is used, the contrast effect can be sufficiently prolonged so that examinations can be performed with a single dose of contrast medium, even under difficult conditions.

Besides contrast agents that distribute nonspecifically in the blood and organs (as Echovist and Albunex), efforts have recently been started to develop organ or cell-specific ultrasound contrast agents. The simplest way is to use the phagocytic capacity of the reticuloendothelial system (RES) to get a selective and, compared with other parts of the body, a higher concentration of the contrast agent in these cells. A prerequisite for this is very stable small particulate scatters of high efficacy which are biodegradable. Such a preparation would lead after i.v. injection firstly to blood flow signal enhancement and secondly, after RES uptake, to enhancement of, for example, liver, spleen, and lymph nodes. The higher concentration of the contrast agent in the RES could lead to a much better distinction between normal and pathologic structures. Other areas of interest for ultrasound contrast agents are more toward functional imaging, like pressure and temperature measurements. The

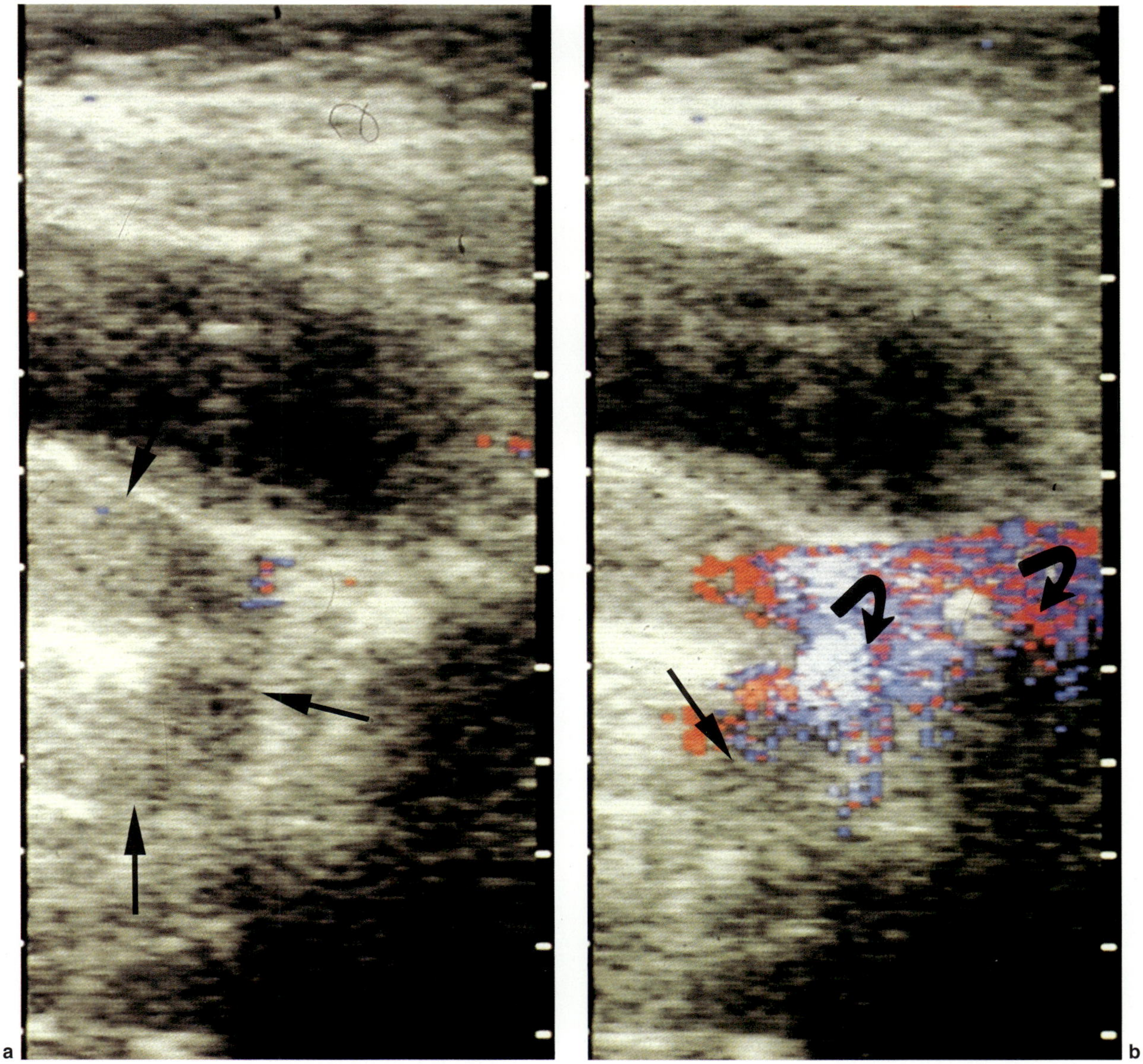

Fig. 16.17 a, b Assessment of tubal patency with CDS imaging. Transverse scan through the lower abdomen with bladder distension
a On the precontrast image, the uterus (arrows) is defined but the tubes are not visualized
b During instillation of the contrast agent (Echovist), conspicuous signals are visible in the uterine cavity (straight arrow) and left uterine tube (curved arrows)

acoustic characteristics of specific contrast medium particles undergo detectable changes which are dependent on the condition of the surrounding tissue.

Color duplex sonography already has become an important, reliable and low-cost diagnostic tool. The combination of CDS with ultrasound contrast agents probably further increases its clinical significance.

16.3 References

Principles and Preclinical Results

1 Anonymous: Shionogi submits NDA of CM for Echocardiography for the first time in the world (in Japanese). Nikkan Yakugyo, Nov. 7 (1991) No. 8267

2 Barnhart, J., E. Levene, E. Villapando, J. Maniquis, J. Fernandez, S. Rice, E. Jablonski: Albunex, Air-filled Albumin Microspheres as an Ultrasound Contrast Agent: Preliminary Findings. Abstracts of MRC '89 Contrast Media Research Symposium, Sydney (1989) S3

3 Barnhart, J. I., H. B. Levene, R. Keen, C. Saravis, J. Maniquis, E. Villapando: Albunex Microsphere Shells, the Unique Feature of a New Ultrasound Contrast Agent. Abstracts of the 2nd International Symposium on Contrast Media, Osaka, Nov. 9–10 (1990) 54

4 Barnhart, J., H. Levene, E. Villapando, J. Maniquis, J. Fernandez, S. Rice, E. Jablonski, T. Gjoen, H. Tolleshaug: Characteristics of Albunex: air-filled albumin microspheres for echocardiography contrast enhancement. Invest. Radiol 25 (1990) 162–164

5 Barnhard, J. L., H. B. Levene, K. J. Widder: Abdominal ultrasound imaging with clearer delineation–using aq. imaging agent contg. micron size clay particles and solubilised hydrocolloid to maintain particles in suspension. United States patent appl. US 660349

6 Berwing, K., M. Schlepper: Echocardiographic imaging of the left ventricle by peripheral intravenous injection of echo contrast agent. Amer. Heart J. 115 (1988) 399–408

7 Bibra, H., F. Hartmann, M. Petrik, R. Schlief, U. Renner, H. Bloemer: Kontrast-Farbdoppler-Echokardiographie verbesserte Rechtsherzdiagnostik nach intravenöser Injektion von Echovist. Z. Kardiol. 78 (1989) 101–108

8 Bleeker, H., K. Shung, J. Barnhart: On the application of ultrasonic contrast agents for blood flowmetry and assessment of cardiac perfusion. J. Ultrasound. Med. 9 (1990) 461–471

9 Burns, P. N., P. Hilpert, B. B. Goldberg: Intravenous Contrast Agent for Ultrasound Doppler In Vivo Measurement of Small Tumor vessel dose response. Annual International Conference IEEE Engineering in Medicine and Biology Society 12 (1990) 0322–0324

10 Carroll, B. A., S. W. Young, J. S. Rasor, R. B. Briller, D. M. Cessel: Ultrasonic contrast enhancement of tissue by encapsulated microbubbles. Radiology 143 (1982) 747–750

11 Chambon, C., R. Kravtzoff, C. Ropars: Contrast medium for imaging circulatory system, vascular organs etc. comprises hydrophilic or hydrosoluble colloidal contrast prods. (e. g. Gd complexes) encapsulated in erythrocytes by lysis resealing. European patent appl. EP0524265

12 Chiang, C. W., F. C. Lin, M. Fu, B. R. Fang, T. S. Hsu, Y. S. Lee: Importance of adequate gas-mixing in contrast echocardiography. Chest 89 (1986) 723–726

13 D'Agincourt: Ultrasound Succumbs to allure of contrast media. Diagn. Imag. July (1990) 119–129

14 De Jong, N., L. Hoff: Simulations and Measurements on Albunex Contrast Agent. Abstracts 9th Symposium on Echocardiography, Rotterdam, June 26–28 (1991) 63–64

15 Dougherty, C., M. Schartl, H. Schmutzler: Quantitative Kontrastechokardiographie bei Patienten mit Vorhofseptumdefekt und Trikuspidalinsuffizienz. Z. Kardiol. 75 (Suppl.) 4 (1986) 41

16 El Mouaaouy, A., T. Riemenschneider: Erweiterung der intraoperativen Lebersonographie mittels Echokontrastmittel. Eine klinische und tierexperimentelle Studie. Ultraschall Klin. Prax. (Suppl.) 1 (1987) 92–93

17 Erbel, R., R. Zotz, V. Krone, M. Magerstadt, A. Walch: Ultrasound Contrast Agent for Diagnosis of Heart and Circulation Disorders–Compromising Microparticles containing Gas and N-Dicarboxylic Acid Derivate of (Poly) Amino Acid-(Poly) Cyclic Imide. European Patent Application EP 458079A2 (1991)

18 Feinstein, S. B., K. Ong, P. M. Shah, H. Staniloff, Y. Fujiyabashi, W. Zwehl, S. Meerbaum, E. Corday: A new standardized, reproducible method for assessing regional myocardial blood flow with sonoicated echo contrast agents. Circulation 70 (Suppl.) II (1984) II–4

19 Feinstein, S. B., M. W. Keller, C. D. Dick, T. R. Bridenstine, R. W. Wissler: Successfull transpulmonary contrast echocardiography in monkeys. J. Amer. Coll. Cardiol. 9 (1987) 111A

20 Feinstein, S. B.: Assessment of myocardial perfusion using contrast echocardiography. Echocardiography 6 (1989) 17–25

21 Feinstein, S., J. Cheirif, F. Ten Cate, P. Silverman, P. Heidenreich, C. Dick, R. Desir, W. Armstrong, M. Quinones, P. Shah: Safety and efficacy of a new transpulmonary ultrasound contrast agent: initial multicenter clinical results. J. Amer. Coll. Cardiol. 16 (1990) 316–324

22 Feßler, B., R. Schlief, W. Fiegler, R. Felix: Verbesserte sonographische Magendarstellung durch Anwendung eines neuen Ultraschallkontrastmittels. Ultraschall Klin. Prax. 1 (Suppl.) 1 (1986) 91

23 Fink, I. J., D. L. Miller, T. H. Shawker, M. Girton, K. Morrish: Lipid emulsions as contrast agents for hepatic sonography: an experimental study in rabbits. Ultrasonic Imag. 7 (1985) 191–197

24 Fobbe, F., J. Siegert, T. Fritzsch, K.-J. Wolf: Ultraschall-Kontrastmittel in der farbkodierenden Duplexsonographie–Neue Möglichkeiten für die gynäkologische und urologische Diagnostik? Ultraschall Klin. Prax. 4 (Suppl.) 1 (1989) 133

25 Fobbe, F., J. Siegert, T. Fritzsch, H.-C. Koch, K.-J. Wolf: Farbkodierte Duplexsonographie und Ultraschallkontrastmittel –Nachweis von renalen Perfusionsdefekten im Tierexperiment. Fortschr. Röntgenstr. 154 (1991) 242–245

26 Fritzsch, T., J. Hilmann, W. Mützel, L. Lange: Right-heart echocontrast in the anesthetized dog after I.V. administration of a new standardized contrast agent. 1st Communication: Dose-response relationship. Arzneimittel-Forsch 36 (1986) 1030–1033

27 Fritzsch, T., W. Mützel, M. Schartl: First experiences with a standardized contrast medium for sonography. In Otto, R. C., C. B. Higgins (Eds.): New Developments in Imaging. Thieme, Stuttgart (1986) 141–149

28 Fritzsch, T., J. Siegert, W. Mützel, W. Bothe: Ein lungenkapillargängiges Echokontrastmittel. In Otto, R. C., P. Schnaars (Hrsg.): Ultraschalldiagnostik 85. Thieme, Stuttgart 1986 (727–728)

29 Fritzsch, T., M. Schartl, J. Siegert: Preclinical and clinical results with an ultrasonic contrast agent. Invest. Radiol. 23 (Suppl.) 1 (1988) 302–305

30 Fritzsch, T., M. Schartl, J. Siegert: Kontrastkardiographie des rechten und linken Herzens nach intravenöser Injektion standardisierter Mikrobläschen. In Grube, E. (Hrsg.): Farb-Doppler und Kontrast-Echokardiographie. Thieme, Stuttgart (1989) 354–367

31 Fritzsch, T., J. Hilmann, M. Kämpfe, N. Müller, C. Schöbel, J. Siegert: SH U 508, a transpulmonary echocontrast agent, initial experience. Invest. Radiol. 25 (Suppl.) (1990) 160–161

32 Fritzsch, T., B. Maaß, B. Müller, C. Schöbel, J. Siegert, K. Stevens: Composition and tolerance of galactose-based echocontrast media. In Katayama, H., R. C. Brasch (Eds.): New Dimensions in Contrast Media. Proceedings of the 2nd International Symposium on Contrast Media, Osaka, Japan, Excerpta Medica Ldt. (1991) 156–162

33 Fritzsch, T., W. Krause, H. J. Weinmann: Status of contrast media research in MRI, ultrasound and X-ray. Europ. Radiol. 2 (1992) 2–13

34 Goldberg, B. B., P. L. Hilpert, P. N. Burns, J. B. Liu, L. M. Newman, D. A. Merton, L. A. Witlin: Hepatic tumors: signal enhancement at Doppler US after intravenous injection of a contrast agent. Radiology 177 (1990) 713–717

35 Goldberg, B. B., Ji-Bin Liu, P. N. Burns, D. A. Merton, F. Forsberg: Galactose-based intravenous sonographic contrast agent: experimental studies. J. Ultrasound Med. (1993) 463–470

36 Goldberg, B. B.: Ultrasound contrast agents. Clin. Diagn. Ultrasound 28 (1993) 35–45

37 Gramiak, R., P. Shah: Echocardiography of the aortic root. Invest. Radiol. 3 (1968) 356–366

38 Gramiak, R., P. M. Shah, D. H. Cramer: Ultrasound cardiography: contrast studies in anatomy and function. Radiology 92 (1969) 939–948

39 Grenier, N., V. Dousset, C. Douws, H. Trillaud: Color Doppler signal enhamcesment of intrarenal vasculature of the rabbit with Perflubron. Europ. J. Radiol. 3 (1993) 156–160

40 Heidelmeyer, C. F., J. B. Brückner, M. Schartl: Myocardial contrast echocardiography: Cardiovascular effects of the contrast medium SH U 454 in dogs. J. Cardiothorac. Anesth. 4 (1990) 60–67

41 Helzel, M. W.: Sonography agent for oral use in ultrasonic diagnosis in the form of suspension of solids in liquid, or of emulsion with particle size 50–2000 microns. German patent DE 3246386

42 Hilpert, P. L., R. F. Mattrey, R. M. Mitten, T. Peterson: Iv injection of air-filled human albumin microspheres to enhance arterial Doppler signal: A preliminary study in rabbits. Amer. J. Roentgenol. 153 (1989) 613–616

43 Hilpert, P. L.: Contrast agents in diagnostic ultrasound. In Rumach, C. M., S. R. Wilson, J. W. Charboneau (Eds.): Diagnostic Ultrasound. Mosby Year Book, St. Louis (1991) 30–42

44 Illum, L., O. Johnson: Solid microspheres for drug delivery systems partic. nasal route also airfilled microcapsules for echo-cardiograph and other ultrasonic imaging. Patent appl. WO 9302712

45 Illum, L., C. Wahington: Hollow microcapsule ultrasound echo-cardiographic diagnostic aid repd. by forming shell around core and removing core, e.g. by evaporation of volatile oil. Patent appl. WO 9112823

46 Keller, M. W., S. B. Feinstein, D. D. Watson: Successful left ventricular opacification following peripheral venous injection of sonicated contrast agent: an experimental evaluation. Amer. Heart J. 114 (1987) 570–575

47 Keller, M. W., W. Glasheen, K. Teja, A. Gear, S. Kaul: Myocardial contrast echocardiography without significant hemodynamic effects or reactive hyperemia: a major advantage in the imaging of regional myocardial perfusion. J. Amer. Coll. Cardiol. 12 (1988) 1039–1047

48 Keller, M. W., W. Glasheen, S. Kaul: Albunex: A safe and effective commercially produced agent for myocardial contrast echocardiography. J. Amer. Soc. Echo. 2 (1989) 48–52

49 Koester, W., W. Kasper, T. Meinertz, T. Hofmann, A. Geibel, P. Billmann, H. Just: Echokontrastphlebographie. Ultraschall Klin. Prax. 1 (Suppl.) 1 (1986) 82

50 Kubale, R., R. M. Schmidt, H. J. Schmitt, A. Irion, A. Seelinger: Kontrastmittelgestützte Darstellung von kleinen Gefäßen am Beispiel des Kaninchens. Ultraschall Klin. Prax. 5 (1990) 235

51 Lange, L., T. Fritzsch, J. Hilmann, G. Kubowicz, W. Mützel: Right-heart echocontrast in the anesthetized dog after I.V. administration of a new standardized sonographic contrast agent. 2nd Communication: Dependence of the intensity of contrast on the interval between preparation of the suspension and its injection. Arzneimittel-Forsch. 36 (1986) 1034–1036

52 Lange, L., T. Fritzsch, J. Hillman, G. Kubowicz, W. Mützel: Right-heart echocontrast in the anesthetized dog after I.V. administration of a new standardized sonographic contrast agent. 3rd Communication: Comparison of various contrast agents employed in contrast echocardiography. Arzneimittel-Forsch. 36 (1986) 1037–1040

53 Lee, F., L. Ginzton: A central nervous system complication of contrast echocardiography. J. Clin. Ultrasound 11 (1983) 292–294

54 Leopold, G. R., W. M. Asher: Deletrious effects of gastrointestinal contrast material on abdominal echocardiography. Radiology 98 (1971) 637 -640

55 Levene, H. B., J. L. Barnhard, E. Villapando, K. J. Widder: New abdominal ultrasound imaging compsn.–contains inorganic particles e.g. kaolin, hydrocolloid e.g. pectin and degassing agent. European patent application EP 5000023

56 Mattrey, R. F.: Perfluorochemicals as liver- and spleen-seeking ultrasound contrast agents. J. Ultrasound Med. 2 (1983) 173–176

57 Mattrey, R. F.: Sonographic enhancement of Doppler signals and perfused tissue with perfluorooctylbromide. Invest. Radiol. 25 (1990) 158–159

58 Monaghan, M. J., J. M. Metcalfe, S. O. Odunlami, S. D. Thomas, A. Waaler, D. E. Jewitt: Digital Radiofrequency in Ultrasound Analysis of Myocardial Contrast Following I.V. Albunex Injection. Abstract of the 9th Symposium on Echocardiology, Rotterdam, June 26–28 (1991) 68

59 Monaghan, M. J., J. P. Quingley, J. M. Metcalfe, S. D. Thomas, D. E. Jewitt: Digital substraction contrast echocardiography: a new method for the evaluation of regional myocardial perfusion. Brit. Heart J. 59 (1988) 12–19

60 Ophir, J., A. Gobuty, R. E. McWhirt, N. F. Maklad: Ultrasonic backscatter from contrast producing collagen microspheres. Ultrasonic Imag. 2 (1980) 67–77

61 Ophir, J., A. Gobuty, N. F. Maklad, T. Tyler, P. Jaeger, R. E. McWhirt: Quantitative assessment of in vivo backscatter enhancement from gelatin microspheres. Ultrasonic Imag. 7 (1985) 293–299

62 Parker, K. J., M. R. Violante, T. A. Tuthill, P. Dentiger: A novel echogenic bubble-particle contrast agent. Ultrasonic Imag. 13 (1991) 194

63 Quay, S. C.: New gaseous ultra-sound contrast media–comprises microbubbles of gas dispersed in aq. soln. Patent appl. WO 9305819

64 Rovai, D., M. Lombardi, A. Distante, A. L'Abbate: Myocardial perfusion by contrast echocardiography. From off-line processing to radio frequency analysis. Circulation 83 (1991) III 97–103

65 Satterfiled, R., M. Tarter, J. Schumacher, P. Tran, R. F. Mattrey: Comparison of different perfluorocarbons as ultrasound contrast agents. Invest. Radiol. 28 (1993) 325–331

66 Schartl, M., T. Fritzsch, W. Friedmann, L. Lange: Quantifizierung myokardialer Perfusionsdefekte mittels zweidimensionaler Kontrastechokardiographie. Z. Kardiol. 73 (1984) 560–567

67 Schartl, M., T. Fritzsch, V. Miszalok: Quantification of Myocardial Perfusion by Contrast Echocardiography. Canad. J. Cardiol. 2 (Suppl.) (1986) 25 A–31 A

68 Schlief, R., G. Grau, H. P. Niendorf: Entwicklungsstand von Ultraschall-Kontrastmitteln. Ultraschall Klin. Prax. (Suppl.) (1989) 132

69 Schlief, R., T. Staks, M. Mahler, M. Rufer, T. Fritzsch, W. Seifert: Successful opacification of the left heart chambers on echocardiographic examination after intravenous injection of a new saccharide based contrast agent. Echocardiography 7 (1990) 61–64

70 Schlief, R., T. Staks, M. Mahler, M. Rufer, T. Fritzsch, W. Seifert: Contrast echocardiographic examination of left-heart chambers after intravenous injection of a new saccharide based contrast agent in humans. J. Amer. Coll. Cardiol. 15 (1990) 18–22

71 Schlief, R., U. Deichert: Hysterosalpingo-contrast sonography of the uterus and fallopian tubes: Results of a clinical trial of a new contrast medium in 120 patients. Radiology 178 (1991) 213–215

72 Schmitt, R. M., H. J. Schmidt, A. Irion: Ultrasonic Characterization of Ultrasound Contrast Agents. IEEE Engineering in Medicine and Biology Society, 11th Annual International Conference Proceedings (1989)

73 Siegert, J., R. M. Schmitt, H. J. Schmidt T, Fritzsch: Application of a Resonance Method for Measuring the Size of Bubbles in an Echocontrast Agent. Proceedings of the IEEE Engineering in Medicine and Biology Society, Boston (1987) 691–692

74 Siegert, J., F. Fobbe, T. Fritzsch: Enhancement of arterial blood flow imaging in color-encoded duplex sonography (CEDS) after intravenous injection of a lung-crossing ultrasound contrast agent. J. Ultrasound Med. 7 (1988) 121

75 Siegert, J., F. Fobbe, T. Fritzsch, K.-J. Wolf: Verstärkte Darstellung von arteriellen Blutflüssen in der farbkodierten Kontrastduplexsonographie (FKKDS) nach i. v. Gabe eines lungenkapillargängigen Ultraschallkontrastmittels. Ultraschall Klin. Prax. 3 (Suppl.) 1 (1988) 68

76 Siegert, J., F. Fobbe, T. Fritzsch, K.-J. Wolf: Ultraschallkontrastmittel im Farbdoppler-Sonogramm. In Flesch, U., Mosler, F., Witt, H.: Qualitätssicherung in der Röntgendiagnostik, Farbdopplersonographie. Schnetztor-Verlag, Konstanz (1990) 166–177

77 Simon, R. H., S. Y. Ho, J. D'Arrigo, A. Wakefield, S. G. Hamilton: Lipid-coated ultrastable microbubbles as a contrast agent in neurosonography. Invest. Radiol. 25 (1990) 1300–1304

78 Skjaerpe, T., L. Hatle: Diagnosis of tricuspid regurgitation. Sensitivity of Doppler ultrasound compared with contrast echocardiography. Europ. Heart J. 6 (1985) 429–436

79 Smith, M. D., O. L. Kwan, H. J. Reiser, A. DeMaria: Superior intensity and reproducibility of SH U 454 a new right-heart contrast agent. J. Amer. Coll. Cardiol. 3 (1984) 992–998

80 Smith, M., O. L. Kwan, S. T. Nissen, J. Elion, D. Rovai, A. Demaria: Left heart opacification after peripheral venous injection: pulmonary transmission of ZK44012, a new echocontrast agent. Circulation, Part II, 72 (Suppl.) III (1985) III–57

81 Stein, M., D. Heldmann, T. Fritzsch, J. Siegert, G. Rössling, U. Speck: Ultraschallkontrastmittel, Verfahren zu deren Herstellung und deren Verwendung als Diagnostika und Therapeutika. European Patent Application EP 0327490 (1989)

82 Tuthill, T. A., M. R. Violante, K. J. Parker: Liver backscatter enhancement with particle uptake. Ultrasonic Imag. 12 (1990) 150–151

83 Tyler, T. D., J. Ophir, N. F. Maklad: In vivo enhancement of ultrasonic image luminance by aqueous solutions with high speed of sound. Ultrasonic Imag. 3 (1981) 323–329

84 Unger, E. C., P. Lund, D. Shen, T. Fritz, L. Fuller: Aerosomes as blood pool and cardiovascular contrast agent for US: In vivo studies. Radiology 188 (Suppl.) (1991) 225

85 Unger, E. C.: Gas-filled liposomes as ultrasound contrast agent for imaging organs – prepd. by use of gaseous precursors by activation or direct induction of gas. European patent appl. EP 0511273

86 Unger, E. C., G. Wu: Contrast media for ultrasonic imaging of gastrointestinal tract contg. biocompatible polyethylene glycol polymer and silicon cpd. e.g. polysiloxane for improved visibility. United States patent appl. US 532213

87 Vanderipe, D. R.: Ultrasound imaging of mammals, after administration of gases that form bubbles to enhance imaging in the blood. Patent appl. WO 9306869

88 Villanueva, F. S., W. P. Glasheen, J. Sklenar, A. R. Jayaweera, W. D. Spotnitz, S. Kaul: Factors affecting successful left ventricular myocardial opacification following right atrial injection of contrast in dogs: preliminary results. J. Amer. Soc. Echo. 4 (1991) 286

89 Vorwerk, D., H. B. Gehl, R. Schlief, A. Nelles, R. W. Günther: Dynamische kontrastmittelgestützte Ultraschallkavographie bei Kavafilterpatienten. Ultraschall Med. 11 (1990) 146–149

90 Wang, X. F., J. Wang, Y. Huang, C. Cai: Contrast echocardiography with hydrogen perioxide – I. Experimental study. Chin. med. J. 92 (1979) 595–599
91 Wang, X. F., Y. Z. Huang, H. R. Chen, C. F. Lu, J. E. Wang, J. K. Zhang: Hydrogen peroxide contrast hepatosonography. Chin. med. J. 104 (1991) 336–342
92 Yeh, H. C., B. S. Wolf: Ultrasonic contrast study to identifiy stomach tap water microbubbles. J. clin. Ultrasound 5 (1977) 170–174
93 Ziskin, M. C., A. Bonakdarpour, D. P. Weinstein, P. R. Lynch: Contrast agents for diagnostic ultrasound. Invest. Radiol. 7 (1972) 500–505
94 Zotz, R., L. Duwe, R. Erbel, P. Frank, R. Brennecke, J. Meyer: Rechtsherzechoventrikulographie mittels Gelifundol. Z. Kardiol. 78 (1989) 95–100

Clinical Application

1 Balen, F. G., C. M. Allen, N. C. Siddle, W. R. Lees: Ultrasound contrast hystersalpingography–eveluation as an outpatient procedure. Brit. J. Radiol. 66 (1993) 592–599
2 Barnhart, J., H. Levene, E. Villapando, J. Maniquis, J. Fernandez, S. Rice, E. Jablonski, T. Gjoen, H. Tolleshaug: Characteristics of Albunex–airfilled albumin microspheres for echocardiography contrast enhancement. Invest. Radiol. 25 (1990) 162–164
3 Becher, H., R. Schlief: Improved sensitivity of color Doppler by SH U 454. Amer. J. Cardiol. 64 (1989) 374–377
4 Becker, A. U., A. Lindner, U. Bogdahn: Imaging of the vertebrobasilar system by trancranial color-coded real time sonography. J. Ultrasound Med. 12 (1993) 395–401
5 von Bibra, H., H. Becher, C. Firschke, R. Schlief, H. P. Emslander, A. Schoemig: Enhancement of mitral regurgitation and normal left atrial color Doppler flow signals with peripheral venous injection of a saccharide-based contrast agent. J. Amer. Coll. Cardiol. 22 (1993) 521–528
6 Bogdahn, U., G. Becker, R. Schlief, J. Reddig, W. Hassel: Contrast-enhanced transcranial color-coded real-time sonography. Stroke 24 (1993) 676–684
7 Fobbe, F., R. Becker, H.-Ch. Koch, J. Hammerstein, K.-J. Wolf: Nachweis der Durchgängigkeit der Tubae uterinae mit der farbkodierten Duplexsonographie. Fortschr. Röntgenstr. 154 (1991) 349–353
8 Fobbe, F., I. Ohnesorge, M. Reichel, P. Dollinger, R. Schürmann, K.-J. Wolf: Farbkodierte Duplexsonographie und Ultraschallkontrastmittel zur Untersuchung peripherer Arterien – Erste klinische Erfahrungen. Ultraschall in Med. 13 (1992) 193–198
9 Rosenkranz, K., W. Zendel, R. Langer, T. Heim, P. Schubeus, A. Scholz, R. Schlief, R. Schürmann, R. Felix: Contrast-emhanced transcranial Doppler UD with a new transpulmonary echo contrast agent based on saccharide microparticles. Radiology 187 (1993) 439–443
10 Schlief, R., T. Staks, M. Mahler, M. Rufer, T. Fritzsch, W. Seifert: Successful opacification on echocardiography examination after intravenous injection of a new saccharide based contrast agent. Echocardiography 7 (1990) 61–64
11 Schlief, R., U. Deichert: Hysterosalpingo-contrast sonography of the uterus and Fallopian tubes: results of a clinical trial of a new contrast medium in 120 patients. Radiology 178 (1991) 213–215
12 Ten Cate, F. J., J. H. Cornel, P. Widimsky, Wim. Vletter, P. Serruys, A. Waaler: Clinical experience with Albunex: A standard echocontrast agent for intravenous and intracoronary use. Amer. J. Cardiac. Imag. 5 (1991) 217–243

17 Physics and Technology of Color Duplex Sonography (CDS)

P.-M. Klews

The correct usage of an ultrasound system and the interpretation of ultrasound gray-scale images, Doppler spectra, and CDS images depends highly on the user's experience and skill. A basic understanding of ultrasound physics and knowledge of the technology used in ultrasound scanners in general is mandatory. In this chapter the ultrasound user and technician are introduced to the basic knowledge needed in understanding the meaning of ultrasound images and Doppler spectra. Many aspects are simplified to achieve a more general understanding of ultrasound. Less stress is put on scientific precision. It is not necessary to go through all the mathematics in this chapter, but the conclusions are of general interest to anyone working in medical diagnostic ultrasound.

17.1 Introduction

Human beings and animals have natural receptors for light and sound. The eyes can evaluate electromagnetic signals only within a very narrow frequency range. Pertaining to sound this is equally valid for the ears. Only after the development of special technologies have the frequency ranges—naturally outside of human detection—been made accessible. Images gained in this way may be called "artificial" images. The quality of the images based on X-(roentgen) rays and ultrasound, for example, are highly dependent on the methods used in data acquisition and image processing. An image is regarded as being "good" if a high spatial resolution can be achieved and at the same time, in gray-scale images, the distribution of the gray values is "pleasing" to the user. Furthermore, a high contrast resolution is expected. Contrast resolution is synonymous with the visualization of minute differences in appearance of objects in gray-scale. (In ultrasound imaging it is possible to say that the contrast resolution is equivalent to the spatial resolution at –40 dB.)

In ultrasound diagnostics the detection of blood flow is continuously growing in importance. In 1842 Christian Doppler described the effect that bears his name. According to this effect, the wavelength of light (and sound) measured by an observer depends on the movement of the source and the observer relative to one another. This effect has been used in medicine since 1959. The introduction of bidirectional Doppler (1966) was followed by pulsed Doppler (1967). Starting around 1981, work has been done on the development of methods for color coding of blood flow in a gray-scale image surrounding. Since 1986 CDS methods that do not rely on the evaluation of the demodulated Doppler signal (4) have been developed.

The color encoding of blood flow in a gray-scale image in real-time is called color flow mapping (CFM) (34, 35). In Europe the name color-coded duplex sonography (CCDS) is used (1) because two different techniques are combined (duplex) to form one image: Doppler signal evaluation and conventional gray-scale amplitude evaluation. The term used throughout this book is color duplex sonography (CDS), omitting the second "C" (coded) for simplicity.

17.2 Ultrasound Imaging in General

Next to conventional radiography, ultrasound is the most frequently used imaging modality in medicine today. Ultrasound images display a two-dimensional slice of a three-dimensional object. All ultrasound imaging methods presented in this book rely on the evaluation of multiple pulse–echo cycles. Individual temporally successive ultrasound pulses are transmitted and the amplitudes, frequencies, and phases of the returning echoes are evaluated separately. With the exception of CW Doppler, all ultrasound methods discussed in this book are time-of-flight methods, i.e., the depth or distance from the transducer, where the echoes originate, is derived from the pulse–echo time of flight. It is generally assumed, that the speed of sound is constant. A unique relationship between the received echoes and the respective transmitted pulse must be assured. For that reason, a new pulse can only be emitted after the arrival at the transducer of the echoes belonging to the previous pulse coming from the greatest possible depth.

In general, an ultrasound scan line or beam is defined as a line in the ultrasound image pointing in the direction in which the ultrasound pulse was emitted. The ultrasound scan lines are directed orthogonally or radially away from the emitting surface of the transducer. (Beam steering on linear array transducers is an exception.) In many cases, such as CDS, more than one pulse–echo cycle is needed to generate a particular ultrasound scan line. Many individual ultrasound scan lines next to one another compose a two-dimensional ultrasound image.

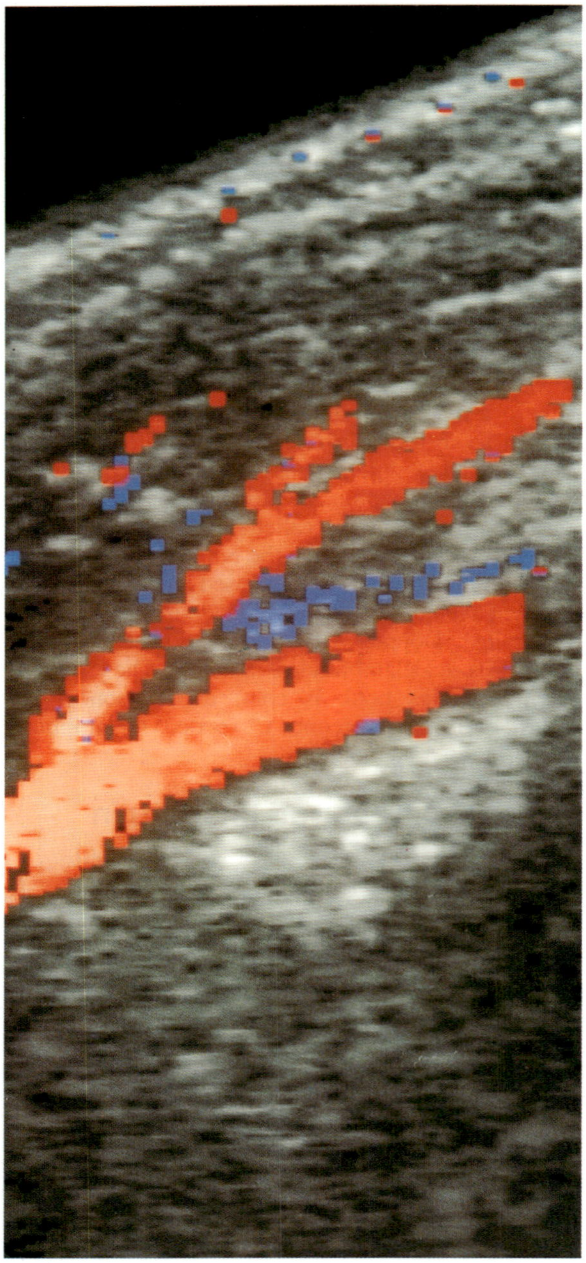

a

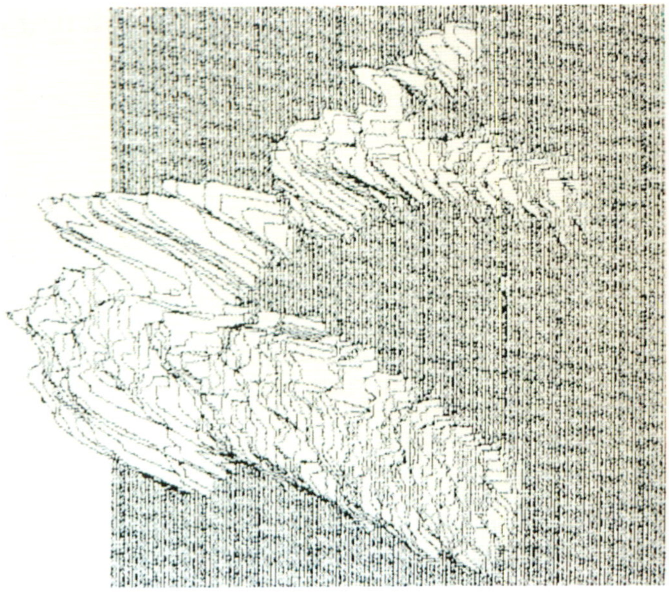

Fig. 17.**1 a, b** Popliteal artery with trifurcation. (**a**) The brighter regions in the vessel on the left side of the image (cranial) designate a higher flow velocity in that region relative to the right side of the image (caudal). Due to the low image acquisition rate and building up the image from right to left, the systolic heart phase is visible on the left while the late diastolic phase of the former heart cycle is still visible on the right side of the image
(**b**) This is also evident in the pseudo three-dimensional reconstruction. The amplitudes are proportional to the local Doppler frequency shifts

It takes a certain amount of time to produce an ultrasound image. This depends on the number of pulse–echo cycles used per line, the number of lines used in one image and on the selected image depth. On the other hand, all picture elements of a normal photograph are created at the same time. The outer lines of an ultrasound image can be separated in time by 0.2 s (at a frame rate of 5 frames per second) and even more. This must be kept in mind, especially when displaying blood flow in color. On the left side of an image for example, the systolic blood pulse might be visible where on the right side of the same image the diastolic flow phase may still be recognizable (Fig. 17.**1 a, b**).

B(brightness)-mode imaging is the most often used imaging modality in medical ultrasound diagnostics. A B-mode image is a pure gray-scale image. Many individual, temporally successive ultrasound scan lines located next to one another are displayed on the monitor as a two-dimensional image. The gray values are proportional to the amplitudes of the ultrasound echoes. The higher the amplitude of the echo, the brighter the displayed shade of gray at the corresponding position in the image. The B-mode image of a kidney can be seen in Figure 17.**2**. A B-mode image shows the structure of an object.

A-mode presentation (amplitude) is seldom used today. B-mode imaging is based on successive A-

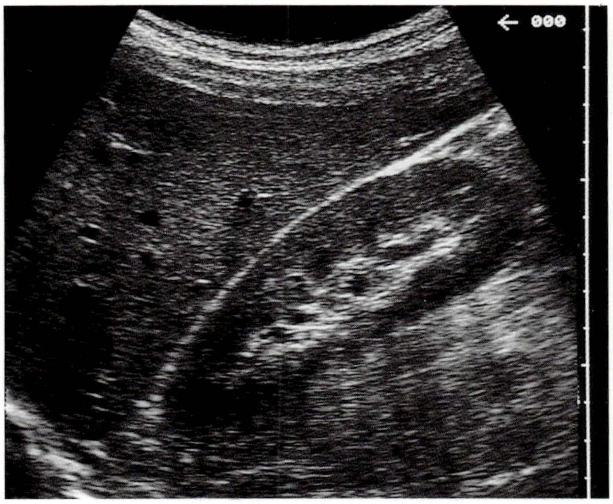

Fig. 17.**2** Long-axis scan of a normal kidney in gray-scale (B-mode image)

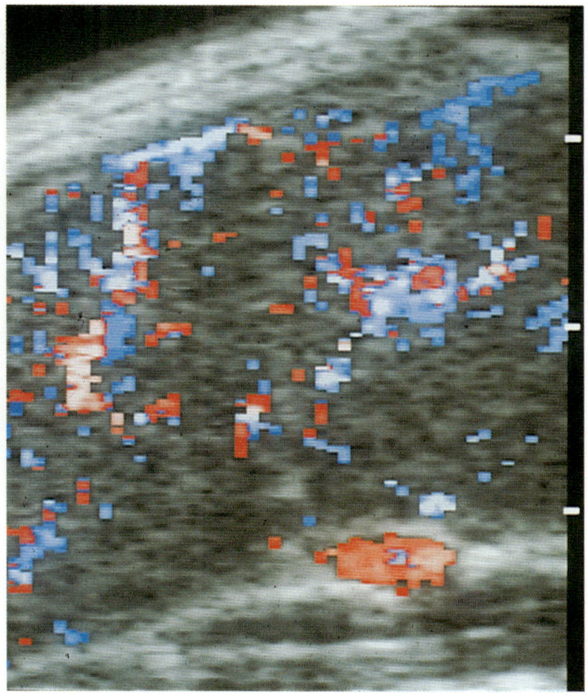

Fig. 17.**3** Thyroid of a patient with Graves' disease (long-axis scan) in CDS. Homogeneous hyporeflexive echo texture and enhanced diffuse perfusion ("red" and "blue" pixels throughout the complete organ)

mode evaluation. A-mode is the graphical presentation of the echo amplitudes (*y*-axis) over time (*x*-axis) of individual ultrasound scan lines. The amplitudes, displayed parallel to the *y*-axis, are proportional in height to the magnitude of the received ultrasound echo amplitudes (Fig. 17.**18**).

Another gray-scale imaging method is called M-(motion)-mode or TM(time–motion)-mode. Ultrasound is pulsed into the body along the same user-selected line of sight. The chosen ultrasound scan line is displayed on the monitor as temporally individual lines next to one another over time, although they belong to the same three-dimensional position in the object. In this way dynamic processes in the body can be monitored. This method is mainly used in cardiology for the diagnosis of valve movement. This is not the topic of this book. The interested reader is referred to the special literature on this topic (19).

In CDS imaging the positions in the image where movement has been detected are color-encoded. Usually the flow of blood is color-encoded. Places in the image without blood flow are displayed in gray-scale. CDS-mode or CFM-mode is a combination of a B-mode image and a color-encoded movement indication (Fig. 17.**3**). The point of reference for the direction of blood flow is the transducer and the direction of the ultrasound scan line. Only the components of movement directed away from or toward the transducer are registered. Usually the different flow directions are displayed in different hues of red and blue. On most systems it is up to the user to decide which flow direction is coded in "blue" and which in "red".

The blood flow velocity displayed by all methods used in color-encoding is the intensity-weighted average velocity or Doppler shift. On most systems the determination of the flow direction and flow velocity is based on the evaluation of the Doppler phase or frequency shift. Today, blood flow can be determined by evaluating the relative time shift of A-mode amplitudes of consecutive ultrasound pulses along the same ultrasound scan line (5). The higher the Doppler shift or the higher the blood flow velocity relative to the transducer, the brighter the shade of the color displayed. In particular, primarily ultrasound systems used in echocardiography also add green to the shades of red and blue to indicate variance. In medicine, variance is looked upon as an indicator of flow turbulance. Variance is actually the possible error of the measurement. Further information on this is also found in books on cardiology (18).

Color M-mode is a combination of a gray-scale M-mode image, and a color-encoded movement indicator displaying flow passing the ultrasound scan line selected by the user (Fig. 17.**4**). The chosen ultrasound scan line is displayed as successive vertical lines drawn next to one another over time along the abscissa used as the time axis. The ordinate is the depth scale, i.e., the distance from the transducer. Color-encoding is done as described above, but in this case only blood flow behavior on one specific ultrasound scan line as a function of time is displayed. Again, color M-mode is primarily used in echocardiography (18). There is also hope of using this method in vascular diagnosis in order to determine the blood flow volume and other flow parameters (14, 21) (see also Section 3.5). Of course, relative indices such as the RI and PI, as well as flow acceleration, can be calculated from a color M-mode image.

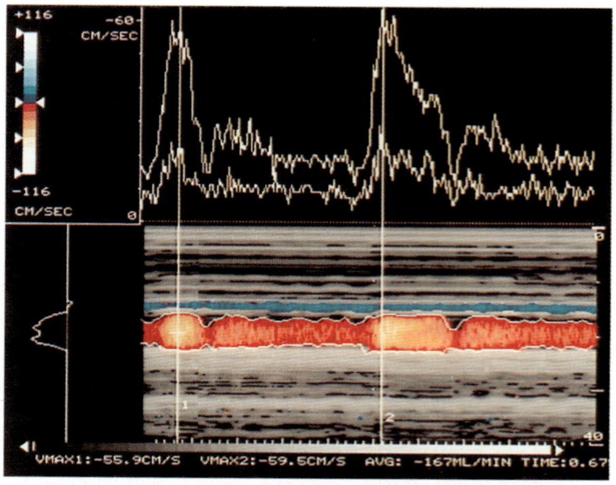

Fig. 17.**4** Color M-mode image of the flow in the common carotid artery (red) and jugular vein (blue). At the top of the image the maximum and minimum flow velocities within the carotid are displayed over time. The velocities displayed in the graph do not have to be situated at the same position in the vessel at all times within the pulse cycle. A flow velocity profile at a certain point in time was drawn on the left side of the image

Spectrum analysis is another method of evaluating ultrasound echoes. Echoes are analyzed according to their frequency distribution. The main interest is directed toward the frequency spectrum of echoes originating from moving scatterers, as for example blood cells. The echo center frequency as well as all other frequencies are Doppler shifted, because of the movement of the blood relative to the transducer. The spectrum is called the Doppler frequency spectrum or the Doppler intensity spectrum and describes, after measuring the Doppler flow angle, the velocity distribution of the blood cells at a user-determined position in the body. The ordinate is the frequency axis. Individual frequency spectra of the Doppler signals are drawn along the abscissa, which represents the time axis. The brightness of the individual dots in the graph is proportional to the intensity or amplitude of the respective frequency or velocity components. In Figure 17.**5**, a medical Doppler spectrum is presented in an unusual manner. The intensity of the individual components is equivalent to the height of the boxes in the graph. In colloquial medical speech the complete temporal–intensity–frequency spectrum is called the Doppler spectrum. For example, the normal Doppler spectrum of a common carotid can be seen in Figure 17.**6 a, b**.

There is a difference between PW (pulsed wave) Doppler and CW (continuous wave) Doppler. In the first case a region of interest called Doppler window, Doppler sample volume, or Doppler gate is positioned by the user within the field of view. Only echoes originating from this window are spectrum analyzed. In the case of CW Doppler, all echoes belonging to one ultrasound scan line are spectrum analyzed and evaluated according to the Doppler shift relative to the reference frequency of the transducer used. There is no axial spatial resolution in CW Doppler.

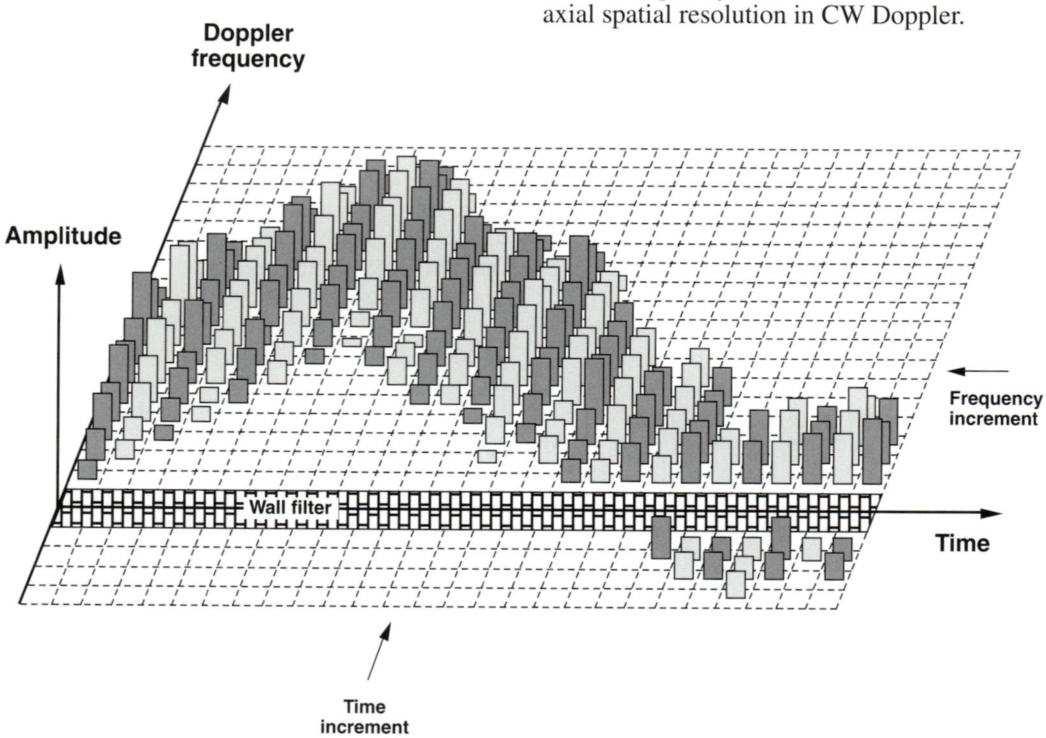

Fig. 17.**5** The complete "three-dimensional" display of the spectrum over time is made up of many individual consecutive Doppler spectra. The height of the boxes correspond to the amplitudes of the respective Doppler frequencies. Usually the amplitudes are displayed in different shades of gray

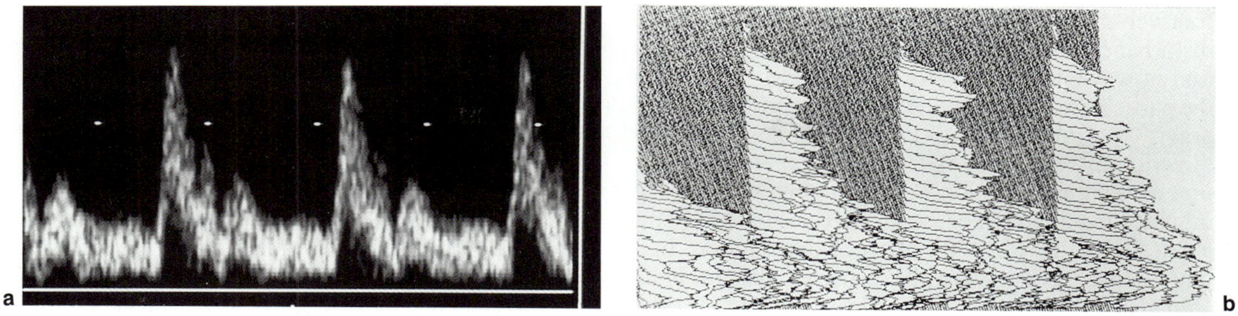

Fig. 17.6 **a, b** Doppler spectrum of a normal common carotid artery (**a**) in the usual gray-scale presentation and (**b**) in the pseudo three-dimensional display

17.2.1 General Physical Aspects

Light and sound have much in common. In both cases one is dealing with wave propagation. That means both phenomena are in general governed by the same laws. Reflection, refraction, interference, diffraction, scattering, and absorption are present in both cases.

Electromagnetic waves and sound waves act according to the laws of wave propagation. The propagation of electromagnetic waves does not rely on the existence of matter. Sound waves can only propagate within a medium, such as air or water for example, but not in a vacuum. That means that it is completely silent in outer space. A sound wave is a pressure (or density) wave, and its propagation is based on the compression and decompression of the surrounding medium. The pressure at a certain location changes over time.

It is necessary to distinguish between transverse and longitudinal wave propagation (Fig. 17.7 **a, b**). A

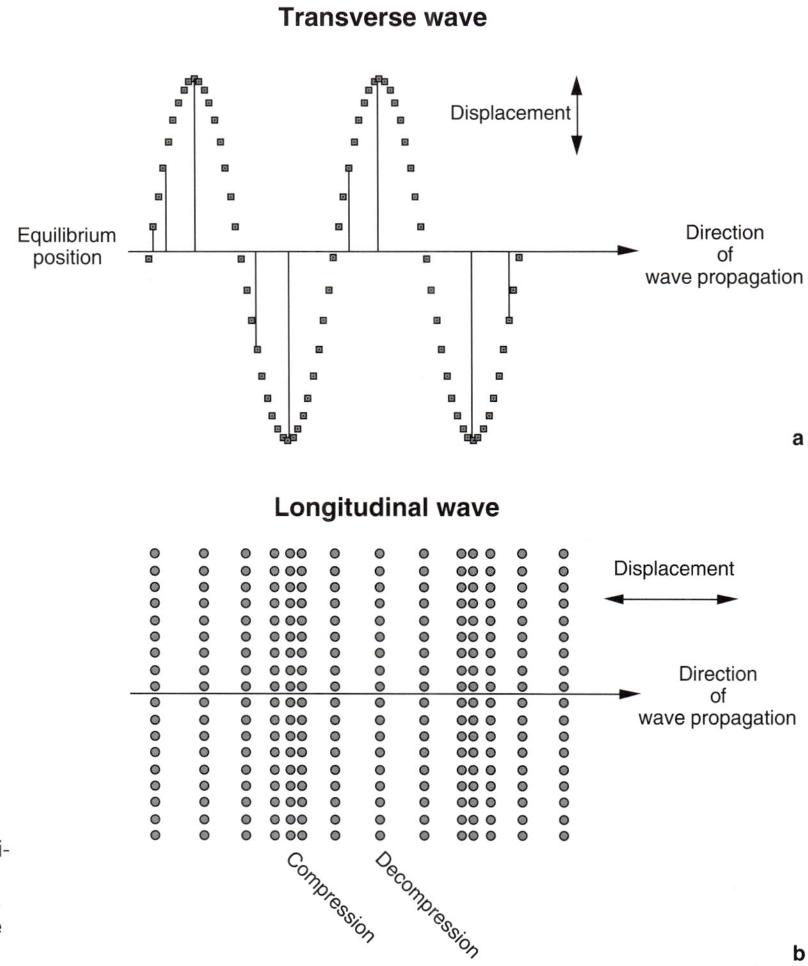

Fig. 17.7 **a, b** The propagation of sound is only possible in matter. In solids both (**a**) transverse and (**b**) longitudinal wave propagation is possible. Only longitudinal waves exist in liquids and gases. In human tissue transverse wave propagation can be neglected

transverse wave is one in which the direction of the disturbance at each point is perpendicular to the direction of wave propagation. In a transverse sound wave the particles oscillate around their respective center of gravity (position of rest or equilibrium position). The direction of oscillation is perpendicular to the direction of wave propagation. A longitudinal wave is one in which the direction of the disturbance at each point is parallel to the direction of wave propagation. In a longitudinal sound wave the particles also oscillate around their respective equilibrium position. The direction of oscillation is parallel to the direction of wave propagation. Energy and momentum are transferred without the particles moving along with the wave, i. e., there is no net transport of matter. Sound waves can be either longitudinal waves or transverse waves. As long as the deformations are reversible (the amplitudes are within the region of validity of Hooke's law), the sound wave is only a passing disturbance of the medium. Only longitudinal waves propagate in liquids and gases because there is practically no shear or tangential stress possible in these media. Apart from bones, humans consist mainly of water. Ultrasound diagnostics is for this reason based on longitudinal wave propagation.

The propagational velocity of a wave c is equal to the product of the wavelength λ times the frequency f:

$$c = \lambda f \qquad (17.1)$$

The speed of sound depends on the compressibility and the density of the medium and so on its temperature. In this case the temperature and the exterior pressure can always be assumed to be constant. This makes the speed of sound a material constant. The speed of sound in a few liquids and different kinds of tissue are listed (48, 49) in Figure 17.**8**.

The average speed of sound in tissue is taken to be 1,540 m/s. The speed of light in tissue is $3.3 \cdot 10^7$ m/s and is a factor $2 \cdot 10^4$ higher than the speed of sound.

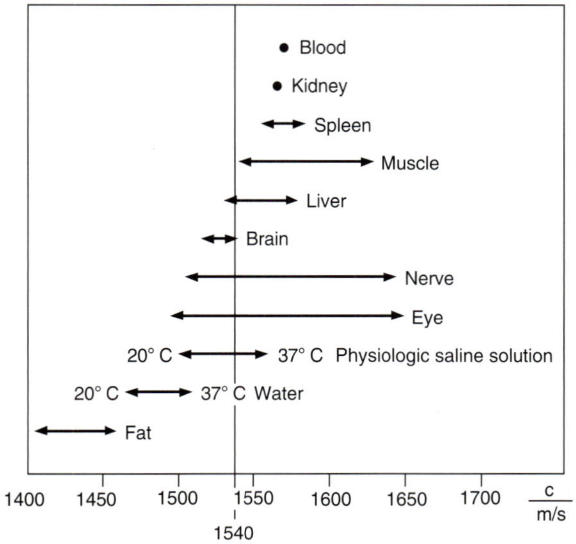

Fig. 17.**8** The speed of sound (longitudinal wave propagation only) in a number of biological materials (see also [49])

This means that at the same frequency the wavelength of sound is shorter by the just mentioned factor c_{EM}/c_{sound} than the wavelength of an electromagnetic wave (Fig. 17.**9a, b**). The relatively low speed of sound is of major importance in understanding how ultrasound images are made.

In ultrasound imaging, an ultrasound pulse is emitted from the transducer and the temporally successive echoes coming from different depths are received by the same transducer. An ultrasound pulse is only a few wavelengths long (Fig. 17.**10**). The larger the lapse of time between the emission of a pulse and the reception of an echo, the longer the time of flight and the greater the distance between the transducer and the reflector from which the sound wave was reflected.

An echo is created at the interface between two media with different sound characteristics. Most important for the magnitude of the echo are the impedances of the different media. Acoustic impedance can be looked upon as a resistance against a sound wave propagating from one medium to the next. Impedance z is equal to the product of the speed of sound c in the medium times the density ρ of the medium:

$$z = c\rho$$

At the boundary between two media, besides reflection, refraction also occurs (Fig. 17.**11**). If the speed of sound in the first medium is higher than in the second medium, then the transmitted wave is refracted toward the vertical (normal) N to the interface in the plane of incidence. In the opposite case the transmitted wave is refracted away from N. Refraction can lead to a misinterpretation of the true position or size of an object or structure (Fig. 17.**12**). Anyone who has tried to pick up an object lying in the water will have witnessed this phenomenon. The object is located at a somewhat different position from that which is expected. This kind of misguidance caused by refraction is only of minor importance in ultrasound diagnostics but should not be altogether forgotten, especially when doing a biopsy.

The intensities I_t and I_r of the transmitted and reflected pulses or echoes, respectively, depend on the individual impedances and respective angles of incidence Θ_e, reflection Θ_r, and refraction Θ_t. The coefficients of reflection R and transmission T at the boundary between medium 1 and medium 2 are:

$$R = \frac{I_r}{I_e} = \frac{(z_2\cos(\Theta_e) - z_1\cos(\Theta_t))^2}{(z_2\cos(\Theta_e) + z_1\cos(\Theta_t))^2}$$

$$T = \frac{I_t}{I_e} = \frac{4z_1z_2\cos(\Theta_e)\cos(\Theta_t)}{(z_2\cos(\Theta_e) + z_1\cos(\Theta_t))^2}$$

Fig. 17.**9 a, b** A comparison of the frequency ranges of (**a**) electromagnetic (EM) waves and (**b**) sound waves. In both cases the equation $c = \lambda \cdot f$ is valid. The speed of light in tissue ($3.3 \cdot 10^7$ m/s) is higher by a factor of $2 \cdot 10^4$ than the speed of sound in tissue (1,540 m/s). That is the reason why at equal frequencies the wavelength of EM waves are longer by this factor compared with the wavelength of the sound waves

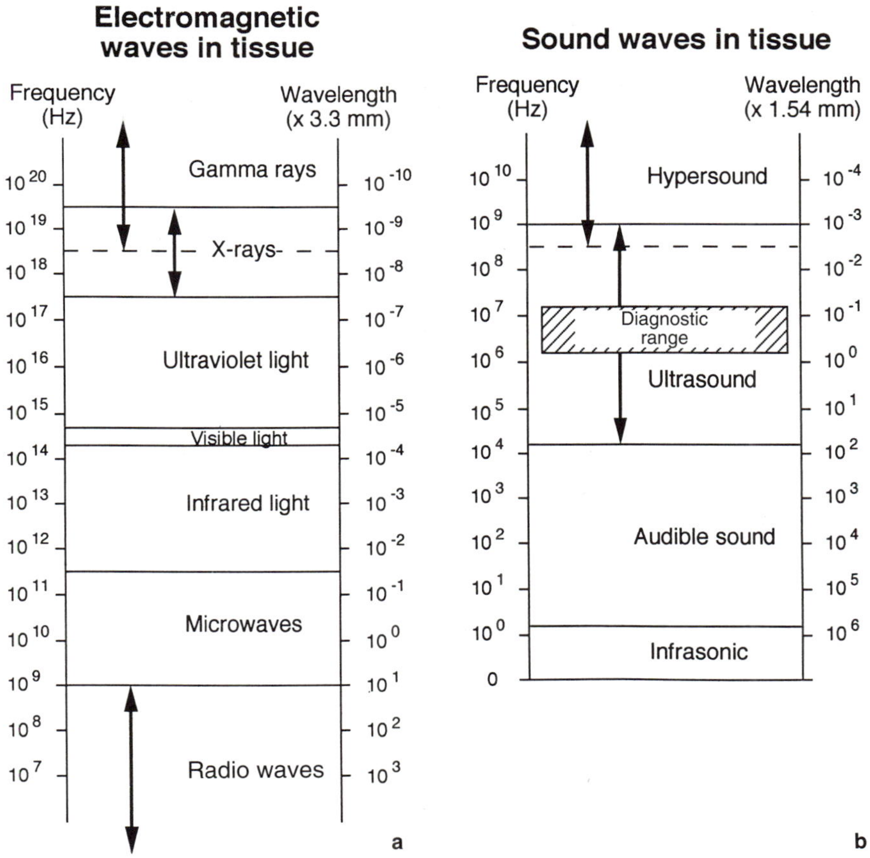

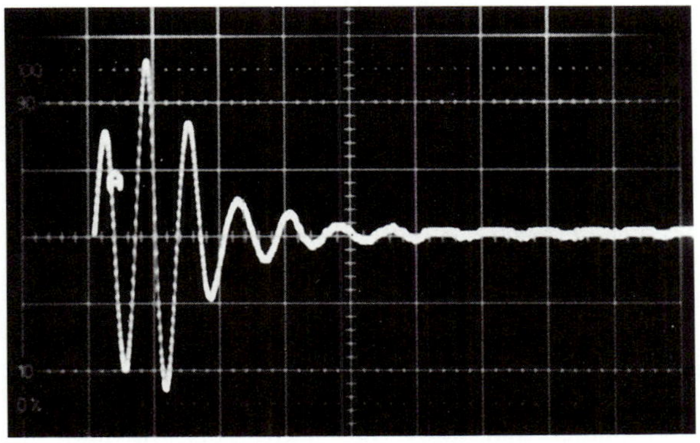

Fig. 17.**10** Image of a 3.17-MHz pulse displayed by an oscilloscope

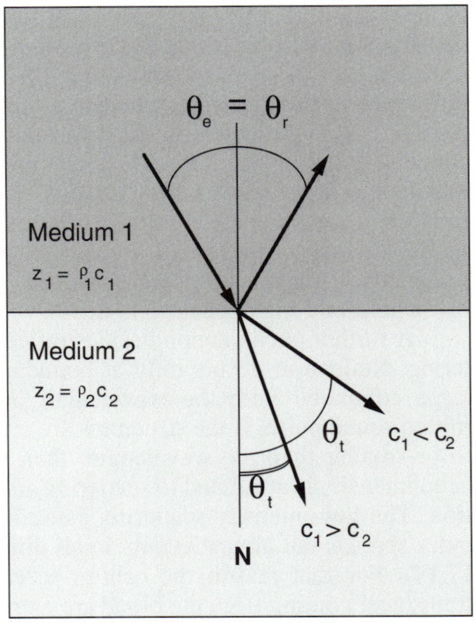

Fig. 17.**11** An ultrasound pulse hits an interface between two different media 1 and 2 at an angle of incidence of Θ_e. A part of the intensity of the pulse is reflected at an angle of reflection of Θ_r and another part of the intensity is transmitted into the second medium at an angle of refraction of Θ_t. The respective speeds of sound in the two media determine whether Θ_t is larger or smaller than Θ_e

In the case of normal incidence at the interface ($\Theta_r = \Theta_t = \Theta_e = 0$) the above equations can be simplified to:

$$R = \frac{I_r}{I_e} = \frac{(z_2 - z_1)^2}{(z_2 + z_1)^2}$$

$$T = \frac{I_t}{I_e} = \frac{4 z_1 z_2}{(z_2 + z_1)^2}$$

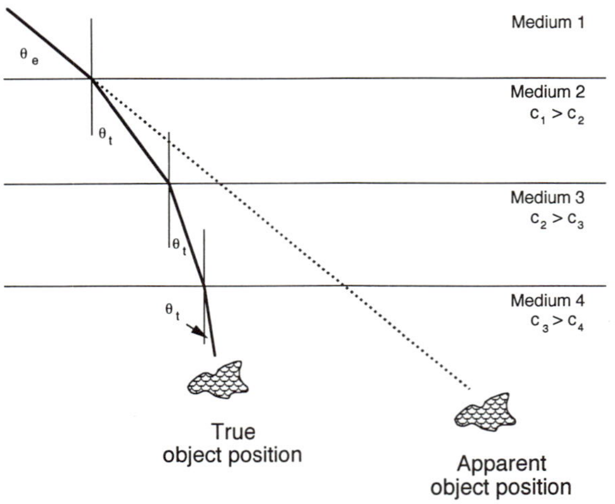

Fig. 17.**12** Caused by refraction the sound pulse may not travel along a straight line as expected but follow a different path

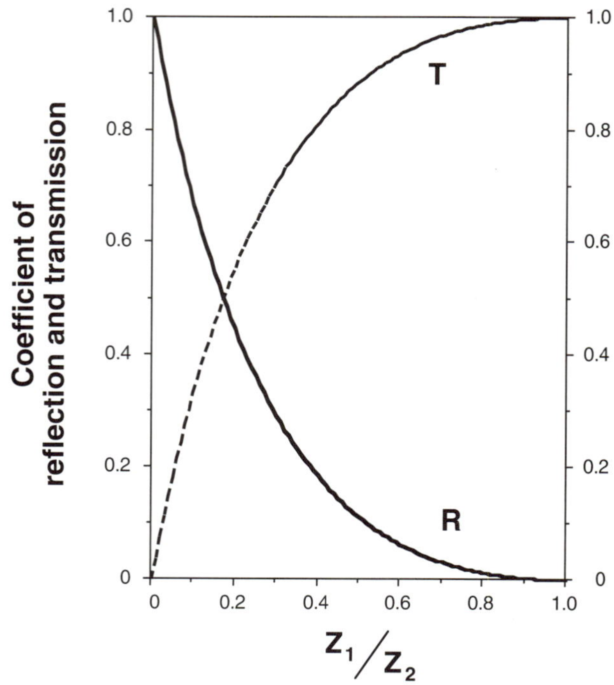

Fig. 17.**13** The coefficient of reflection R and transmission T in the case of an angle of incidence of 0° as a function of the impedances of the two media

As can be seen in Figure 17.**13**, in the presence of a large impedance jump, transmission is minute and the major part of the intensity is reflected. The impedance of air is about $0.0004 \cdot 10^6$ kg/m²s caused by the low density of air and the low speed of sound, whereas the impedance of tissue is roughly $1.62 \cdot 10^6$ kg/m²s. The difference in impedance is equal to a factor of about 4,050. This automatically calls for the use of an aqueous coupling medium when making ultrasound examinations because, otherwise only a very small fraction of the intensity would be transmitted into the body. Owing to the small impedance changes in tissue, only weak echoes are produced, resulting in the benefit of a high penetration depth.

A further phenomenon besides reflection is scattering. Reflection occurs only at boundaries that are large compared with the wavelength of the transmitted sound pulse. If the structures are similar in size to or smaller than the wavelength, then most of the echo intensity is attributed to scattering and not reflection. The low-intensity scattering caused by erythrocytes spreads out almost evenly in all directions (Fig. 17.**14**). For that reason the echoes received by the transducer coming from the blood are extremely weak and blood vessels in a B-mode image are, compared with tissue in which scattering and reflection occur, much darker at the same depth. Tissue also scatters much more intensity in all directions than blood particles do because the effective scattering cross section of tissue is much larger. The scattered intensity is proportional to the fourth power of the frequency of the ultrasound waves (16, 38). Absorption increases with frequency (see below). The scattered intensity of a 7.5-MHz signal is higher by a factor of 21 than that of a 3.5-MHZ signal. Using a 5-MHz signal still results in an increase in scattering by a factor of 4 compared with a 3.5-MHz signal. Intensive scattering at higher frequencies can partially compensate for the loss of intensity caused by the absorption in tissue. Scattering plays the dominant role in ultrasound imaging and in Doppler analysis. Small structures of different densities are the origin of scattering in the body. This is especially true for erythrocytes, whose larger diameter is about 7 μm and whose smaller diameter is roughly 2 μm. In evaluating blood flow the scattering characteristics of blood are of major importance. It is regrettable that they are extremely difficult to measure in vivo.

Two waves passing through the same region of space at the same time can influence one another (Fig. 17.**15**). This is called interference. Depending on the respective phases of the individual waves within the zone of interaction, the resulting amplitudes will be either larger or smaller than the amplitudes of the individual waves.

Diffraction is responsible for the nonlinear propagation of waves. Using the Huygens' principle, the ultrasound field starting at the transducer can be qualitatively described. Huygens' principle states that each point in space hit by a wavefront becomes the origin of a secondary wave. The envelope of these secondary waves determines the characteristics of the wavefront

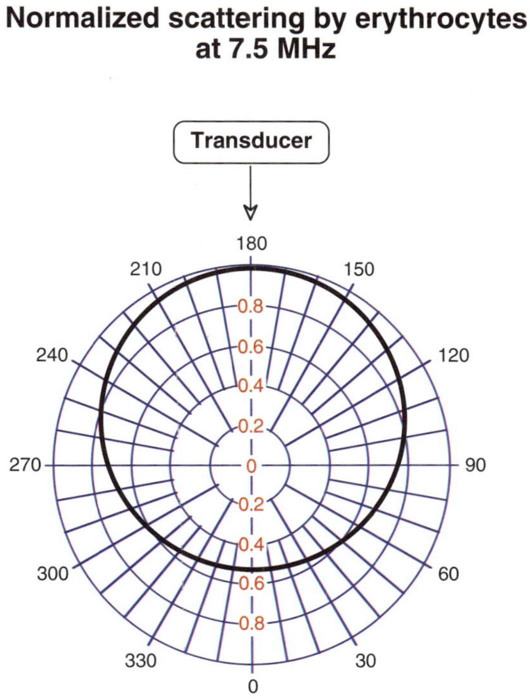

Fig. 17.**14** Ultrasound is scattered by erythrocytes in all directions with a slight preponderance of backward scattering (16, 38)

at a later point in time. Without diffraction it would not be possible, for example, to hear sounds coming from behind an obstacle. Diffraction and interference determine the characteristics of the sound field.

The penetration depth of an ultrasound pulse is limited by attenuation. During the time of flight of the pulse–echo signal, caused by absorption, the energy stored in the ultrasound signal is converted to heat except for the energy that is reflected or scattered. Attenuation partially caused by absorption reduces the initial intensity I_0 of the ultrasound pulse. The intensity decreases exponentially as a function of the distance s traveled. The coefficient of attenuation α is a material constant.The total loss of intensity as a function of distance caused by absorption (transformation to heat), reflection, scattering, geometrical losses, and other effects leads to the following equation:

$$I = I_0\, e^{-\alpha s} \qquad (17.2)$$

The terms absorption and attenuation are often erroneously used synonymously when describing the reduction of intensity caused by many different effects.

The human body is definitely not a homogeneous medium, but can be more or less described as a stratified medium. Different types of organic material such as fat, muscle, blood, tendons, as well as individual organs have their own special coefficient of attenuation (13, 42). The average coefficient of attenuation (24) is in the range of 0.3 to 0.6 dB/MHzcm. This results in a value between 0.6 and 1.2 dB/MHzcm for the round trip pulse–echo system. Taking the coefficient of attenuation to be equal to 1.0 dB/MHzcm simplifies the calculations.

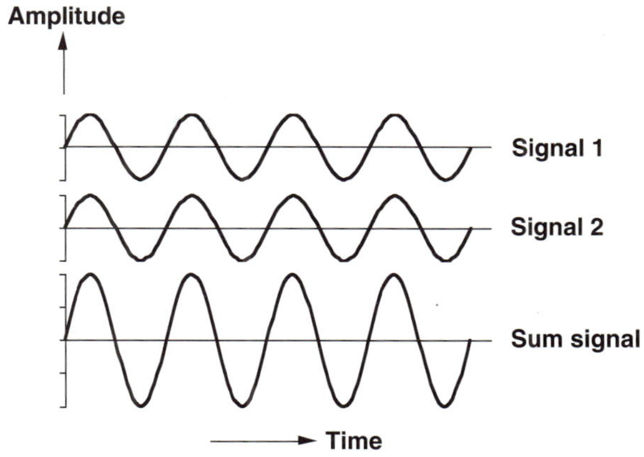

Fig. 17.**15** Interference of two waves with equal frequencies and phases leads to a wave with an amplitude equal in magnitude to the sum of the amplitudes of the two waves. If the waves were phase shifted by π (half a wavelength), the sum of the amplitudes would be zero

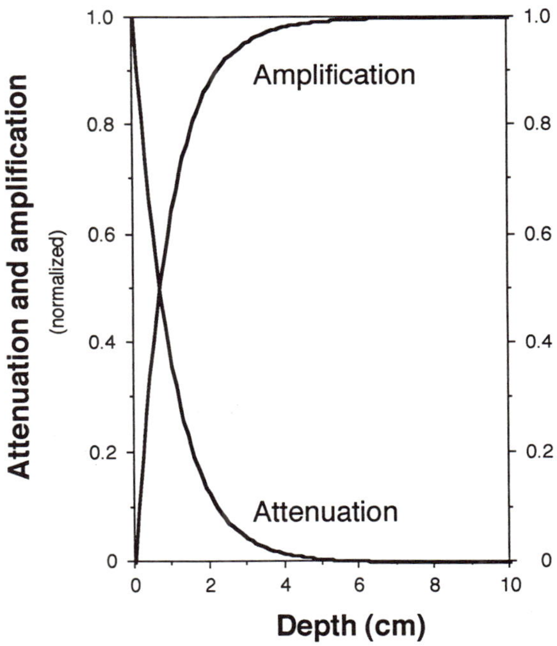

Fig. 17.**16** Depth-dependent gain compensation is necessary to correct for the attenuation of the ultrasound pulse and echo in tissue

Attenuation is accounted for by varying the amount of amplification applied by the ultrasound system to the echo signals (see Fig. 17.**16**). Depth-dependent amplification is a combination of the user-selected TGC (time gain compensation), also called swept gain or DGC (depth gain compensation), and the general overall amplification (gain) applied. Due to differences in tissue-dependent attenuation from one place to another and also between different persons, the local amplification has to be optimized for each and every image.

As stated above, attenuation is frequency-dependent. The higher the frequency the stronger the attenuation and—with a given maximum transmit power output and maximum accessible amplification—the smaller the depth from which an interpretable ultrasound signal can be attained. Furthermore, the center frequency of the ultrasound signal is shifted with depth to lower values caused by the greater attenuation of higher-frequency components compared with lower-frequency components in the ultrasound signal. This can be a problem when interpreting Doppler spectra coming from deep within the body. This is especially so when using short (broad band) signals in order to achieve small Doppler sample volumes. The use of broad-band transmit pulses in Doppler analysis is not especially sensible anyway, as will be explained in Sections 17.2.4 and 17.3.3. The narrower the bandwidth of the signal, the less the importance of this effect. In the case of CW Doppler this effect can be ignored completely. (See Section 17.2.4 for the explanation of bandwidth.)

The dynamic range of the signal is of major importance for the penetration depth. The dynamic range of an echo signal is defined as the difference between the maximum usable echo amplitude and the minimum amplitude that can be separated from the total noise background. The absolute maximum transmit amplitude depends on the ultrasound intensity that can be transmitted into the body without harm. Near the transducer a dynamic range of about 110 dB

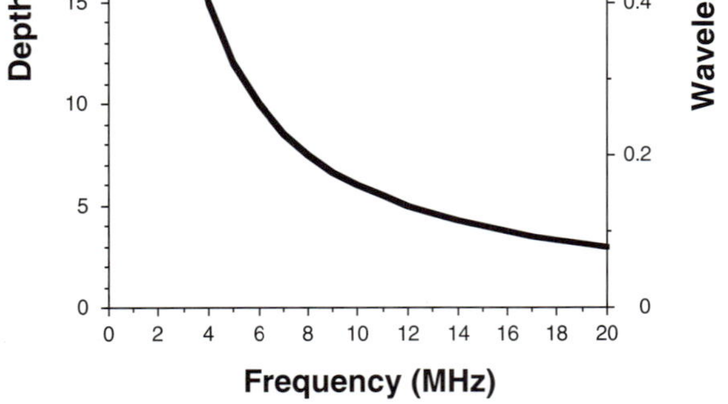

Fig. 17.**17** The wavelength and the average penetration of ultrasound in tissue as a function of the transducer center frequency using an expected attenuation coefficient of 0.9 dB/MHz cm for the pulse–echo round-trip distance

is possible. The dynamic range decreases with depth because of absorption.

The spatial resolution, especially the axial resolution, is tied to the wavelength (see Section 17.2.4). The higher the frequency, the shorter the wavelength according to equation 17.1 and the better the spatial resolution. In order to be able to work with the best possible resolution in all applications, ranging from the abdomen to the thyroid—due to the frequency-dependence of the penetration depth—a couple of transducers working at different center frequencies are needed. Present-day "multifrequency" transducers offer only a minute advantage for the user (see Section 17.2.3). The relationship between penetration depth and wavelength as a function of transmit frequency has been drawn in Figure 17.**17**. The penetration depth can only be estimated because it is very patient–dependent. The fat layer beneath the skin causes a great deal of scattering, also, total reflection at the boundary to air pockets, for example, and local attenuation play a dominant role here.

17.2.2 The Importance of the Speed of Sound in Imaging

An ultrasound image is based on multiple pulse–echo cycles composing the individual ultrasound scan lines. The speed of sound in human tissue is taken to be constant. By measuring the time span between the emission of an ultrasound pulse and the reception of an echo, the distance from the transducer at which the echo was created can be calculated. In order to be able to uniquely designate an echo to the specific place where it was created, all possible echoes belonging to a certain pulse must have arrived at the transducer before the next pulse may be emitted. Actually a couple of microseconds are needed for initialization processes within the machine itself before the next pulse is emitted from the transducer. The maximum penetration depth from which echoes can be registered depends on the attenuation (equation 17.2) and scattering characteristics of the medium and also on the transmit and receive characteristics as well as the signal-to-noise ratio of the ultrasound machine.

The distance s traveled by the sound pulse within time t is:

$$s = ct \tag{17.3}$$

The average speed of sound in human tissue is generally accepted in ultrasound diagnostics to be equal to c = 1,540 m/s (see Fig. 17.**8**). This value is used by all producers of ultrasound imaging equipment. Since imaging is based on the evaluation of multiple pulse–echo cycles, the distance s traveled by the pulse and the echo together is twice as long as the distance d between the transducer and the reflector displayed in the image. First the pulse must reach the reflector and then the echo must travel back along the same path to the transducer. The displayed distance after a time of flight t is equal to:

$$d = \frac{ct}{2} \quad (17.4)$$

The maximum allowed distance d_{max} is called the penetration depth or image depth. From the above it follows that for a given penetration depth and, requiring a unique mapping of the echoes to well-defined distances from the transducer, the maximum pulse repetition frequency f_{PRFmax} is:

$$f_{PRFmax} = \frac{c}{2d_{max}} \quad (17.5)$$

An A-mode ultrasound image is made up of just one ultrasound line. The echo amplitude is displayed as a function of time (see Fig. 17.**18**). More than one pulse–echo cycle is required in all other imaging modes. Many ultrasound scan lines located next to one another are needed to make one B-mode image. When selecting only one transmit focus, one pulse–echo cycle corresponds to one ultrasound scan line. In CDS, as will be explained later, more than one pulse–echo cycle per ultrasound scan line is always needed to acquire the flow information.

The speed of sound determines the relationship between the frame rate and the line density relative to the displayed image depth (Fig. 17.**19**). This can best be explained by looking, for example, at a CDS image with one transmit focus.

A frame rate of 20 images per second is desired, for example. That means, that there are 0.05 s available to acquire one image frame. According to equation 17.3, the total distance the sound may travel within this span of time is then equal to 77 m. Since imaging relies on multiple pulse–echo cycles, the total displayed distance according to equation 17.4 is only

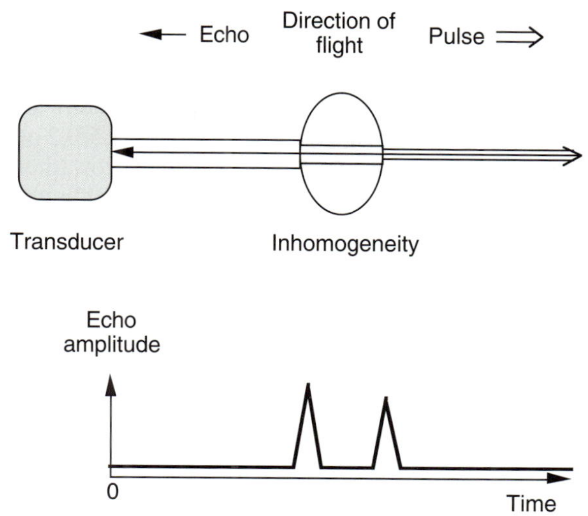

Fig. 17.**18** An ultrasound pulse passes interfaces between different media. A part of the energy is reflected, creating echoes that travel back to the transducer where they are registered. At the bottom of the figure the echo amplitudes are displayed as a function of time (A-mode image). The starting point of the temporal display is defined by the emission of the pulse

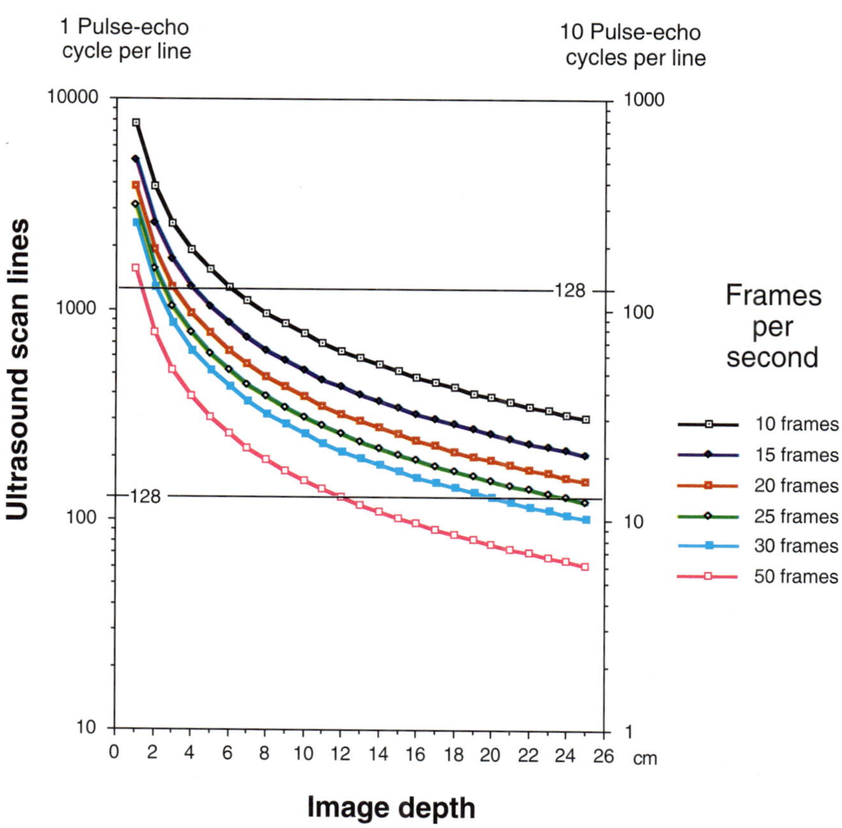

Fig. 17.**19** By selecting a certain frame rate and penetration depth the maximum possible number of pulse–echo cycles per image can be calculated. When using multiple transmit focusing or in CDS imaging more than one pulse–echo cycle per scan line is needed. The calculations in this example are based on either 1 *(left)* or 10 *(right)* pulse–echo cycles per scan line

half the above distance and is equal to 38.5 m. The image depth will, in this example, be limited to 20 cm. This at once makes it possible to calculate the maximum number of ultrasound scan lines that can be used in one B-mode image. In this case 192 lines (38.5/0.2 m) are possible. If the image must also display flow, then the number of ultrasound scan lines is reduced by the number of pulse–echo cycles needed per line to acquire the flow data. For example, at 10 pulse–echo cycles per line the maximum number of ultrasound scan lines possible is reduced to 19. By choosing more than one transmit focus, the number of lines is further reduced by the number of transmit focuses selected, because one pulse–echo cycle is needed for each individual transmit focus.

Most ultrasound machines on the market work with 64 to 192 ultrasound scan lines per image. The lateral spacing of the real ultrasound scan lines in a B-mode image should not exceed the equivalent of 3 to 4 wavelengths. On a 3.5-MHz transducer the lateral distance between the lines is then equal to $3 \cdot 0.44 = 1.32$ mm, equivalent to a line density of 7.58 lines per centimeter. If a higher line density is wanted, the frame rate is automatically reduced. As an alternative, the image width can be reduced by reducing the number of lines used. In this case, there is no degrading of image quality. The latter is often used in CDS mode. The selection of the width of the color window is left up to the user. The width of the gray-scale part of the image (total image width) is kept constant (see Fig. 17.**20**). Changing only the length (= depth) or the position of the color window does not influence the frame rate because the number of color lines is not changed. This is only valid if the pulse repetition frequency is not optimized according to the depth of the color box. In general, this is not the case.

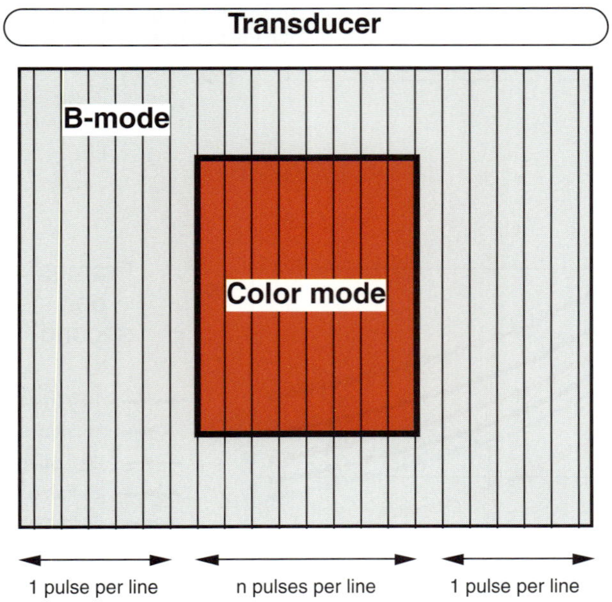

Fig. 17.**20** A CDS image is composed of a number of scan lines. More than one pulse–echo cycle is needed per scan line. In the pure B-mode image, using only one transmit focus, only one pulse–echo cycle per scan line is needed. The width of the color window is user-selectable in order to optimize the frame rate required for the actual application

The low speed of sound in tissue also limits the velocity range in Doppler spectrum analysis. Since uniqueness regarding the location of the origin of the signals used in pulsed Doppler spectrum analysis is to be maintained, all echoes coming from the region of interest must be received before the next pulse can be emitted. As explained later in Section 17.3.1, Doppler shifts can be uniquely determined only up to a maximum of one-half the pulse repetition frequency (Nyquist limit). Doppler shifts above this limit cannot be unambiguously determined without some additional assumptions. The pulse repetition frequency depends on the image depth, and this means that it is directly related to the speed of sound.

17.2.3 The Transducer

An ultrasound system is made up of a central control unit and at least one transducer. The image quality of the whole system depends a great deal on the transducers. This of course sounds very logical, but is often forgotten in everyday usage.

Electronic linear (LA), curved (CA) and phased-array transducers are used as well as mechanical transducers. Mechanical transducers may contain a single piezoelement (fixed focus) or multiple piezoelements (annular array). In multielement (up to about 12) annular-array transducers, the elements are basically created by subdividing a large circular element into concentric rings.

The image created using an LA transducer is rectangular. The maximum image width is defined by the width of the transducer (= total width of all the piezoelements). The image field of phased-array and mechanical transducers have the shape of a sector of a circle. LA and phased-array transducers are composed of one long rectangular piezoelement subdivided into adjacent individual small rectangles. LA and phased-array transducers differ in size and in the way the individual elements in the transducers are electronically steered over time. The width of the individual piezoelements in a phased-array transducer must not exceed one-half the wavelength of the ultrasound center frequency used. This limitation is not necessarily valid in the case of LA transducers.

A CA transducer is very similar to an LA transducer with the exception that the individual piezoelements are positioned in a row in the same plane along a certain radius of curvature. The shape of the image field can be looked upon as a combination of an LA and a sector-shaped image field. Near the transducer, the image field of a CA transducer is comparable in width to an LA transducer. The width of the image field increases with increasing distance from the transducer and then resembles that of a sector transducer.

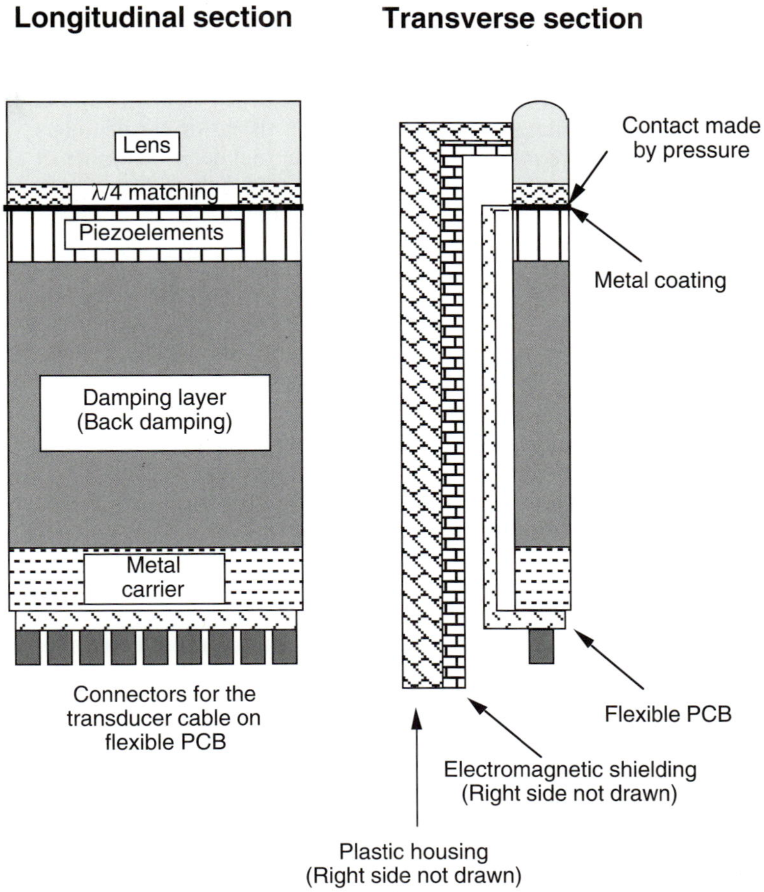

Fig. 17.**21** All transducers are basically very similar. A linear array transducer is shown in longitudinal and transverse cross section

On electronic transducers the direction of the ultrasound beam (the direction of flight of the ultrasound pulse) depends on the way the individual elements are electronically excited to emit an ultrasound pulse. On sector transducers the complete acoustic assembly must be rotated in a specific direction for the emission of an ultrasound pulse and reception of the echoes for each individual ultrasound scan line.

Emission of sound is based on the reverse piezoelectric effect. Applying a voltage between certain planes of special types of crystals produces a mechanical elongation or shortening of the crystal proportional to the polarity and amplitude of the voltage applied. In the opposite case, applying a mechanical force or pressure to the same crystal results in electric charges appearing on the surfaces of the crystal. The applied force distorts the crystal structure in such a way that the position of the positive and negative charges are changed relative to one another. This effect is called the piezoelectric effect. The resulting electric voltage, which is proportional to the magnitude of the force applied, can be measured. Crystals having a polar axis and no center of symmetry show piezoelectric properties. Quartz is, for example, a piezoelectric material. In transducers used in ultrasound imaging lead–zirconate–titanate–oxide ceramics called PZT are used ($PbZiTiO_2$). The ceramics are polarized in a strong electric field and in this way receive their piezoelectric properties (28). There are one or more piezoelements in every transducer. Recently, experiments with piezoelectric polymers called polyvinylidenflouride (PVDF) have been conducted. These polymers show excellent properties on receive such as a large bandwidth and a high sensitivity, but are not usable as transmitters of ultrasound (12). Work is also being done on composites, where piezoelectric materials such as PZT are enclosed in a passive polymer matrix. Such transducers are already being used in medical imaging, but at present are not superior to well-built PZT transducers. This may improve in the future.

Figure 17.**21** shows the general design of the acoustic module of a transducer. A linear array has been chosen as an example. In general, all transducers show the same basic construction. From top to bottom, the acoustic lens is followed by the quarter-wave matching layer, the piezoelements, the backdamping material, and finally, in arrays, a metal or plastic plate used for support. The shape and the specific material properties determine the acoustic characteristics of the transducer. To limit electromagnetic emission and interference, the acoustic module is inclosed in a grounded metal foil used for shielding. The outsides of a transducer are formed by a tightly sealed plastic cover.

The resonance frequency of a transducer element is determined by the thickness of the piezoelements. The thickness of the piezoelements is equal to one-half of the wavelength at resonance frequency in the piezoelectric material itself (and not in tissue or water). In “multifrequency” transducers the thickness of the piezoelements cannot be changed. The piezoelements are only excited at frequencies within the range of the bandwidth of the piezo assembly, usually equal to about 40–70% of the center frequency. To improve the electrical connection and to make sure that the voltage is applied evenly to the piezoelements, they are coated with a thin metal film of aluminium or silver. One wire is connected (bonded) to each individual piezoelement. Either a ground wire is contacted to the front of the piezoelements, or the backdamping layer is capable of conducting an electric current and then used for grounding as a whole. This is done, for example, by adding tungsten powder to the material.

The properties of the backdamping material have to be tailored to the planned usage of the transducer. This material is often composed of an epoxy resin containing in some cases tungsten or aluminium particles (23). In a pure CW pencil probe, the material is not supposed to damp the oscillations of the piezoelement and in this way create a narrow band ultrasound transmit signal. On transducers used purely for imaging, the damping should be very high in order to have an extremely short pulse length. The shorter the pulse, the broader the bandwidth of the transducer. Regrettably, the higher the damping, the lower the sensitivity of the transducer elements. Transducers used in duplex sonography for imaging and in Doppler analysis must have a broad bandwidth and a small bandwidth at the same time. This is of course a contradiction in itself. A compromise solution must be found favoring one specific application.

The piezoelements are coated with an antireflex layer. This coating has the same function as the antireflex coating on glasses. It is supposed to reduce the losses caused by reflection at the interface between the transducer and the tissue. The thickness of the coating is equal to one-quarter of the wavelength ($\lambda/4$) of the ultrasound frequency used and should have an impedance equal to $Z_{layer} = \sqrt{Z_{piezo} \cdot Z_{tissue}}$.

Array transducers contain a linear (or linear curved) array of individual mechanically and electronically divided piezoelements. A (for the chosen application) geometrically suited piezo-“plate” is subdivided into individual piezoelements by cutting the plate with a diamond saw or a laser. The number and width of the elements depend on the application and on the number of elements that can be addressed separately by the electronics of the central unit. In phased-array transducers, usually 32 to 128 independent elements are used. In LA and CA transducers, between about 64 and 192 elements are used. This has nothing to do with the number of electronic channels that determine the transmit and receive aperture. The aperture is usually a subset of the number of piezoelements in the transducer. The number of mechanically separate elements in a transducer can be twice or even four times as large as stated above. Mechanically subdividing the elements but using these subdivided elements electronically as one element helps in suppressing side lobes. This method is called “subdicing.” The number of elements also depends on the geometry of the transducer.

The outer top cover of array transducers is used as an acoustic lens. The lens is glued directly onto the quarter-wave matching layer. Silicon rubber with certain additional chemicals is often used as a lens material. The lens is supposed to bundle the sound waves and in this way focus the transducer in the direction normal to the image plane, because out-of-plane electronic focusing is not possible today. Because the elements are all in one row, out-of-plane focusing is only possible by refraction. The focal depth is defined by the manufacturer of the transducer. The focus position depends on the geometry of the lens and on the index of refraction of the chosen material. In-plane focusing is done electronically. Composite piezoelements can be the solution to this problem in the future. Thin, individually eletronically excitable piezorods embedded in an epoxy matrix are a possible type. Electronic steering of the sound emission might then be possible in all directions (44). Today’s composites are still one-row array elements. Industrial manufacturing of the kind of elements mentioned above will probably not be possible in the very near future.

Mechanical transducers are built somewhat differently from electronic transducers because of the necessity of an exact mechanical positioning of the acoustic block. The acoustic block itself also contains a quarter-wave matching layer followed by one (fixed-focus) or more (annular-array) piezoelements and a backdamping layer suited for the selected application. The acoustic block is moved with the help of some kind of motor-driven positioning system. The rotational velocity of the acoustic block including the piezoelements depends mainly on the image depth. The greater the image depth, the slower the piezoelements have to be rotated. The piezoelements are moved within a special oil which usually shows only low acoustic damping. The outer cap of the transducer must be strong enough to withstand the force applied to the transducer by the user during scanning, in order not to disturb the movement of the transducer element.

Focusing on mechanical transducers is done differently on fixed-focus and annular-array transducers. Electronic focusing is possible in all directions on annular-array transducers and not just in-plane as on other array transducers. On fixed-focus elements, focusing is achieved by giving the piezoelement a concave shape. The focus is defined by the manufacturer of the transducer and cannot be changed by the user.

17.2.4 The Ultrasound Field

One of the most commonly used types of transducers is the linear-array transducer (Figs. 17.**22** and 17.**23**). What is said in this section about the LA transducer is also valid, or at least very similar, in the case of a CA or phased-array transducer. In all these cases the piezoelements are evenly spaced in one row next to one another. The elements are always grouped together electronically to transmit and receive an ultrasound signal. In Figure 17.**23** the complete sound field of a linear-array transducer has been drawn schematically. The piezoelements are situated in the x,y-plane. Sound is emitted in z-direction, i. e., parallel to the z-axis. An ultrasound B-mode or CDS-mode image is composed of many individual ultrasound scan lines next to one another in y-direction. The resulting image is not the image of the infinitely thin y,z-plane but a two-dimensional representation of the three-dimensional ultrasound field varying in thickness depending on depth. The quality of an ultrasound image is equally dependent on transmit focusing and receive focusing. Furthermore, the complete analog and digital imaging chain is of extreme importance.

The width of the sound field in x-direction, also called slice thickness, is defined by the shape and acoustic characteristics of the lens (see Section 17.2.3). The shape of the ultrasound field in this direction is determined by the manufacturer of the transducer and cannot be electronicly influenced. The aim is to produce an ultrasound field that is as narrow as possible over the whole image depth in order to achieve a high depth of field. Focusing in y-direction is dependent on the way the individual piezoelements are controlled electronically. What is important in transmit is looked at first. Transmit and receive are, with few exceptions, physically and technically very similar.

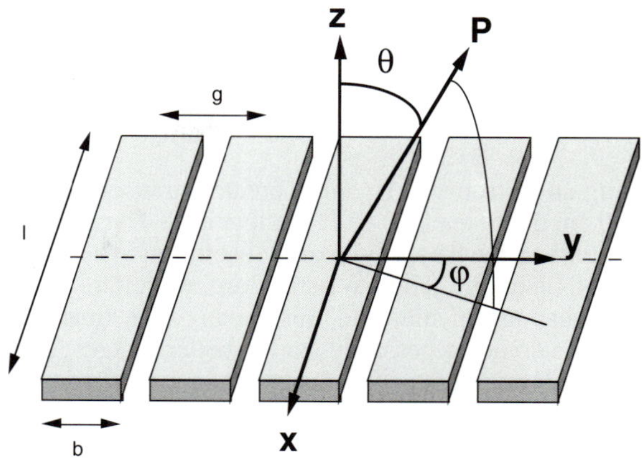

Fig. 17.**22** Reference system used on a linear-array transducer: l = length and b = width of a single piezoelement, g = pitch of the elements, θ and φ are the polar coordinates

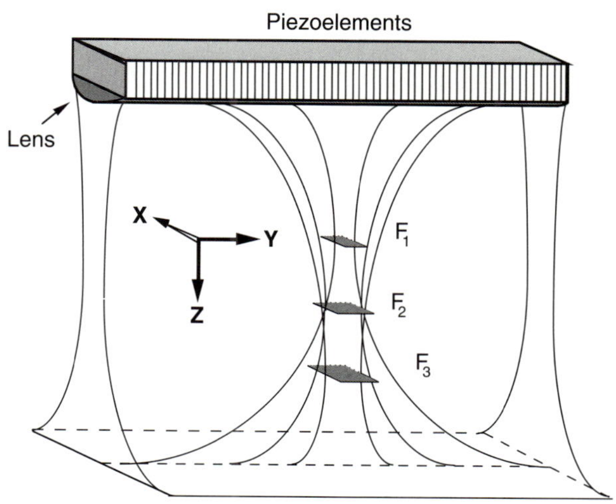

Fig. 17.**23** Ultrasound field of a linear-array transducer with three transmit focuses F_1, F_2, F_3

Transmit

The size of the group of piezoelements used in transmit depends on the selected distance of the transmit focus position from the transducer and on the electronics of the system, i. e., how many individual channels can or should be grouped together in transmit. The number of usable channels cannot exceed the number of piezoelements. It must not be forgotten that only one transmit focus can be selected for each transmit pulse (axiconal focusing is not discussed here). Using more than one transmit focus automatically leads to a frame rate reduction. When using more than one transmit focus per ultrasound scan line, the focus farthest away from the transducer is usually internally selected first. After that the other focus positions are aimed at in reverse order of their distance from the transducer. On frame rate optimized systems, at the time the last echo from the individual focus zone reaches the transducer, the next pulse is fired. The echoes originating closer to the transducer are much stronger than echoes coming from farther away from it. The underlying acoustic noise caused by echoes from outside of the focal (image) zone can usually be neglected. In this way the reduction in frame rate caused by multiple transmit focusing can be somewhat limited. The received and evaluated echoes are assigned to the individual focus zones resulting in one complete ultrasound scan line.

Three transmit focuses F_1, F_2 and F_3 are used in Figure 17.**23**. The closer the position of the transmit focus to the transducer, the less elements are used to produce the focused ultrasound pulse. Terminology from photography and having a similar meaning there is used. The aperture A is defined in ultrasound as the width of the group of elements used to transmit each individual pulse and definitely not the total length of all transducer elements in the transducer. The “F-number” (focal ratio in photography) is obtained by dividing the distance z_t of the focus from the transducer by the aperture used at that distance:

$$F = \frac{z_t}{A}$$

Using an aperture of 10 cm to create a transmit focus at 20 cm depth leads to an *F*-number of 2. The smaller the number, the better the spatial resolution in a homogeneous medium. Human beings are, regrettably, not homogeneous media, and this means that small *F*-numbers do not necessarily lead to better images (26). A small *F*-number can be an advantage in obstetrics in case the placenta is located on the far side of the body,

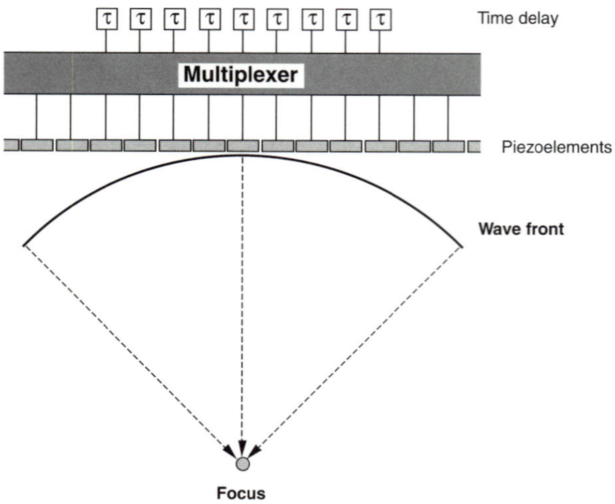

Fig. 17.**24** A focused wave front is created by time-delayed excitation of the individual elements. The position of the transmit focus is defined by the choice of the time delays τ. With the help of a multiplexer the group of piezoelements used for transmission and reception are selected

away from the transducer. This will most likely not be so in the abdomen with its many different tissue layers and air-filled regions. Owing to differing velocities of sound in different tissue types, the time of flight of the ultrasound pulse and echo will not be the same throughout the ultrasound field. The time of flight of the ultrasound pulse and echo along the line of sight between the outer left piezoelement of a focus group and an object and the outer right piezoelement and the same object may be very different. A theoretical point focus will then have an elliptical shape. The tissue-dependent absorption has not even been taken into account in this case. Furthermore, scattering and diffraction may also disrupt the image quality. Many ultrasound systems use an *F*-number of 6 at greater depths in abdominal applications.

As stated above, and shown in Figure 17.**23**, the aperture used in transmit and receive increases with depth. This kind of function is called aperture growth and is implemented on all high-quality ultrasound systems. The F-number is still a function of the distance from the transducer.

Focusing is technically achieved as shown in Figure 17.**24** by delaying the excitation of the individual piezoelements of a transmit group by a certain amount of time relative to one another. The outer elements of the group are excited first and, depending on the position of the selected focus, the time delay grows in magnitude toward the center elements. The phase-corrected or time-of-flight corrected summation of the elementary waves leads to the resulting wave front as depicted in Figure 17.**25**. On linear and curved arrays the time delay is symmetrical relative to the center element, except for the outer ultrasound scan lines. On phased arrays the deflection of the ultrasound beam is facilitated by precise control of the time delays (Fig. 17.**26**). The method is called beam steering. In this case there is no symmetry, which calls for an increase in the complexity of the electronics.

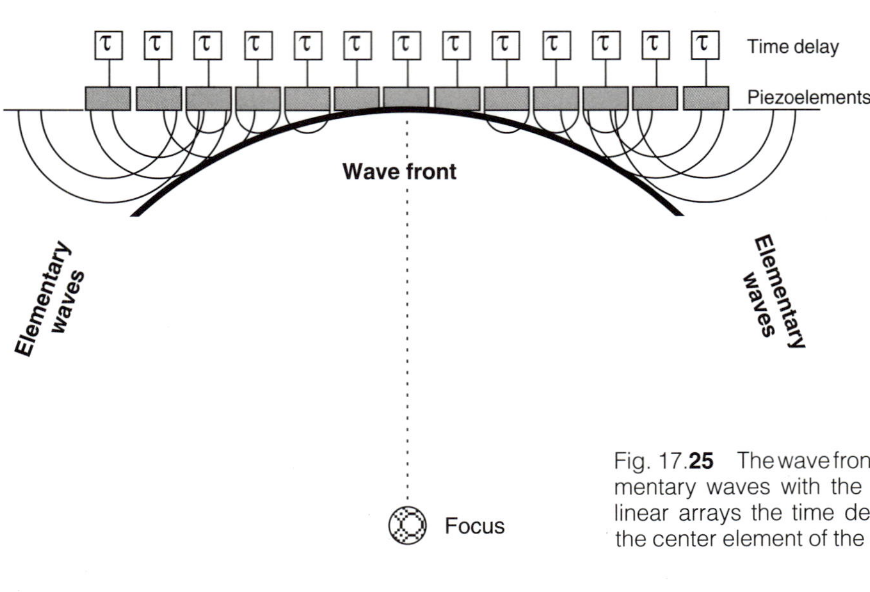

Fig. 17.**25** The wave front can be constructed from the elementary waves with the help of Huygens' principle. On linear arrays the time delays are symmetrical relative to the center element of the chosen piezo group.

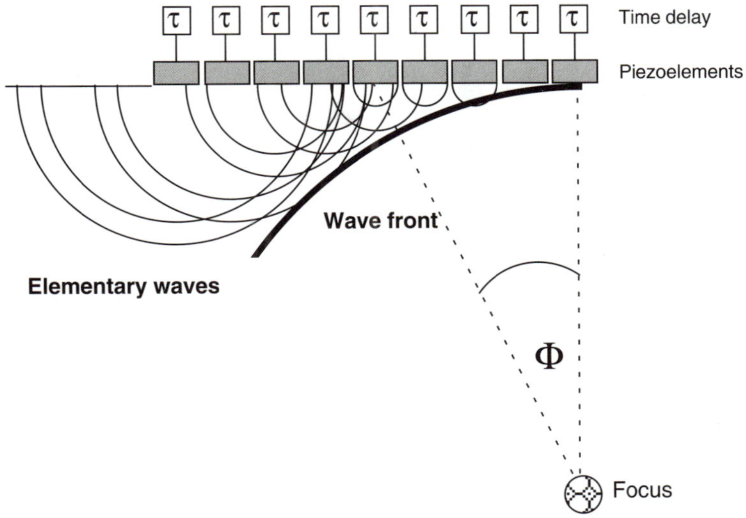

Fig. 17.**26** The steering angle ϕ on phased arrays is defined by the time delays τ. On this kind of transducer all elements are used to create the desired wave front

When using large angle deflection, the electronic circuitry needed to achieve the much larger time delays when compared to linear arrays is far more complex. On color-encoded systems the beam is often steered at an angle of 10^0 to 20^0 in order to achieve a more advantageous Doppler angle (small angle deflection). This is done on linear-array transducers in exactly the same way as on phased arrays. Actually, the phased array is a special kind of linear array.

The piezoelements are selected with the help of a multiplexer. For example, elements number 25 to 56 are selected (32 elements). These elements are then electrically excited with a certain time delay relative to each other. This results in a focused ultrasound wave front propagating through the tissue. After reception of the echoes coming from the greatest possible depth, the transmit piezo group is then switched by one element to elements 26 to 57. This will then deliver the next ultrasound scan line. With the help of the multiplexer, the line density can easily be increased by a factor of 2 without any additional electronic circuitry. By alternately selecting an odd number of N piezoelements and then for the next ultrasound scan line an even number of elements (N–1), the ultrasound scan lines will be switched laterally by half the width of a piezoelement. By increasing the line density, the frame rate is automatically decreased by the same amount. In this way, on a 128-element transducer for instance, one can easily increase the number of ultrasound scan lines from 128 to 256. The number of ultrasound scan lines per image is not directly coupled to the number of electronic channels in the system. The number of channels used, combined with the piezoelement spacing, determines the aperture size and in this way also the F-number.

In the case of LA and CA transducers, a problem naturally arises at the end of the piezo arrays. Symmetrical focusing is not always possible here. Sometimes additional piezoelements are added to the arrays, in this way increasing the array length. The length of the piezo array then exceeds the image width. Alternatively, the ultrasound intensities at the end elements must be weighted differently than in the symmetrical case. Often the image is somewhat poorer at the edges than in the center. This is especially true on phased-array transducers. The reason for this is different, as will be explained later.

An ultrasound image is composed of a certain number of individual ultrasound scan lines. Each line represents one pulse–echo cycle when only one transmit focus is used. In the case of multiple transmit focusing, each line corresponds to a number of pulse–echo cycles equivalent to the number of transmit focuses used.

Spatial and Frequency Resolution

Spatial resolution defines the ability to visualize two neighboring objects as separate, individual entities. A point object is displayed as a disk in a B-mode image. The brightness decreases to the sides of the image. An ultrasound pulse is displayed in Figure 17.**10**. It must not be forgotten that besides the transmit characteristics the receive characteristics and especially the dynamic range of the ultrasound system is of importance. Additionally, the ability of the eye to discriminate differences in brightness also influences the perceived spatial resolution. The dynamic range of the human eye is about 30 dB. Around 35 different grayscale values can be discriminated (37). Often an image width of a "point" object at an intensity of –6 dB (half-width) is used to define the shortest distance between the two objects at which they can still be recognized as being separate. The envelope of two images of neighboring objects at the –6 dB distance will then show a visible intensity minimum of –0.7 dB between the images of the two (Fig. 17.**27**). Furthermore, the ultrasound signal dynamic range decreases with depth because of the loss of intensity caused by attenuation and by the shift of the center

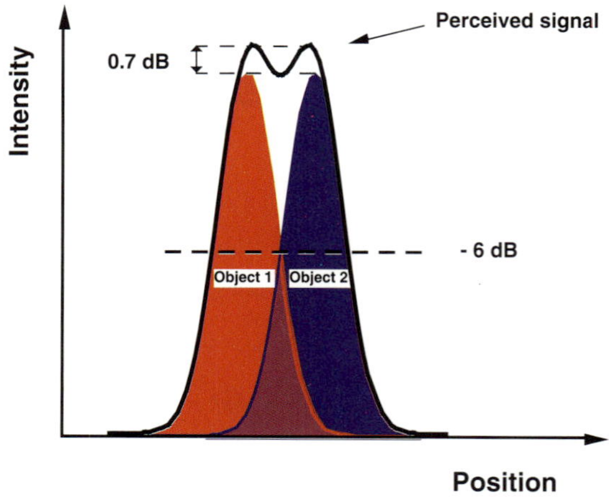

Fig. 17.**27** Two objects can be distinguished from one another if the position of maximum intensity of the image of one object is located at the position of minimum intensity of the image of the other object. Usually the diameter at half-width intensity is used to define the size of the image. The perceived total signal of two objects separated by the half-width distance results in an intensity minimum between the objects of only about 0.7 dB

frequency toward lower frequencies (see Section 17.2.1). This will also lead to a depth-dependent spatial resolution.

The axial spatial resolution Δz depends on the temporal length τ of the ultrasound pulse and on the pulse shape. The following relation is valid:

$$\Delta z = \frac{\tau c}{2} \qquad (17.6)$$

The temporal pulse length must be defined in order to determine the axial resolution. The pulse length depends, among other things, on the center frequency used. The higher the center frequency at constant relative pulse length, the better the axial spatial resolution. An ultrasound pulse has been schematically drawn in Figure 17.**28**. The perceived pulse length depends on the intensity differences that can be recognized by an observer. If a drop in signal intensity of –6 dB is used, then the spatial resolution in axial direction would be seemingly very good. If a reduction in signal intensity down to –40 dB is allowed, the pulse length is much longer, and the perceived axial resolution decreases a great deal. Often the –6 dB, –20 dB and –40 dB values are stated by the manufacturers of ultrasound diagnostic equipment. The truly achievable and visible spatial resolution depends on the conditions during each and every examination. The change in perceived spatial resolution can easily be observed on a wire phantom by changing the signal receive gain. When using the –6 dB signal, an axial resolution equivalent to the wavelength at the center frequency used can be observed.

The pulse bandwidth B (Fig. 17.**29**), which is very important for Doppler frequency resolution (see Section 17.3.3), is directly coupled to the temporal pulse length τ. $\tau_{-6\,dB}$ and $B_{-6\,dB}$ represent the temporal half-width and the pulse bandwidth respectively. The bandwidth is:

$$B_{-6dB} = \frac{1}{\tau_{-6dB}} \qquad (17.7)$$

Introducing this equation into equation 17.6 results in:

$$\Delta z_{-6dB} = \frac{c}{2B_{-6dB}} \qquad (17.8)$$

The bandwidth of an ultrasound pulse defines the frequency range where the amplitudes of individual frequencies exceed a certain limit. Normally the –6 dB amplitude range is used. The bandwidth is often expressed as a percentage of the center frequency. If, for example, the –6 dB values on both sides of the center frequency of 5.0 MHz are 3.75 MHz and 6.25 MHz, equivalent to a range of 2.5 MHz, the bandwidth, in

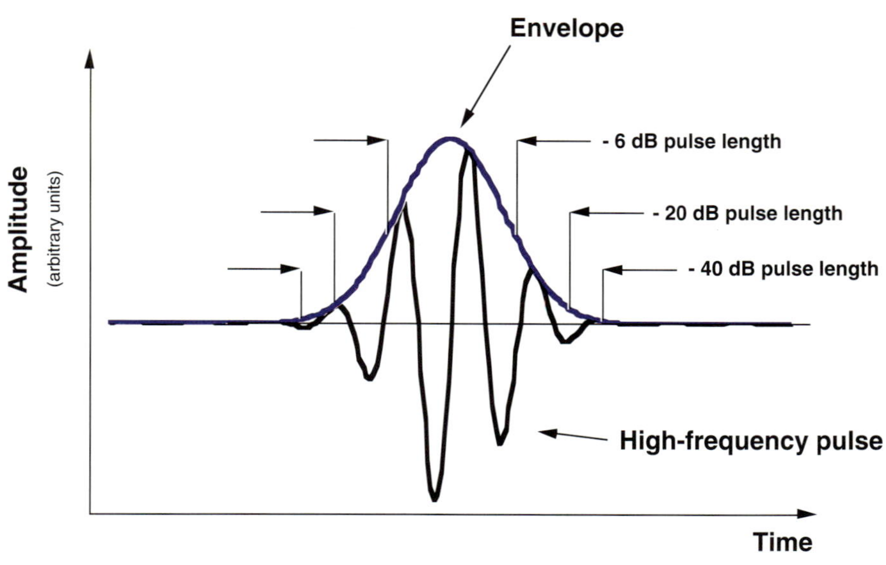

Fig. 17.**28** Time domain representation of a pulse. The length of an ultrasound pulse depends on the selected cutoff signal intensity

Fig. 17.**29** Frequency domain representation of a pulse. The bandwidth of an ultrasound pulse is defined by frequencies whose amplitudes exceed a certain magnitude. Often the full width at half maximum (−6 dB) is used. The bandwidth is often stated as a percentage of the center frequency

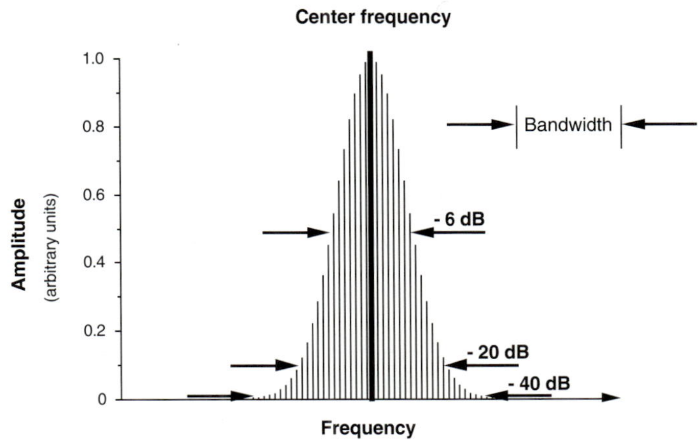

this case, would be equal to 50%. The bandwidth of the ultrasound pulse is also especially important in Doppler spectrum analysis.

In order to be able to perform a good spectrum analysis, in determining the Doppler frequency shift, a very narrow band pulse is needed, i. e., the bandwidth must be small. The longer the span of time available for performing the measurements, the better the frequency resolution. This means, according to equation 17.7, the pulse length τ must be long. It would be ideal if the pulse length were infinite as in the case of CW Doppler. The bandwidth of a CW Doppler is practically zero. The axial length of the Doppler gate in PW Doppler is determined by the length of the ultrasound pulse and the time duration during which the ultrasound system is in receive mode. The length of the gate is usually user-selectable. In order to make sure that the scatterer does not leave the Doppler sample volume during measurement, the ultrasound field should also be very wide. This will result in a poor lateral resolution compared with gray-scale imaging. A small Doppler sample volume will result in a poorer frequency resolution. The relative frequency resolution $\Delta f_d/f_d$ is inversely proportional to the length of the pulse train in the Doppler gate that can interact with the scatterers being observed. The effect involved is called intrinsic spectral broadening (17). This immediately results, according to equation 17.8, in a poorer spatial resolution for all Doppler methods compared with B-mode imaging as long as a precise frequency resolution is desired. High spatial resolution in B-mode imaging relies on a short, wide band pulse, with a narrow lateral ultrasound field width. To achieve a high-frequency resolution, the total Doppler sample volume must be very large. Contrary to general opinion, focusing is not advantageous in this case, except in order to raise the pulse intensity in the vicinity of the selected sample volume. As in many other cases, the developer of an ultrasound system, especially in CDS, must find some kind of compromise.

A closer look at this is necessary. The scatterer should remain within the sample volume for as long a period of time as possible. Scatterers leaving or entering the Doppler sample volume during the time of measurement will lead to a broader frequency spectrum. Their dwell time within the sample volume is short. Figuratively speaking, it is impossible to distinguish between a short time of residence caused by the high speed of a particle or because of the particle's delayed entry into the sample volume or its leaving the sample volume before the measurement has been completed. This cause of spectral broadening is based on the transit time effect. The effect reduces the frequency resolution. A Doppler shift f_d with an uncertainty of Δf_d is the result. The following explanations are based on a presentation by Angelsen (27, 32). Δf_d corresponds to the bandwidth of equation 17.7 and leads to

$$\Delta f_d = \frac{1}{T_t}$$

According to Figure 17.**30**:

$$T_t = \frac{L}{v}$$

where T_t = transit time of the scatterer passing through the Doppler gate
L = path length of the scatterer within the Doppler gate
v = velocity of the scatterer

This leads to:

$$v = \frac{L}{T_t} = L\,\Delta f_d \qquad (17.9)$$

According to equation 17.12 the following expression is valid for the Doppler shift and the center frequency f_0 at a Doppler angle of α:

$$v = \frac{f_d}{2f_0}\;\frac{c}{\cos(\alpha)}$$

Combining equation 17.9 and the above equation to eliminate v and then performing a simple transformation results in

$$\frac{\Delta f_d}{f_d} = \frac{c}{f_0 2L\cos(\alpha)}$$

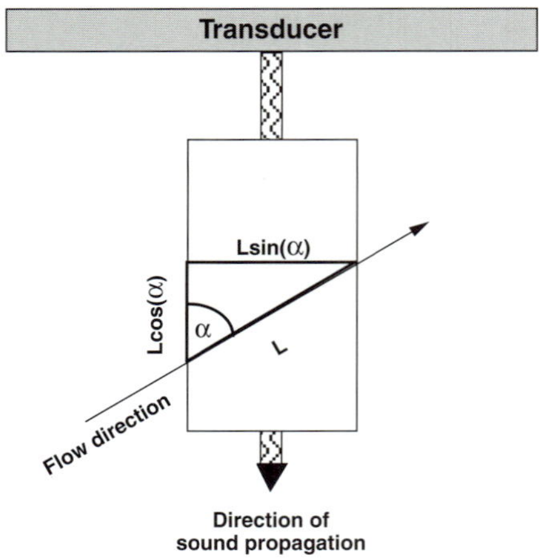

Fig. 17.**30** A particle passes through the Doppler sample volume along path L. The angle α is the angle between L and the direction of propagation of the ultrasound signal

Rewriting equation 17.1 to receive the wavelength λ and inserting the resulting expression leads to the relative Doppler frequency resolution

$$\frac{\Delta f_d}{f_d} = \frac{\lambda}{2L\cos(\alpha)}$$

The longer the scatterer remains in the region under observation, i. e., the larger the length of the Doppler window L, the better the frequency resolution. Making the pulse length smaller leads to a smaller L and an improvement in the axial spatial resolution but also leads to a deterioration of the Doppler frequency resolution. An improvement in spatial resolution leads to poorer frequency resolution and vice versa. Furthermore, the closer the Doppler angle gets to 90°, the poorer the frequency resolution.

Of course blood contains not merely one scatterer but is composed of many. The scattering characteristics are not constant but vary considerably over time. Furthermore, the Doppler sample volume is not homogeneously insonated. The sound intensity varies throughout the Doppler window. All in all, this leads to a smoothing (averaging) of the spectrum and to a reduction in frequency resolution.

A closer look at the ultrasound field reveals that the sound intensity depends heavily on the position in the field and is much more complex then one would think at first. Owing to interference and diffraction, among other phenomena, the pressure changes constantly. A complete analytical solution exists for a flat disk element (36) along the acoustic axis of the transducer.

$$\left|\frac{p}{p_0}\right| = 2\left|\sin\left(\frac{\pi}{\lambda}\left(\sqrt{a^2 + z^2} - z\right)\right)\right| \qquad (17.10)$$

where $\frac{p}{p_0}$ = normalized pressure
a = outer radius of the piezoelement
λ = wavelength of the signal
z = distance from the piezoelement along the z-axis

This function has been drawn in Figure 17.**31**. In addition to the monochromatic solution above, the polychromatic case has been calculated and drawn. The monochromatic case corresponds to CW Doppler. The polychromatic case has to be used in all pulsed ultrasound applications such as PW Doppler, B-mode imaging, and CDS. A bandwidth of 50% and a Gaussian intensity distribution of frequencies were used. Today, very good state-of-the-art multielement transducers exhibit a bandwidth of about 70%.

The near-field or Fresnel zone extends from the surface of the piezoelement to the last maximum of the function at a distance a^2/λ (assuming $a \gg \lambda$). From then on, in the far field or Frauenhofer zone, the intensity drops continuously. It is important to note that in the near field in the case of CW Doppler many pressure maxima and minima exist. In other words, there are regions from which only low-intensity Doppler

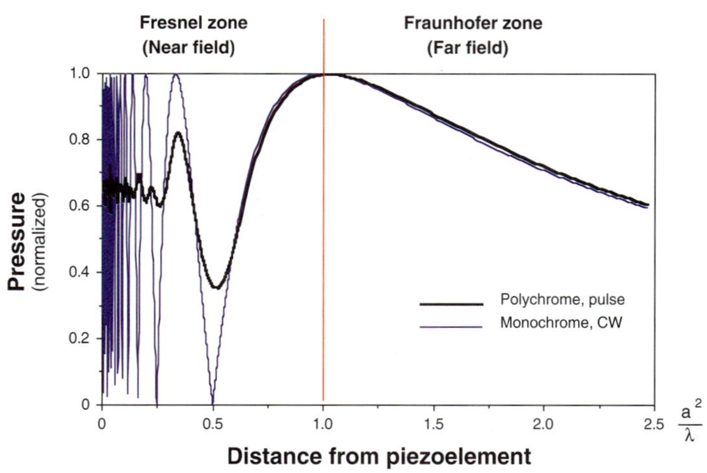

Fig. 17.**31** Sound intensity along the acoustic axis of a flat disk element according to equation 17.10. The monochromatic and polychromatic (50% bandwidth) cases were calculated. The center frequencies are the same in both cases

Table 17.**1** Length of the near-field zone in case of flat disk unfocused transducers at different center frequencies and different piezo diameters.

Frequency (MHz)	Piezo diameter (mm)	Near-field length (mm)
3.0	10	49
	15	110
	20	195
5.0	5	20
	10	81
	15	183
7.5	5	30
	7.5	69
	10	122

signals will come. In the polychromatic case in PW Doppler and B-mode imaging, the near-field intensities vary much less. In both cases the transition between near and far field occurs at the same distance from the transducer. The position of the last maximum on the acoustic axis has been calculated for some special cases in Table 17.**1**. It is immediately apparent that ultrasound imaging is mostly done in the near field. When focusing and aperture growth are taken into account, this is generally not the case.

Owing to the shape of the ultrasound field, the lateral spatial resolution in x- and y-direction is not as good as the axial resolution. As stated above, the lateral resolution depends on the distance of the structures under observation from the transducer. Huygens' principle is used in constructing and calculating the ultrasound field. According to Huygens' principle, every point hit by a light wave front (sound wave front) may be regarded as the origin of secondary waves. The envelope of these secondary waves determines the position of the wave front at a later point in time. Using this principle, the sound field and the effects of focusing on all kinds of transducers can be demonstrated very effectively. This principle was used in Figures 17.**25** and 17.**26**. Using a simplified model, the far field of an array transducer resembles the field of an optical diffraction grating. Using this model, the field results by superimposing the diffraction pattern of a single rectangular slit (single piezoelement) and the interference pattern produced by a grating of many parallel rectangular slits (many piezoelements). According to this highly simplified model (pulsing is not included), the intensity I (actually the directivity) of the ultrasound field in the far field in the x,y-plane ($\varphi = 0$, see Fig. 17.**22**) may be expressed as (8):

$$I = \frac{b^2 L}{\lambda} \cdot \left(\frac{\sin(q)}{q}\right)^2 \cdot \left(\frac{\sin(mp)}{\sin(p)}\right)^2$$

where $p = \frac{\pi}{\lambda} g \sin(\Theta)$,

$q = \frac{\pi}{\lambda} b \sin(\Theta)$

m = number of piezoelements used

In the case of phased arrays or beam steering on linear arrays, $\sin(\Theta)$ is substituted for $(\sin(\Theta) - \sin(\Phi))$. Φ is the steering angle of the ultrasound beam.

Calculating the intensity as a function of the in-plane takeoff angle Θ defines the transmit characteristics of the transducer. In Figures 17.**32** and 17.**33** the transmit characteristics (directivity) of two different linear-array transducers have been drawn.

It is easy to see that the transmit field intensity is not simply cone-shaped, but is composed of many "lobes." The absolute maximum or main lobe is situated at 0° and the less intensive side lobes are found at angles other than 0° (LA and CA transducers). The center piezoelement of the transmit group is used as the point of reference. On phased arrays this is somewhat different. The beam is steered in a different direction for every ultrasound scan line. In all cases, except along the central ultrasound image line, the steering angle Φ is not equal to zero (LA case without beam

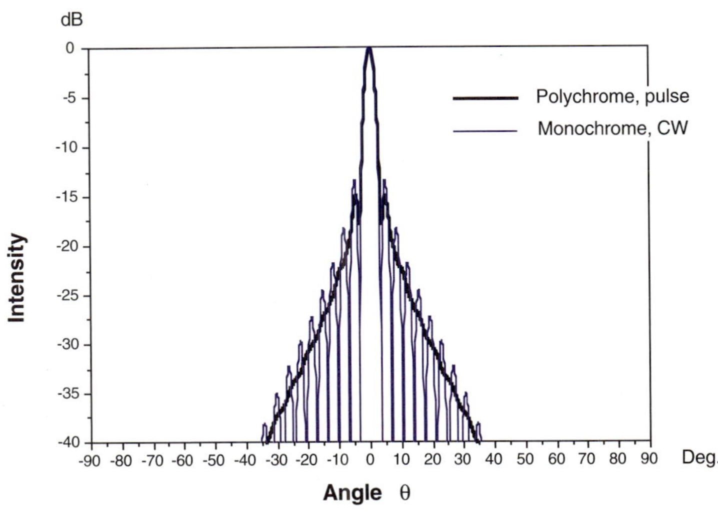

Fig. 17.**32** Directivity function of a 5-MHz linear-array transducer with m = 12 elements, b = 0.38 mm, g = 0.43 mm, and l = 10 mm (see Fig. 17.**22**). The monochromatic and polychromatic (50% bandwidth, Gauss weighting) cases were calculated

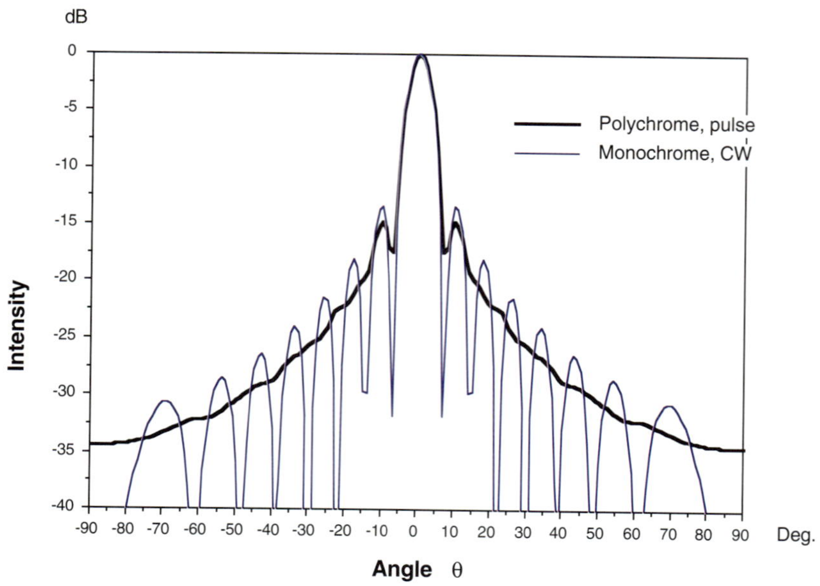

Fig. 17.**33** Directivity function of a 5-MHz linear-array transducer with m = 16 elements, b = 0.15 mm, g = 0.154 mm, and l = 10 mm (see Fig. 17.**22**). The monochromatic and polychromatic (50% bandwidth, Gauss weighting) cases were calculated

steering). This results in a poorer lateral resolution compared with a linear or curved array because the main lobe becomes wider when steered at large angles. Comparing Figures 17.**33** and 17.**34** shows that when steering at 40°, the −6 dB intensity value of the main lobe is spread by 2°. The first intensity minimum is shifted 6° to one side. The larger the steering angle, the smaller the difference between side lobe and main lobe intensities, and also the poorer the lateral resolution. This is also the case during small angle steering on LA transducers. The effective transmit transducer area also decreases when steering proportionally to the cosine of the steering angle. On electronic transducers, the piezoelements are not rotated in beam direction. This means that only the projection of the piezo area in the direction steered can be used for transmit and receive. This results in a reduction of signal intensity and dynamic range. Electronic compensation by raising the transmit power at large steering angles is only partially possible.

The size of the side lobes can be reduced. This is achieved on transmit by sending different transmit voltage amplitudes to the individual piezoelements of a transmit group. A Gauss or Hamming weighting of the applied amplitudes is used. This leads, if done correctly, to a significant reduction of the side lobe intensity but also results in a broadening of the main lobe. This method is called apodization. The developer of an ultrasound imaging device must decide whether the additional expensive electronics is really worth the effort. Another possibility is to subdivide the piezoelements mechanically but not electronically. This also leads to a side lobe reduction and is done on high-quality equipment.

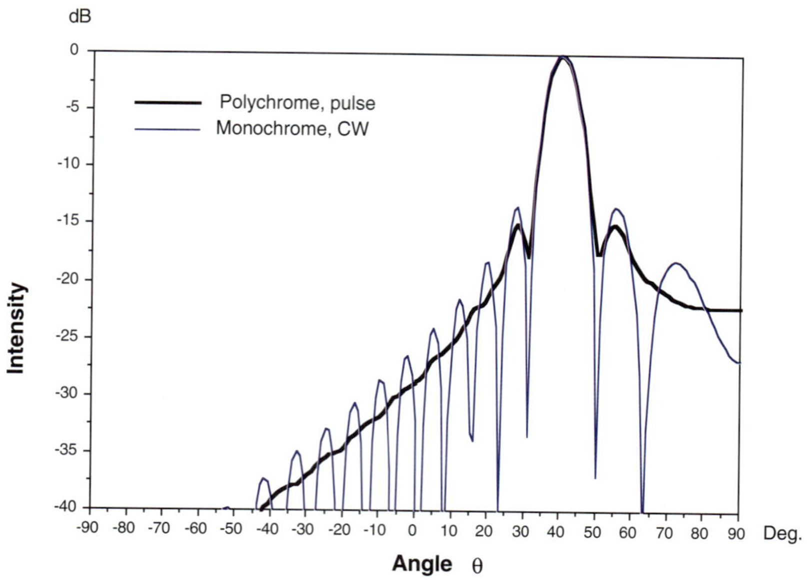

Fig. 17.**34** Directivity function of a 5-MHz phased-array transducer with m = 16 elements, b = 0.15 mm, g = 0.154 mm, and l = 10 mm (see Fig. 17.**22**). The monochromatic and polychromatic (50% bandwidth, Gauss weighting) cases were calculated. The steering angle ϕ is 40°

Focusing was excluded in the above discussion of lateral resolution. An analytical solution does not exist in the case of focusing. A numerical solution must be sought in every individual case (43). Nevertheless, the above results are the foundation of ultrasound imaging. With the help of focusing and aperture growth, the position at which the near field ends and the far field begins can be changed along with the beam width. On the one hand, the spatial lateral resolution within the focal zone can be improved by focusing. On the other, the depth of field is decreased by focusing. Here again a compromise must be found. This is the reason for increasing the electronic complexity of the system to be able to achieve multiple transmit focusing. In order to improve the lateral resolution, the user has to take into account the reduced frame rate in multiple-transmit focusing mode. The more exact the time delays can be set in transmit and receive focusing, the better the focusing capability. This is especially important for the image quality in the near field close to the transducer. As a rule of the thumb, the precision should be as high as 0.1 wavelengths. For example, on a 5.0-MHz transducer, the achievable time delay differences between individual elements should be about 20 nsec ($20 \cdot 10^{-9}$ = 20 billionth of a second!).

Receive

After the ultrasound pulse has been transmitted, the system immediately switches to receive. A continuous stream of echoes with differing amplitudes reaches the transducer. The echoes are partially phase and frequency shifted.

The ultrasound transmit signal is scattered and reflected from objects within the sound field. The signals returning from an object reach the individual transducer elements at different points in time, depending on the distance between the object and each piezoelement. It is taken for granted that the speed of sound along all paths from the scatterer to the piezoelements is the same. Figuratively speaking, one imagines a spherical wave front moving away from the scatterer toward the transducer. This assumption is in the abdomen, for example, not always correct because the speed of sound is tissue-dependent. A large aperture can be a disadvantage, especially in abdominal scanning. The inner elements of the receive piezo group are reached first by the scattered wave and the outer elements last. This is almost never true for phased arrays and during beam steering on LA transducers. The relations are more complex there. The spherical wave front model is used in all cases. In order to sum up the right signals belonging to the same object, the individually received signals have to be delayed in time before summation. The greater the distance between the outer and inner elements, the longer the signals received by the inner elements have to be delayed (Fig. 17.**35**). In this way, selected echoes are added together, and the resulting signal is passed on for further evaluation. Without implementing aperture growth on high quality large aperture systems, the wrong signals coming from side lobes or other objects might be included in the sum.

In receive there is one very important advantage compared with transmit. Focusing can be changed continuously or dynamically without a loss in frame rate. By continuously changing the time delays in correspondence to the depth from which the echoes are coming, the scatterers are always in the focal plane. In photography this corresponds to continuously changing the focus in order to always have a sharp picture of an object although it is moving away from the camera. In reality, the change of the receive focus does not take place continuously in most ultrasound systems but in small jumps. Sixteen focal zones is a typical number and usually sufficient. Switching from one focal zone to another can cause disturbances in the image. There are a few ways to suppress this. Dynamic focusing and aperture growth are two of the

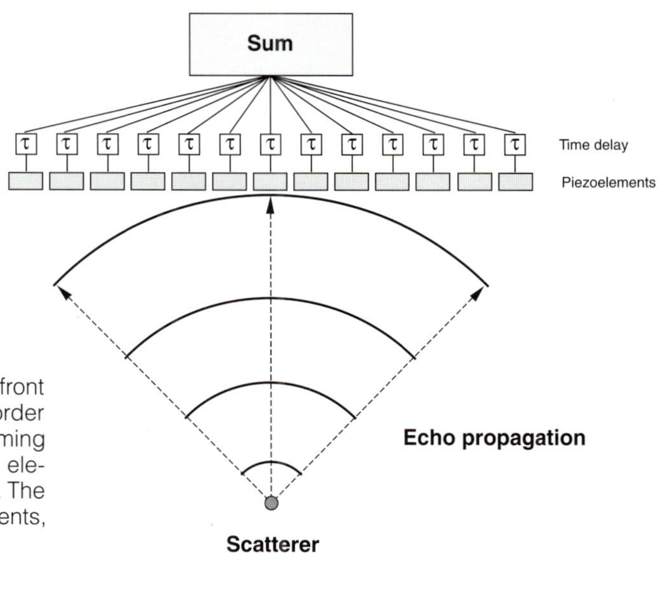

Fig. 17.**35** During receive the spherical wave front reaches the center elements of a linear array first. In order to be able to add up the intensities of the signals coming from the same source the signals at the individual elements have to be delayed in time by a certain amount. The farther away the elements are from the center elements, the smaller the time delays of those signals

major advantages of array transducers when compared with mechanical fixed-focus transducers.

Piezoelements can only register the pressure component normal to the piezo surface (surface waves are not discussed here). For this reason the amplitudes of the spherical wave front detected by the outer elements are lower than those measured by the inner elements. On phased arrays this can be a serious problem.

Another problem with large apertures is the poor image quality in the region close to the transducer. The outer elements receive a higher side lobe intensity than the central elements. The side lobes are emitted to the side of the main lobe as explained above. As in transmit, apodization helps to reduce the side lobes on receive by weighting the received amplitudes differently, depending on their position. The value of the signals at the outer elements is weighted less than the signal at the center elements. Dynamic aperture growth is also used to improve the near-field image. The number of elements is increased as the transmit pulse moves away from the transducer.

With the help of a water path or standoff, the transducer is moved away from the skin. This helps in improving the image in the skin region. If the standoff is wedge-shaped, this also helps to improve the Doppler angle when looking at superficial vessels. From a purely physical point of view it is better to use a standoff than applying beam steering. In a few medical applications it is sometimes easier and more beneficial to use beam steering.

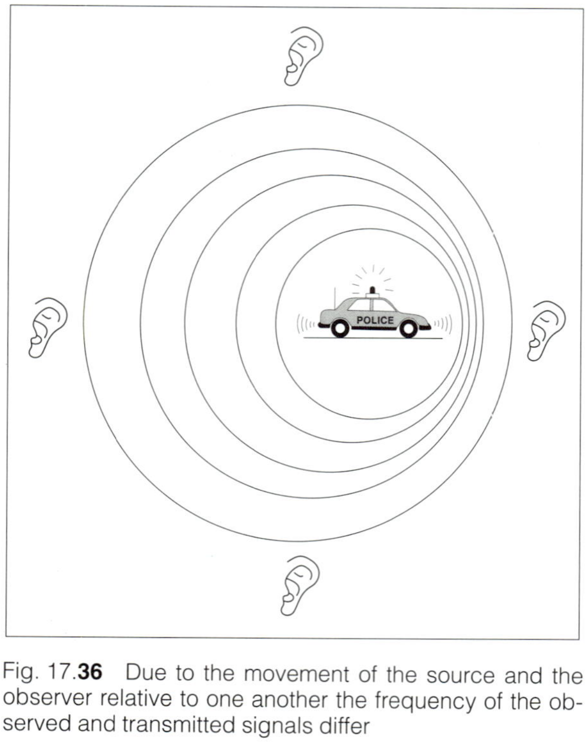

Fig. 17.**36** Due to the movement of the source and the observer relative to one another the frequency of the observed and transmitted signals differ

17.3 The Doppler Effect

If an observer and a sound-emitting source are moving relative to one another, the frequency measured by the observer will be different from the frequency measured by a—relative to the source—stationary observer. If source and observer are moving away from each other, the frequency measured by the observer will be lower than the frequency detected by the stationary observer. If they are moving toward each other, the frequency will be higher. This effect was first observed by Christian Doppler in 1842 and was named after him. In medicine it is used to determine blood flow velocity.

In daily life everyone has probably already noticed the Doppler effect (Fig. 17.**36**). The sound coming from the siren of a police car moving toward an observer is at a higher pitch than the sound measured by another observer when the police car is moving away from him. When the car is passing an observer, a sudden jump in the sound frequency can be clearly heard. Exactly the same thing would be noticed in the opposite case, where an observer is moving toward a stationary sound source, passes it, and then moves away from the source. If the emitter and the observer are moving toward one another, the perceived wavelength is shortened, resulting in the perception of a higher frequency. If the emitter and the observer are moving away from one another, the perceived wavelength is longer than in the stationary case, resulting in the perception of a lower frequency.

In general

$$f_B = f_0 \frac{c + v_{observer}}{c - v_{source}}$$

where f_B = observed frequency
f_0 = true emitted frequency (in this chapter the reference frequency of the transducer)
$v_{observer}$ = velocity of the observer
v_{source} = velocity of the source
c = speed of sound

In this case the velocities are equal ($v_{observer} = v_{source} = v$) and the above equation changes to:

$$f_B = f_0 \frac{c + v}{c - v}$$

Expanding this function in a Taylor series and assuming $v \ll c$ and also ignoring higher order terms results in:

$$f_B = f_0 (1 + \frac{2\,v}{c}) \quad \text{or} \quad f_B - f_0 = 2f_0 \frac{v}{c}$$

The difference $f_B - f_0$ is equal to the Doppler shift f_d. If the source and the observer are not moving directly away from or toward each other but at an angle α, the last equation has to be modified to

$$f_d = 2f_0 \frac{v}{c} \cos(\alpha) \qquad (17.11)$$

Only the component vertical to the transducer, i. e., parallel to the ultrasound beam, is detected (see Fig. 17.**37**). In the following, the angle α is called the Doppler angle for short. The Doppler shift can be positive or negative. This corresponds to a movement toward the transducer or away from it. The reference frequency used in this chapter is—for clarity—always the transducer center frequency, although this is by no means necessary. Any frequency within the bandwidth of the transducer may be used as a reference frequency. In most diagnostic ultrasound systems, a referency frequency about 25% lower than the center frequency is used in order to improve the penetration and the velocity range.

Solving equation 17.11 for v results in:

$$v = \frac{f_d}{2f_0} \frac{c}{\cos(\alpha)} \qquad (17.12)$$

Equation 17.11 and the derived equation 17.12 are the two most important equations in the medical usage of the Doppler effect. Equation 17.11 is often called the Doppler formula. When interpreting the measured Doppler shifts it must never be forgotten that the effect is angle- and reference frequency-dependent. Just stating the measured Doppler shift alone is of no value whatsoever. Only by naming the Doppler angle, the reference frequency used, and the Doppler shift can the blood flow velocity be calculated. The measurement is only then understandable in general terms (Fig. 17.**38**). When using systems with selectable reference frequencies on the same transducer, completely different Doppler shifts are measured although the blood flow velocity is the same. The same thing happens when varying the Doppler angle (Fig. 17.**39 a, b**).

The angle dependency of the effect is very impressively visible in CDS. This can easily lead to a misinterpretation of the true hemodynamics at bifurcations or in vessels that do not pass through the image in a straight line. The bifurcation of the superficial femoral artery and the profunda is shown in Figures 17.**40 a** and **b**. The seemingly apparent flow acceleration visualized by the light red area in the picture disappears immediately after angle correction.

A Doppler shift at a Doppler angle of 90° is not detectable because the measured Doppler shift depends on the cosine of the Doppler angle. It makes no difference whether or not there is any flow present because the cosine of 90° is zero. The cosine changes most rapidly in the region around 90°. For that reason

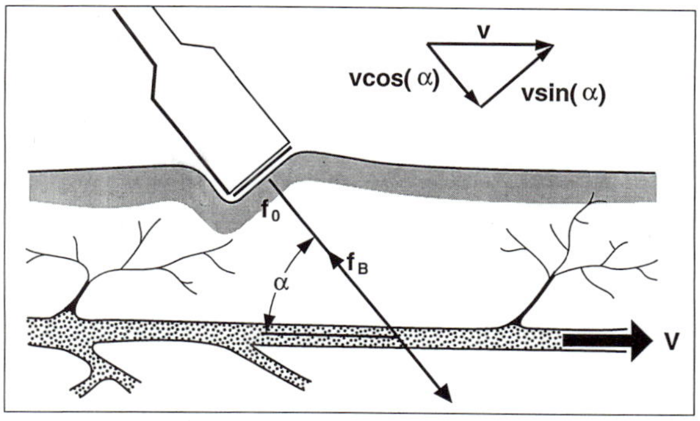

Fig. 17.**37** Definition of the Doppler angle α

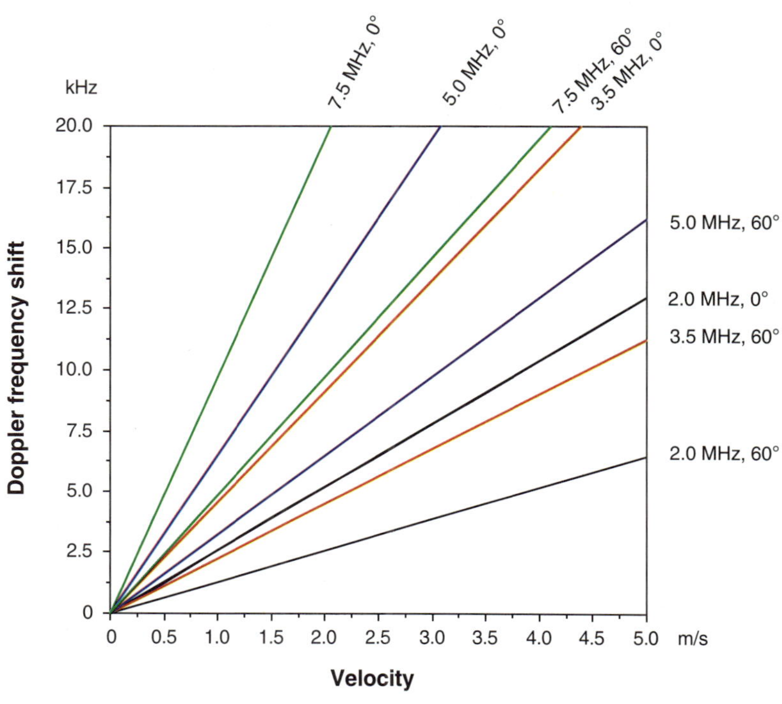

Fig. 17.**38** The observed Doppler frequency shift depends on the reference frequency and the Doppler angle

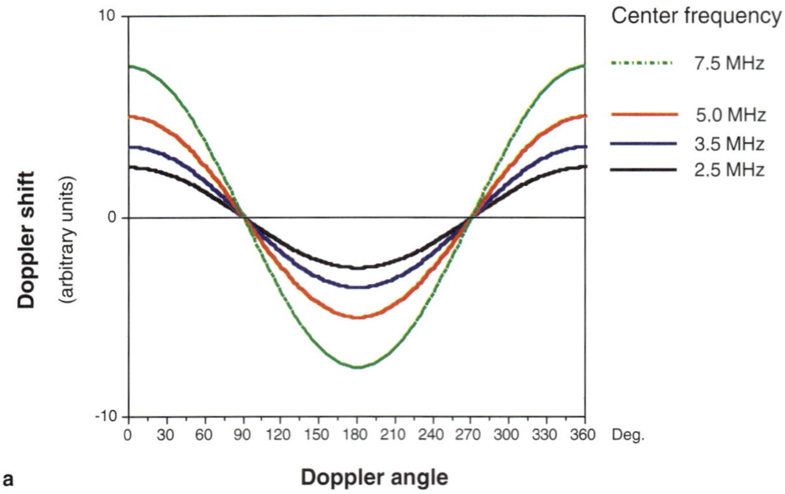

a

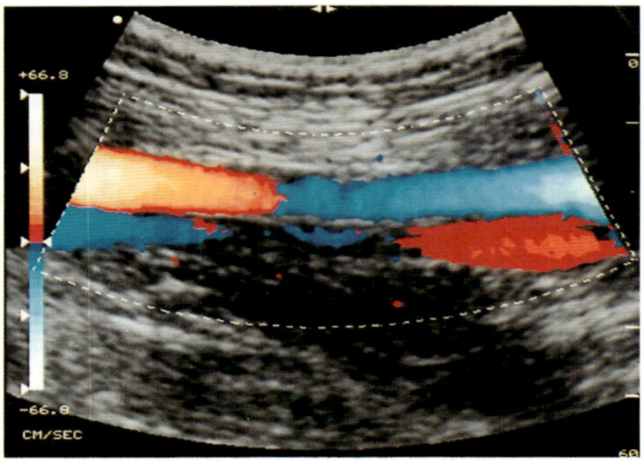

b

Fig. 17.**39** Angle dependency of the Doppler frequency shift at different reference frequencies (**a**). CDS image of blood flow in two tubes. In the top tube blood is flowing from left to right. In the bottom tube blood is flowing from right to left. Blood is flowing at constant velocity in both tubes. The flow velocity is roughly 10 times higher in the upper tube. Since a CA transducer was used, the Doppler angle changes continuously during a scan. Without angle correction this results in the display of different flow velocities and directions throughout the image. "Red" designates flow toward the transducer and "blue" away from the transducer (**b**)

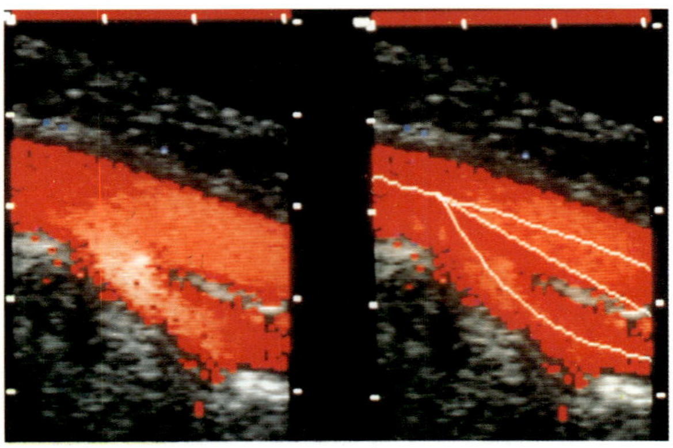

a b

Fig. 17.**40 a, b** Bifurcation of the superficial femoral artery and the profunda. The visible flow acceleration in the left image (**a**) disappears immediately after flow angle correction in the right image (**b**)

the measurement of blood flow velocity is highly dependent on a very precise angle measurement when the Doppler angle is near 90°. At an angle of 90° the flow velocity would be infinite. As long as the flow direction is visible in the image, determining the angle to within ±2° should be possible. Missing the true angle by ±2° at Doppler angles above 70° leads to an error in the calculated blood flow velocity of more than 10%. One should try to keep the Doppler angle as low as possible (Fig. 17.**41**). For anatomic reasons this is seldom achieved.

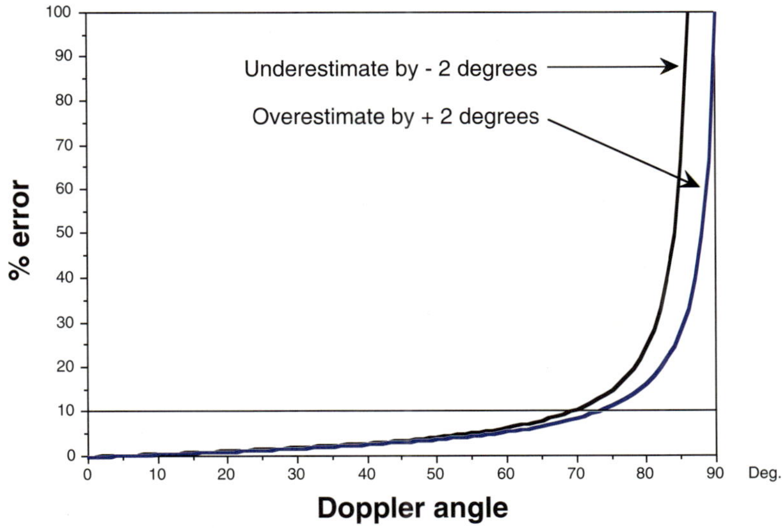

Fig. 17.**41** Error in calculating the flow velocity when the Doppler angle is off by ± 2°

17.3.1 Aliasing

Doppler shifts above a certain limit are not correctly represented in the Doppler spectrum displayed. Aliasing is the name for this phenomenon. Aliasing is well known from motion pictures. A film is composed of a series of separate pictures that have been taken at a certain frame rate. In Figure 17.**42** the wheel of an accelerating car is first turning clockwise and then, seemingly, counterclockwise and then again clockwise and so forth. The velocities where the movement is reversed are proportional to multiples of one-half the sampling frequency, which is equal to the frame rate in this example. If "sampling" were done continuously, aliasing would not occur.

Two different Doppler methods exist: CW (continuous wave) Doppler and PW (pulsed wave) Doppler. In CW Doppler, ultrasound waves of a certain

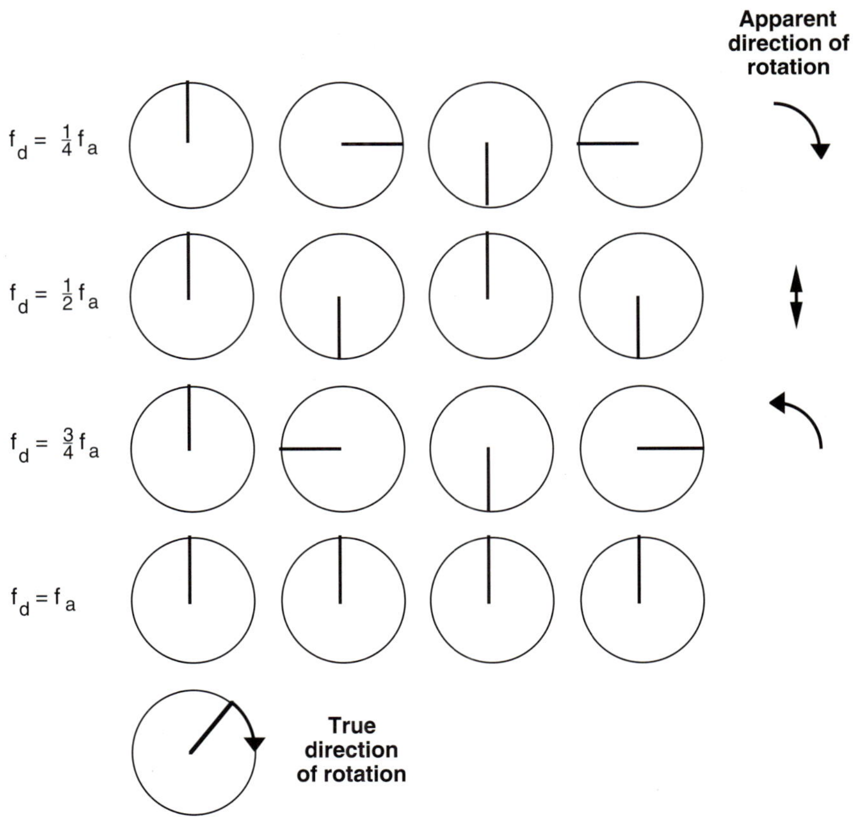

Fig. 17.**42** The position of a rotating wheel is measured at different intervals (frequencies) f_a. The true rotational direction and frequency f_d of the wheel is constant. When looking at the individual snap shots one has the impression that the wheel is turning in different directions. At $f_d = {}^1/_2 f_a$ the wheel seems to be flipping back and forth. At $f_a = f_d$ the wheel seems to be standing still

frequency are continuously emitted from the transducer and at the same time continuously received by the (same) transducer. With this method it is not possible to tell from which depth the echoes are coming. In PW Doppler, only short ultrasound pulses are emitted from the transducer. Since the speed of sound is known, so is the origin of the received echoes, i. e., the image depth from which the echoes are coming. For this reason all CDS methods are based on PW Doppler. The CW method is not applicable here. Principally, there is no aliasing in CW Doppler. Methods based on sampling are always limited by aliasing. The most important characteristics of the different Doppler methods are summarized in Table 17.**2**.

The example of Figure 17.**42** clarifies the fact that an erroneous measurement based on aliasing is possible. As just stated, in PW Doppler only short ultrasound pulses are emitted from the transducer. In pulsed spectral Doppler the ultrasound system only goes into receive mode to evaluate signals coming from a user-defined position (Doppler gate, Doppler sample volume) in the image. The machine only takes well-defined samples of all the incoming echoes. The Doppler signal has to be constructed from these samples. In color duplex sonography the machine automatically opens up many gates and then attaches the received samples correctly to a certain gate. The Doppler frequency shift f_d, which is only in the order of magnitude of about 0.1% or less of the transducer reference frequency, is sought. Only the low-frequency Doppler shift is registered. It is not possible to attain a Doppler curve from one single short pulse. Only one single discrete value per pulse can be gathered. Many discrete samples are needed in order to construct the complete Doppler signal. The more and faster the samples are gathered, the better the Doppler signal can be constructed. The pulse repetition frequency f_{PRF} or sampling frequency defines the temporal distance between the samples.

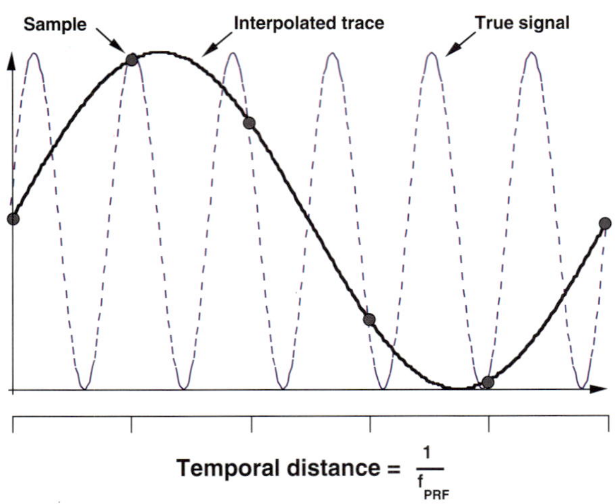

Fig. 17.**43** If the sample frequency f_{PRF} is less than twice the frequency of the signal being measured, the true signal cannot be reconstructed from the samples correctly

Table 17.**2** Comparison of the Doppler methods

	PW Doppler	CW Doppler
Aliasing	yes	no
Depth resolution	yes	no
Lateral resolution	yes	yes
Used in CDS	yes	no

Sampled values gathered at regular intervals – which are actually the phases of the Doppler signal – have been drawn in Figure 17.**43**. Connecting the samples results in the trace drawn. Since in this example f_{PRF} is smaller than the frequency of the true signal, a low-frequency interpolated trace is produced. The true signal is not reproduced correctly. In order to be able to reproduce the true signal correctly, the following requirements must be fulfilled:

$$\left|f_d\right| < \frac{1}{2} f_{PRF} \quad \text{or} \quad f_{PRF} > 2\left|f_d\right| \qquad (17.13)$$

The frequency $\frac{f_{PRF}}{2}$ is called the Nyquist frequency or Nyquist limit. If the Doppler shift is above the Nyquist limit, the uniqueness of the result is lost.

The wheel analogy of Figure 17.**42** will be used again in order to understand what happens when the Doppler frequency is just above $\frac{f_{PRF}}{2}$. It must not be forgotten that from the start the observer does not know in which direction the wheel is actually turning. In the first case the wheel rotates clockwise almost half a turn—except for a small amount δ—between the first and second measurement (sample). It is then rotating with almost the highest uniquely measurable frequency. In the second case the wheel rotates clockwise half a turn plus a small amount δ between the first and second sample. To the observer it seems as if the wheel were rotating counterclockwise with almost the highest uniquely measurable frequency. In other words: If the Nyquist limit is surpassed, the displayed Doppler shift jumps from the highest possible positive Doppler shift to the highest possible negative Doppler shift and vice versa (Figs. 17.**44** and 17.**45 a, b**). If the velocity of the object under observation continues to grow, the displayed Doppler shift decreases until the full f_{PRF} (twice the Nyquist frequency) is reached. Then the displayed Doppler shift increases in the opposite direction again. Every time a full multiple of the Nyquist frequency is reached, the direction of motion seems to change.

In the above explanation of aliasing, implicitly only the absolute value of the Doppler shift was used. Actually, Doppler shifts between $-\frac{f_{PRF}}{2}$ and $+\frac{f_{PRF}}{2}$ can be uniquely displayed. The range of uniqueness is equal to $2 \cdot \frac{f_{PRF}}{2} = f_{PRF}$. This frequency range can be

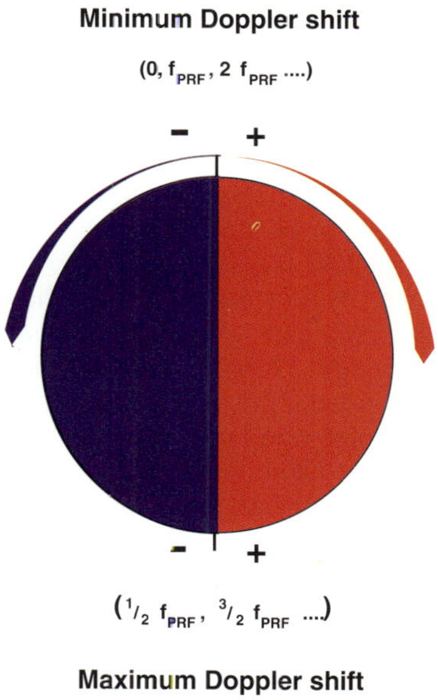

Fig. 17.**44** When the signal frequency passes the Nyquist limit, the displayed Doppler frequency shift jumps from the highest positive Doppler shift to the highest negative Doppler shift and vice versa

manually and freely divided into a forward and reverse flow region by a so-called zero-point or baseline shift. It must be emphasized that the size of the complete range of uniquely measurable frequencies cannot be augmented (Figs. 17.**45 a, b** and 17.**46**). Accordingly, the forward flow component can comprise the complete range of frequencies up to f_{PRF}. The drawback is that in such a case the reverse flow region is compressed to zero, i.e., reverse flow cannot be uniquely identified. In order to be able to do this the user must have some knowledge about the expected flow velocities and direction. In this particular case it must be certain that no reverse flow is present.

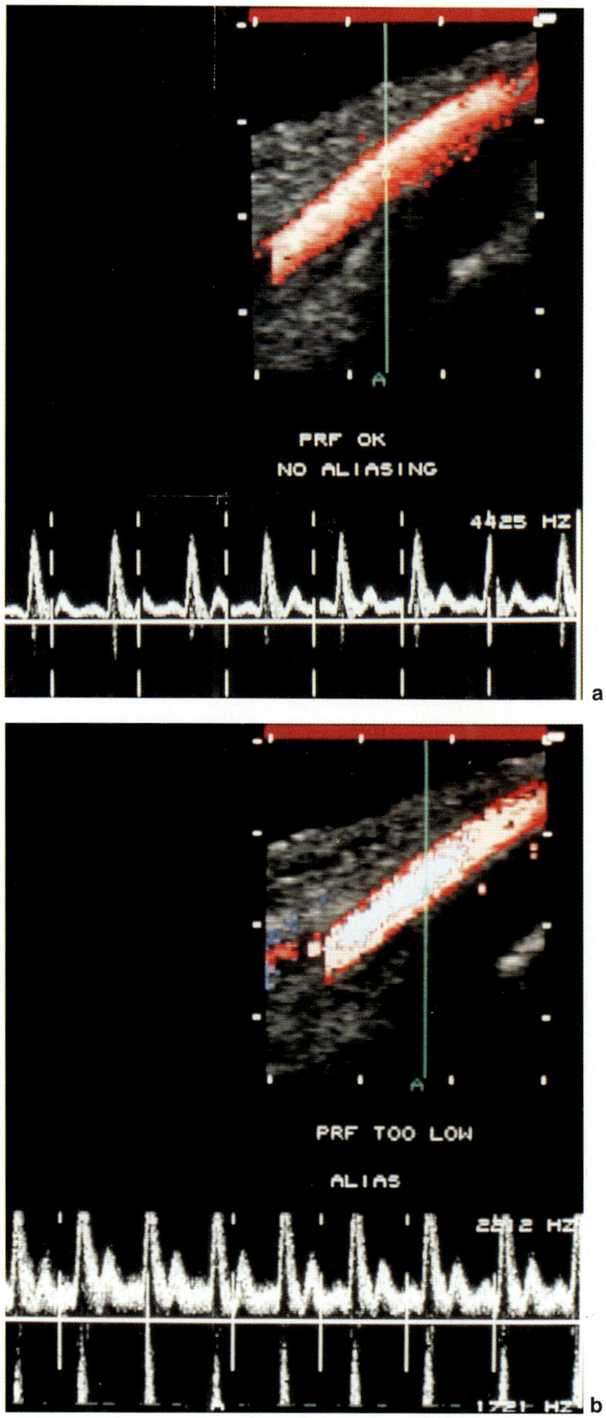

Fig. 17.**45** CDS images of the CCA. (**a**) Aliasing disappears after increasing f_{PRF} by a factor of 2. (**b**) The Doppler frequency spectrum and the color display shows aliasing

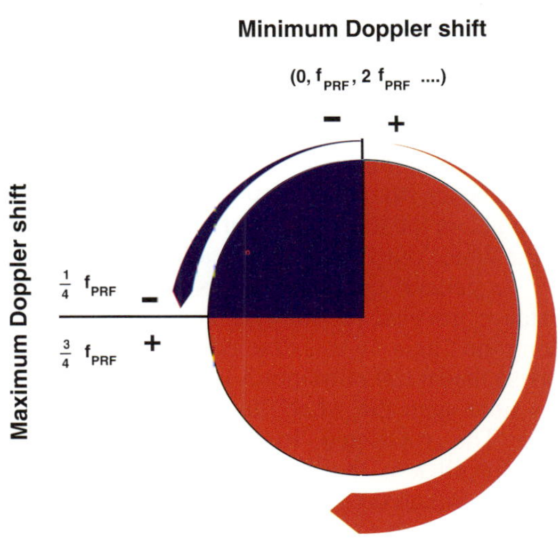

◀ Fig. 17.**46** The size of the positive and negative Doppler frequency ranges without aliasing can be changed manually by a baseline shift. The size of the total unique Doppler frequency range does not change after a baseline shift

The pulse repetition frequency cannot be raised freely. It was explained in Section 17.2.2 that the return of the last echo of the previous pulse has to be awaited until a new pulse may be emitted from the transducer. The pulse repetition frequency is limited in the same way by the position of the Doppler gate set by the operator. The farther the sample gate is positioned away from the transducer, the lower f_{PRF}.

Multiplying equations 17.12 and 17.4 leads to

$$vd = \frac{f_d}{2f_0} \frac{c}{\cos(\alpha)} \frac{ct}{2} \qquad (17.14)$$

where d = Doppler gate position (distance from the transducer)

t = round-trip time of flight, transducer–Doppler gate–transducer

It is:

$$t = t_{PRF} = \frac{1}{f_{PRF}} \qquad (17.15)$$

The highest uniquely detectable Doppler shift without a baseline shift according to equation 17.13 is $f_d < f_{PRF}/2$. Introducing these results into equation 17.14 leads to

$$v_{max}d < \frac{c^2}{8f_0} \frac{1}{\cos(\alpha)}$$

After isolating v_{max}, the highest uniquely measurable flow velocity is

$$v_{max} < \frac{c^2}{8df_0} \frac{1}{\cos(\alpha)}$$

v_{max} has been evaluated in Figure 17.**47** for a few of the most often used reference frequencies. A Doppler angle of 0° was used.

In CDS, d is equal to the greatest displayed image depth or, if the system gathers gray-scale and color information separately, d is equivalent to the maximum depth of the color region.

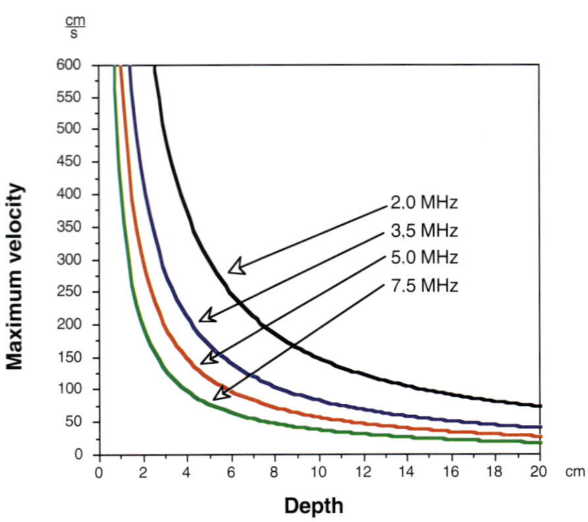

Fig. 17.**47** The maximum uniquely measurable velocity at different reference frequencies as a function of the depth of the Doppler sample volume. The Doppler angle is 0° in all cases

A short look will be taken at HPRF Doppler (high pulse repetition frequency). This is a special pulsed Doppler method in which the pulse repetition frequency is higher than equation 17.5 allows. This means, the position of the Doppler gate is no longer uniquely defined. If f_{PRF}, for example, were twice as high as allowed by equation 17.5, then there would be a second Doppler gate at the halfway distance between the (primary) Doppler gate and the transducer. It cannot be decided if the data is coming from the first or second Doppler gate because the echoes reach the transducer at the same time. If f_{PRF} is raised even more, additional gates are created. The advantage of the method is that the aliasing-free frequency range is larger than in standard PW Doppler. The disadvantage is the loss of the ability of precisely knowing from which depth the Doppler data is coming, i. e., uniqueness of position.

17.3.2 Amplitude, Frequency, Phase

At least a basic idea of the meaning of the terms amplitude, frequency, and phase is necessary in order to be able to understand the different Doppler evaluation methods. These terms are explained with the help of Figure 17.**48**.

The continuous rotational movement of point a on the rim of a single-spoked wheel is transferred to a graph with a linear time axis t. The angle between the spoke S and the positive t-axis is called the phase angle or phase for short. The phase φ (t) changes continuously with time. After the spoke has completed one revolution of 360°, the spoke is again positioned parallel to the t-axis and a new revolution may begin. In the time graph the trace also crosses the t-axis at 0°, 180°, and 360° (every 180°). The rotational velocity of the wheel and spoke defines the number of revolutions per second. The number of 360° revolutions (of the wheel) per second is called (the wheel's rotational) frequency. The vertical distance A between point a and the t-axis varies over time. This is equal to the elongation of A following point a in the time graph. The maximum elongation of A is equal to the length of the spoke S. Point a in the time graph describes a wave-shaped trace. The elongation of A(t) is called the amplitude of the wave and is a function of time. The length of the (vertical) projection of the path of point a in the time graph during one 360° revolution of the wheel onto the t-axis is called the wavelength.

In general the velocity c is equal to the straight distance traveled (at constant velocity) per unit time along the t-axis. In this case point a in the time graph travels the straight distance λ within the time t. Within this time span the wheel has completed one revolution. The rotational frequency is $f = 1/t$. The wavelength λ is the distance between two adjacent points at which the phases, at the same instant, are the same. This leads to the fundamental equation 17.1 stat-

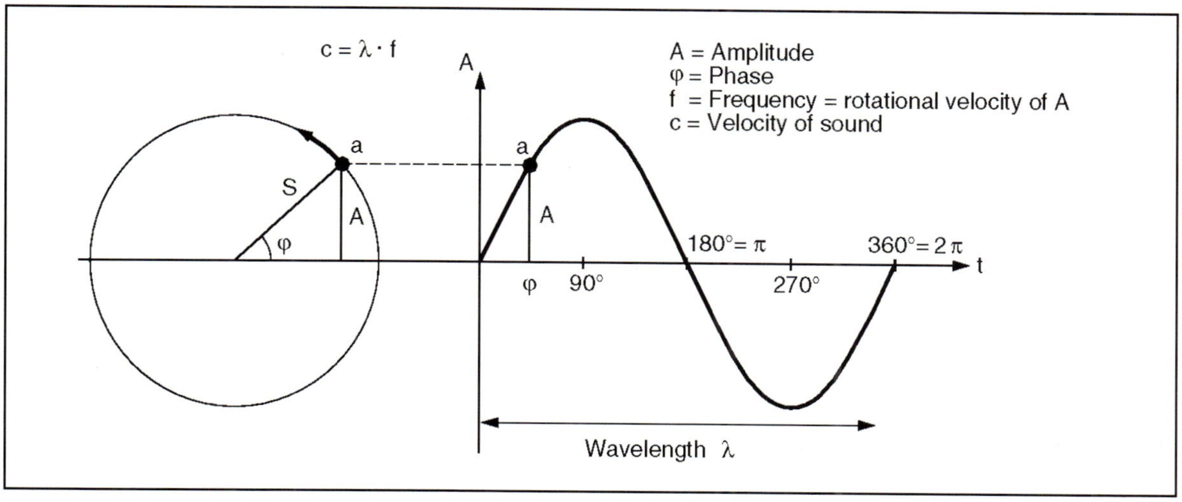

Fig. 17.**48** Definition of the terms amplitude A, frequency f, phase φ, and wavelength λ. In general, the speed of sound is $c = \lambda \cdot f$

ing that the speed of sound is equal to the product of wavelength times frequency:

$$c = \lambda f$$

In the next step, two waves having different frequencies will be compared with one another (Fig. 17.**49**). Both waves are excited at exactly the same time. At the time $t = 0$ both waves are in phase $[\varphi_1(t{=}0) = \varphi_2(t{=}0) = 0]$. Wave number 2 lags behind wave number 1 in time. Imagine that the phase angles $\varphi_1(t_1)$ of wave 1 and $\varphi_2(t_2)$ of wave 2 are equal. Wave 1 passes through phase $\varphi_1(t_1)$ earlier than wave 2 phase $\varphi_2(t_2)$. In other words, wave 1, having the shorter wavelength, reaches a certain phase earlier than wave 2 having the longer wavelength. Since wave 1 passes through all phase states more quickly than wave number 2, it not only has a shorter wavelength than wave 2 but also a higher frequency than wave 2. This means, that it is possible by phase comparison to detect a difference in wavelength and frequency of two waves. In Doppler analysis this means that by phase comparison one can detect a phase shift and from that deduct a frequency shift and also a change in wavelength. In general, the relation between phase and frequency may be written as

$$\varphi(t) = 2\pi f t \qquad (17.16)$$

It will now be shown how the Doppler frequency can be calculated directly from the phase difference. The phase of the Doppler signal results from quadrature demodulation as will be explained in Section 17.3.4.

The distance d between the transducer and the reflector displayed on the monitor was defined in equation 17.4 as

$$d = \frac{ct}{2}$$

where c is the speed of sound and t is the pulse–echo time of flight. In the time t_0 the first pulse and echo travel the distance d_0 to the moving object and back. In the time t_n the n-th pulse and echo travel the distance d_n to the moving object and back.

$$d_0 = \frac{ct_0}{2} \quad \text{and} \quad d_n = \frac{ct_n}{2} \qquad (17.17)$$

The distance the blood has moved between the first and the n-th pulse–echo cycle is Δd. Δd is equal to the product of the blood flow velocity v_{blood} and the pulse interval. The temporal distance between the measurements is nt_{PRF} which is n times the time span between two consecutive pulses (the pulse interval).

$$\Delta d = v_{blood}\, n\, t_{PRF} \qquad (17.18)$$

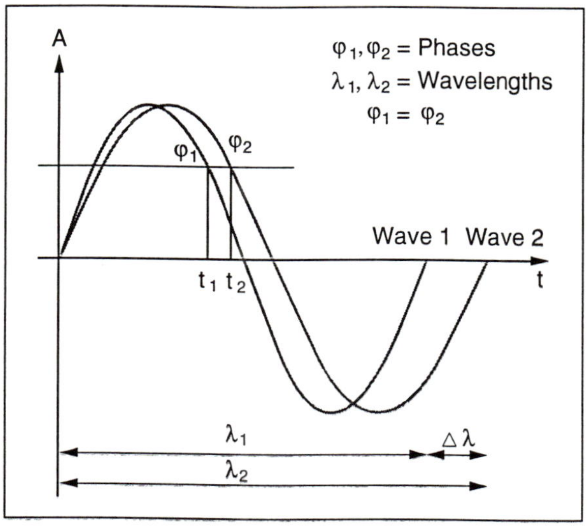

Fig. 17.**49** Two waves 1 and 2 having different frequencies pass through the same phase $\varphi_1(t_1) = \varphi_2(t_2)$ at different points in time

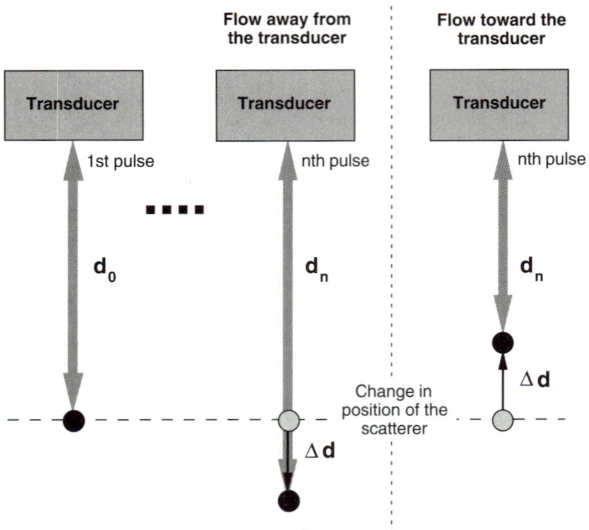

Fig. 17.**50** Determining the movement of a scatterer. d_0 and d_n are the distances between the scatterer and the transducer at different points in time. Δd is the difference between the two distances

If flow is directed toward the transducer according to Figure 17.**50**

$$d_0 = d_n + \Delta d$$

If flow is directed away from the transducer, then

$$d_0 = d_n - \Delta d \qquad (17.19)$$

The two equations differ only in the sign of Δd. In the following, only flow directed away from the transducer will be discussed. The angle relative to the ultrasound beam (Doppler angle) is always 0°. The opposite direction results automatically by changing the sign. Substituting the components of equation 17.19 as given by equations 17.17 and 17.18 one obtains

$$t_n = \frac{2}{c}(d_0 + v_{blood} n t_{PRF})$$

Entering this expression into equation 17.16 results in

$$\varphi_n = 2\pi f_0 \frac{2}{c}(d_0 + v_{blood} n t_{PRF})$$

where f_0 is the transducer reference frequency.

Furthermore $\varphi_0 = 2\pi f_0 t_0 = 2\pi f_0 \frac{2d_0}{c}$

Combining the above two equations leads to:

$$\varphi_n = \varphi_0 + 2\pi f_0 \frac{2}{c}(v_{blood} n t_{PRF})$$

The Doppler formula 17.11 was derived earlier. Using a Doppler angle of 0° and then substituting equation 17.11 into the above expression, the following equation results

$$\varphi_n = \varphi_0 + 2\pi f_d\, n t_{PRF}$$

According to equation 17.15, t_{PRF} is the reciprocal of the pulse repetition frequency f_{PRF}. This changes the above expression to

$$\varphi_n = \varphi_0 \pm 2\pi n \frac{f_d}{f_{PRF}}$$

The upper (plus) sign is valid for movement away from the transducer and the lower (minus) sign indicates flow toward the transducer.

Subtracting the phases φ_n and φ_{n+1} from each other results in

$$\Delta\varphi = \varphi_{n+1} - \varphi_n = \pm 2\pi \frac{f_d}{f_{PRF}}$$

Solving for the Doppler frequency shift f_d leads to:

$$f_d = \mp \Delta\varphi \frac{f_{PRF}}{2\pi} \quad \text{or}$$

$$f_d = \mp(\varphi_{n+1} - \varphi_n) \frac{f_{PFR}}{2\pi} \qquad (17.20)$$

In this way it is possible to calculate the Doppler frequency shift by performing two phase measurements. It is clearly visible from the last equation that the Doppler shift cannot unambiguously exceed $\frac{f_{PRF}}{2}$ because a phase shift of more than π is not uniquely defined. This fits in perfectly with the discussion in Section 17.3.1, Aliasing. The flow direction can at once be determined by looking at the sign of the above equation.

It is not all that simple to measure the phase of the Doppler shift. On the other hand, most Doppler methods are based on the evaluation of the phase shift. This also holds true for CDS. For a better understanding of the Doppler methods, the model used in Figure 17.**48** has to be improved. This is done in Figure 17.**51**.

The same construction that was used in Figure 17.**48** in order to introduce wave motion will be used a second time in Figure 17.**51** along an additional axis vertical to the first t-axis. Along the new axis the amplitude B(t) reaches its maximum value at the time t = 0. All in all the traces along the two axes are identical except for a phase shift of 90°.

The t-axis of Figure 17.**48** is now called the imaginary axis (Im). The equation describing the curve is a sine function, $A(t)\sin(\omega t + \varphi)$. It is $\omega = 2\pi f$. The new additional axis is called the real axis (Re). The equation describing this curve is a cosine function, $B(t)\cos(\omega t + \varphi)$. Combining the real and imaginary parts with the imaginary unit $i = \sqrt{-1}$, yields the complex equation of wave motion (17.21)

$$Y(t) = Re + Im$$
$$= B(t)\cos(2\pi f_0 t + \varphi) + iA(t)\sin(2\pi f_0 t + \varphi)$$

where f_0 is the reference frequency of the transducer and

$$f_0 = \frac{\omega_0}{2\pi}$$

In general, the real amplitude A is equal to

$$A = \sqrt{Re^2 + Im^2} \qquad (17.22)$$

and the phase φ is

$$\varphi = \text{arc tg}\,\frac{Re}{Im} \qquad (17.23)$$

With the help of this simple transformation it is now possible to calculate the phase and the amplitude at any given time.

17.3.3 The Origin of the Doppler Spectrum—The Fourier Transform

Those who have already worked with a Doppler spectrum will have probably heard of the term FFT. The FFT (fast Fourier transform) is a mathematical algorithm used in order to quickly accomplish a Fourier transform. It is not the aim of this section to explain how a fast Fourier transform is performed, but a general understanding of what a Fourier transform is and does is important. There are a few interesting results that will help in understanding Doppler spectra. Nowadays special integrated circuits (ICs, chips) exist that are capable of quickly performing an FFT. There are a number of books available on the fast Fourier transform and the Fourier transform (for example [9, 20, 46]). The more interested reader is referred to these excellent but definitely not basic books.

First of all the term spectrum must be explained a bit more precisely. In this section the velocity distribution of blood flow over time displayed on the monitor of an ultrasound diagnostic unit is not meant by the term Doppler spectrum, but rather the spectrum analysis of the Doppler signal displayed as the intensity of the spectral components as a function of frequency. This corresponds to one vertical line in the "medical" Doppler spectrum. The velocity distribution of blood flow over time, usually called Doppler spectrum in medicine, is in reality the display of many temporally consecutive spectrum analyses of the demodulated Doppler signals—the true intensity spectrum, meant in this section. In a 128-point FFT the Doppler signal is divided into 128 frequencies within a bandwidth equal to the pulse repetition frequency. With the help of a mathematical algorithm, the amplitudes of the individual frequencies are calculated. The Doppler signal is looked at as being constant and periodic over the complete measurement period. The method of Fourier analysis will be explained below. It should become evident why the method is of major importance.

Any arbitrary periodic function can be generated by the superposition of a number of sine and cosine functions (Fig. 17.**52**). It is important to note that the amplitudes (coefficients) a_i and b_i may be different and that the frequencies are integral multiples of a fundamental frequency $\omega = 2\pi f$. (The reason behind this is that the measurement must be completed within a finite span of time.) $n\omega$ are the harmonic frequencies,

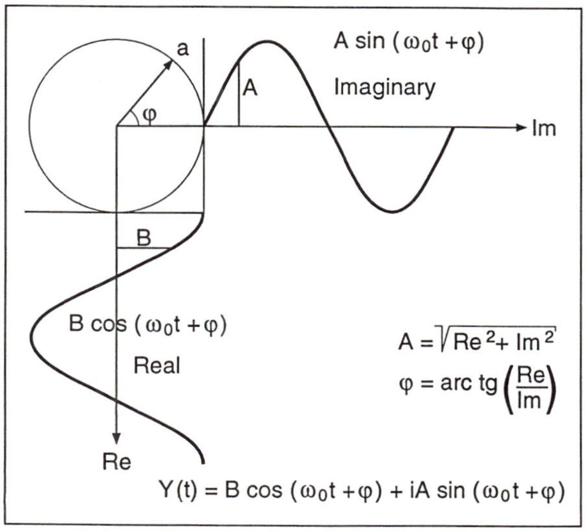

Fig. 17.**51** Complex wave description using the real and imaginary components

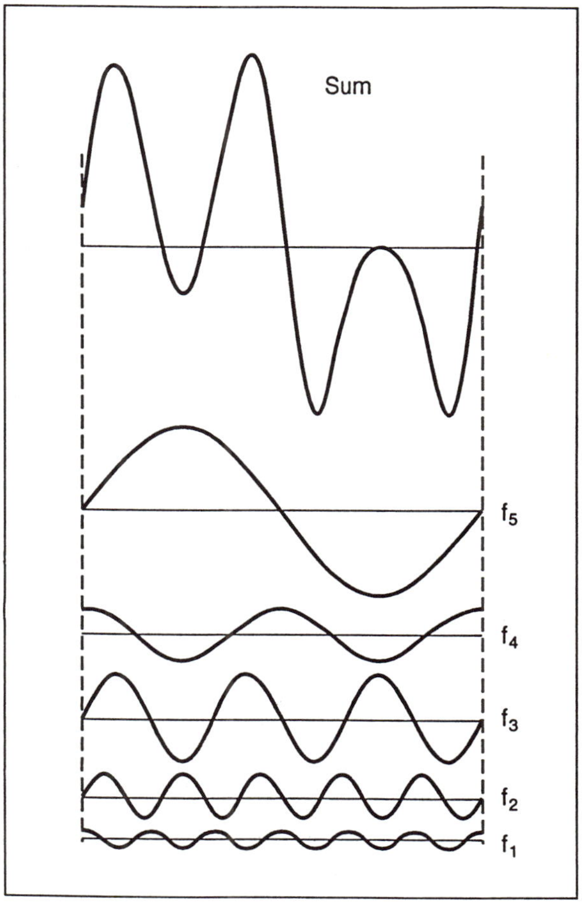

Fig. 17.**52** Any periodic function can be created by adding individual sine and cosine functions with different frequencies and amplitudes

also called harmonic overtones. In Doppler spectrum analysis, due to the Nyquist limit, the highest possible frequency ($n\omega = \frac{f_{PRF}}{2}$) is defined by the pulse repetition frequency f_{PRF}. To be exact, the Doppler shifts are calculated in two steps for the two separate regions $-\frac{f_{PRF}}{2}$ to 0 and 0 to $+\frac{f_{PRF}}{2}$.

According to equation 17.13 the highest uniquely measurable frequency is $\frac{f_{PRF}}{2}$. The Fourier series may be expressed as (a function of time, f(t))

$$f(t) = \frac{a_0}{2} + a_1\cos(\omega t) + b_1\sin(\omega t) + a_2\cos(2\omega t) + b_2\sin(2\omega t) + \ldots + a_n\cos(n\omega t) + b_n\sin(n\omega t) + \ldots$$

or $$f(t) = \frac{a_0}{2} + \sum_{n=1}^{\infty} [a_n\cos(n\omega t) + b_n\sin(n\omega t)]$$

The Fourier series is needed in the complex format and not in the real format. Furthermore the Euler relation is always valid for any complex number:

$$e^{i(n\omega t)} = \cos(n\omega t) + i\sin(n\omega t)$$

It is possible with the help of the above equation to construct the sine and cosine functions:

$$\cos(n\omega t) = \frac{e^{i(n\omega t)} + e^{-i(n\omega t)}}{2} \quad \text{and}$$

$$\sin(n\omega t) = \frac{e^{i(n\omega t)} - e^{-i(n\omega t)}}{2i}$$

Substituting these expressions into f(t) results in:

$$f(t) = \frac{a_0}{2} + \sum_{n=1}^{\infty} [a_n \frac{e^{i(n\omega t)} + e^{-i(n\omega t)}}{2} + b_n \frac{e^{i(n\omega t)} - e^{-i(n\omega t)}}{2i}]$$

A rather complex transformation leads to (33):

$$f(t) = \sum_{-\infty}^{\infty} A_n e^{i(n\omega t)}$$

where $$\left|A_n\right| = \frac{1}{2}\sqrt{a_n^2 + b_n^2} \quad \text{and}$$

$$\varphi_n = n\omega t = \text{arc tg}\,\frac{b_n}{a_n}$$

The last two expressions are equivalent to the equations 17.22 and 17.23 respectively, and have already been explained in Section 17.3.2.

The summation in the last equation for f(t) can be converted to an integral, where the integral is taken as the limit of the sum of the individual terms:

$$f(t) = \int_{-\infty}^{\infty} F(\omega)e^{i\omega t}d\omega$$

It must be integrated (summated) over all frequencies. There were only discrete frequencies $n\omega$ present in summation. Now integration must be performed over all frequencies within the continuous region from $-\infty$ to $+\infty$. The amplitudes A_n belonging to the frequencies of the individual harmonic waves are now also a function of frequency $F(\omega)$. $F(\omega)$ the Fourier transform of f(t) is sometimes also called the Fourier spectral distribution or Fourier spectrum of f(t). The absolute value $|F(\omega)|$ is called the amplitude spectrum, power spectrum, or frequency spectrum and its square $|F(\omega)|^2$ is the intensity spectrum of f(t).

The above integral is the inverse Fourier transform. In spectrum analysis exactly the opposite is sought. A certain waveform resulting from the measured Doppler shifted echoes has to be analyzed. (To be exact, this pertains to the low-frequency Doppler signal after demodulation: see Section 17.3.4.) The waveform to be analyzed is defined by its amplitude behavior over time (time domain). The amplitude as a function of frequency is to be determined (frequency domain). That means that $F(\omega)$ is sought. Expressed in the discrete form, the amplitudes A_n belonging to the discrete frequencies $n\omega$ of the individual sine and cosine functions, that by superposition add up to the waveform being analyzed, must be calculated. This is exactly what the Fourier transform does. This is a transformation from the amplitude–time domain to the amplitude–frequency domain (Fig. 17.**53**). The graphical presentation of the intensities (squares of the amplitude values) of the individual frequencies is exactly the Doppler spectrum as defined in the beginning of this section. Typically, the higher the intensity, the brighter the frequency value presented in the "medical type" graphic display. Mathematically, the Fourier transform is written as

$$F(\omega) = \frac{1}{2\pi}\int_{-\infty}^{\infty} f(t)e^{-i\omega t}dt$$

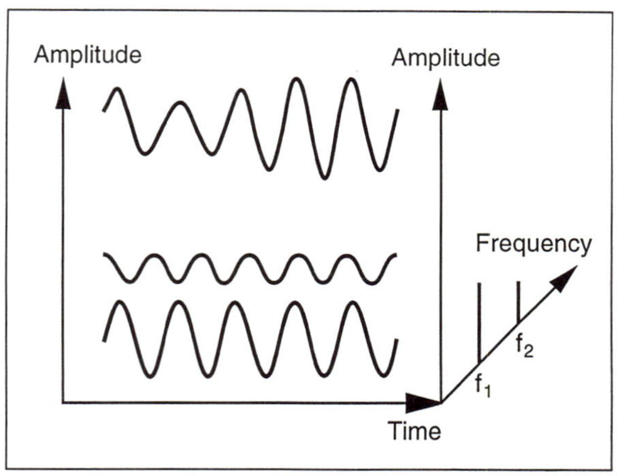

Fig. 17.**53** Transformation from the amplitude–time domain to the amplitude–frequency domain

The intensity spectrum $|F(\omega)|^2$ of the Doppler signal f(t) is sought.

Actually the Fourier transform is based on integration over an infinite span of time. This is not possible in ultrasound and especially not in pulsed Doppler. This results in a limitation of the frequency resolution of the Doppler spectrum and in the division of the continuous spectrum into discrete, equidistant Doppler frequencies. The resolution is inversely proportional to the total amount of time used to produce the Doppler signal being evaluated $\frac{1}{Nt_{PRF}}$.

The PW Doppler signal is finite in time and based on discrete sampled data. Instead of the above equation utilizing the FFT algorithm, the discrete Fourier transform (DFT) may also be used. The DFT is based on the evaluation of discrete data. According to Figure 17.**54a, b**, every pulse contributes one discrete piece of sampled data to the Doppler signal.

The DFT and the inverse DFT are respectively

$$F(nf) = \sum_{k=0}^{N-1} f(kt)e^{-i\frac{2\pi kn}{N}}$$

where $n = 0, 1, 2, \ldots, N-1$

and

$$f(kt) = \frac{1}{N}\sum_{n=0}^{N-1} F(nf)e^{i\frac{2\pi kn}{N}}$$

where $k = 0, 1, 2, \ldots, N-1$

where $f = \frac{\omega}{2\pi}$

The real and imaginary parts of F(nf) are evaluated separately. The intensity spectrum $|F(nf)|^2$ is equal to the sum of the squares of the real and imaginary components of F(nf). These are the I- and Q-components of the Doppler signal (explained in Section 17.3.4) multiplied by the exponential functions of the DFT. The exponential functions of the DFT are used as weight functions.

The DFT works on samples, and the sum includes all N samples. The individual samples are equally spaced over time. The spacing t is equal to the reciprocal of the pulse repetition frequency f_{PRF}:

$$t = t_{PRF} = \frac{1}{f_{PRF}}$$

A short pulse automatically having a large bandwidth leads to a poor frequency resolution Δf because the

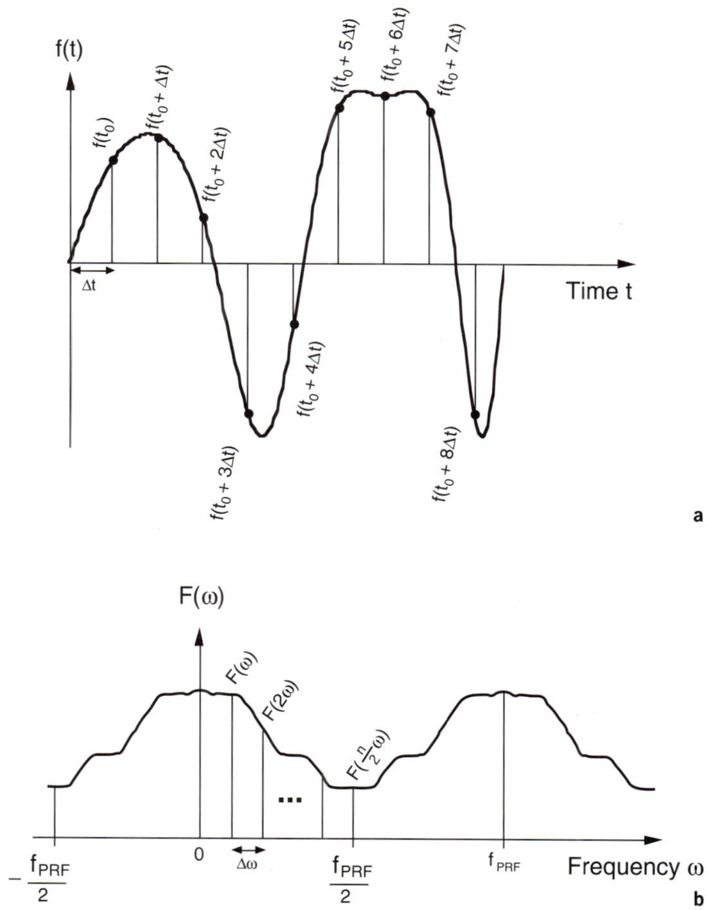

Fig. 17.**54** Explanation of the DFT. (**a**) A Doppler signal f(t) including the sample points at regular intervals is drawn (time domain). (**b**) The periodic (f_{PRF}) Fourier transform F(ω) is displayed (frequency domain)

frequency resolution is equal to the reciprocal of the temporal pulse length T_t.

$$\Delta f = \frac{1}{T_t}$$

The separation of the frequencies within the intensity spectrum is equal to the frequency increment f. This is equal to the pulse repetition frequency divided by the number of samples per spectrum. This is equivalent to saying: The spectral resolution of the Fourier transform is inversely proportional to the total amount of time T needed to collect the complete data set for spectrum analysis.

$$f = \frac{1}{T} = \frac{1}{Nt_{PRF}} = \frac{f_{PRF}}{N}$$

At an f_{PRF} of 15 kHz, for example, the temporal increment t_{PRF} is equal to 1/15,000 = 66.7 μs. Using 128 samples per spectrum, for example, the smallest Doppler frequency shift from which the amplitude is calculated with the help of the DFT (or FFT) is equal to $f = \frac{1}{128\,t_{PRF}} = 117$ Hz. On the other hand, the total amount of time needed to collect the data set in this case is 128 · 66.7 μs, which is equal to 8.54 ms. The reciprocal of this value is again 117 Hz. Normally the mathematical algorithm used is the FFT because it saves a lot of calculation time (see Section 17.4.2). In this case one would say that a 128-point FFT was used.

It is evident that by using a higher number of samples per spectrum, the number of available Doppler frequencies goes up and the spectral resolution is improved. Furthermore, spectral resolution is also improved by reducing the pulse repetition frequency. At the same time this also leads to a reduction of the aliasing-free, unique frequency (velocity) range. This means that an improved spectral resolution automatically leads either to a reduction in the size of the region of frequency unambiguity or a reduction in the number of Doppler spectra that can be calculated per second. It is of course necessary to ensure that the desired spectral resolution is not disrupted by spectral broadening caused by the transit time effect (see Section 17.2.4) or a too short transmit pulse, for example.

It is also taken for granted that blood flow is constant during data collection for the spectra. The total time needed for sampling in the above example of a 128-point FFT was 8.5 ms. Looking at a vessel in 15 cm depth reduces the maximum pulse repetition frequency to 5.13 kHz. The total time needed for sampling is then 0.02 s. It is at least questionable whether the flow velocity during systole is truly constant over this period of time. At this depth only 40 spectra per second using a 128-point FFT are possible. It is also arguable whether the temporal resolution of the flow dynamics is sufficient for diagnosis in this case. It may be sensible to reduce the number of samples per spectrum in order to raise the number of spectra per second. Reducing the number of samples by a factor of ½ to 64 points increases the number of spectra that can be acquired per second by a factor of 2 to 80 per second in this example.

17.3.4 Isolating the Doppler Signal—Demodulation

As already stated in Section 17.3.1 (Aliasing), Doppler frequency shifts are low-frequency alterations of the transmitted ultrasound signal. The low-frequency Doppler signal (Hz to kHz) can be visualized as being superimposed upon the high-frequency (MHz) ultrasound signal. This is technically called "modulation" (Fig. 17.**55 a–d**). The same thing happens in radio. The receiver displays the high-frequency carrier signal (MHz). Music or just speech is the low-frequency modulation (Hz to kHz) of the carrier. The signal is demodulated in the radio receiver, i. e., the carrier is eliminated. The modulation is what is left. Exactly the same kind of demodulation is performed by the ultrasound system. In CW Doppler this could be done continuously. In PW Doppler and in CDS, only individual samples of the Doppler signal are obtained, creating the problem of aliasing. After demodulation, the Doppler signal is spectrum analyzed. Of course, as in radio, demodulation is possible at any (reference) frequency and not only at the center frequency of the transmitted signal. Related to Doppler, this is also the meaning behind "multi-frequency" transducers.

In order to get rid of the carrier a method called coherent demodulation (Fig. 17.**56**) is used. This method multiplies the received echo signal with a signal having the same frequency as the carrier but no modulation. The resulting signal is then low-pass filtered, allowing only signals in the frequency range of the Doppler shifts to pass.

If demodulation is done as described above, information regarding the direction of flow is lost. This information is retained if this kind of demodulation is done twice in parallel. Along one channel, the echo signal is demodulated with a $\cos(\omega_t t)$ signal, and along the other channel a $\sin(\omega_t t)$ signal is used. ω_t is the frequency of the carrier. The results are exactly the same except for a phase shift of 90°. They are called the I- (direct or cosine) and Q- (quadrature or sine) components of the Doppler signal. Depending on the flow direction, one component leads the other in time, or one might also say, one signal lags behind the other. This kind of coherent demodulation in parallel is called quadrature demodulation. From here on the signal paths are different for CDS and the Doppler sound and spectrum (Fig. 17.**57**). Time domain processing in CDS works differently and is described in Section 17.4.3.

In PW Doppler spectrum analysis, the I- and Q-signals pass through a time gate. This gate is only open for signals coming from the Doppler sample volume positioned by the user. Afterward the signals are passed through an inverter that is activated by the user in order to invert the spectrum, for example when displaying the arterial signals positive (above the time axis) and the venous signals negative (below the time axis). The inverter is often omitted and the function is realized by inverting the digital signals read from

Fig. 17.**55 a–d** The carrier is amplitude (**b**) and frequency modulated (**c**). The Doppler signal (**d**) has to be extracted from the received echo signal (**a**)

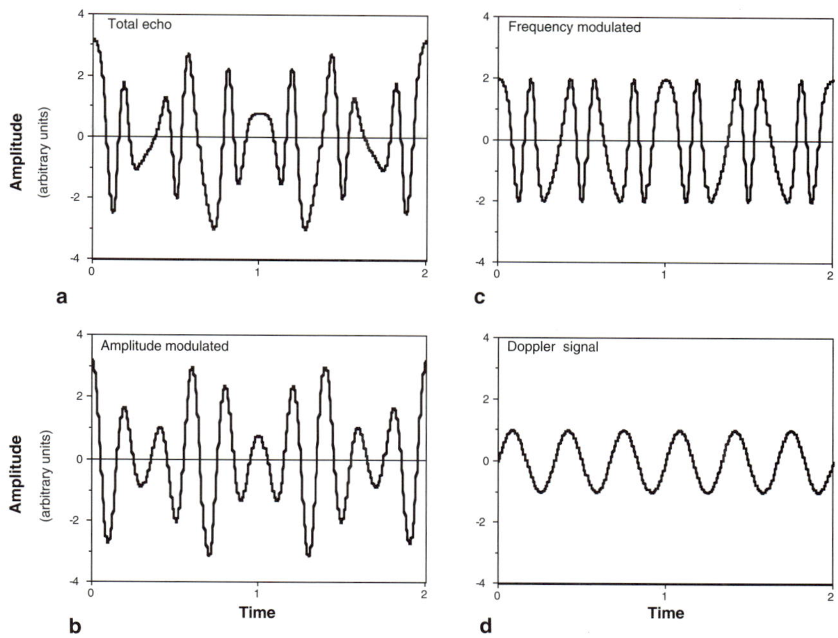

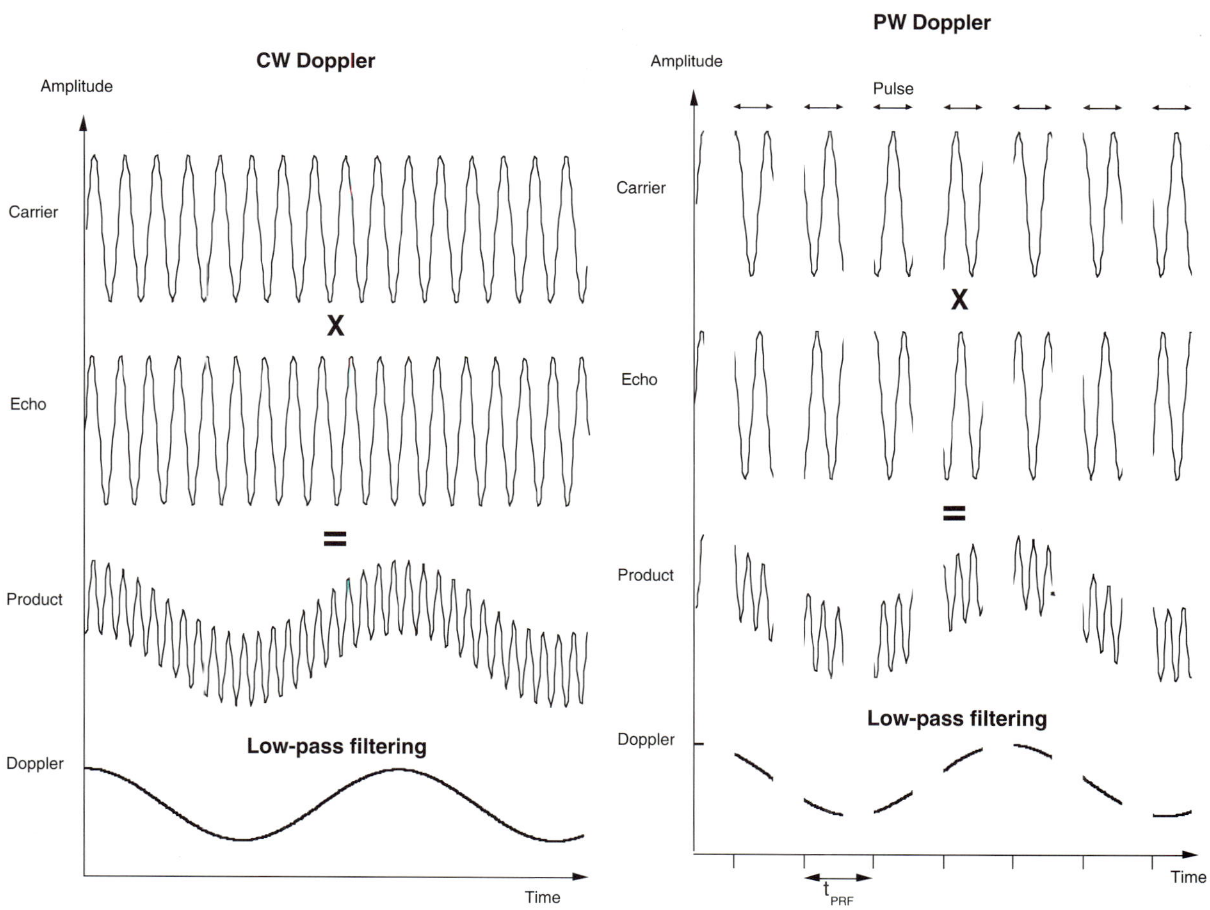

Fig. 17.**56** The Doppler signals are isolated by coherent demodulation (see text). CW Doppler is shown on the left and PW Doppler on the right. The modulation frequency and the sample frequency ($1/t_{PRF}$) are in general at least a factor of 10^3 lower than the carrier frequency. In case of PW Doppler in reality only individual points (phases) of the modulation are registered and not short wave forms. The true relationship cannot be correctly displayed here

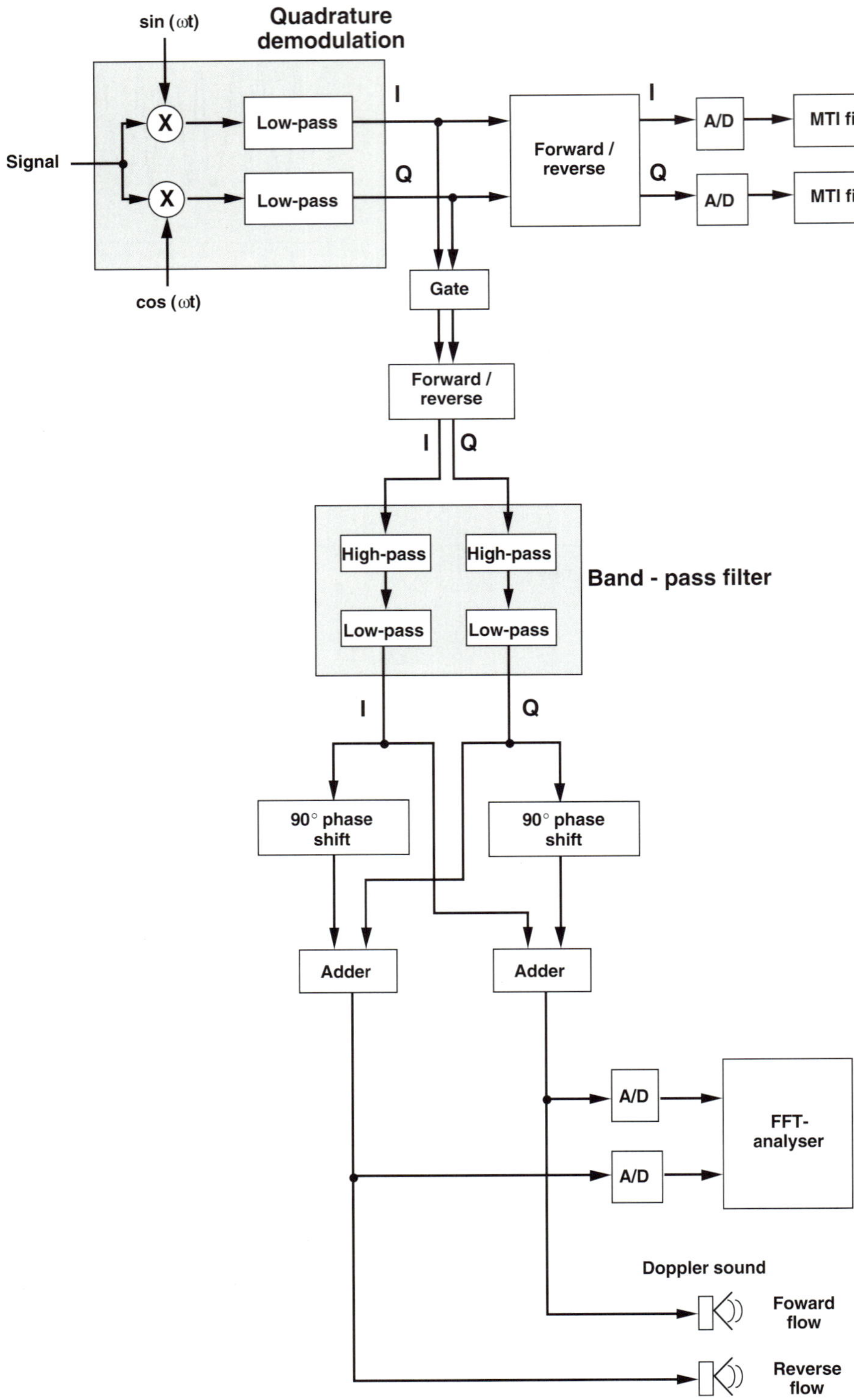

Fig. 17.**57** Block diagram of the methods of evaluating the echo signals in CDS (autocorrelation), frequency analysis by FFT as well as Doppler audio

memory after FFT analysis. The inverter has been included here in order to complete the signal path. The following band-pass filter is composed of a high-pass and a low-pass filter. The function of the low-pass filter is to eliminate signals above one-half the pulse repetition frequency above which aliasing occurs. This is called an anti-aliasing filter. The high-pass or "wall" filter eliminates signal frequencies below a certain user-defined value. The selectable cutoff frequencies are usually 50 Hz, 100 Hz, 200 Hz, 400 Hz, or 800 Hz.

The I- and Q-flow components have to be cleaned up for FFT Doppler spectrum analysis and Doppler stereo sound output. Each signal must be completely free of flow components of the other. After a phase shift of each component of $\pi/2$ or 90°, the signals are added. Each phase-shifted signal is added to the others nonphase-shifted signal, resulting in a distinct separation of forward and reverse flows. In the case of forward flow, the reverse flow signal should now be zero and vice versa. This last method of signal processing is called phase domain processing. Afterwards the signals are either analog to digital (A/D) converted and then passed on to a digital FFT analyzer, or they are prepared for Doppler stereo acoustic output by loudspeakers.

Crosstalk between channels when using this method is about –40 dB. Crosstalk is the reason why in some cases an (inverted) mirror spectrum is sometimes displayed along with the true spectrum. This occurs only when strong Doppler-shifted echoes, usually coming from the near-field, are received. This is a well-known artifact in Doppler ultrasound diagnostics. This artifact can be reduced or eliminated by reducing the transmit power or the Doppler receive gain.

Demodulation, as shown in Figure 17.**57** and explained above, is used in color duplex sonography (autocorrelation and DFT methods). After quadrature demodulation the signals pass through a user-accessible flow inverter. This leaves it up to the user to define which flow directions are coded "red" and "blue."

The received signal is not only frequency modulated by blood flow but also by the movement of vessel walls, for instance. The signals are also amplitude modulated by stationary objects. The signal components coming from these objects are much stronger than the weak signals coming from the blood. Besides the carrier, these unwanted signals must also be eliminated. The "clutter canceler" follows after quadrature demodulation. The so-called MTI (moving target indicator) filter is often a part of the clutter canceler. This filter is also called a delay-line filter. In medicine the first name is more common. In the simplest case the filter works as described in Figure 17.**58**. The echoes coming from two consecutive pulses along the same ultrasound scan line are correctly subtracted from one another. Correctly means that only echo signals coming from the same depth along the same ultrasound scan line are subtracted from one another. This results in the elimination of signals coming from stationary objects because these signals are identical. Echoes from moving objects are phase shifted relative

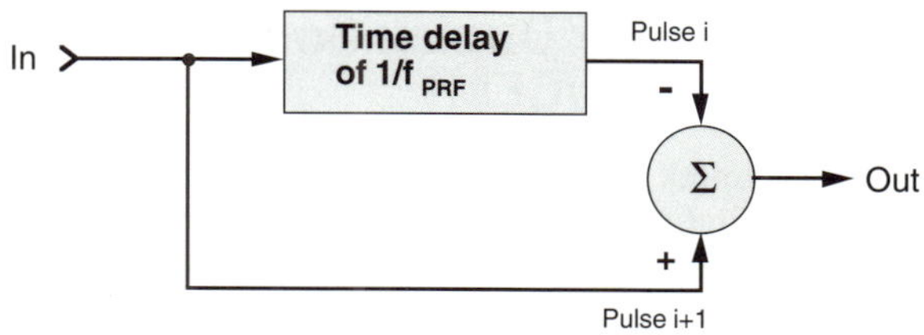

Fig. 17.**58** Wall or MTI filter used in CDS. Signals from stationary objects are eliminated by correctly subtracting two consecutive echo signals from one another

to one another, leading to a non-zero result of the subtraction. In order to eliminate the strong echoes coming from moving vessel walls an advanced clutter canceler, taking the signal amplitudes into account, is needed (39).

The negative side effect of the MTI filter is a reduction of the number of signals available for Doppler analysis by one signal. That means that after MTI filtering 9 pulse–echo cycles, for example, lead to only 8 signals that can be evaluated by the respective Doppler analyzer used in CDS.

Depending on the method used, the autocorrelator or DFT-analyzer, where the Doppler shifts are analyzed, follows after the movement filter. The most common method is the autocorrelation method. Basically this can be looked upon as a phase analyzer. In Figure 17.**51** the cosine component in the complex wave description was called the real part and the sine component the imaginary part of the complex wave function. It was also explained, that the phase of a function can be calculated by combining its real part (Re) and its imaginary part (Im). Consequently the phase of the Doppler signal can be calculated with the help of the I- and Q-signals originating from the quadrature demodulator.

$$\varphi = \text{arc tg}\,\frac{\text{Re}}{\text{Im}} = \text{arc tg}\,\frac{\text{I}}{\text{Q}}$$

As explained in Section 17.3.2, the Doppler frequency shift can be calculated from the phase difference of two consecutive echoes coming from the same region. The actual autocorrelation method does work somewhat differently but this is sufficient for a basic understanding. The method will be more thoroughly described in Section 17.4.1.

Besides the autocorrelation method, a method based on the discrete Fourier transform (40) is used. Both methods evaluate the demodulated Doppler signals. A new method is now coming into use which evaluates the high-frequency signals directly. This method is called time domain processing (5). It must not be mistaken for the direction-sensing method of evaluating Doppler signals of the same name (2).

17.4 Color Duplex Sonography (CDS/CFM)

In color duplex sonography (CDS), also called color flow mapping (CFM), every point in the image is assigned either a gray value or a color value. The grayscale part of the image (B-mode) contains morphological information, and the color-encoded part indicates blood flow. Color represents only one component of the Doppler spectrum. It is the intensity-weighted average Doppler shift. By stating the Doppler angle, this is equivalent to the intensity-weighted average blood flow velocity. This is roughly the velocity at which most of the blood flows at the specific position within the image field.

One might ask why straightforward Doppler spectrum analysis by FFT is not used in CDS. The reason behind this is the desire to have a real-time imaging method for visualizing blood flow. Assume that a frame rate of 20 frames per second has to be achieved. The penetration depth is 20 cm. The number of ultrasound scan lines to be used per frame is 50 in this example. The amount of time allowed to complete one ultrasound image frame is 1/20 s = 0.05 s. The maximum time allowed for the acquisition of one ultrasound scan line is then 0.05/50 s = 1 ms. At the given penetration depth only 4 pulse–echo cycles per ultrasound scan line can be used at a maximum f_{PRF} of 4 kHz. When using the Fourier spectrum analysis method, the resolution is equivalent to 1 kHz. The best possible frequency resolution in this case is, of course, not sufficient. It must be pointed out that this has nothing to do with the computational speed of the computer used.

In CDS only one single value per picture element (pixel) is needed and not a complete spectrum. Average velocity methods are in this case more promising and display a very high accuracy.

17.4.1 Color Duplex Sonography using Autocorrelation

In general two methods are used in color-encoded Doppler blood flow analysis by evaluation of the demodulated echo signals. In one case it is a special application of the discrete Fourier analysis. This method has already been basically explained in Section 17.3.3. The method will be dealt with in more detail in Section 17.4.2. The autocorrelation method used by most manufacturers will be described here. The mathematics used in this section are somewhat more difficult. It is not necessary to follow up all the calculations. It is sensible, though, for the user to get acquainted with the assumptions and limitations of the method.

Kasai and Namekawa proposed the use of the autocorrelation function. The method was developed by them around 1982 and published in 1985 (34, 35).

A correlation R(t) is defined in general as:

$$R(t) = g(t) \cdot h(t) = \int_{-\infty}^{+\infty} g^*(\tau)h(\tau + t)d\tau \qquad (17.24)$$

In this case g(t) and h(t) are two continuous functions that are to be correlated with one another. That is, they are displaced by the shift t relative to and multiplied with one another, and then the result is integrated from $-\infty$ to $+\infty$. $g^*(t)$ is the complex conjugate of g(t). The result obtained is the value of the correlation at the time t.

If g(t) and h(t) are the same functions, R(t) is called the autocorrelation function. If they differ the term cross-correlation function is used for R(t). The cross-correlation function will be the topic of the section dealing with the time-of-flight analysis method. A very good introduction to this subject can be found in (10).

In general the "intensity-weighted" average Doppler frequency shift $\bar{\omega}$ ($\omega = 2\pi f$) (as well as any other average) can be written in the form:

$$\overline{\omega} = \frac{\int_{-\infty}^{+\infty} \omega P(\omega)d\omega}{\int_{-\infty}^{+\infty} P(\omega)d\omega}$$

$P(\omega)$ is the power spectrum of the Doppler signal (see Section 17.3.3). $\bar{\omega}$ is called the average or arithmetic mean Doppler shift. As in the case of FFT analysis, a constant signal (velocity) behavior during the complete measurement period is assumed.

Furthermore, the precision of the method is of interest. The square of the standard deviation or variance σ^2 can be calculated. It is interesting to note that the result of this calculation is added in green to the different shades of red and blue and is then called "turbulence indicator" in medicine. The variance of any value is equal to the difference between the average of the square $(\overline{\omega^2})$ and the square of the average $(\bar{\omega})^2$ of the value. The general definition of variance σ^2 related to this case is:

$$\sigma^2 = (\overline{\omega^2}) - (\overline{\omega})^2 = \frac{\int_{-\infty}^{+\infty} (\omega - \overline{\omega})^2 P(\omega)d\omega}{\int_{-\infty}^{+\infty} P(\omega)d\omega}$$

For proof of validity see (45).

Finally the following relation is still needed:

$$R(t) = \int_{-\infty}^{+\infty} P(\omega)e^{i\omega t}d\omega$$

This means that the inverse Fourier transform of the Doppler power spectrum is equal to the autocorrelation function. For proof see (11).

Kasai and Namekawa have derived the first and second derivatives of the above function:

$$\dot{R}(t) = i\int_{-\infty}^{+\infty} \omega P(\omega)e^{i\omega t}d\omega$$

$$\ddot{R}(t) = -\int_{-\infty}^{+\infty} \omega^2 P(\omega)e^{i\omega t}d\omega$$

The functions at $t = 0$ are equal to:

$$R(0) = \int_{-\infty}^{+\infty} P(\omega)d\omega$$

$$\dot{R}(0) = i\int_{-\infty}^{+\infty} \omega P(\omega)d\omega$$

$$\ddot{R}(0) = -\int_{-\infty}^{+\infty} \omega^2 P(\omega)d\omega$$

This results in $\overline{\omega}$ being equal to:

$$\overline{\omega} = -i\frac{\dot{R}(0)}{R(0)}$$

and for σ^2 one obtains:

$$\sigma^2 = \left(\frac{\dot{R}(0)}{R(0)}\right)^2 - \frac{\ddot{R}(0)}{R(0)}$$

With the help of the derivatives of the autocorrelation function at the nonshifted position $t = 0$, the mean Doppler shift $\bar{\omega}$ and the variance σ^2 can be calculated. The method can be simplified technically.

Using the exponential form of a complex value the function $R(t)$ (as any other complex value) can be written as:

$$R(t) = |R(t)|e^{i\varphi(t)}$$

$|R(t)|$ is the absolute value and $\varphi(t)$ is the phase of the function. Kasai and Namekawa also obtained the derivatives of the autocorrelation function as stated above and calculated the value of the function at $t = 0$ under the supposition that $|R(t)|$ is an even function and $\varphi(t)$ is an odd function. In case of an even function $f(-x) = f(x)$ and in the case of an odd function $f(-x) = -f(x)$. The results were introduced into the above equation and the following approximations were derived:

$$\overline{\omega} \cong \frac{\varphi(T) - \varphi(0)}{T} = \frac{\varphi(T)}{T} \qquad (17.25)$$

and

$$\sigma^2 \cong \frac{2}{T^2}\left(1 - \frac{|R(T)|}{R(0)}\right) \qquad (17.26)$$

where $T = \frac{1}{f_{PRF}}$ denotes the temporal distance between two pulses (the pulse interval) and $|R(T)|$ is equal to the absolute value of the autocorrelation function shifted by T. That it is possible to derive the Doppler shift from the phase difference was already explained in Section 17.3.2 (Amplitude, Frequency, Phase). Equations 17.20 and 17.25 coincide in principle but are applied to different functions. Variance σ^2 is the associated error in calculating the mean Doppler shift. The variance depends on the relationship between $|R(T)|$ and $R(0)$. The more similar $R(T)$ and $R(0)$, the smaller the variance. This is equivalent to stating that the more uniform the flow is over time, the more precisely the mean Doppler shift can be calculated. One can also say the greater the amount of flow turbulence, the less reliable the resulting average flow velocity value is. The longer the integration time, i. e., the greater the number of pulse–echo cycles used per color line, the higher the precision of the results.

$\bar{\omega}$ and σ^2 are calculated by complex multiplication. The general definition of a complex number $a + ib$ is used: A complex number is equal to the sum of its real part a and its imaginary part b multiplied by the imaginary unit $i = \sqrt{-1}$ (equation 17.21). The function $g(t)$ is displaced by the shift T. Autocorrelation is carried out according to equation 17.24:

$$\begin{aligned} g^*(\tau) &= x(t) - iy(t) \\ \text{and} \quad h(\tau + T) &= x(t + T) + iy(t + T) \\ g^*(\tau)h(\tau + T) &= x(t)x(t + T) + y(t)y(t + T) + \\ &\quad i[x(t)y(t + T) - y(t)x(t + T)] \\ &= Re + Im \end{aligned}$$

When working on discrete samples, the integration is replaced by a summation of all N echoes coming from the respective depth. The integration time is NT.

$$R(T,t) = R_r + R_i = \sum_{n=1}^{N} Re + \sum_{n=1}^{N} Im$$

The absolute value of a complex number $|R(T,t)|$ is according to equation 17.22:

$$|R(T,t)| = \sqrt{R_r^2 + R_i^2}$$

The phase $\varphi(T)$ is derived from equation 17.23:

$$\varphi(T,t) = \text{arc tg}\,\frac{R_r}{R_i}$$

In the nonshifted case $R(0,t)$ is obtained with the help of the above equation:

$$R(0,t) = \sum_{n=0}^{N}[x^2(t) + y^2(t)]$$

In order to calculate $\bar{\omega}$ and σ^2 all that is left to be done is to enter the above results into equations 17.25 and 17.26. The demodulation of the Doppler signal was described in Section 17.3.4. The I- and Q-signals are equivalent to $x(t)$ and $iy(t)$ respectively. That means that in principle the electronic circuit is now well defined (Fig. 17.**59**).

It must be kept in mind that the whole calculation has to be performed for each and every pixel. Only one electronic circuit exists, of course. The individual I- and Q-values of all pixels of each ultrasound scan line have to be stored until the final results have been calculated. The pixels are worked on one after the other. Then the next ultrasound scan line is examined until all the ultrasound scan lines of one image have been covered. After all this is done, one (!) single image frame can be displayed on the monitor.

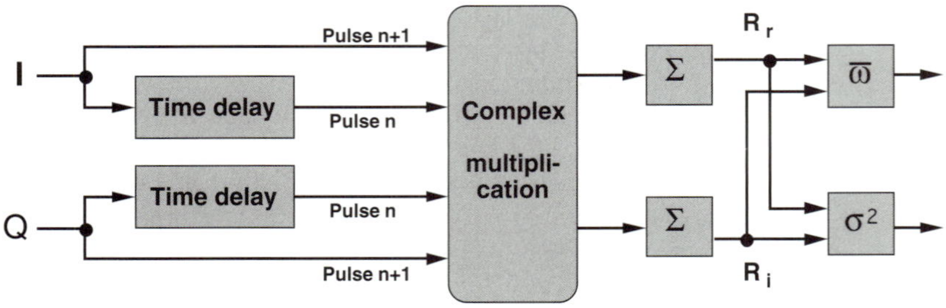

Fig. 17.**59** Block diagram of the autocorrelation method used in calculating $\bar{\omega}$ and σ^2 in CDS (see text)

17.4.2 Color Duplex Sonography using the Discrete Fourier Transform

As explained in Section 17.4 it is not advisable to use the straightforward fast Fourier transform (FFT) algorithm in CDS because—where real-time imaging is involved—the frequency and/or temporal resolution of the received spectrum would be too poor. The frequency resolution is equal to $\frac{f_{PRF}}{N}$ where f_{PRF} is the pulse repetition frequency and N is the number of samples used. Since only one frequency per pixel is sought in CDS, it is possible to use the FFT or discrete Fourier transform (DFT) in combination with a (spatial,) temporal, or frequency-averaging method. The FFT or DFT methods are of course applied to the demodulated signal after MTI filtering and not to the high-frequency RF signal.

The FFT algorithm is just a quick way of calculating a Fourier transform when using many sample points. There are only N · ld N (ld = base 2 logarithm) calculations needed compared to N^2 calculations involved in a DFT. If there are only a few samples involved, the DFT has its advantages. First of all the FFT is a base 2 algorithm. The DFT can use any number of sample points. If only a well-defined number of samples is used, the calculation of the DFT can be simplified tremendously. Because of the required temporal resolution it is not sensible to use more than 16 samples in the DFT analysis. The DFT function F(nf) was explained in Section 17.3.3 where nf are the individual frequencies of the Doppler shift. The DFT is defined as:

$$F(nf) = \sum_{k=0}^{N-1} f(kt) e^{-i\frac{2\pi kn}{N}}$$
$$\text{where } n = 0, 1, 2, \ldots, N-1$$

The exponential function $e^{-i\frac{2\pi kn}{N}}$ is a weight function and can be precalculated for all cases involved and stored in memory. This will technically speed up the calculation process. The Doppler signal contains not only one single frequency but a whole frequency spectrum. Only the magnitudes of the discrete amplitudes f(kt) of the complex Doppler I (direct)- and Q (quadrature)-signals have to be measured in order to calculate the amplitudes of the Doppler frequencies F(nf). The frequencies nf are, as explained earlier (Section 17.3.3), evenly spaced over the whole unique, aliasing-free frequency range. Technically it is possible to apply a sort of band-pass filter at each DFT frequency. The result of the calculations are the amplitudes at each possible Doppler frequency. The magnitudes of the complex amplitudes are calculated according to equation 17.22.

After calculating the amplitudes of the discrete frequencies, the frequency having the highest amplitude may be selected. Alternatively, the intensity-weighted average value can be calculated (see the definition of average in Section 17.4.1). By interpolating it is possible to precisely calculate the intensity-weighted average Doppler frequency with the help of the calculated amplitudes at the known Doppler frequencies. This seemingly increases the number of possible frequencies from 16 to 64 or more.

In any case, the received value should be filtered by including the average of the surrounding pixel values. Using a spatial averaging method eliminates "color dropouts" thus creating a smoother image impression. A block diagram of the DFT method including the MTI filter and quadrature demodulation is shown in Figure 17.**60**.

The DFT method of evaluating the demodulated signals including interpolation is a very elegant way of doing real-time CDS imaging. By lowering the pulse repetition frequency, Doppler frequency resolution is improved by the same factor. At the same time the unambiguous frequency range also decreases by exactly the same factor (see Sections 17.3.1 and 17.3.3). Because of range ambiguity, the pulse repetition frequency cannot exceed a maximum image depth-dependent value.

17.4.3 Color Duplex Sonography using Time-of-Flight Analysis

Another method used in calculating the intensity-weighted average flow velocity is called time domain processing (TDP) or Color Velocity Imaging (CVI). It was mainly developed by O. Bonnefous and P. Pasqué and published in 1986 (4, 5). It is expected that this method will be increasingly implemented on new ultrasound machines. This method does not look for the Doppler frequency or phase shift of the echoes in respect to the transmit pulse. It is a new formulation of the Doppler effect in the (space) time domain. This

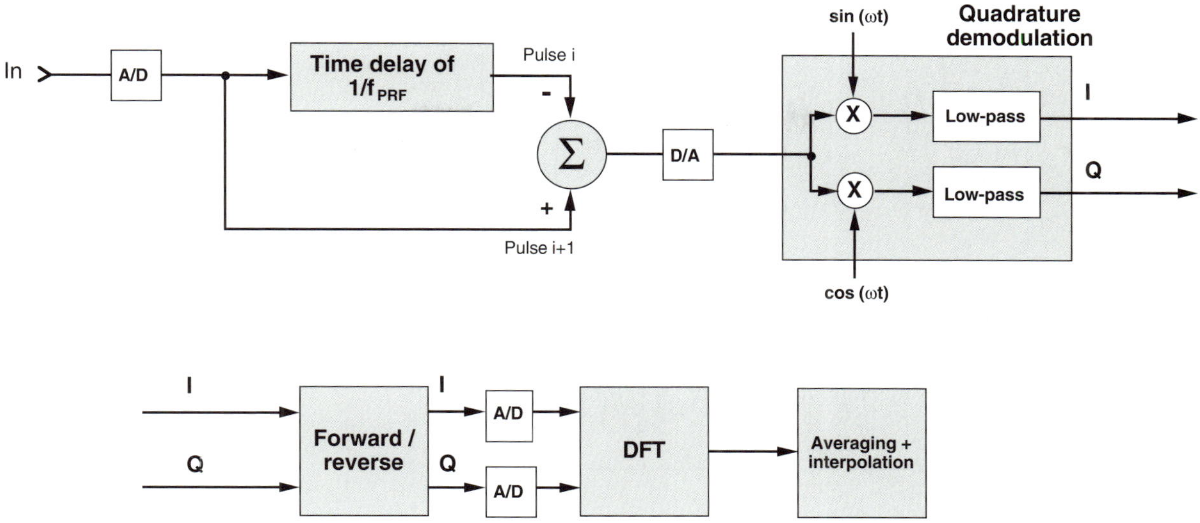

Fig. 17.**60** Block diagram of the DFT method used in calculating the Doppler frequency shift in CDS (see text)

new formulation describes the Doppler shift of consecutive pulse–echo cycles as a relative time delay or shift caused by the movement of the scatterers.

The velocity-dependent change of position of the characteristic echoes is determined. In other words, the change in position of the amplitudes of an A-mode line in the time between 2 pulse–echo cycles is analyzed. This relies on the recognition of individual echoes, requiring a good signal-to-noise ratio (> 6dB) (29, 30). In contrast to the methods evaluating the Doppler frequency or phase shift, the received echo signal is not demodulated. The high-frequency echo series are analog-to-digital converted in real-time and then compared with one another.

For a better understanding look at Figure 17.**61**. A high-frequency nondemodulated RF–echo signal coming from groups of erythrocytes is shown. Due to the moving erythrocytes this signal is of course Doppler shifted. In Figure 17.**62** the echo signals of two consecutive pulse–echo cycles along the same ultrasound scan line have been drawn. Within the window the first echo series has been superimposed on the second echo series (dashed line). It can easily be seen that the amplitudes of both signals show the same behavior but are shifted in time relative to each other. The magnitude of the time shift is proportional to the velocity of the erythrocytes under observation.

To quantify this method look at Figure 17.**63**. As already described earlier (see Section 17.2.4), the sound field is not infinitely small but has a finite lateral dimension. Lateral movement within the field is not detectable, but only axial movement can be registered. A scatterer travels the distance $S_{1,2}$ in the time t_{PRF} between two pulses. The distance Δd is measured. Angle-corrected, the velocity v_{blood} resulting from the two measurements is:

$$v_{blood} = \frac{\Delta d}{t_{PRF} \cos\alpha} \qquad \text{(assuming } v_{blood} \ll c\text{)}$$

The received echoes of the scatterers are coming from different image depths and are shifted by the difference in time of flight $t_v = t_2 - t_1$ of the two pulse–echo cycles. That is, they are received at an earlier or later point in time relative to the instant of the respective pulse emission from the transducer. t_v is positive

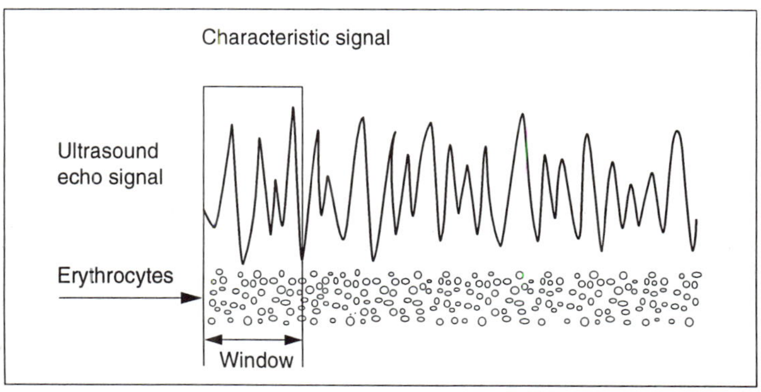

Fig. 17.**61** Ultrasound echo signal coming from the blood

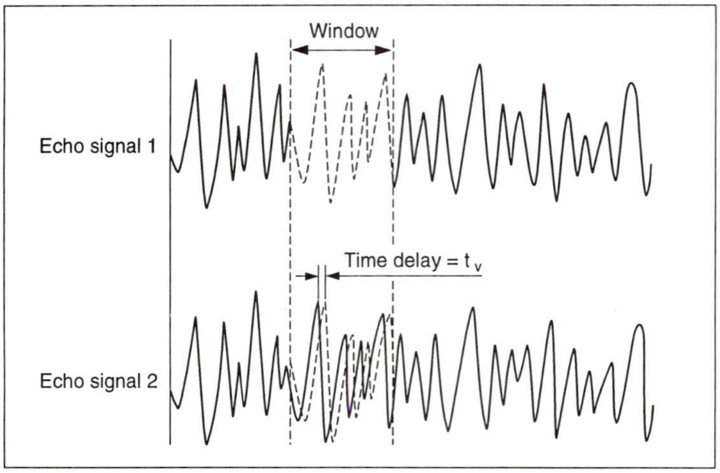

Fig. 17.**62** Comparison of two echo signals

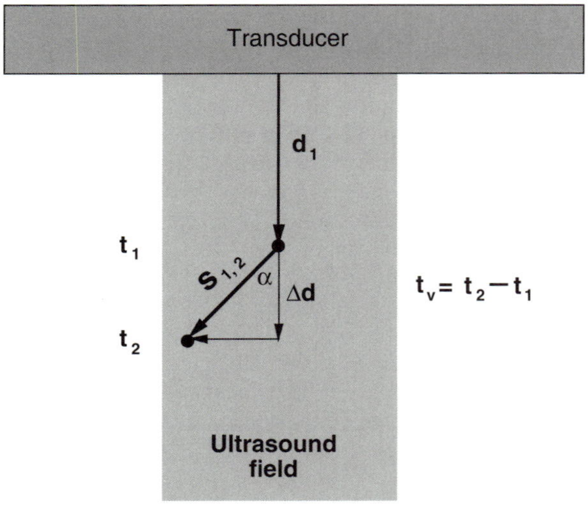

$$v = \frac{S_{1,2}}{t_{PRF}} = \frac{\Delta d}{t_{PRF} \cos\alpha} = \frac{c}{2}\,\frac{t_v}{t_{PRF} \cos\alpha}$$

Fig. 17.**63** Determining the velocity v of a scatterer using two pulses (see text)

if the movement is directed away from the transducer and negative in the other direction. Combining equation 17.4 and the above equation results in:

$$v_{blood} = \frac{c}{2}\,\frac{t_v}{t_{PRF}\cos\alpha} \quad (17.27)$$

From now on it will be assumed that the pulses used to calculate the time shift are separated in time by t_{PRF}, i.e., temporal successive pulses are evaluated. In order to augment the time between two pulses when measuring slow flow velocities, it is sensible to evaluate a few ultrasound scan lines in parallel. In this way the frame rate will not drop off too much. The lines 1, 2, and 3 can, for example, be evaluated in parallel by pulsing along the respective ultrasound scan lines in the order 1, 2, 3, 1, 2, 3, . . . , 1, 2, 3. In this way the frame rate will remain constant, although the time interval between two measurements of the same line is increased by a factor of 3. Using this simple trick, the velocity resolution is improved by a factor of 3 (see below). Other ways of doing this are also possible. Figuratively speaking, with the help of this simple method the scatterers are given time to change their position.

The problem lies in the recognition of a specific signal shape. Two consecutive echo series g(t) and h(t) belonging to the same ultrasound scan line have to be compared, and the position of maximum conformity must be found. Literally speaking, the maximum correlation between the echo of signals g(t) and h(t) has to be found. Expressed mathematically, one is looking for the maximum of the cross-correlation function R(t) of equation 17.24:

$$\begin{aligned}\max[R(t)] &= \max[g(t)\cdot h(t)]\\ &= \max\left[\int_{-\infty}^{+\infty} g(\tau)h(\tau + t)d\tau\right]\end{aligned}$$

Since one is only dealing with real functions here, $g^*(t)$ was replaced by g(t). The mathematical method is the same as in the case of autocorrelation. Two continuous functions are displaced by the time shift t relative to each other and multiplied by one another. Then the result is integrated from $-\infty$ to $+\infty$. The result obtained is the value of the cross-correlation at the time t. Then the maximum amplitude of the cross-correlation function R(t) for all time shifts t is sought. The maximum of the cross-correlation function is found at $t = t_v$. It must be kept in mind that in contrast to the former cases (Sections 17.4.1 and 17.4.2) the demodulated signals are not used here but instead the true high-frequency echo signals are evaluated.

The analog echo signal is converted to digital at the sample frequency or sample rate f_s. The series are then divided into discrete segments of equal length

(Fig. 17.**64**). There are N discrete samples, equidistant in time, in each segment s_i. The size of the segments is a compromise between a high spatial axial resolution and the accuracy in determining the flow velocity within a segment. The segment length L is:

$$L = c\frac{N}{f_s} = cNt_s$$

The smaller the segment, the lower the accuracy of the determined velocity (29), but the higher the axial spatial resolution. The larger the segment, the poorer the axial spatial resolution, but the higher the accuracy of the velocity resolution. The discrete cross-correlation function is given by:

$$R(n,s_i) = \sum_{k=0}^{N-1} g(k + s_iN)h(k + s_iN + n)$$

By going to discrete digital values one obtains $g(\tau) \rightarrow g[(k+s_iN)t_s]$ and $h(\tau+t) \rightarrow h[k+s_iN+n)t_s]$. The temporal separation of the values is constant and equal to $\frac{1}{f_s} = t_s$. This factor was omitted. One starts with segment zero and then goes through all i segments down to the last segment s_i. $h(k+s_iN+n)$ is shifted by *n* in each of the summations below. It seems sensible to vary $h(k+s_iN+n)$ within the range $-N \leq n \leq +N$. In this way the respective center segment is moved stepwise over the two neighboring segments. The first and last segments form special cases and must be treated separately.

$(2N+1)f_s$ multiplications and additions have to be carried out per second. After that the maximum value of $R(n,s_i)$ has to be found in each segment. The position where the functions show maximum similarity defines the time shift $t_v = n_v t_s$ and, according to equation 17.27, also the flow velocity in each segment respectively. n_v is the number of digital samples by which the signals are shifted relative to one another to achieve the best fit.

$$R(n,0) = \sum_{k=0}^{N-1} g(k + 0)h(k + 0 + n)$$

$$R(n,1) = \sum_{k=0}^{N-1} g(k + N)h(k + N + n)$$

$$\vdots$$

$$R(n,s_i) = \sum_{k=0}^{N-1} g(k + s_iN)h(k + s_iN + n)$$

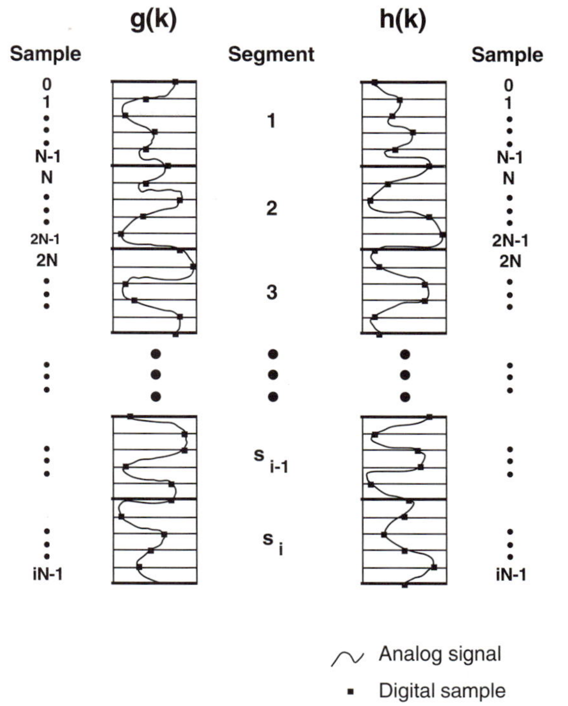

Fig. 17.**64** Segmentation of the A-mode lines in time domain processing (see text)

A block diagram has been drawn in Figure 17.**65** showing how flow velocity is calculated by the time shift method discussed here.

Jensen (29) states that the digital series of samples describe the analog signal correctly if

$$f_s > 4\,(f_0 + \frac{B}{2})$$

where B = bandwidth and f_0 = center frequency of the signal.

If the chosen sample frequency is too low, the result of the calculations might not be unique (see Section 17.3.1). In the case of a 5-MHz transducer with 50% bandwidth, f_s should be, according to the above explanation, at least 25 MHz. In any case, $f_s \geq 4f_0$ must be achieved where the high-frequency components at the upper band limit are then neglected. In the case of the 5-MHz transducer, f_s should then at least be equal to 20 MHz.

The axial spatial resolution Δz of the method using two pulse–echo cycles is equivalent to half the

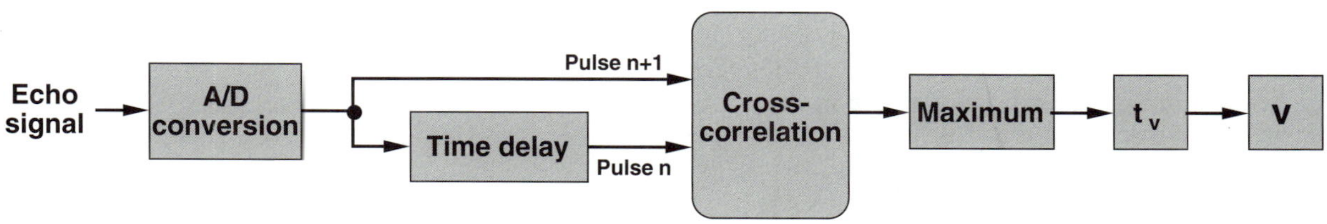

Fig. 17.**65** Block diagram of the time-of-flight method used in calculating the flow velocity in CDS (see text)

segment length chosen (see Section 17.2.2, equation 17.4):

$$\Delta z = \frac{c}{2}\frac{N}{f_s} = \frac{c}{2}Nt_s$$

The lowest detectable velocity v_{min} and the highest detectable velocity v_{max} are, respectively:

$$v_{min} = \frac{c}{2}\frac{f_{PRF}}{f_s} \quad \text{and} \quad v_{max} = \frac{c}{2}N\frac{f_{PRF}}{f_s}$$

Foster et al. (21, 14) described a system using a 5-MHz transducer with $N = 40$ and $f_s = 50$ MHz. An 8-bit A/D converter was used. On this system $4 \cdot 10^9$ (4 billion!) calculations per second would have to be realized in order to have the system work in real-time. The axial resolution would then be 0.616 mm equivalent to two wavelengths. On that system the maximum pulse repetition frequency was $f_s = 30$ kHz. When using an f_{PRF} of 30 kHz, the smallest detectable velocity would then be 46.2 cm/s and the highest detectable velocity 1,848 cm/s. Selecting an f_{PRF} of 2.5 kHz gets v_{min} down to 3.85 cm/s and decreases v_{max} to 154 cm/s. If 3 ultrasound scan lines are evaluated in parallel as described above, an improvement of the velocity resolution by a factor of 1/3 can be achieved allowing v_{min} to go down as far as 1.3 cm/s.

In order to obtain a confident result, it is sensible to use more than just 2 pulse–echo cycles per ultrasound scan line and then average the results. Only discrete flow velocity values are possible. By averaging the results from many pulse–echo cycle comparisons to find the true flow velocity per segment, the level of confidence improves. The true flow velocity can then also be located between these discrete levels. Using 5 pulse-echocycles instead of 2 increases the number of velocity values by a factor of 4 (29).

Using 8 or more bits for the correlation calculation is expensive. For that reason Bonnefous and Pasqué proposed using only the sign of the data for the multiplication. Still, the A/D conversion has to be done with as high an accuracy as possible using 8 to 12 bits, but the subsequent calculations can be done with one single bit representing the sign of the amplitude. This makes the electronics much cheaper. The loss of precision is only minor and in some cases it surprisingly even improves (29, 30).

Jensen (29, 30, 31) has carefully examined the method and comes to the following conclusions: The signal-to-noise ratio has the greatest influence on the method. It must be higher than 6 dB in any case. This immediately limits the penetration depth which has been explained in Section 17.2.1. The shorter the emitted pulse, i.e., the larger the bandwidth, the higher the probability of getting the correct results. The bandwidth must be greater than 20%. It is interesting to note that the level of confidence of the calculated flow velocity is practically velocity-independent. The more pulse–echo cycles used, the higher the reliability of the resulting velocity.

In the above discussion the transit time effect and other limiting effects were not included (see Section 17.2.4). Unfortunately one is not dealing with one scatterer alone but with many scatterers, most of them being erythrocytes. Erythrocytes are only within the sample volume during a finite amount of time depending on the segment length, the lateral width of the sound field, and the flow velocity. Erythrocytes in real blood vessels move at different velocities at the same time within the sample volume. This was examined by O. Bonnefous (6). She came to the conclusion that these real features of blood flow reduce the magnitude of the maximum of the cross-correlation function but do not lead to invalid results. She also described how variance can be calculated within this model. This will not be discussed here because, at the moment, machines where time domain processing has been implemented do not display variance.

Time domain processing compared with other Doppler methods working on the demodulated Doppler signal has a number of advantages. There is no real physical limit to the velocity range, i.e., to the highest or lowest velocities that can be measured. Aliasing, observed on these machines, originates from the limited technical feasibility of a much higher sample rate. If the true absolute maximum of the cross-correlation function is outside the range of the evaluated time shifts defined by n, the relative maximum is automatically found by the above algorithm. This leads to a phenomenon similar to aliasing. This has nothing to do with the Nyquist limit as described before in the case of the demodulated signal, although it is a problem of sampling fast enough. A limitation imposed by the pulse repetition frequency does exist and must not be forgotten. The penetration depth needed by the user limits the pulse repetition frequency.

Furthermore, there is no longer a contradiction between the aim of having a good gray-scale image with high spatial resolution and a high-velocity resolution in color at the same time. Where Doppler methods based on the phase and frequency analysis of the demodulated signals require a narrow-band pulse, the time-of-flight method as well as the gray-scale image require a wide-band pulse. An increase in penetration depth in comparison with the other methods is, unfortunately, not to be expected. Most likely, frequency-dependent attenuation in tissue that may lead to misleading results in the case of the phase and frequency analysis methods is of no importance here. The time domain method does not require as many pulse–echo cycles per ultrasound color line as the other methods do. This makes it possible for the manufacturer or the user to choose between a higher frame rate by using the same number of color lines as with the other methods or a higher lateral resolution by using more color lines.

17.5 Image Processing

As mentioned at the beginning of this chapter, human beings cannot see, feel, hear, or in any other way sense signals in the ultrasound frequency range. Ultrasound images are not a part of our natural environment. Additionally, the time of flight of the ultrasound signals limits the number of pulse–echo cycles that can be used per image in real-time imaging. This means that the quality of the ultrasound images depends on the signal and image processing applied. Regrettably, only a few interesting aspects can be discussed here. Interested readers are referred to the special literature on this topic (for example [22, 41]).

It is taken for granted that the user has done everything physically necessary to optimize the image. This means that the correct transducer needed for the specific application has been chosen and the TGC and total gain have been optimized. The transmit focus or focuses have been positioned correctly, and a sufficient amount of ultrasound gel has been applied.

A gray-scale image is a two-dimensional array of pixels (*pic*ture *el*ements). After the echoes have been received by the transducer, the signals are amplified, rectified, and A/D converted. Then they are stored in a digital memory (RAM = *r*andom *a*ccess *m*emory). Every pixel is assigned a gray value proportional to the amplitude of the echo coming from that particular position of the image field.

The color values are calculated and also stored in a digital memory, in most cases separate from the gray-scale values. Gray-scale and color values are read from their respective positions in memory and are then D/A converted. Usually color values have a write priority. In color systems three separate D/A converters are necessary for the three colors red, green, and blue (RGB colors). In the case of a gray value, all the D/A converters are loaded with the same number. According to the numeric value, the respective pixel is displayed darker or brighter on the monitor, where zero is often defined as absolute black and white corresponding to the largest possible gray value. In the case of a color pixel, different numerical values are sent to the individual D/A converters.

Assigning the raw data values to the correct pixels in the two-dimensional display is a general problem. The monitor coordinates are cartesian coordinates (y, z) that are generally well known from school. The y-axis runs parallel to the top of the monitor from left to right for positive values. The z-axis is on the left side of the image, pointing downward toward higher positive values. Every pixel on the monitor corresponds to a coordinate pair (y_i, z_k). The number i defines the column and k the row in which the pixel can be found. Using a simplified model in the case of a linear array, a pulse is transmitted along column $i = 0$, and the amplitude values of the successive returning echoes are assigned the coordinates (y_0, z_0), (y_0, z_1), (y_0, z_2), . . ., (y_0, z_n). Depending on the sampling frequency, there usually are 128, 256, or 512 different values (pixels) per column. After the first pulse–echo cycle has been terminated, the next column is filled with data. This data is assigned the coordinates (y_1, z_0), (y_1, z_1), (y_1, z_2), . . ., (y_1, z_n). This is done for all m pulse–echo cycles per image. The last column of the image is assigned the coordinates (y_m, z_0), (y_m, z_1), (y_m, z_2), . . ., (y_m, z_n).

The pulses and echoes are, except in the case of beam steering, emitted and received along a line vertical to the transducer surface. The time of flight is proportional to the distance r between reflector and transducer. The ultrasound scan lines are all parallel to one another on a linear array. If another kind of transducer is used, the ultrasound scan lines are offset by an angle φ. The pixel coordinates or addresses are then (r_i, φ_k). r_i is a distance or length from the transducer and φ_k is an angle. This coordinate system is called the polar coordinate system. A coordinate transformation from the raw data polar coordinates to the cartesian coordinates of the monitor has to be performed, and the data must be transferred to the right addresses. This kind of data processing is done by the scan converter in real-time (see Fig. 17.**66a, b**). Normally this is not a one-to-one conversion, i.e., for every address in polar coordi-

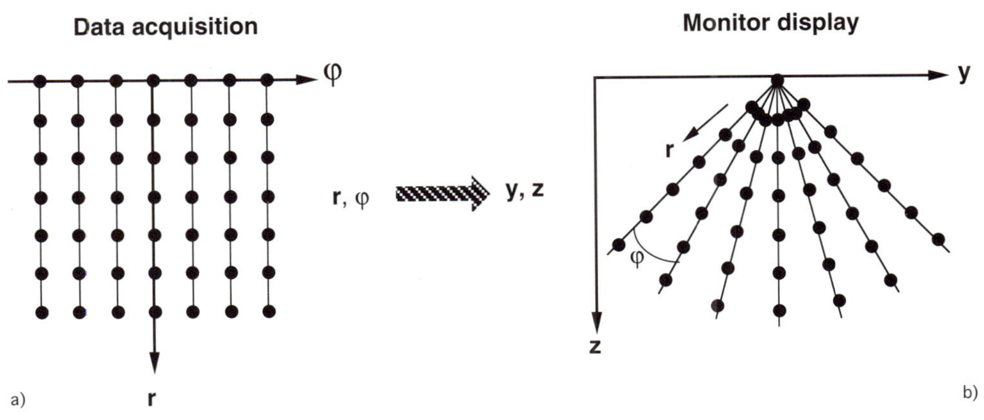

Fig. 17.**66** Transformation of the polar coordinates of the line memory (**a**) to the cartesian coordinates (**b**) of the video display

nates there will not be a corresponding address in cartesian coordinates and vice versa, where in both cases the addresses are composed of two integers. In those cases, the closest address is chosen. The transformation will, especially in the near field, map more than one (r_i, φ_k) address to a single (y_i, z_k) address and, especially in the far field, some (y_i, z_k) addresses will not receive any data at all. After or during coordinate transformation, data interpolation will ensure that all (y_i, z_k) addresses receive appropriate data. If the transformation and interpolation are not done correctly, a superimposed line structure will appear on the screen (Moiré).

An often applied and very simple interpolation method used in vector transformation is just copying the same data to the empty addresses to the left or right of the address hit by transformation. As soon as an angle of about $\pm 45°$ has been reached, this kind of interpolation tends to create dark and bright horizontal lines in the image and in this way blurs the image near the outer left and right sides. The simple method just described that is used in most systems is of course not adequate for doing straightforward 360° scans.

In some top class systems a different method, called back transformation or rho-theta-conversion, is used. A (y_i, z_k) address in the video (screen) memory calls up the appropriate (r_i, φ_k) address in the line memory (raw data memory). The distance r is calculated with the help of the Pythagorean theorem ($r = \sqrt{x^2 + y^2}$). The angle φ is calculated by $\varphi = \mathrm{arctg}(x/y)$. The operations square root and arc tangent normally do not deliver integers as results, even if they are applied to integer values (y_i, z_k). This means that an approximation method must also be applied here because all addresses have integer coordinates. In the simplest case only rounding is used and the value from the calculated line memory address is transferred to the video memory address. In more sophisticated systems the data from all integer addresses surrounding the calculated line memory coordinates are used. With the help of a weighted bilinear interpolation method a new pixel value is calculated and stored in the video memory address. Weighting depends on the linear distance between the calculated line memory coordinates and the surrounding coordinates considered. This real-time method can well handle 360° scans. At the same time a read zoom and image flip of the frozen image is possible. The selection of a ROI (region of interest) is possible. This last method is difficult to realize and very expensive.

Because ultrasound imaging must be done in realtime, very few real ultrasound scan lines can be used per image. Normally used line numbers are 64, 96, 128, 192, and, rarely, 256. The axial resolution is limited by the wavelength of the ultrasound signal and the finite sampling rate. Usually only 128, 256, or 512 samples per ultrasound scan line are used. A PAL video image (50 Hz) contains 625 lines (rows). The horizontal resolution is about 240 lines (columns). S–VHS systems can resolve about 400 lines (3). In other words: The number of columns and rows or pixels displayed on a video monitor is clearly larger than the complete set of real ultrasound data. This immediately calls for some kind of interpolation to calculate the missing data needed for video presentation. For example, a weighted bilinear interpolation method can be used. The pixels in between two real data values are calculated from the neighboring pixels.

By raising the sampling frequency on high end systems using linear arrays, interpolation is not necessary parallel to the direction of the ultrasound scan line. Interpolation is then only necessary in scan direction, parallel to the transducer surface. It is even easier to just copy the same data to the empty addresses to the left or right and above or below the actually existing ultrasound data until the next real data address is reached. It is easy to imagine that interpolation in the case of a pure read zoom is rather difficult. In read zoom no additional ultrasound data is gathered. The image is simply rescaled and additional pixels are calculated by interpolation. In the case of a write zoom, the ultrasound line density and/or the sampling frequency increases.

There are ultrasound systems on the market using 16, 32, 64, 128, and 256 digital shades of gray. The human eye can only differentiate about 35 shades of gray (37) (see Fig. 17.**67a–d**).

The digital values are D/A converted on being read from memory and transferred to the monitor. The look-up tables used for translating the digital grayvalues to analog signals are not necessarily linear, but are corrected according to monitor characteristics and the sensitivity of the eye (γ-correction). The image can then be seen on the monitor. The picture tube is coated with a light-emitting substance (phosphor). The light emission decreases over time. This, by itself, has an averaging effect. Often the signal amplitudes are smoothed on being sent to the monitor or somewhere else in the image chain.

Almost every ultrasound system gives the user the option of smoothing the images. Smoothing is often called scan correlation (SCC). The aim is to suppress unavoidable electronic and acoustic noise. This is facilitated, for example, by adding the values of corresponding pixels of two or more images and then dividing the resulting values by the number of images used. This is the simplest way of smoothing digital images. In some cases on high-quality systems the pixel values are weighted in order to reduce motion artefacts.

Most systems also allow for some kind of edge enhancement. This can be done easily before A/D conversion by adding the derivative of the analog echo signal to the signal itself. The changes in the grayscale image are enhanced by changing the analog signal. This feature is often called "enhance" on ultrasound systems.

Image processing is also applied to the color part of an image. Depending on the method used for color coding, between about 5 and 17 pulse–echo cycles per ultrasound scan line are used. If this were done for as many ultrasound lines as used in gray-scale imag-

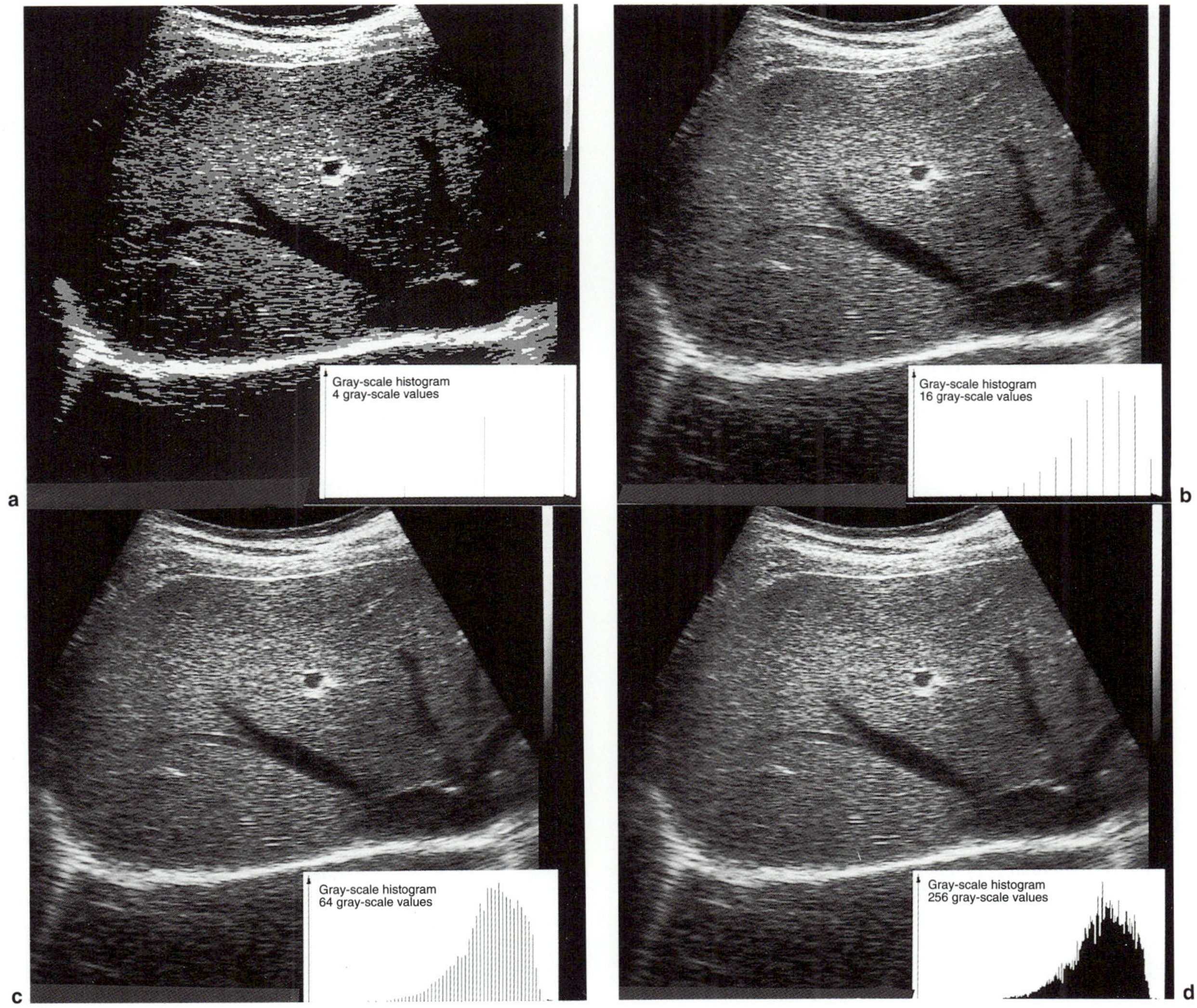

Fig. 17.**67a–d** The same image of the liver using 4, 16, 64 and 256 gray-scale values. The respective gray-scale histograms are displayed on the bottom right of each image

ing, real-time imaging in color would not be possible. Instead, fewer lines are used and additional color pixel values between the real color lines are created by interpolation. This can be done in the same way as on gray-scale images.

Also special filters such as a median filter can be used. A median filter replaces the color value of a pixel by the median color value in the surrounding area and not by the average value. This filter smooths out sudden changes or single color pixel dropouts but only slightly influences color edge detection. An example using a 3×3 median filter is shown below. The 9 pixel values are:

$$\begin{Bmatrix} 25 & 30 & 10 \\ 30 & 100 & 35 \\ 25 & 40 & 25 \end{Bmatrix}$$

The center pixel value (100) is to be replaced. The pixel values are listed in order of magnitude:

10, 25, 25, 25, *30,* 30, 35, 40, 100

The center or median value is 30. The average is $320/9 = 35.56 \rightarrow 36$. In this case 100 is replaced by 30 and not 36.

Many other filters are possible, as long as they can be used in real-time imaging. For more information, read the specialized literature on this topic (for example [22, 41]).

17.6 References

1 Abstracts of the Drei-Länder-Treffen in Lausanne, Ultraschalldiagnostik 91, Oct 16–19, 1991, Ultraschall Klin. Prax. 6, No. 3 (1991)
2 Atkinson, P., J. P. Woodcock: Doppler Ultrasound and its Use in Clinical Measurement. Academic Press (1982) 69–70
3 Bahr, H.: Alles über Video. Hüthig-Verlag (1991) 169
4 Bonnefous, O., P. Pasqué: Time Domain Formulation of Pulse-Doppler Ultrasound and Blood Velocity Estimation by Cross Correlation. Ultrasonic Imaging, Vol. 8, Academic Press (1986) 73–85
5 Bonnefous, O., P. Pasqué, X. Bernard: A New Velocity Estimator for Color Flow Mapping. IEEE Ultrasonics Symposium (1986) 855–860

6 Bonnefous, O.: Statistical Analysis and Time Correlation Processes applied to Velocity Measurement. IEEE Ultrasonics Symposium (1989) 887–892

7 Born, M.: Optik. Springer-Verlag (1985) 142–147

8 Born, M.: Optik. Springer-Verlag (1985) 162–170

9 Brigham, E. O.: The Fast Fourier Transform. Prentice-Hall (1974)

10 Brigham, E. O.: The Fast Fourier Transform. Prentice-Hall (1974) 50–75

11 Brigham, E. O.: The Fast Fourier Transform. Prentice-Hall (1974) 66–68

12 Chatigny, J. V.: Piezofilm– ein Sensorik-Basismaterial. Elektroniker 7 (1988)

13 Chivers, R. C., F. Santosa: Numerical Considerations for Interface Reflections in Medical Ultrasound. Phys. Med. Biol. 31, No. 8 (1986) 819–837

14 Embree, P. M., W. D. O'Brien: Volumetric Blood Flow via Time-Domain Correlation: Experimental Verification. IEEE Transactions on Ultrasonics, Ferroelectrics and Frequency Control, Vol. 37, No. 2, (1990) 176–189

15 Evans, D. H., W. N. McDicken, R. Skidmore, J. P. Woodcock: Doppler Ultrasound. John Wiley (1991) 3

16 Evans, D. H., W. N. McDicken, R. Skidmore, J. P. Woodcock: Doppler Ultrasound. John Wiley (1991) 118–122

17 Evans, D. H., W. N. McDicken, R. Skidmore, J. P. Woodcock: Doppler Ultrasound. John Wiley (1991) 127–130

18 Fehske, W.: Praxis der konventionellen und farbkodierten Doppler-Echokardiographie. Verlag Hans Huber (1988)

19 Feigenbaum, H.: Echokardiographie, Beiträge zur Kardiologie, Bd. 12. Perimed Fachbuch-Verlagsges. mbH (1986)

20 Föllinger, O.: Laplace- und Fourier-Transformation. AEG-Telefunken (1982)

21 Foster, S., P. M. Embree, W. D. O'Brien: Flow Velocity Profile via Time-Domain Correlation: Error Analysis and Computer Simulation. IEEE Transactions on Ultrasonics, Ferroelectrics and Frequency Control, Vol. 37, No. 2 (1990) 164–175

22 Gonzalez, R. C., P. Wintz: Digital Image Processing, 2nd ed. Addison-Wesley (1987)

23 Grewe, M. G., T. R. Gururaja, T. R. Shrout, R. E. Newnham: Acoustic Properties of Particle/Polymer Composites for Ultrasonic Transducer Backing Applications. IEEE Transactions on Ultrasonics, Ferroelectrics and Frequency Control, Vol. 37, No. 6 (1990) 506–514

24 510(k) Guide for Measuring and Reporting Acoustic Output of Diagnostic Ultrasound Medical Devices (FDA). Appendix D, Center for Devices and Radiological Health (12.1985) D4

25 Haerten, R.: Technische Kenngrößen von Ultraschalldiagnosegeräten und ihre Bestimmung. Ultraschall 1 (1980) 1–11

26 Harris, R. A., D. H. Follett, M. Halliwell, P. N. T. Wells: Ultimate limits in Ultrasonic Imaging Resolution. Ultrasound Med. Biol. 17, No. 6 (1991) 547–558

27 Hatle, L., B. Angelsen: Doppler Ultrasound in Cardiology. Lea & Febiger (1982) 194–199

28 Jaffe, B., W. R. Cook, H. Jaffe: Piezoelectric Ceramics. Academic Press (1971)

29 Jensen, J. A.: Artefacts in Velocity Estimation using Ultrasound and Cross-Correlation. Submitted to IEEE Transactions on Medical Imaging (7. 91)

30 Jensen, J. A.: Stationary Echo Canceling in Velocity Estimation by Time Domain Cross-Correlation. Submitted to IEEE Transactions on Medical Imaging (8. 91)

31 Jensen, J. A.: Implementation of Ultrasound Time Domain Cross-Correlation Blood Velocity Estimators. Submitted to IEEE Transactions on Biomedical Engineering (8. 91)

32 Jones, S. A., D. P. Giddens: A Simulation of Transit Time Effects in Doppler Ultrasound Signals. Ultrasound Med. Biol. 16, No. 6 (1990) 607–619

33 Kaplan, W.: Advanced Calculus, 2nd ed. Addison-Wesley (1973) 509–511

34 Kasai, C., K. Namekawa: Real-Time Two-dimensional Blood Flow Imaging using an Autocorrelation Technique. IEEE Ultrasonics Symposium (1985) 953–985

35 Kasai, C., K. Namekawa, A. Koyano, R. Omoto: Real-Time Two-Dimensional Blood Flow Imaging using an Autocorrelation Technique. IEEE Transactions on Sonics and Ultrasonics, Vol. SU-32 (1985) 458–463

36 Krautkrämer, J., H. Krautkrämer: Werkstoffprüfung mit Ultraschall. Springer-Verlag (1961) 62

37 Krestel, E. (Ed.): Bildgebende Systeme für die medizinische Diagnostik, 2nd ed. Siemens A. G. (1988) 213

38 Millner, R. (Ed.): Ultraschalltechnik. Physik Verlag (1987) 41–48

39 Omoto, R. (Ed.): Color Atlas of Real-Time Two-Dimensional Doppler Echocardiography, 2nd ed. Lea & Febiger (1987) 14–15, 20–21

40 Powis, R. L.: A New Real-Time Look at the Vascular System. Appl. Radiol. 1 (1986)

41 Pratt, W. K.: Digital Image Processing. John Wiley (1978)

42 Safety Standard for Diagnostic Ultrasound Equipment, AIUM/NEMA Standards Pub. No. UL1–1981. J. Ultrasound Med. (Suppl.) 2, No. 4 (1983) 21

43 Schwarz, H. P., W. Gebhardt: Optimierung des Fokusschlauches von Phased-Arrays für die Impulsechoprüfung an dickwandigen Komponenten, Fraunhofer-Gesellschaft, Inst. f. zerstörungsfreie Prüfverfahren. Report No. 820219-TW, 1982

44 Smith, W. A., B. A. Auld: Modeling 1–3 Composite Piezoelectrics: Thickness-Mode Oscillations. IEEE Transactions on Ultrasonics, Ferroelectrics and Frequency Control. 38, No. 1 (1991) 40 –47

45 Sommerfeld, A.: Vorlesungen über theoretische Physik, Band V, Thermodynamik und Statistik. Verlag Harri Deutsch (1977) 240–241

46 Spiegel, M. R.: Fourier-Analysis, Schaum's Outline. McGraw-Hill (1976)

47 Turnbull, D. H., F. S. Foster: Beam Steering with Two-Dimensional Transducer Arrays. IEEE Transactions on Ultrasonics, Ferroelectrics and Frequency Control. 38, No. 4 (1991) 320–333

48 Wassenaar, D.: Ultrasound Basic Training Course, p. 10. Philips Medical Systems (1988) Print 4522 984 14301/794 1988–08

49 Wells, P. N. T.: Biomedical Ultrasonics. Academic Press (1977) 124–125

18 Glossary

P.-M. Klews

Absorption: The conversion of (mechanical, kinetic) energy (of an ultrasound signal) to heat and thus reducing the (mechanical) energy of the signal.

Acoustic power output: Energy emitted by the transducer per unit time.

Aliasing: Doppler shifts above the Nyquist limit (= half the pulse repetition frequency) are displayed at the wrong frequency. The displayed frequency is off by an integer multiple of the pulse repetition frequency. At high flow velocities above the Nyquist limit, the flow appears to be flowing in the wrong direction.

A-mode system: Ultrasound system that displays the amplitudes of the ultrasound echoes as a function of echo time of flight or the distance of the echogenic structure from the transducer. The display is similar to an oscilloscope trace. Interfaces with a large impedance jump produce a high-amplitude deflection, and interfaces with a small impedance change produce a low-amplitude deflection.

Amplitude display in Doppler frequency analysis: See Frequency analysis.

Annular-array transducer: Mechanical sector transducer in which the ring-shaped piezoelectric elements are concentrically arranged.

Apodization: Suppression of side lobes by different weighting of the signals at the individual piezoelectric elements in a transmitting and/or receiving array.

Attenuation: A loss of energy (of an ultrasound signal) caused by many different factors such as absorption, scattering, reflection, . . .

Axial resolution: Spatial resolution in the direction of propagation of the sound waves.

B-mode, B-mode image, B-mode display: Two-dimensional gray-scale ultrasound image (B = brightness) in which the brightness of each pixel (spot) in the sectional image is proportional to the echo intensity (amplitude) at that location.

Bandwidth: An ultrasound pulse contains not only a single frequency but a range of frequencies grouped around a center frequency. The bandwidth equals the difference between the upper and lower cutoff frequencies, i.e., usually the frequencies above and below the center frequency whose amplitudes are half that of the center frequency.

Baseline: The line in a Doppler display that represents the non-Doppler shifted frequency (zero shift). This line generally serves as the time axis.

Baseline shift (zero point shift): Upward or downward shift of the baseline to expand the aliasing-free frequency (velocity) range in one direction, producing an equal reduction of the frequency (velocity) range displayed in the other direction.

Beam steering: Electronically controlled ultrasound beam deflection in a linear-array transducer. The same technique is basically used in phased-array transducers.

Cavitation: The production of minute gas bubbles by the action of ultrasound waves (in the negative pressure phase).

Center frequency: The frequency in an ultrasound pulse (often) having the highest amplitude (see also bandwidth).

Color Doppler: Refers to the methods of phase, time-of-flight, and frequency analysis used in color-encoded (Doppler) imaging. The results are displayed in different colors instead of gray levels. Usually the term is used synonymously with color duplex sonography.

Color duplex sonography (CDS), color-coded duplex sonography (CCDS), color duplex, color flow mapping (CFM): Method allowing the simultaneous visualization of soft-tissue structures and blood flow. The color-encoded flow information is superimposed on the gray-scale image (= soft-tissue structures). When motion is detected, the gray-scale value displayed at that location is replaced by the appropriate color value. Most systems encode motion in red or blue, each color representing a direction of movement relative to the transducer. Velocity (frequency shift) is represented by color shades, with lighter shades indicating higher velocities (frequency shifts). Slow blood flow toward the transducer, for example, may be encoded in dark blue while rapid flow away from the transducer is encoded in light red.

Crosstalk damping: Separation of two directional channels so that little if any signal in one channel interferes with the signal in the other channel. Similar to channel separation (undesired coupling of channels) in stereo radio.

Cursor, marker: A marker in an image that can be used for measurement purposes or as a pointer.

Curved-array transducer (CA): Transducer with a curved surface owing to the curved arrangement of its adjacent piezoelectric elements (in one row). The image field has the approximate shape of a trapezoid.

CW Doppler (continuous-wave Doppler): Measurement of the frequency (phase) shifts or wavelength changes of a sound wave that is continuously emitted and received. The process has no axial resolution in terms of the site from which a Doppler signal is acquired. There is no physical upper limit (Nyquist limit) imposed on the unambiguous determination of Doppler shifts in CW Doppler systems.

Demodulation: Method of eliminating the carrier wave (in MHz) to obtain the desired information (Doppler signal in diagnostic ultrasound, music in a radio).

Depth resolution: Axial spatial resolution.

Diffraction: Nonlinear propagation of waves resulting from the presence of inhomogeneities (obstacles).

Directional channels: Two separate signal paths are used to process and display the Doppler signals according to whether the blood is moving toward or away from the transducer.

Doppler angle: Angle between the direction of sound propagation (sound beam) and the flow direction (e.g., direction of the moving erythrocytes).

Doppler effect, Doppler shift: Frequency (phase) shifts or wavelength changes produced in a signal by the motion of the source (scatterer, reflector) and observer (transducer) relative to each other. The magnitude of the frequency shift is proportional to the observed velocity.

Doppler formula: $F_d = (2\ F_0\ v \cos \alpha)/c$, where F_d = measured frequency shift, F_0 = transducer reference frequency, v = velocity of the measured object, α = angle between the direction of propagation of the sound wave and the direction of motion of the measured object, c = speed of sound in tissue.

Doppler gate, Doppler sample volume: The region in an image field from which the Doppler signal of interest originates. In most instruments the operator can define the size and position of the sample volume within the image field.

Doppler information: The measured Doppler shifts in an ultrasound signal presented to the examiner in the form of audible signals, a Doppler spectrum, or other type of display.

Doppler reference frequency: The frequency used in demodulation of the RF-signal for the analysis of the Doppler frequency shift. This is usually not the center frequency of the transducer but, in most cases, a lower frequency in order to achieve a higher penetration depth. This frequency is designated F_0 in the Doppler formula.

Doppler signals: The Doppler-shifted components of the echo signals (= frequency and phase shift).

Doppler spectrum: Frequencies (velocities) and amplitudes determined by spectrum analysis of Doppler signals displayed over time.

Duplex sonography, duplex scanning: In general, the capability of accomplishing two tasks at the same time, for example, B- + M-mode imaging, B-mode + color-encoded imaging, . . . etc. Especially, the ultrasound technique with the combined capacity for acquiring and displaying a B-mode image (to detect soft-tissue structures) and a Doppler spectrum (to detect flow) is meant. The flow information is displayed in the form of a spectral trace outside the B-mode image field.

Duty factor: Ratio of the pulse duration to the temporal pulse interval which is equal to the product of the pulse duration and the pulse repetition frequency.

Dynamic focusing: Process in which the receive focus is continuously automatically varied over the image depth to keep the received echoes constantly in focus.

Dynamic range: Ratio, in decibels (dB), of the strongest to the weakest ultrasound signals that can be detected in a system.

Fast Fourier transform (FFT): Mathematical algorithm used in calculating the amplitudes of the (Doppler) frequency components in a periodic (Doppler) signal.

Flow direction: The direction of blood flow relative to the direction of propagation of the sound wave. Doppler systems measure only the velocity components of blood flow that are parallel to the direction of the sound beam. Thus, flow that is perpendicular to the sound beam, or parallel to the transducer surface (cosine 90° in the Doppler formula), cannot be detected.

Focal distance: Distance from the transducer surface to the focal plane in the direction of propagation of the sound wave.

Focal length: Depth range around the focus in which the cross-sectional area of the sound field does not exceed a specified value (generally four times the cross-sectional beam area in the focal plane).

Focal plane: The plane perpendicular to the direction of propagation of the sound wave that contains the focus.

Focal region: See Focal length.

Frame rate, image repetition frequency: Number of complete images (frames) generated by the ultrasound instrument per unit time (second).

Freeze mode: System mode in which all real-time functions are paused.

Frequency: Number of events (oscillations, cycles) per unit time. The fundamental unit is hertz, Hz = 1/s.

Frequency analysis, spectrum analysis: Measurement and display of the individual frequency components and corresponding amplitudes that by superposition compose the (Doppler) signal (analogous to the prismatic dispersion of light, decomposing white light into colors).

Frequency resolution: The smallest Doppler shift that is still detectable. In Doppler frequency analysis using the Fourier transform, frequency resolution is equal to the pulse repetition frequency divided by the number of measurements.

Gain: The electronic amplification applied to the received signals. (See also Time gain compensation.)

Gray scale, gray levels: Analog echo amplitudes are converted to digital values (A/D conversion) and displayed as bright spots on a monitor. The brightness levels are proportional to the echo amplitudes.

Gray-scale image: See B-mode.

High-pass filter: A filter that allows only frequencies above a designated cutoff frequency to pass through. It eliminates low-frequency disturbances such as the Doppler shifts caused by motion of the vessel wall.

HPRF Doppler (high pulse repetition frequency): Technique for expanding the unambiguously detectable Doppler frequency range by increasing the pulse repetition frequency (PRF). The unique unambiguous axial location of the origin of the Doppler signals is sacrificed.

Image memory: Digital memory (RAM = random access memory) in which the digitized gray-level values in an image are stored pixel by pixel.

Impedance (acoustic): Mathematically, the product of the material-dependent speed of sound and density. Impedance is a material constant and characterizes the resistance to sound propagation from one medium to another. The larger the impedance difference at an interface, the greater the amount of reflected incident energy.

Index of refraction: The ratio of the velocities of sound propagation in two media.

Insonation angle: The angle between the sound beam and the structure of interest (e.g., a blood vessel). The insonation angle is always between 0° and 90°. At 0° the flow direction is parallel to the sound beam. At 90° the flow direction is perpendicular to the sound beam. According to the Doppler formula (see above), a frequency shift cannot be measured when the insonation angle equals 90°.

Intensity: Sound intensity refers to the energy (energy flux of the sound beam) that passes through a given area perpendicular to the direction of the sound beam per unit time (1 second). (Sound energy per unit time is called acoustic power. Intensity is power per unit area.) Intensity is commonly measured in milliwatts per square centimeter (mW/cm^2). The maximum instantaneous intensity is $I_{moment} = \frac{P^2}{\varrho c}$, where P = instantaneous acoustic pressure, ϱ = density, and c = speed of sound in the medium. Many different definitions of intensity are used. Their difference pertains to the time and/or area over which the intensity is averaged:

– I_M: intensity of the sound pulse time-averaged over one pulse half-cycle.

– I_{SAPA} **(spatial average–pulse average):** Pulse average intensity averaged over the pulse cross-sectional area.

– I_{SATA} **(spatial average–temporal average):** Temporal average intensity averaged over the pulse cross-sectional area.

– I_{SATP} **(spatial average-temporal peak):** Temporal peak intensity averaged over the pulse cross-sectional area.

– I_{SPPA} **(spatial peak–pulse average):** Spatial peak of the pulse average intensity.

– I_{SPTA} **(spatial peak–temporal average):** Spatial peak of the temporal average intensity.

– I_{SPTP} **(spatial peak–temporal peak):** Spatial peak of the temporal peak intensity.

– **Pulse average intensity:** Time average of the instantaneous intensity averaged over the pulse duration.

– **Temporal average intensity:** Time average of the instantaneous intensity averaged over the scan interval.

Interface: The boundary surface between two media (with different impedances).

Lateral resolution: Spatial resolution in a plane perpendicular to the direction of sound propagation. Generally denotes resolution parallel to the transducer surface in scan direction.

Linear-array transducer (LA): Transducer with a linear arrangement of adjacent piezoelectric elements in one row. The image field is rectangular.

Longitudinal wave (sound): Wave propagation in which the particles oscillate around their equilibrium position parallel to the direction of propagation of the wave.

Lower cutoff frequency: The lowest frequency in a Doppler signal that can still be detected or displayed by an instrument.

Low-pass filter: A filter that allows only frequencies below a designated cutoff frequency to pass through. It eliminates high-frequency signals above a certain limit and is used as an anti-aliasing filter in Doppler analysis and gray-scale imaging.

M-mode, M-mode image, M-mode display, TM-mode, TM-mode image: A gray-scale ultrasound imaging mode (time–motion mode) in which the movement of tissue structures along a selected ultrasound scan line is displayed as a function of time. The brightness of each image pixel is proportional to the echo signal amplitude at that location at a particular point in time. The display progresses along the abscissa, which represents the temporal axis. The ordinate represents the depth of the echo-generating structures. This mode is used chiefly in echocardiography.

Nominal frequency: The transducer frequency stated by the manufacturer and distributor. All transducers are manufactured to specific tolerances and emit sound waves at a certain (center) frequency that is close to the nominal frequency. For simplicity, a transducer with a true center frequency of 3.4 MHz, for example, is said to have a nominal frequency of 3.5 MHz.

Nyquist limit: The frequency beyond which Doppler shifts can no longer be unambiguously determined (see Aliasing). It is equal to half the pulse repetition frequency.

Phase: Instantaneous state of oscillation.

Phased-array transducer: Transducer with a single-row linear array of adjacent piezoelectric elements that produce a sector-shaped image field. Deflection of the sound pulse is produced by a relative time delay in the activation of individual elements that are electronically grouped together to transmit a pulse (beam steering).

Piezoelectric element: The smallest unit in a transducer that converts electrical signals to mechanical energy (emission of sound waves) and mechanical deformation to an electrical voltage (arrival of sound waves at the receiver).

Pixel: Picture element.

Preprocessing: Signal-processing operations that are carried out before the signals are stored in memory and can no longer be performed after the image has been frozen. Many preprocessing functions can also be carried out (emulated) digitally in postprocessing.

Postprocessing: Signal-processing operations that are carried out after the signals have been stored in image memory.

Pressure: Force per unit area (pascal = Pa).

Pulse: (The emission of) a short burst of energy.

Pulse duration: Time from the beginning to the end of a pulse (depends on the allowed amplitude).

Pulse interval: Time from the beginning of one pulse to the beginning of the next. Reciprocal of the pulse repetition frequency.

Pulse repetition frequency (PRF, f_{PRF}): The frequency at which individual ultrasound pulses are emitted from the transducer. The reciprocal of the PRF is the pulse interval. The PRF is a function of the desired imaging depth.

PW (pulsed wave) Doppler, pulsed Doppler: Frequency (phase) shifts or wavelength changes in a sound pulse based on the Doppler effect. Because the transmitted pulses are of short duration, this technique can be used to interrogate flow at a specified depth. An upper limit (Nyquist frequency) is imposed on the Doppler frequency shift that can be unambiguously determined in a pulsed Doppler system. The lowest detectable frequency is equal to the pulse repetition frequency divided by the number *n* of samples used (*n*-point FFT).

Quadrature (-phase) demodulation: Special method for eliminating the carrier wave (in MHz) to obtain direction-dependent Doppler information (Hz to kHz).

Reflection: Reversal of the direction of wave propagation at the interface between two media (angle of incidence = angle of reflection). The interface must be larger than the sound wavelength.

Refraction: Change in the direction of sound passing through the interface between two media.

Resolution: See Axial resolution, Frequency resolution, Spatial resolution, Temporal resolution.

Sample volume: The user-defined region in PW Doppler from which echoes are selectively received for Doppler evaluation.

Scan: An ultrasound image sweep comprised of individual ultrasound scan lines, in which all the scan lines are successively evaluated.

Scan converter: Electronic assembly in which the polar coordinates of the raw data pixels used with convex and sector transducers are converted to cartesian coordinates for display. The image memory is often erroneously referred to as being a part of the scan converter.

Scan correlation: Time-weighted method of image (frame) averaging.

Scan direction: Direction of the line-by-line generation of the ultrasound image.

Scan line: A line in the ultrasound image that represents the ultrasound beam. There are usually more video lines than scan lines in the images. The additional pixels are calculated by interpolation of the samples along and between the scan lines.

Scattering: In general, the change in direction of particles or waves caused by a collision with another particle or system. Diffuse reflection, refraction, and diffraction of sound on encountering structures (interfaces, irregularities) that are smaller than the sound wavelength.

Sector scanner, sector transducer: An electronic or mechanical transducer whose image field has the shape of a sector of a circle.

Side lobes, grating lobes: Sound–pressure maxima that travel out in directions different from the main pressure maximum of the sound field.

Signal processing: The images obtained with ultrasound depend on the technique used for data acquisition and image processing. The entire chain from the reception of an echo to its display on the monitor involves a sequence of signal manipulations. The most familiar signal manipulations (processing steps) include edge enhancement and time gain compensation.

Slice thickness resolution: The lateral spatial resolution perpendicular to both the transducer and the scan direction.

Sound field: The space occupied by the emitted sound waves.

Sound wave: The propagation of mechanical oscillations. Particles are induced to oscillate around their resting or equilibrium position (center of gravity). The local pressure (density) changes periodically. The wave transports energy and momentum. Basically, only longitudinal waves occur in tissue, fluids, and gases.

Spatial resolution: The smallest distance between two points that can still be identified as separate points in the image.

Spectral components: The individual frequencies with their amplitudes in frequency analysis.

Spectrum: Graphic representation of the amplitudes of the individual frequency components in a (Doppler) signal. The temporal progression of many consecutive (Doppler) signals is of interest in medical diagnosis. This time-varying representation is referred to simply as the Doppler spectrum.

Speed of sound: The velocity of propagation of sound is material-dependent and is approximately 1,540 m/s ± 10% in tissue. In medical ultrasound devices, a constant velocity of propagation of sound equal to 1,540 m/s is assumed.

Stereo acoustic output: Doppler signals are processed in two separate channels, depending on whether the blood is moving toward or away from the transducer, and are relayed to two loudspeakers for stereo output.

Temperature rise: Inevitably absorption of sound energy in tissue can lead to a rise in temperature in the area being insonated.

Temporal resolution: The smallest measurable time interval between two successive events. In Doppler frequency analysis, temporal resolution refers to the time that is required to produce a Doppler spectrum. It equals the product of the pulse interval times the number of pulse–echo cycles used per spectrum. Temporal resolution is not limited by digital signal analysis in modern systems.

Time gain compensation (TGC), depth gain compensation (DGC), swept gain: Range-dependent electronic amplification of the received echo signals after conversion of the received echoes to electrical signals in the transducer. Signals returning from structures farther away from the transducer are amplified more than signals from structures close to the transducer. This type of signal amplification creates an image in which the shade of gray of the object under observation is independent of its location within the image field.

Transducer: The component of an ultrasound system that emits the sound and receives the returning echoes. The individual piezoelectric elements of the transducer convert electrical signals to acoustic signals and vice versa.

Transducer frequency: The center frequency of the transmitted ultrasound signal.

Transverse wave (sound): Wave propagation in which the particles oscillate perpendicular to the direction of propagation of the wave.

Unambiguous velocity range: Aliasing (Nyquist limit) limits the velocity range that can be unambiguously evaluated in pulsed Doppler systems. Velocities (Doppler frequency shifts) outside the unambiguous range can no longer be uniquely assigned to a specific velocity or frequency shift.

Wall filter: High-pass filter (see above) that can be adjusted by the examiner.

Wavelength: The distance between two identical states, e.g., in propagating sound waves. The wavelength is the ratio of the speed of sound to frequency (e.g., 0.3 mm for a 5-MHz-transducer).

Index

O

P

Q

R

S

T

U

V

W